MASTER TECHNIQUES IN ORTHOPAEDIC SURGERY

■

FRACTURES

Second Edition

MASTER TECHNIQUES IN ORTHOPAEDIC SURGERY

■

Editor-in-Chief
Bernard F. Morrey, M.D.

Founding Editor
Roby C. Thompson, Jr., M.D.

Volume Editors

SURGICAL EXPOSURES
Bernard F. Morrey, M.D.

THE HAND
James Strickland, M.D.
Thomas Graham, M.D.

THE WRIST
Richard H. Gelberman, M.D.

THE ELBOW
Bernard F. Morrey, M.D.

THE SHOULDER
Edward V. Craig, M.D.

THE SPINE
David S. Bradford, M.D.
Thomas L. Zdeblick, M.D.

THE HIP
Robert L. Barrack, M.D.

RECONSTRUCTIVE KNEE SURGERY
Douglas W. Jackson, M.D.

KNEE ARTHROPLASTY
Paul A. Lotke, M.D.
Jess H. Lonner, M.D.

THE FOOT & ANKLE
Harold B. Kitaoka, M.D.

FRACTURES
Donald A. Wiss, M.D.

PEDIATRICS
Vernon T. Tolo, M.D.
David L. Skaggs, M.D.

SOFT TISSUE SURGERY
William Cooney, M.D.
Steven L. Moran, M.D.

FRACTURES
Second Edition

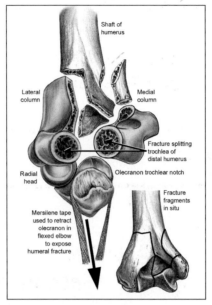

Shaft of humerus

Lateral column

Medial column

Fracture splitting trochlea of distal humerus

Radial head

Olecranon trochlear notch

Mersilene tape used to retract olecranon in flexed elbow to expose humeral fracture

Fracture fragments in situ

Editor

DONALD A. WISS, M.D.
Southern California Orthopaedic Institute
Van Nuys, California

Illustrators

Carolyn M. Capers, M.S.M.I., C.M.I.
Christopher Blake Williams, M.A.

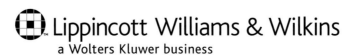

Lippincott Williams & Wilkins
a Wolters Kluwer business

Philadelphia · Baltimore · New York · London
Buenos Aires · Hong Kong · Sydney · Tokyo

Acquisitions Editor: Robert Hurley
Managing Editor: Michelle LaPlante
Project Manager: Nicole Walz
Senior Manufacturing Manager: Ben Rivera
Marketing Director: Sharon Zinner
Creative Director: Doug Smock
Cover Design: Andrew Gatto
Production Services: Maryland Composition Inc
Printer: Quebecor World Bogota

The publisher is not responsible (as a matter of product liability, negligence or otherwise) for an
injury resulting from any material contained herein. This publication contains information relating
to general principles of medical care which should not be constructed as specific instruction for
individual patients. Manufacturer's product information should be reviewed for current information,
including contraindications, dosages, and precautions.

Printed in Colombia

Library of Congress Cataloging-in-Publication Data
Fractures / editor, Donald A. Wiss; illustrators, Carolyn M. Capers, Christopher Blake Williams.—2nd ed.
    p. ; cm. — (Master techniques in orthopaedic surgery)
      ISBN 13: 978-0-7817-5290-9
      ISBN 10: 0-7817-5290-6
      1. Fracture fixation—Atlases.   I. Wiss, Donald A.   II. Series: Master techniques in orthopaedic
    surgery (2nd ed.)
    [DNLM: 1. Fractures, Bone—surgery.   2. Fracture Fixation, Internal—methods. WE 185
    E7988 2006]
  RD103.F58F73   2006
  617.1'5—dc22

                                                         2005034098

The publishers have made every effort to trace copyright holders for borrowed material. If they have
inadvertently overlooked any, they will be pleased to make the necessary arrangements at the first
opportunity.

To purchase additional copies of this book, call our customer service department at (800) 638-3030 or
fax orders to (301) 223-2320. International customers should call (301) 223-2300.

Visit Lippincott Williams & Wilkins on the Internet at http://www.lww.com. Lippincott Williams &
Wilkins customer service representatives are available from 8:30am to 6:30pm, EST, Monday through
Friday, for telephone access.

10 9 8 7 6 5 4

To my wife, Deborah,
my sons, Jeremy and David,
and my parents, Dorothy and William,
whose guidance, love, and support made this book a reality

■

ACKNOWLEDGMENTS

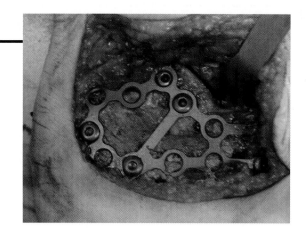

Master Techniques in Orthopaedic Surgery: Fractures was edited in Southern California between 2003 and 2006 while I was practicing at the Southern California Orthopaedic Institute (SCOI). It reflects nearly 25 years of study and treatment of fractures and their sequelae. Anyone undertaking such a work will incur debts of gratitude to a number of people who worked on this project with considerable commitment and little public recognition.

I am particularly grateful to Carolyn M. Capers, the medical illustrator of this text, for her magnificent artwork depicting complex fractures and their fixation. The drawings show greater detail and improved three-dimensional reality.

I would like to acknowledge and extend my gratitude to Eleanor O'Brien, who typed and retyped virtually all of the manuscripts during the inevitable revision process. This book would have been enormously more difficult without her editorial and organizational talents, as well as her cheerful and patient attitude. Pam Swan, my practice coordinator, also handled many of the details with the authors and their staffs, as well as the publishing team at Lippincott Williams & Wilkins. Thanks are due to Michelle LaPlante and her staff at Lippincott Williams & Wilkins for editorial assistance, support, and patience while completing the second edition of the *Master Techniques in Orthopaedic Surgery: Fractures*.

Finally, my heartfelt thanks and appreciation to each of the contributing authors who answered the "bell" once again with yet another academic request for their precious time. Their willingness to share their considerable expertise and to explain the details and nuances of fracture care will unequivocally benefit orthopaedic surgeons everywhere who treat patients with musculoskeletal trauma.

TABLE OF CONTENTS

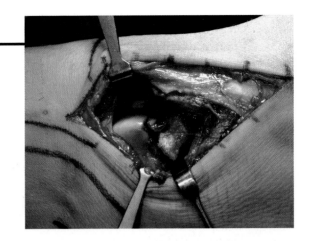

[†]Deceased.

SECTION IV   MISCELLANEOUS TOPICS

CONTRIBUTORS

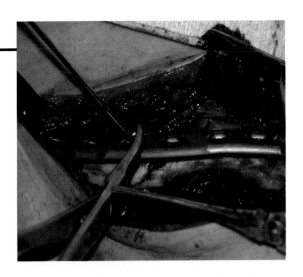

Jeffrey O. Anglen, M.D.
Professor and Chairman
Department of Orthopaedics
Indiana University
Indianapolis, Indiana

Sean F. Bak, M.D.
Shoulder, Elbow and Sports Medicine Fellow
Department of Orthopaedic Surgery
New York Orthopaedic Hospital
Columbia-Presbyterian Medical Center
New York, New York

Craig S. Bartlett, M.D.
Department of Orthopaedic Surgery and Rehabilitation
University of Vermont
McClure Musculoskeletal Research Center
Burlington, Vermont

Michael R. Baumgaertner, M.D.
Associate Professor of Orthopaedic Surgery
Yale University School of Medicine
Chief, Orthopaedic Trauma
Department of Orthopaedics
Yale-New Haven Hospital
New Haven, Connecticut

Stephen K. Benirschke, M.D.
Department of Orthopaedics
Harborview Medical Center
Seattle, Washington

Louis U. Bigliani, M.D.
Frank E. Stinchfield Professor and Chairman of
  Orthopaedic Surgery
Chief, The Shoulder Service
New York Orthopaedic Hospital
Columbia-Presbyterian Medical Center
Columbia University
New York, New York

Brett R. Bolhofner, M.D.
Director, Orthopaedic Trauma
Bay Front Medical Center
All Florida Orthopaedic Associates
St. Petersburg, Florida

Joseph Borrelli, Jr., M.D.
Associate Professor of Orthopaedic Surgery
Chief of Orthopaedic Trauma Service
Washington University School of Medicine
Barnes-Jewish Hospital
St. Louis, Missouri

Bruce D. Browner, M.D.
Gray-Gossling Professor and Chairman
Department of Orthopaedic Surgery
University of Connecticut Health Center
John Dempsey Hospital
Farmington, Connecticut

Andrew E. Caputo, M.D.
Department of Orthopaedics
University of Connecticut Health Center
Farmington, Connecticut

Anikar Chhabra, M.D., M.S.
Fellow, Orthopaedic Surgery
Center for Sports Medicine
University of Pittsburgh
Pittsburgh, Pennsylvania

Peter A. Cole, M.D.
Associate Professor of Orthopaedic Surgery
University of Minnesota
Minneapolis, Minnesota
Medical Director, Orthopaedic Surgery
Regions Hospital
St. Paul, Minnesota

George S.M. Dyer, M.D.
Resident in Harvard Combined Orthopaedic Surgery
Massachusetts General Hospital
Boston, Massachusetts

Eric D. Farrell, M.D.
Associate Director of Orthopaedic Trauma
Cooper University Hospital
Camden, New Jersey

Paul T. Fortin, M.D.
William Beaumont Hospital
Royal Oak, Michigan

Michael J. Gardner, M.D.
Senior Resident
Weill-Cornell University Medical Center
Senior Clinical Associate of Orthopaedic Surgery
Hospital for Special Surgery
New York, New York

Paul B. Gladden, M.D.
Assistant Professor of Orthopaedic Surgery
University of Florida
Chief of Orthopaedic Trauma Surgery
The Bone and Joint Institute
Jacksonville, Florida

Steven S. Goldberg, M.D.
Associate Staff Physician
Department of Orthopaedic Surgery
Cleveland Clinic Florida
Naples, Florida

Mark T. Gould, M.D.
Department of Orthopaedics
Harborview Medical Center
Seattle, Washington

Michael W. Grafe, M.D.
Attending Surgeon
Redwood Orthopaedic Surgery Group
Santa Rosa, California

Jonathan C. Haas, M.D.
Assistant Professor of Orthopaedic Surgery
University of Minnesota
Faculty, Department of Orthopaedic Surgery
Hennepin County Medical Center
Minneapolis, Minnesota

George J. Haidukewych, M.D.
Orthopedic Traumatologist and Adult Reconstructive
  Surgeon
Florida Orthopedic Institute
Tampa General Hospital
University of South Florida
Tampa, Florida

David J. Hak, M.D., M.B.A.
Associate Professor
Vice Chair and Residency Program Director
Department of Orthopaedic Surgery
University of California, Davis
Sacramento, California

Christopher D. Harner, M.D.
Blue Cross of Western Pennsylvania Professor and
  Director
Center for Sports Medicine
University of Pittsburgh Medical Center
Pittsburgh, Pennsylvania

David L. Helfet, M.D.
Professor of Orthopaedic Surgery
Weill Medical College of Cornell University
Director of Orthopaedic Trauma Service
Hospital for Special Surgery
New York Presbyterian Hospital
New York, New York

James J. Hutson, Jr., M.D.
Orthopaedic Traumatology
Department of Orthopaedics and Rehabilitation
University of Miami
Miami, Florida

Eric E. Johnson, M.D.
Professor of Orthopaedic Surgery
University of California at Los Angeles Medical Center
Los Angeles, California

Jesse B. Jupiter, M.D.
Hansjorg Weiss AO Professor of Orthopaedic Surgery
Harvard Medical School
Director of Orthopaedic Hand Surgery
Massachusetts General Hospital
Boston, Massachusetts

Enes M. Kanlic, M.D., M.S., Ph.D.
Associate Professor of Orthopaedic Surgery and
  Rehabilitation
Texas Tech University Health Sciences Center in El Paso
El Paso, Texas

Paul D. Kim, M.D.
Fellow in Orthopaedic Surgery
Columbia University Medical Center
New York, New York

Kenneth J. Koval, M.D.
Professor of Orthopaedic Surgery
Dartmouth Hitchcock Medical Center
Lebanon, New Hampshire

Richard F. Kyle, M.D.
Professor of Orthopaedic Surgery
Department of Orthopaedic Surgery
University of Minnesota
Chairman, Department of Orthopaedic Surgery
Hennepin County Medical Center
Minneapolis, Minnesota

Mark A. Lee, M.D.
Assistant Professor of Orthopaedic Trauma
UC Davis Medical Center
University of California, Davis
Sacramento, California

Dean G. Lorich, M.D.
Assistant Professor, Department of Orthopaedic Surgery
Weill Medical College of Cornell University
Attending Physician, Department of Orthopaedic Surgery
Hospital for Special Surgery
New York, New York

Lawrence J. Maciolek, M.D.
Chief Administrative Assistant
Department of Orthopaedic Surgery
Medical College of Wisconsin
Milwaukee, Wisconsin

Arthur L. Malkani, M.D.
Department of Orthopaedic Surgery
University of Louisville
Louisville, Kentucky

Joel M. Matta, M.D.
The John C. Wilson Professor of Orthopaedic Surgery
University of Southern California
Hospital of the Good Samaritan
Los Angeles, California

Augustus D. Mazzocca, M.D.
Department of Orthopaedics
University of Connecticut Health Center
Farmington, Connecticut

Michael D. McKee, M.D., F.R.C.S.C.
Associate Professor of Surgery
University of Toronto
Staff, Department of Surgery, Division of Orthopaedics
St. Michael's Hospital
Toronto, Ontario, Canada

Berton R. Moed, M.D.
Professor and Chairman of Orthopaedic Surgery
Saint Louis University School of Medicine
St. Louis, Missouri

Steven J. Morgan, M.D.
Associate Professor of Orthopaedics
University of Colorado School of Medicine
Denver Health Medical Center
Denver, Colorado

Sean E. Nork, M.D.
Associate Professor of Orthopaedic Surgery
Harborview Medical Center
University of Washington
Seattle, Washington

Peter J. O'Brien, M.D., F.R.C.S.C.
Associate Professor of Orthopaedics
University of British Columbia
Vancouver Hospital and Health Sciences Center
Vancouver, British Columbia, Canada

Robert F. Ostrum, M.D.
Professor of Surgery
UMD-NJ Robert Wood Johnson Medical School
Director of Orthopaedic Trauma
Cooper University Hospital
Camden, New Jersey

Hector O. Pacheco, M.D.
Assistant Professor of Orthopaedic Surgery and
*   Rehabilitation*
Texas Tech University Health Sciences Center in El Paso
El Paso, Texas

Mark C. Reilly, M.D.
Assistant Professor of Orthopaedics
Co-Chief, Orthopaedic Trauma Service
New Jersey Medical School
Newark, New Jersey

Sharad Rhaban, M.D.
Resident in Plastic and Reconstructive Surgery
Keck School of Medicine
University of Southern California
Los Angeles, California

David Ring, M.D.
Assistant Professor of Orthopaedic Surgery
Harvard Medical School
Hand and Upper Extremity Service
Department of Orthopaedic Surgery
Massachusetts General Hospital
Boston, Massachusetts

Craig S. Roberts, M.D.
Professor of Orthopaedic Surgery
University of Louisville School of Medicine
Louisville, Kentucky

Derek E. Robinson, M.B. Ch.B., F.R.C.S.
Consultant Orthopaedic Surgeon
Royal United Hospital
Bath, Somerset, United Kingdom

Melvin P. Rosenwasser, M.D.
Carroll Professor of Orthopaedic Surgery
Columbia University Medical Center
Director of Hand, Microvascular, and Orthopaedic
*   Trauma*
New York Presbyterian Hospital
New York, New York

M. L. Chip Routt, Jr., M.D.
Professor of Orthopaedic Surgery
University of Washington
Harborview Medical Center
Seattle, Washington

Thomas A. Russell, M.D.
Professor of Orthopaedic Surgery
University of Tennessee
Campbell Clinic
Memphis, Tennessee

Nicholas Sama, M.D.
Orthopaedic Trauma Fellow
Hospital for Special Surgery
New York, New York

Roy W. Sanders, M.D.
Chief, Department of Orthopaedics
Tampa General Hospital
Director, Orthopaedic Trauma Services
Florida Orthopaedic Institute
Tampa, Florida

Bruce J. Sangeorzan, M.D.
Department of Orthopaedics
Harborview Medical Center
Seattle, Washington

Edward Rainier G. Santos, M.D.
Assistant Professor of Orthopaedics
University of Minnesota
Minneapolis, Minnesota

Emil H. Schemitsch, M.D.
Professor of Surgery
University of Toronto
Chief of Orthopaedic Surgery
St. Michael's Hospital
Toronto, Ontario, Canada

Gregory J. Schmeling, M.D.
Associate Professor of Orthopaedic Surgery
Residency Program Director
Department of Orthopaedic Surgery
Medical College of Wisconsin
Milwaukee, Wisconsin

Andrew H. Schmidt, M.D.
Associate Professor of Orthopaedic Surgery
University of Minnesota
Faculty and Attending Physician
Department of Orthopaedic Surgery
Hennepin County Medical Center
Minneapolis, Minnesota

S. Andrew Sems, M.D.
Clinical Instructor of Orthopaedic Surgery
Mayo Medical School
Senior Associate Consultant
Department of Orthopaedic Surgery
Mayo Clinic
Rochester, Minnesota

Milan K. Sen, M.D.
Orthopaedic Trauma Fellow
Hospital for Special Surgery
New York, New York

Shane T. Seroyer, M.D.
Resident Physician
Department of Orthopaedic Surgery
University of Pittsburgh Medical Center
Pittsburgh, Pennsylvania

Randy Sherman, M.D.
The Audrey Skirball Kenis Professor and Chair
Division of Plastic and Reconstructive Surgery
Keck School of Medicine
University of Southern California
Los Angeles, California

James P. Stannard, M.D.
Associate Professor of Surgery
University of Alabama at Birmingham
Chief of Orthopaedic Trama Surgery
University of Alabama at Birmingham Hospital
Birmingham, Alabama

Marc F. Swiontkowski, M.D.
Professor and Chairman of Orthopaedic Surgery
University of Minnesota
Attending Orthopaedic Surgeon
University of Minnesota Medical Center at Fairview
Minneapolis, Minnesota

Sudeep Taksali, M.D.
Orthopaedic Resident
Department of Orthopaedics and Rehabilitation
Yale University School of Medicine
New Haven, Connecticut

J. Charles Taylor, M.D.
Specialty Orthopedics, P.C.
Memphis, Tennessee

David C. Templeman, M.D.
Associate Professor of Orthopaedic Surgery
University of Minnesota
Department of Orthopaedic Surgery
Hennepin County Medical Center
Minneapolis, Minnesota

Paul Tornetta, III, M.D.
Professor of Orthopaedic Surgery
Boston University School of Medicine
Director of Orthopaedic Trauma
Boston University Medical Center
Boston, Massachusetts

Andrew P. Van Houwelingen, M.D.
Orthopaedic Surgery Resident
Division of Orthopaedic Surgery
St. Michael's Hospital and the University of Toronto
Toronto, Ontario, Canada

Brent M. Walz, M.D.
Chief Resident in Orthopaedic Surgery
University of Louisville School of Medicine
Louisville, Kentucky

J. Tracy Watson, M.D.
Professor of Orthopaedic Surgery
Saint Louis University School of Medicine
Chief, Division of Orthopaedic Traumatology
Saint Louis University Health Science Center
St. Louis, Missouri

Patrick J. Wiater, M.D.
William Beaumont Hospital
Royal Oak, Michigan

John H. Wilber, M.D.
Professor of Orthopaedic Surgery
Case Western Reserve University
Director of Orthopaedic Trauma
University Hospitals of Cleveland
MetroHealth Medical Center
Cleveland, Ohio

Robert A. Winquist, M.D.
Attending in Orthopedic Surgery, Trauma and Joint
  Reconstruction
Clinical Professor
University of Washington Medical School
Seattle, Washington

Jonathan G. Yerasimides, M.D.
Chief Resident in Orthopaedic Surgery
University of Louisville School of Medicine
Louisville, Kentucky

Patrick Yoon, M.D.
Assistant Professor of Orthopaedic Surgery
University of Minnesota
Faculty, Department of Orthopaedic Surgery
Hennepin County Medical Center
Minneapolis, Minnesota

Daniel M. Zinar, M.D.
Chair and Director
Orthopaedic Trauma Service
Harbor-UCLA Medical Center
Torrance, California

Gary L. Zohman, M.D.
Director of Orthopedic Trauma
Department of Surgery
Kern Medical Center
Bakersfield, California

SERIES PREFACE

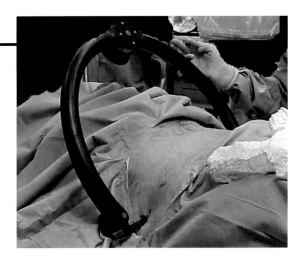

Since its inception in 1994, the Master Techniques in Orthopaedic Surgery Series has become a well-accepted "must" for surgeons in training and in practice. The user-friendly style of providing and illustrating authoritative information on a broad spectrum of orthopaedic techniques has filled a void in orthopaedic education materials. The exceptional success of the series may be traced to the leadership of the original series editor, Roby Thompson, whose clarity of thought and focused vision sought "to provide direct, detailed access to techniques preferred by orthopaedic surgeons who are recognized by their colleagues as 'masters' in their specialty" (Series preface, Volume I). The essential elements of success are clear. In addition to the careful selection of the master volume editor, the format of the presented material has almost become classic. I am personally rewarded by numerous comments by both residents and practicing orthopaedic surgeons regarding the value of these volumes to their training or in their practice. The format has become a standard against which others are to be compared, "A standardized presentation of information replete with tips and pearls through years of experience with abundant color photographs and drawings to guide you step by step through the procedures" (Series preface, Volume II).

Ten second edition volumes are currently in print. Building on the success of the current ten-volume series, we are in the process of expanding the texts to include an even broader range of relevant orthopaedic topics. New volumes will appear on surgical exposures as well as peripheral nerve surgery. Other topics are being actively explored with an ex-

pectation that the series will expand to 15 titles over the next several years.

I am honored to be assuming the responsibility of the series editor. The true worth of this endeavor will be measured by the ongoing and ever-increasing success and critical acceptance of the series. I am indebted to Dr. Thompson for his inaugural vision and leadership as well as to the Master Series editors and to the numerous contributors who have been true to the style and to the vision. Ultimately, as is stated by the Mayo brothers, "The best interest of the patient is the only interest to be considered." It is hoped that the information in the Master Series equips the surgeon to realize this patient-centric view of our surgical practice.

Bernard F. Morrey, M.D.
Series Editor

PREFACE

American medicine remains in the midst of a profound and wrenching transformation. The government, Wall Street, third party payers, and patients have demanded improved medical care at lower cost. Better medicine (orthopaedics) occurs when doctors practice medicine consistently on the basis of the best scientific evidence available, set up systems to measure performance, analyze results and outcomes, and make this information widely available to patients and the public. Reduced costs have been achieved partially through a wholesale shift to health maintenance organization, capitation, and managed care.

Trauma is a complex problem where initial decisions often dramatically determine the ultimate outcome. Death, deformity, and medicolegal entanglements may follow vacillation and error. When treatment is approached with confidence, planning, and technical skill, the associated mortality rate, preventable complications, permanent damage, and economic loss may be significantly reduced. Uncertainty, inactivity, and inappropriate intervention by physicians are all detrimental to patient care. Certain traditional concepts and fixation techniques need to be abandoned and new approaches learned.

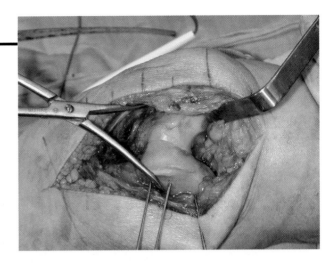

This text attempts to address society's mandate to our profession: better orthopaedics at reduced cost. It provides residents and practitioners with surgical approaches to 46 common but often problematic fractures that, when correctly done, have proven to be safe and effective. It is my hope that the second edition of this textbook remains a valuable fixture in the catalog of literature on fracture management.

Donald A. Wiss, M.D.

Upper Extremity

1

Clavicular Fractures: Open Reduction Internal Fixation

Andrew P. Van Houwelingen, Michael D. McKee, and Emil H. Schemitsch

Fractures of the clavicle account for approximately 4% of all fractures and 35% of fractures in the shoulder region (1). The majority of clavicular fractures can be treated by nonoperative methods, which have been traditionally thought to have fewer complications than surgery. This reasoning probably has prevailed because internal fixation methods are typically reserved for severe fractures.

Nonoperative management usually involves either a simple arm sling or a figure-of-eight harness. Until recently, nonoperative treatment of clavicular fractures was thought to be associated with high rates of union and a low probability of complications. The deformity that often accompanies conservative care of these fractures was thought to be of cosmetic concern only and that full function was typically observed after healing (2). However, many of the reports regarding clavicular fractures have included data from children and adolescents who have the capability for rapid healing and remodeling of residual deformities (2,3). Complication rates following displaced clavicular fractures in adults and elderly patients show that outcomes in these patients are much less satisfactory than for the young. Nonunion or malunion of a clavicular fracture can lead to a variety of undesirable outcomes including pain, deformity, weakness, neurovascular symptoms, and decreased function (4). The increasing recognition of adverse outcomes following fracture has led to a renewed interest in internal fixation of displaced clavicular fractures in adults.

A thorough knowledge of the basic anatomy and biomechanics of the clavicle and shoulder is essential if rational treatment is to be provided. The clavicle has an S-shaped configuration, and when viewed from medial to lateral, it has an anterior convex to concave curvature. The medial portion of the clavicle is cylindrical, but the lateral portion is relatively flat. The typical medullary canal is very small due to the thick cortical bone that surrounds it. Medially, the clavicle is held in position by three very strong ligaments: the sternoclavicular, costoclavicular, and interclavicular ligaments. On the lateral end, the acromioclavicular and the two coracoclavicular ligaments, the conoid and the trapezoid, serve to anchor the clavicle to the scapula. The osseous surface of the clavicle serves as the origin for many of the important muscles of the upper limb including the platysma, sternocleidomastoid, pectoralis major, subclavius, deltoid, and trapezius. Furthermore, the clavicle shields important underlying neurovascular structures such as the brachial plexus and the subclavian vessels. It also holds the distinction of being the only bone that connects the upper limb to the axial skeleton. Biomechanically, the clavicle acts as a strut that holds the shoulder girdle away from the thorax. Surgical excision of part or the entire clavicle results in decreased strength and stability of the shoulder girdle, especially when the patient is reaching across his or her body (5).

Several classification systems have been proposed to describe the wide variety of clavicular fractures. The most commonly used system was proposed by Allman (6) and is used to divide fractures into three basic categories: group I, middle third fractures; group II, lateral third fractures; group III, medial third fractures. Neer (7,8) subdivided group II fractures into separate subgroups based on the extent of the associated ligamentous injury: In type I fractures, the coracoclavicular ligaments remain intact; in type II fractures, disruption of the coracoclavicular ligaments is associated with a corresponding upward displacement of the medial fragment; type III fractures involve the articular surface of the acromioclavicular joint. However, most physicians base treatment on the direction and degree of fragment displacement.

Epidemiological studies have shown that 80% of clavicular fractures occur in the middle third (group I) (1). This correlates with biomechanical studies that have shown that the weakest point of the clavicle lies at the transition region between the curves where the bone is found to be thinnest and lacks any muscular or ligamentous support (9). Of the remaining fractures, 15% occur in the distal third and less than 5% involve the medial third of the clavicle.

Several studies have shown a bimodal distribution of clavicular fractures with the peaks found in data obtained from people in the second/third and sixth/seventh decades of life (1,10). This specific pattern can be explained if the mechanism of injury is taken into consideration. Most of the fractures occurring in the second and third decades of life are found in males, and they usually result from violent or high-energy injuries (e.g., bicycle and motor vehicle accidents as well as sports injuries). In these cases, direct trauma to the point of the shoulder causes the compressed clavicle to fail (9). For patients over 60 years, the majority of clavicular fractures is in osteoporotic bones and is the result of simple falls from a standing height onto an outstretched hand.

INDICATIONS/CONTRAINDICATIONS

Although nonoperative care results in high-union rates for most clavicular fractures, surgery is indicated in certain circumstances. In these particular situations, operative fixation is thought to yield the best clinical results in terms of alignment, union, and early mobilization. The main indication for internal fixation of a clavicular fracture is displacement and/or shortening greater than 15 to 20 mm in young, healthy, active individuals (11). Although the clavicle has good healing and remodeling capabilities, significantly displaced fractures have been shown to cause pain and decreased patient satisfaction due to cosmetic deformity and functional limitations (11). Relative indications for internal fixation of clavicular fractures include the following:

- open fractures;
- associated vascular injury;
- progressive neurological deficits;
- gross displacement with skin tenting that will likely lead to skin breakdown;
- significant medialization of the shoulder girdle;
- torn coracoclavicular ligaments with distal fracture;
- ipsilateral fractures of the clavicle and scapula (floating shoulder);
- multiply injured patients;
- bilateral clavicular fractures; and
- complex, ipsilateral, upper-extremity fracture.

Contraindications to surgical management of clavicular fractures include compromised soft tissue, active infection at or near the operative site, an unreliable or noncompliant patient, and pathologic or severely osteopenic bone that prevent adequate surgical fixation (12).

PATIENT EVALUATION AND PREOPERATIVE PLANNING

As with any musculoskeletal injury, a complete history and physical examination should be performed. Specific information should be obtained regarding the mechanism of the injury, the degree or magnitude of pain, paresthesia, or loss of function. A proper physical examination should include a thorough inspection of the injured shoulder for signs of swelling, ecchymosis, deformity, skin tenting, or compromise (Fig. 1.1). Shoulder asymmetry may or may not be detected when comparing the injured and contralateral sides. Typically, a displaced clavicular fracture can be diagnosed by observation and be based on clinical deformity. Palpation along the entire length of the clavicle is very accurate as the fracture site is very tender and a step-off deformity can often be appreciated.

One must also examine the sternoclavicular and acromioclavicular joints as well as the scapula and shoulder joint for focal areas of tenderness that may reveal associated injuries. Due to the close proximity of numerous other important structures, the physical examination should include a careful assessment of neurovascular or lung pathology. Brachial plexus injuries, while rare, can occur in conjunction with clavicular fractures (13,14) and can be detected through detailed neurological testing in the upper limb. The upper extremity must also be assessed for evidence of vascular compromise by comparing the temperature, color, peripheral pulses, and blood pressure of the injured limb to those characteristics of the contralateral extremity. If the comparison yields no differences, then vascular damage did not occur. An angiogram should be obtained if the physician suspects vascular injury associated with the clavicular fracture. In patients with high-energy injuries, physical examination of the lung fields and a chest x-ray should be performed because pneumothorax occurs in 3% of patients (2).

Ultimately, the diagnosis of a clavicular fracture is confirmed with a radiograph of the injured shoulder. Usually, a standard anteroposterior (AP) view of the clavicle is enough to establish the definitive diagnosis (Fig. 1.2). It is important that the AP radiograph includes the sternoclavicular and acromioclavicular joints so that any disruption or fracture of these joints can be ruled out. An apical oblique view, with the x-ray beam angled 20 to 60 degrees cephalad, minimizes the interference of the thoracic cage and improves visualization of the clavicle (Fig. 1.3) (15). To better analyze the integrity of the coracoclavicular ligaments in clavicular fractures of the lateral third, physicians should view the effect of weight-bearing radiograph (4.5 kg) (3).

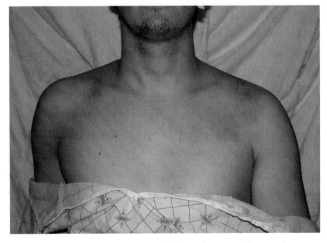

Figure 1.1. Clinical photograph showing swelling and ecchymosis over the left clavicle.

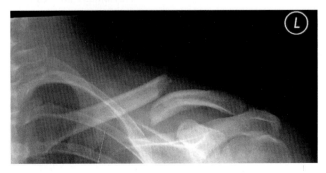

Figure 1.2. Preoperative AP radiograph demonstrating a midclavicular fracture with shortening and overriding of the fracture.

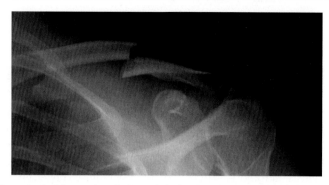

Figure 1.3. An apical oblique view helps minimize interference of the thoracic structures when viewing the fracture.

Medial clavicular fractures, although rare, require special attention if any posterior displacement or intra-articular extension is found. Because it will provide the optimal visualization of the fracture and sternoclavicular joint, a computed tomography (CT) scan is often helpful when a complex, medial, clavicular fracture is present.

Careful preoperative planning based on the fracture characteristics is essential to any orthopedic surgical procedure. Although the emphasis of this chapter is on plate fixation of acute clavicular fractures, other surgical procedures, with varying results, have been described. Intramedullary pins or nails are a viable treatment alternative because they allow for limited exposure and soft-tissue disruption. However, numerous case reports have been cited regarding pin migration out of the bone and into the lung (16), ascending aorta (17), pulmonary artery (18), abdominal aorta (19), and even the spinal canal (20). Although rare, the potential for migration still exists, even when precautionary measures such as using threaded pins or bending the pin at the end, are used.

In our opinion, plate fixation is a better surgical option for clavicular fractures than pin fixation for several reasons. First and foremost, intramedullary fixation fails to provide rotational control at the fracture site. Plate fixation controls both length and rotation as well as providing compression in length stable fracture patterns. The stable construct obtained after plate fixation allows for early use of the upper extremity, unlike the postoperative immobilization that is often required after intramedullary pin fixation.

SURGICAL TECHNIQUE

Acute Clavicular Fracture

Surgery is performed with the patient under general anesthesia. Some surgeons advocate a regional nerve block in combination with general anesthesia for postoperative pain control. The patient is placed in a beach-chair (semisitting) position with a small pad behind the shoulder blade and the involved upper extremity tucked into the side (Fig. 1.4) and square draped (Fig. 1.5). We have found that in typical circumstances the arm need not be free draped to obtain or maintain a fracture reduction. The opposite iliac crest is square draped if autologous bone grafting will be required in patients with severely comminuted fractures.

The proximal and distal ends of the clavicle are marked on the skin and an incision is centered over the fracture site (Fig. 1.6). An oblique incision is made along the superior surface of the clavicle. The skin and subcutaneous tissue are raised as a flap, protecting any obvious cutaneous nerve branches, and reflected upward allowing the underlying myofascia to be identified (Fig. 1.7). This layer, including the deltopectoral muscle attachment, is raised as contiguous flaps and is preserved so that a two-layered closure can be achieved over the plate (21).

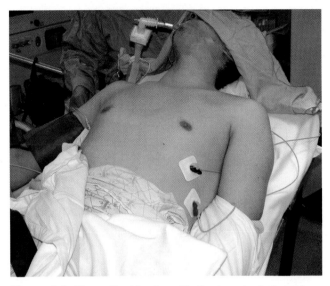

Figure 1.4. The patient is placed in the beach-chair position with a small pad behind the involved shoulder. The arm is draped at the side.

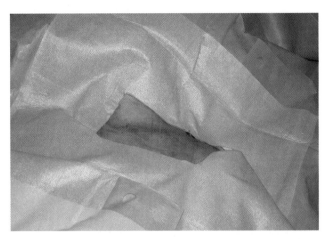

Figure 1.5. Placement of a sterile covering over the patient with an appropriate sized opening to address the clavicle fracture.

Next, the fracture site is identified by fully exposing the proximal and distal fragments (Fig. 1.8), which are held with reduction forceps, and the clavicle is realigned (Figs. 1.9 and 1.10). As little soft-tissue dissection as possible is used to allow correct repositioning and apposition of the fracture.

Following reduction, the fracture can be temporarily fixed with a 2.0-mm Kirschner wire aimed perpendicular to the fracture line (Fig. 1.11). A 3.5-mm limited-contact dynamic-compression (LCDC) plate with a minimum of 6 holes (10-hole maximum) is applied superiorly and held in position with a reduction clamp (Fig. 1.12). The first screw is inserted in a hole on the side of the fracture site opposite where the K wire and the reduction clamp are positioned (Fig. 1.13). Extreme care should be taken in drilling and placing the screws to avoid injury to the subclavian structures and the lung. It is generally advisable to place a protective instrument along the inferior surface of the clavicle to prevent the drill from inadvertently damaging any vital structures. A minimum of three screws should be placed on either side of the fracture such that purchase is achieved through all six cortices of bone.

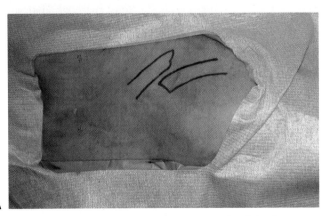

A

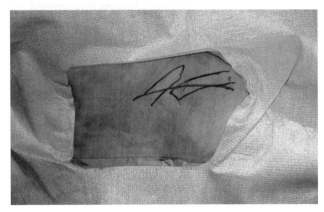

B

Figure 1.6. A. The proximal and distal ends of the fracture are marked on the skin. **B.** The skin incision is then performed between these two points.

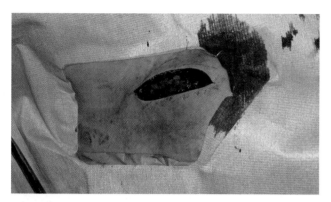

Figure 1.7. The subcutaneous tissues are incised, revealing the myofascial layer underneath, which is dissected as a contiguous flap superiorly and inferiorly and preserved for later closure.

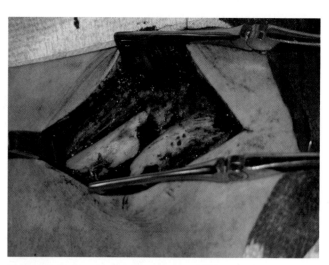

Figure 1.8. The fracture site is exposed.

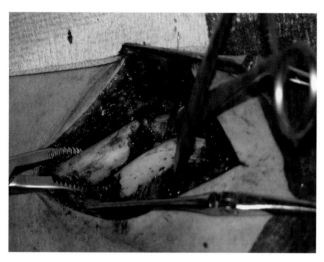

Figure 1.9. The proximal and distal fragments are mobilized with small-fragment reduction forceps.

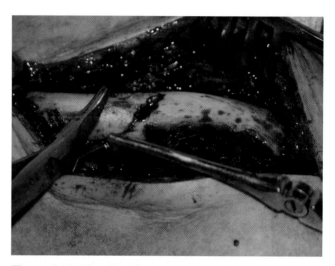

Figure 1.10. The distal fragment is distracted, elevated, and derotated, and the fragments are reduced. A small defect is present in the center due to fracture comminution.

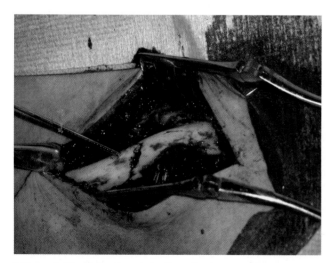

Figure 1.11. Following reduction, the fracture site is temporarily fixed with a 2.0-mm K wire aimed perpendicular to the fracture line.

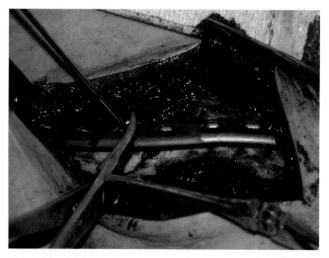

Figure 1.12. After temporary transfixion with a 2.0-mm K wire, a precontoured plate is applied. The use of a precontoured plate saves operative time and reduces soft-tissue irritation at the proximal and distal ends.

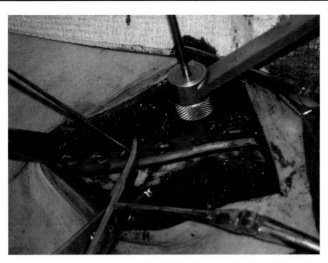

Figure 1.13. The first screw should be positioned in a hole on the opposite side of the fracture where the K wire and the reduction clamp are securing the plate.

It is easier to contour a 3.5-mm LCDC plate to the S-shaped clavicle than it is to contour a standard compression plate, as has been previously described (22), and the LCDC plate is stronger than a similarly sized pelvic-reconstruction plate. More recently, we have used anatomic plates precontoured to fit the clavicle. Use of precontoured plates saves time, as extensive intraoperative contouring is not required, and their low-profile anatomic shape minimizes prominence, especially medially where a straight plate tends to project anteriorly (Fig. 1.14). Because the most common fracture pattern for midshaft clavicular fractures is transverse, the plate is applied in the compression mode to maximize compression.

Once all of the screws have been inserted and the stability of the construct insured, the field is copiously irrigated with normal saline (Fig. 1.15). A standard closure is then performed in layers with use of no. 1 absorbable sutures for the myofascia, no. 2–0 absorbable sutures for the subcutaneous tissue, and clips or a subcuticular stitch for the skin

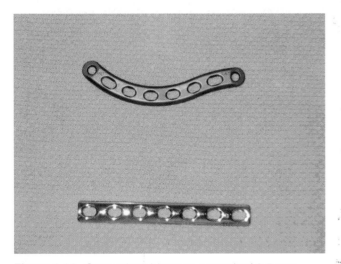

Figure 1.14. Comparison between a standard 3.5-mm LCDC plate and an anatomic plate contoured to fit the clavicle. A precontoured plate saves operative time and minimizes the prominence of the hardware.

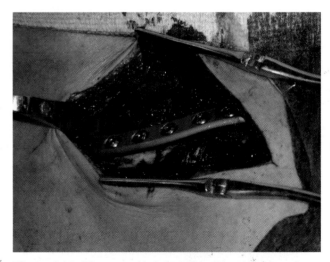

Figure 1.15. The wound is irrigated and local bone graft can be packed around the fracture site both anteriorly and posteriorly (if needed). Care is taken to avoid placing excessive amounts of bone inferiorly, where it may interfere with the thoracic outlet.

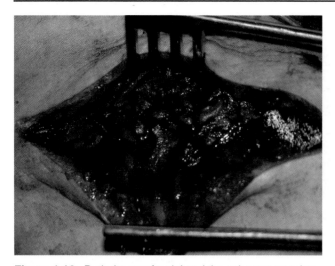

Figure 1.16. Both the myofascial and the subcutaneous layers are closed with interrupted absorbable sutures.

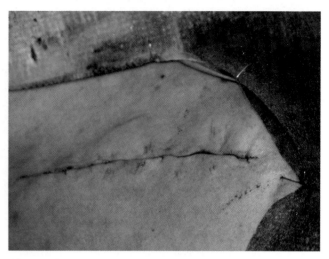

Figure 1.17. The skin layer is closed with clips or a subcuticular stitch.

(Figs. 1.16 and 1.17). Secure wound closure is essential to insure adequate soft-tissue coverage of the bone as well as a decreased incidence of wound hematoma. Drains are not used. Infiltration with long-acting local anesthetic may be used at this time to help manage postoperative pain (Fig. 1.18). After the surgery, the arm is placed in a sling or shoulder immobilizer (Fig. 1.19).

Malunion and Nonunion

When a clavicular fracture is initially managed nonoperatively but fails to unite, indications for repair include (10)

- malunion or nonunion with shortening (>15 mm, often 2 to 3 cm);
- angulatory deformity (>30 degrees at the fracture site) or translation (>1 cm);

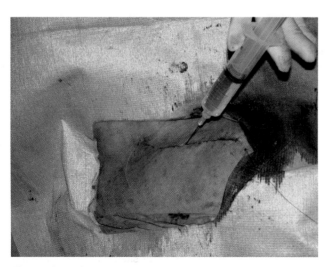

Figure 1.18. Long-acting local anesthetic may be injected to help manage postoperative pain.

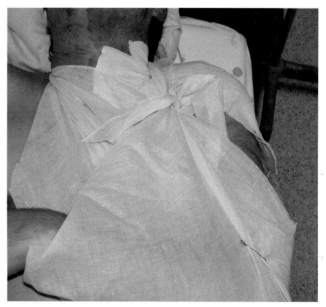

Figure 1.19. After the surgery, the arm is placed in a conventional sling.

- symptoms consistent with thoracic outlet syndrome;
- chronic pain with repetitive, overhead, or resisted activity;
- pain when using shoulder straps or backpacks;
- dissatisfaction with the appearance or asymmetry of the shoulders; or
- substantial disability detected on patient-oriented limb specific health measures.

For these patients, thorough preoperative planning, based on clinical and radiographic data, is used to identify the amount and degree of deformity as well as the correction that will be required. Also, if the malunion or nonunion caused shortening, then length should be restored. If the clinical and radiographic data show that shortening exceeds 1 cm, an intercalary bone graft may be required to compensate for bone loss. In patients with symptomatic malunions, an osteotomy must often be performed through the extensively remodeled fracture. In these patients, a combination of osteotomes and a microsagittal saw (cooled continually with irrigation throughout the cutting) is used to re-create the original fracture line. The medullary canal is opened with a 3.5-mm drill bit in each fragment. An intercalary bone graft can then be placed where necessary. A small notch should be made with the saw in each fragment prior to the corrective osteotomy as a means to measure the clavicular length. The distal fragment is typically rotated anteriorly, such that its flat, superior surface faces anteriorly rather than superiorly. Malrotation is best corrected by redirecting superiorly the flat, superior surface of the distal fragment, creating similar clavicular surfaces on both sides of the osteotomy. Caution should be taken to protect the underlying neural and vascular structures, and no attempt should be made to explore or formally decompress the brachial plexus.

For patients whose clavicular fractures have failed to unite, plate fixation is an excellent treatment option. With atrophic nonunions, the iliac crest is draped for supplemental autologous bone graft. In hypertrophic nonunions, augmentation of the nonunion site with iliac crest bone graft is unnecessary because abundant local bone, which is resected from the bone ends, may be used for this purpose. When packing the osteotomy or nonunion site with local callus or autologous bone graft, care should be taken not to place an abundant amount of bone graft inferiorly because the formation of a large callus could impinge on the underlying neurovascular structures.

POSTOPERATIVE MANAGEMENT

Most patients are discharged with their arm immobilized in a sling or shoulder immobilizer for comfort. Patients begin pendulum exercises during the first postoperative week and active-assisted motion at 2 weeks. Immediate motion of the elbow and shoulder are encouraged to improve function and to restore patient independence. The sutures or staples are generally removed in 10 to 14 postoperative days.

Patients are followed at 2 to 4 week intervals during the first 8 weeks with standard radiographs to ensure that the reduction is maintained and that the hardware has not loosened or changed position. Often, the standard AP view of the clavicle may not provide adequate visualization of the fracture because the overlying hardware obscures the fracture site. Riemer et al (23) recommended an abduction-lordotic view, with the shoulder abducted to 135 degrees and the x-ray beam angled 25 degrees cephalad. This results in the superior rotation of the clavicle so the plate no longer obstructs the view of the fracture site. By combining this view with a standard AP view, one can visualize almost 90 degrees of the clavicle for an accurate assessment of fracture healing.

At 4 weeks, if radiographs show no loss of reduction (Fig. 1.20), full active and passive motion is initiated and the patient is weaned from the sling. Resistance and strengthening activities are allowed when radiographs reveal union, typically at 6 to 8 weeks postinjury. Complete shoulder rehabilitation is recommended before the patient resumes any throwing, racquet, contact, or collision sports.

Several studies have examined the rates of union following plate osteosynthesis of acute clavicular fractures. Early studies suggested that open reduction and internal fixation of clavicular fractures were associated with a high-nonunion rate (2,3). However, more recent

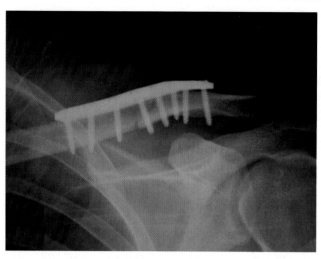

Figure 1.20. Postoperative radiograph demonstrating correction of the deformity, apposition of the bone ends, and accurate placement of the plate.

reports using modern small-fragment implants have shown vastly improved outcomes. The first of these studies involved a small number of patients and reported 100% union rates following primary plate fixation of midclavicular fractures (2,24). In a larger study (122 patients), Poigenfurst et al (21) achieved union in 96% of patients treated with plating for acute clavicular fractures. The five nonunions healed after re-operation and secondary plating. Bostman et al (26) studied 103 patients with midclavicular fractures treated with primary plate fixation. They documented a union rate of 97.1% with only 3 nonunions and 3 delayed unions. More recently, Shen et al (27) conducted the largest research project involving plate fixation of acute clavicular fractures in which 232 patients were followed for a minimum of 3 postoperative years. They reported a union rate of 97% with the mean time to union 10 weeks; no patients were shown to have any impairment in their shoulder strength and range of motion. Overall, the results of these studies demonstrate that internal fixation of acute clavicular fractures leads to high rates of union and very good functional results. To our knowledge, no randomized, controlled trials have been published in which nonoperative treatments were compared to internal fixation of acute clavicular fractures.

COMPLICATIONS

Complications following the plating of a clavicular fracture are uncommon. Vascular injuries, ranging from acute lacerations to trauma-inducing thrombosis or aneurysm, are rare but limb-threatening injuries. Brachial plexus injuries tend to be mostly traction neurapraxia from which the patient usually recovers within 3 to 4 months of injury. Excessive callus formation at the fracture site has been associated with thoracic outlet syndrome (28,29). Although rare, chronic impingement of the neurovascular structures between the callus and the underlying first rib can lead to symptoms of arm pain, paresthesia, and weakness.

Bony complications associated with clavicular fractures include malunion, nonunion, and posttraumatic arthritis of the sternoclavicular and acromioclavicular joints. Malunion of the clavicle after plating is very rare and is the result of hardware failure or technical error. If a clavicular fracture fails to unite by 4 to 6 months following the surgery, it can be classified as a nonunion (21,23,25–27). Although the exact cause of a nonunion is unknown, several systemic and local factors have been implicated in its development. Systemic factors include smoking, alcoholism, poor nutrition, and the presence of a chronic systemic disease. Poorly reduced or insecurely fixed fractures can also contribute to the development of a nonunion. Schwarz and Hocker (30) reported a nonunion rate of 12% following surgical fixation of clavicular fractures with 2.7-mm dynamic compression plates. They attributed their high failure rate to using plates of inadequate length and size and concluded that a minimum of three screws or six cortices must be placed on either side of the fracture site to achieve adequate stabilization. The development of symptomatic arthritis of the sternoclavicular or acromioclavicular joints following a clavicle fracture is dependent on the initial fracture pattern. Even with accurate surgical fixation of the clavicle, patients with intra-articular fractures are at risk for developing posttraumatic degenerative arthritis

As with any surgical procedure, plate fixation of a clavicular fracture carries a small risk of infection, blood loss, and hardware-related prominence or failure. Deep infection can lead to loosening of the hardware, soft-tissue ulceration, and the development of a nonunion. However, the incidences of postoperative infection following clavicular plating remain few. In their study of 103 patients, Bostman et al (26) reported that only five patients developed deep infection requiring re-operation and removal of the hardware, and only three patients developed superficial infection, which subsided in each case with the use of antibiotic therapy. With similar results to Bostman (26), Shen et al (27) reported only a single case of deep infection and four cases of superficial infection in their 232 patient population.

The treatment of deep infection associated with plate fixation requires early recognition and aggressive treatment. Although a long-term antibiotic regimen and local debridement are the standard treatments, hardware removal is also necessary to control the infection in the majority of patients. Superficial infections can be managed with local irrigation and debridement along with a short course of oral antibiotic therapy.

Perhaps the most common but easily avoidable complication remains shoulder stiffness after prolonged immobilization. Close follow-up with a physician or physiotherapist is necessary to insure that the patient is performing range-of-motion exercises. Most patients regain full shoulder range of motion and strength.

Other important postoperative complications include hardware failure and soft-tissue irritation with possible wound dehiscence. Hardware failure is a rare occurrence when appropriate issues are addressed in the selection and insertion of the plate. Loosening and breakage of the plate can often be predicted by insufficient purchase of the screws during the procedure or selection of an inadequately sized plate (30).

Due to the paucity of soft tissues and prominence of the plate and screws, many patients require later hardware removal. Shen et al (27) reported that 171 of their 232 patients had their hardware removed, with two of these patients suffering a refracture after hardware removal. Generally, refracture after plate removal is rare as long as 12 months have passed since the fixation of the fracture.

RECOMMENDED READINGS

1. Nordqvist A, Petersson C. The incidence of fractures of the clavicle. *Clin Orthop* 1994;300:127–132.
2. Rowe CR. An atlas of anatomy and treatment of midclavicular fractures. *Clin Orthop* 1968;58:29–42.
3. Neer CS. Nonunion of the clavicle. *JAMA.* 1960;172:1006–1011.
4. McKee MD, Schemitsch EH, Stephen DJ, et al. Functional outcome following clavicle fractures in polytrauma patients [abstract]. *J Trauma* 1999;47:616.
5. Craig EV. Fractures of the clavicle. In: Rockwood CA, Matsen FA, eds. *The Shoulder* Philadelphia: WB Saunders; 1990:367–412.
6. Allman FL. Fractures and ligamentous injuries of the clavicle and its articulation. *J Bone Joint Surg Am* 1967;49A:774–784.
7. Neer CS. Fractures of the distal clavicle with detachment of the coracoclavicular ligaments in adults. *J Trauma* 1963;3:99–110.
8. Neer CS. Fractures of the distal third of the clavicle. *Clin Orthop* 1968;58:43–50.
9. Stanley D, Trowbridge EA, Norris SH. The mechanism of clavicular fracture: a clinical and biomechanical analysis. *J Bone Joint Surg Br* 1988;70B:461–464.
10. Robinson CM. Fractures of the clavicle in the adult: epidemiology and classification. *J Bone Joint Surg Br* 1998;80B:476–484.
11. Hill JM, McGuire MH, Crosby LA. Closed treatment of displaced middle-third fractures of the clavicle gives poor results. *J Bone Joint Surg Br* 1997;79B:537–539.
12. McKee MD, Wild LM, Schemitsch EH. Midshaft malunions of the clavicle. *J Bone Joint Surg Am* 2004;86A(suppl 1):37–43.
13. Barbier O, Malghem J, Delaere O, et al. Injury to the brachial plexus by a fragment of bone after fracture of the clavicle. *J Bone Joint Surg Br* 1997;79:534–536.
14. Rumball KM, Da Silva VF, Preston DN, et al. Brachial-plexus injury after clavicular fracture: case report and literature review. *Can J Surg* 1991;34:264–266.

15. Weinberg B, Seife B, Alonso P. The apical oblique view of the clavicle: its usefulness in neonatal and childhood trauma. *Skeletal Radiol* 1991;20:201–203.
16. McCaughan JS, Miller PR. Migration of Steinmann pin from shoulder to lung. *JAMA* 1969;207:1917.
17. Nordback I, Markkula H. Migration of Kirschner wire from clavicle into ascending aorta. *Acta Chirop Scand* 1985;151:177–179.
18. Leonard JW, Gifford RW. Migration of a Kirschner wire from clavicle into pulmonary artery. *Am J Cardiol* 1965;16:598–600.
19. Naidoo P. Migration of Kirschner wire from clavicle into the abdominal aorta. *Arch Emerg Med* 1991;8:292–295.
20. Norrell H, Llewellyn RC. Migration of a threaded Steinmann pin from an acromioclavicular joint into the spinal canal. *J Bone Joint Surg Am* 1965;47A:1024–1026.
21. Poigenfurst J, Rappold G, Fischer W. Plating of fresh clavicular fractures: results of 122 operations. *Injury* 1992;23:237–241.
22. McKee MD, Seiler JG, Jupiter JB. The application of the limited contact dynamic compression plate in the upper extremity: an analysis of 114 consecutive cases. *Injury* 1995;26:661–666.
23. Riemer BL, Butterfield SL, Daffner RH, et al. The abduction lordotic view of the clavicle: a new technique for radiographic visualization. *J Orthop Trauma* 1991;5:392–394.
24. Ali Khan MA, Lucas HK. Plating of fractures of the middle third of the clavicle. *Injury* 1978;9:263–267.
25. O'Rourke IC, Middleton RW. The place and efficacy of operative management of fractured clavicle. *Injury* 1975;6:236–240.
26. Bostman O, Manninen M, Pihlajamaki H. Complications of plate fixation in fresh displaced midclavicular fractures. *J Trauma* 1997;43:778–783.
27. Shen WJ, Liu TJ, Shen YS. Plate fixation of fresh displaced midshaft clavicle fractures. *Injury* 1999;30:497–500.
28. Connolly J, Dehne R. Nonunion of the clavicle and thoracic outlet syndrome. *J Trauma* 1989;29:1127–1133.
29. Fujita K, Matsuda K, Sakai Y, et al. Late thoracic outlet syndrome secondary to malunion of the fractured clavicle: case report and review of the literature. *J Trauma* 2001;50:332–335.
30. Schwarz N, Hocker K. Osteosynthesis of irreducible fractures of the clavicle with 2.7-mm ASIF plates. *J Trauma* 1992;33:179–183.

2

Scapula Fractures: Open Reduction Internal Fixation

Peter A. Cole

INDICATIONS/CONTRAINDICATIONS

In 1938, Wilson recorded a 1% incidence of scapula fractures in a comprehensive review of 4,390 broken bones. It is estimated that scapula fractures account for 3% to 5% of all fractures about the shoulder girdle. The well-endowed parascapular musculature, the oblique plane mobility of the scapula on the thorax, and the surrounding skeletal structures (which usually yield first) explain the relative rarity of scapula fractures. However, increased recognition of shoulder morbidity after high-energy trauma as well as improving familiarity with surgical approaches to the scapula have clarified the indications for nonoperative versus surgical treatment.

Fractures of the scapula follow a bimodal pattern of injuries based on the vector and mechanism of force to the shoulder. Low-energy and sporting accidents often lead to partial articular fractures that usually involve the anterior glenoid process and are commonly associated with anterior shoulder dislocations. These fractures are often referred to as bony Bankart lesions and may be characterized by anterior shoulder instability. If shoulder instability is present either clinically or on radiographic examination, then operative intervention in an appropriate surgical candidate is recommended. These criteria are usually present with fractures involving more than 20% of the articular surface.

A second variety of scapula fractures involves the glenoid neck and body, and they generally occur as a result of high-energy trauma. These fractures may or may not involve the glenoid articular surface. Because of the mechanism causing the fracture, associated injuries occur in many of these patients. In seriously injured patients, diagnosis and subsequent treatment of a scapula fracture are often delayed due to treatment of other life-threatening or limb-threatening conditions. According to a common misconception, scapulothoracic dissociation frequently occurs in the setting of scapula fractures; however, scapulothoracic injury results from a violent traction force to the upper extremity, which is quite the opposite mechanism of a typical scapula fracture.

Displaced scapular fractures that extend into the glenoid articular surface often require surgical treatment. Articular fractures should be treated with open reduction and internal fixation (ORIF) if a step off of 3 to 4 mm is encountered and more than 20% of the joint is involved (Fig. 2.1). Lesser degrees of articular step off, gap, and percentage of joint involvement, must be placed into the context of the patient's occupation, age, activity level, physiologic status, and hand dominance.

The optimal treatment of displaced extra-articular scapular fractures remains controversial. Recent studies support internal fixation of scapula neck fractures since large displacement or angulation leads to compromise of shoulder function. Ada and Miller have recommended ORIF of scapular neck fractures when the glenoid is medially displaced more than 9 mm or angular displacement exceeds 40 degrees. Their recommendation is based on a review of 16 patients treated nonoperatively: 50% had pain, 40% had exertional weakness, and 20% had decreased motion at a follow-up of 15 months or later. Eight patients in this same study were treated operatively, and all achieved a painless range of motion.

In the experience of other authors, medialization of the glenoid up to 1 cm has been well tolerated in most patients. Therefore, ORIF should be considered when medialization of the glenohumeral joint measures more than 15 mm, angular deformity in the semicoronal plane is more than 25 degrees, or fracture translation exceeds 100% at the lateral border of the scapula (Fig. 2.2). The indications for surgery are even stronger when two or more of the noted severity criteria are met.

In 1993, Goss described the superior shoulder suspensory complex (SSSC), an osseoligamentous ring made up by the acromion, coracoid, clavicle, and glenoid (Fig. 2.3). Goss theorized that if two disruptions are found in the ring structures, including their capsuloligamentous connections, then the glenohumeral joint would be "floating," a condition that describes discontinuity between the axial and appendicular skeleton (Fig. 2.4). Although this theory has been challenged by some authors, Goss advocated surgery if two or more components of the SSSC are injured simultaneously. Further studies have suggested that surgery is indicated when the SSSC complex structures are displaced and unstable. Somewhat arbitrarily, if each SSSC injury causes displacement of more than 1 cm, the floating shoulder condition warrants surgery in an appropriate candidate. Most commonly, the decision-making process leads to surgical fixation of both injuries, which facilitates early rehabilitation.

Isolated fractures to the acromion or coracoid process are less common. Acromion process and spine fractures occur as a result of direct and concentrated blows to the superior shoulder region, whereas coracoid process fractures result from traction injuries through the biceps and coracobrachialis. If either an acromion or coracoid fracture is displaced more than 10 mm, ORIF may be indicated in a physiologically young and active patient. If the acromion fracture is displaced, then a supraspinatus-outlet x-ray should be evaluated for acromial depression, which may contribute to impingement syndrome, and therefore warrant operative correction.

Surgery is contraindicated when an extra-articular scapular fracture is displaced less than 10 mm and angulated less than 25 degrees because the outcomes of nonoperative treatment for even moderately displaced scapula fractures are uniformly good. Active mobility of the elbow and wrist are encouraged immediately, but a sling and rest are indicated for 10 to 14 days. Scapula fractures heal rapidly due to the rich blood supply in the shoulder girdle. Active range of motion can be started by 4 weeks and maximized quickly. Resistive exercises are begun by 8 weeks, and return to full activities is usually possible by 12 weeks.

CLASSIFICATION

Only a few classifications have been developed for scapula fractures. The classification of Ada and Miller, as well as that of Hardegger et al, are anatomically defined and comprehensive. The classification scheme developed by Mayo et al is a reorganized version of the Ideberg classification and is based on a consideration of the imaging and operative findings of 27 intra-articular glenoid fractures. The latter classification is helpful in directing surgical decision making, and it takes into account the associated scapula body and process fractures (Fig. 2.5). The Orthopaedic Trauma Association (OTA) Classification System is an alphanumeric system in which both intra-articular and extra-articular variants are classified (Fig. 2.6).

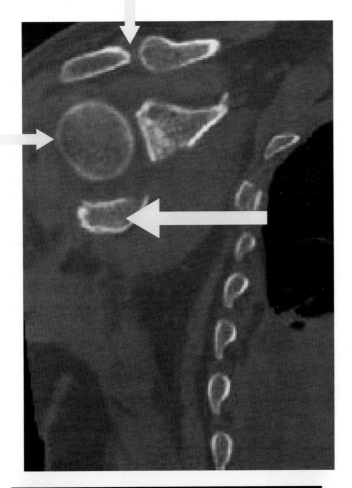

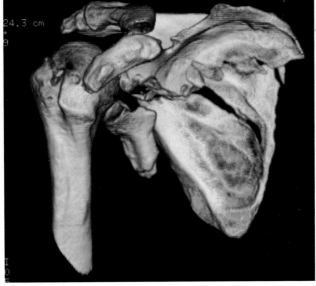

Figure 2.1. A. A 2D-CT view, reformatted in the semicoronal plane, demonstrating the displacement between superior and inferior glenoid fragments. Most superior is the acromioclavicular joint (*downward arrow*), beneath which is the humeral head articulating with the superior glenoid fragment (*rightward arrow*). Below the articulating head is the smaller glenoid fragment (*leftward arrow*). **B.** A 3D-CT image for the same patient as shown in **(A)**. It is easier to interpret relationships of key fragments with a 3D-CT; however, the 2D-CT is necessary because volume averaging causes three-dimensional reconstructions to miss minor fracture lines.

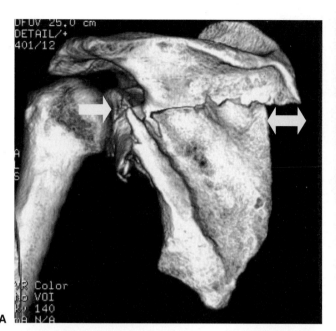

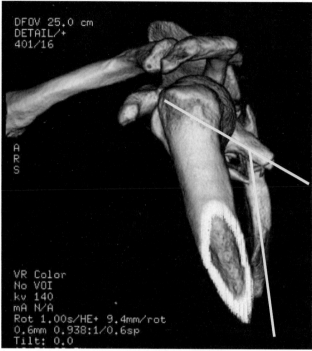

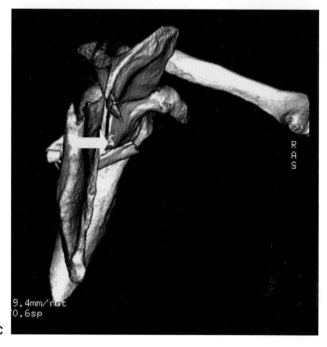

Figure 2.2. **A.** Medialization: a 3D-CT AP image of a scapula demonstrating medialization of the glenoid relative to the scapula body as seen both at the lateral border (*rightward arrow*) and at the superomedial angle at the vertebral border (*two-way arrow*). **B.** Angulation: a 3D-CT image of the same scapula in a plane parallel to the body mimicking the scapula Y x-ray view. Here the two lines marking the lateral borders on the two fragments create a 45-degree angle to each other. **C.** Translation: a 3D-CT image of the same scapula and in the same plane as **B**, but imaging has been taken from the medial side instead of from the lateral side. The amount of translation of the scapula borders, as indicated by the *yellow two-way arrow*, is easy to appreciate.

PREOPERATIVE PLANNING

History

As with many fractures, indications for surgery can be less than distinct. Manual laborers who work with heavy loads and high-demand athletes may need surgery with relatively few indications. Also, if the injury occurs in the dominant extremity of an active individual, or if a patient requires engagement in significant overhead activity, then ORIF may be an attractive alternative treatment. However, injuries more than 3 weeks old, in elderly patients, and in individuals with multiple confounding co-morbidities, nonoperative treatment is likely the best choice.

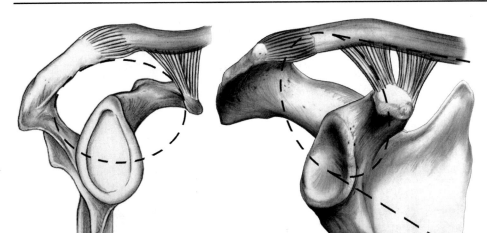

Figure 2.3. This illustration depicts the SSSC, which is an osseoligamentous ring made up of the structures along the broken line circle in this illustration. Goss theorized that if two structures in the ring are disrupted, then a floating shoulder lesion, without osseous or ligamentous continuity between the axial skeleton and the forequarter, would exist. A case of a floating shoulder lesion is illustrated at the end of this chapter (Figs. 2.17 to 2.26).

Physical Examination

The physical examination in the multiply injured patient should follow the advanced trauma life support (ATLS) guidelines. In less seriously injured patients, inspection of the shoulder in a standing or sitting patient is helpful (Fig. 2.7). Medial and caudad displacement of the shoulder may be obvious and cause asymmetry, and it correlates well with the degree of medialization and depression of the glenoid found on radiographs. Because of pain, patients with displaced scapula fractures, particularly when associated with multiple rib or clavicle fractures, cannot voluntarily forward elevate or externally rotate their shoulders to any significant degree.

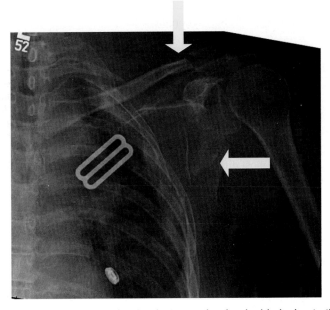

Figure 2.4. An AP x-ray of a shoulder that has sustained a double lesion to the SSSC, which has resulted in a floating shoulder. Note the distal clavicle fracture (*downward arrow*) and glenoid neck fracture (*leftward arrow*), which are both substantially displaced.

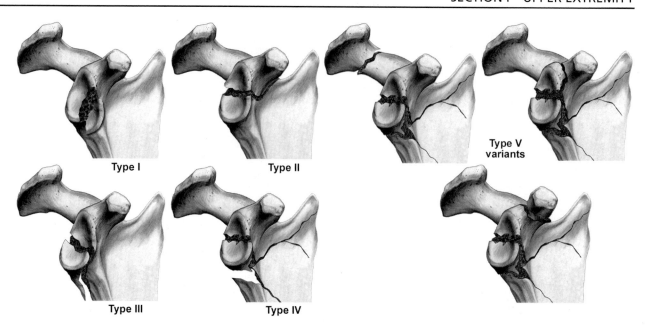

Type I

Type II

Type V variants

Type III

Type IV

Figure 2.5. This image depicts the Ideberg classification as it was modified by Mayo et al. The classification is specific for intra-articular glenoid fractures, and it allows for consideration of the commonly associated fractures of the body and processes. It is helpful for determining the surgical approach; for example, an Ideberg I, II fracture should be addressed via an anterior deltopectoral approach, but the Ideberg IV and V injury is best approached posteriorly because the surgeon needs to stabilize the lateral border.

Ipsilateral, concomitant, neurovascular injuries, while uncommon, require a careful assessment of the brachial plexus and distal limb perfusion. Brachial-plexus injuries occur in up to 10% of patients with scapula fractures and may at times be subtle. Axillary nerve sensation should be documented; however, motor assessment is frequently impossible with displaced fractures. The integrity of the skin should be assessed because abrasions are common after the typical direct-blow mechanism to the shoulder that causes scapula fractures (Fig. 2.8). If the circulation in the upper extremity is questionable, vascular surgery consultation and angiography is strongly recommended.

Radiographic Studies

Three plain x-ray views should be evaluated before proceeding to other studies, which include anteroposterior (AP), scapula Y, and axillary views. The AP x-ray of the scapula should be taken 35 degrees off the sagittal plane to correspond with the same angular position of the scapula on the thorax. The orthogonal scapula Y view is 90 degrees to the AP. The axillary lateral is the most difficult to obtain because of patient discomfort, but it is extremely important.

If an intra-articular glenoid fracture is detected on any x-ray view, then a two-dimensional computed tomography (2D-CT) scan with 1 mm axial cuts, together with coronal and sagittal reconstructions, are helpful to delineate articular displacement, comminution, and fracture location (Fig. 2.9). If more than 1 cm of fracture displacement is found at the scapula neck in any x-ray view, then an opposite shoulder AP radiograph and a three-dimensional (3D)-CT scan should be obtained to better define the fracture displacement. Being misled with an AP view of the injured shoulder is common because the glenoid may be significantly angulated through the lateral border so that visualization of the glenohumeral joint (clear space) is impossible. In these circumstances, a 3D-CT scan is helpful in evaluating angular deformity and medialization of the glenoid.

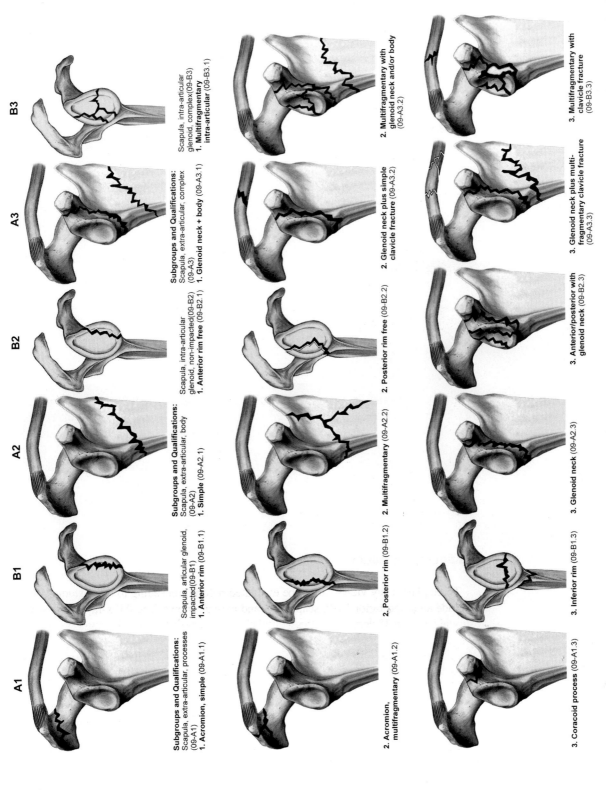

Figure 2.6. This figure shows the AO/OTA classification for scapula fractures. Though it provides a systematic way of classification, I have found it to be inadequate in classifying 15 out of 40 fracture patterns on which operations were performed consecutively between 1999 and 2002. Furthermore, the types of A, B, and C assigned to scapula fractures do not correspond with extra-articular, partial articular, and complete articular variants as they do for other long-bone articulations. The AO/OTA is currently reviewing and revising this classification scheme to address these concerns.

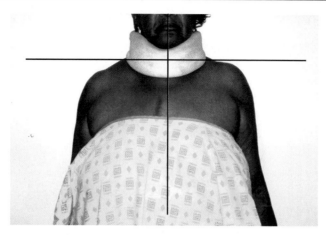

Figure 2.7. This image illustrates why a patient should be properly disrobed for an examination. The dramatic depression and medialization (*black lines*) of the forequarter can occur with high-energy injury.

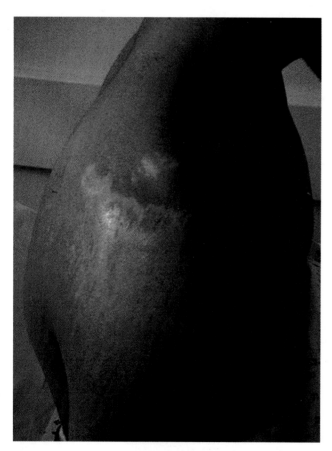

Figure 2.8. Severe scarring resulted from abrasions that occurred during impact of the patient's forequarter. The injury mechanism was caused by a motorcycle crash, and one can imagine the shoulder hitting the gravel embankment at the roadside. To decrease the chance of infection, this patient's operation was delayed 2.5 weeks until the skin re-epithelialized.

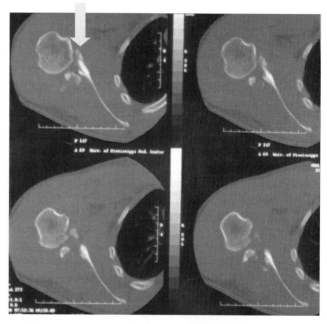

Figure 2.9. This 2D-CT image illustrates the importance of such a study for the intra-articular variants. The surgeon can appreciate the extensive comminution of the joint and that best access and buttress plating will require a posterior approach. The *top arrow* depicts the anterior glenoid.

Surgical Considerations

The scapula is part of a suspensory mechanism of the shoulder, which attaches the upper extremity to the axial skeleton through the clavicle. Eighteen muscular origins and insertions on the scapula aid in providing a stable base for glenohumeral mobility. The goal of surgery is to restore this stable base as well as the relationship of the axial and appendicular skeleton and thus allow for early rehabilitation.

Although fracture-specific exceptions exist, two surgical approaches are used in the vast majority of patients with displaced scapula fractures: the anterior deltopectoral and posterior Judet approaches. Patient positioning and draping, implant selection, cosmesis, and surgical risks are all affected by the approach.

Isolated, anterior, glenoid fractures, as well as the associated transverse fracture extending in a coronal plane from the superomedial angle or scapula vertebral border through the glenoid, are best treated through a deltopectoral approach. In these injuries, the superior glenoid is detached with the coracoid, as in the Mayo Type II fracture. In most other fractures involving the scapula (scapula neck or body fracture with or without glenoid involvement), a posterior approach is preferred. Rarely, combined anterior and posterior approaches are necessary; for example, they may be required in the case of concomitant, anterior articular fractures combined with scapula neck and body variants. The clavicle or acromioclavicular joint may require a separate approach for fixation when indicated.

Viewed from the anterior perspective, the coracoid process is a curved osseous projection off the anterior neck. It is the origin for five anatomic structures and an important surgical landmark. The glenoid process, under the acromion, contains the pear-shaped glenoid fossa, which is approximately 39 mm in a superior-inferior direction and 29 mm in an anterior-posterior direction (in the lower half).

Viewed from posterior, the scapula is a triangular flat bone with a thin translucent body surrounded by thick borders that are well developed as points of muscular origins and insertions. The lateral border of the scapula sweeps up from the inferior angle, forming the thickest condensation of bone, which ends in the neck of the glenoid process. The scapula borders and the glenoid neck provide the best bone for reduction and fixation with plates and screws.

SURGERY

Anterior Approach

The patient is placed in a beach-chair position with an arm board attached to support the extremity. Positioning an x-ray plate behind the shoulder during the setup will help to obtain an intraoperative film following reduction and fixation. A small towel roll under the ipsilateral shoulder helps thrust the shoulder forward. Direct visualization of the joint will minimize the need for intraoperative fluoroscopy; however, the surgeon should evaluate a single, AP, shoulder x-ray after fixation.

An incision is made from the palpable coracoid to a point just lateral to the axillary fold, commonly named the "deltopectoral groove" (Fig. 2.10). This incision is deepened to the deltopectoral interval where the cephalic vein is identified and retracted laterally with the deltoid and protected in the flap. The interval between the deltoid and pectoralis major is developed down to the clavipectoral fascia, which covers the coracobrachialis and subscapularis tendon. This fascia is incised and retractors are placed superiorly and inferiorly. The humerus should be externally rotated to create tension on the subscapularis tendon and to improve visualization of the lesser tuberosity. With the humerus in a neutral position, the subscapularis tendon should be cut 1 cm from its insertion for later repair. For an accurate closure, the surgeon should dissect the subscapularis from the capsule as a distinct layer; this approach is particularly helpful for an anterior glenoid fracture because the surgeon needs to work on both sides (intra-articular and extra-articular) of the capsule. The anterior, circumflex, humeral vessels are at the inferior margin of the subscapularis.

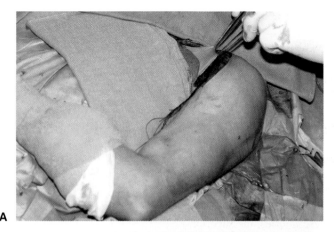

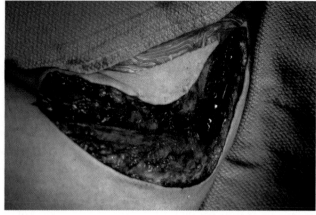

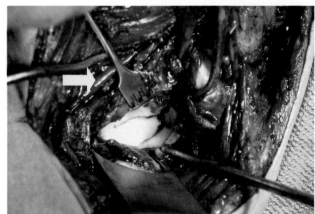

Figure 2.10. **A.** A patient in the beach-chair position has an incision to address a clavicle and ipsilateral glenoid fracture (a common pattern). The isolated, anterior, glenoid fractures and Ideberg II fractures are best approached from this approach. In normal circumstances, a deltopectoral incision runs from the coracoid toward the deltoid insertion, but in this case, it was curved proximally and medially over the anterior clavicle. **B.** The same patient shown in **(A)** after fixation of the clavicle fracture with a 2.7-mm dynamic compression plate. The orientation is the same in **(A)** and **(C)** with the axilla to the left. **C.** The exposure of the glenoid fracture is shown. The sutures are tagging the infraspinatus, and a Fakuda retractor is inside the joint retracting the humeral head. One can see the interval developed between the deltoid and the infraspinatus as landmarked by the cephalic vein (*yellow arrow*).

Below this leash of vessels is the axillary nerve. Stay sutures are placed on each side of the subscapularis muscle to assist in closure and to avoid damage to the axillary nerve.

The joint capsule is cut longitudinally just off the palpable glenoid rim and tagged, or the surgeon can work through the fracture to wash out the joint (see Fig. 2.10C) and then obtain an indirect articular reduction by working extra-articularly with the fragment. Fracture reduction can be improved with a dental pick or small bone hook, and provisional fixation is obtained with Kirschner (K) wires. Depending on the size of the fragment or the degree of comminution, implant (screw) choices may range from 2.0 to 3.5 mm. Most frequently, a mini buttress plate on the anterior-inferior edge is appropriate.

Closure of the capsule and subscapularis is done with no. 2 braided suture. The subcutaneous tissue is approximated with no. 2-0 suture. The skin is closed with a monofilament, subcuticular, absorbable suture.

Posterior Approach

Cervical and thoracic spine injuries are associated with high-energy scapula fractures in 10% to 20% of cases. Treatment requires careful intraoperative patient position. Whenever possible, the injured vertebral segments should be internally stabilized first to insure protection of the spinal cord. However, if nonoperative spine management is chosen, halo traction is preferable to a cervical collar in terms of patient safety.

The patient is positioned in the lateral decubitus position, flopping slightly forward on a beanbag with an axillary roll well placed. The affected upper extremity should be positioned on an arm board or Mayo stand to support the extremity in a 90-degree forward-flexed and slightly abducted position (Fig. 2.11). The entire shoulder, chest wall, and neck should be prepped and draped to allow for manipulation of the shoulder. The planned incision is drawn on the skin with a sterile marker. It is made by following the prominent pos-

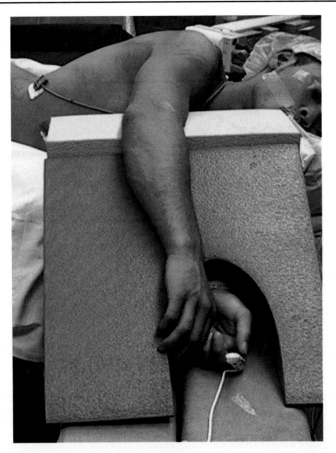

Figure 2.11. This image demonstrates appropriate positioning of the patient when the surgeon is performing a posterior approach to the scapula. Soft-positioning wedges allow for a supportive working surface while protecting the downside arm. The body, positioned on a beanbag, should be allowed to flop forward. The entire arm should be prepped free to allow for manipulation and motion of the glenohumeral joint during the procedure.

terolateral acromion and extending medially to the superomedial angle of the scapula, and then the incision turns caudad along the vertebral border.

"Shucking" the shoulder with one hand, as if to protract and retract the shoulder to create scapulothoracic excursion, the surgeon feels the bony landmarks with his/her opposite hand. A Judet posterior incision is planned along these landmarks. The incision should be 1 cm caudad to the acromial spine and 1 cm lateral to the vertebral border, which allows closure over a plate and improves lateral retraction of the flap during surgery (Fig. 2.12).

The incision is deepened onto the bony ridge of the acromial spine, splitting the interval between trapezius and deltoid insertions. The incision curves distally around the superomedial angle and down the vertebral border. For access to the lateral border of the scapula, the incision must be generous enough to allow for flap mobilization should the surgeon require a more extensile approach. Properly executed, the fascial incision along the acromial spine and medial border should provide a cuff of tissue that is sutured back to its bony origin at the end of the procedure.

The depth of the dissection depends on the need for limited or complete exposure of the posterior scapula; this should be determined in the preoperative plan. Limited windows can be used to access fractures at the lateral border, acromial spine, and vertebral border (Fig. 2.13). An extensive approach can be executed to expose the entire posterior scapula by elevating all musculature off the infraspinatus fossa (Fig. 2.14). The extensile approach preserves the entire subscapularis-muscular sleeve on the anterior surface of the scapula, and of course, the elevated flap respects vascular planes because the surgeon raises it on its neurovascular pedicle (suprascapular artery and nerve) (see Fig. 2.14B). I find it most helpful to utilize an extensile approach for fractures over a week old by elevating the deltoid, infraspinatus, and teres minor

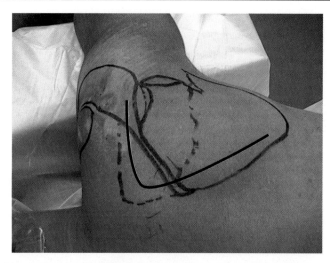

Figure 2.12. The patient is allowed to flop forward, and the scapula landmarks are detailed along with the fracture pattern. The healed abrasion is directly over the fractured posterior spine of the acromion. The incision depicted by the black line is slightly caudad to the acromial spine and lateral to the vertebral border of the scapula.

in a single flap. Also, for complex patterns, the extensive approach is useful when there are more than three exit points around the ring of the scapula. The extensile exposure allows the surgeon adequate control of the fracture at multiple points to effect the reduction and mobilize the fracture by breaking up intervening callus. It will not allow for exposure of the glenoid due to the large flap, which cannot be retracted sufficiently lateral for joint exposure.

If limited windows are desired, tactically created intervals around the scapula perimeter can be used to access specific fracture locations. The muscle plane entered at the acromial

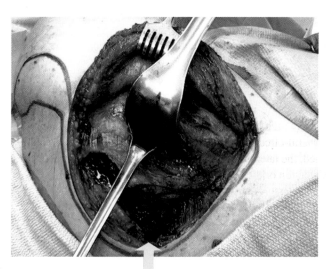

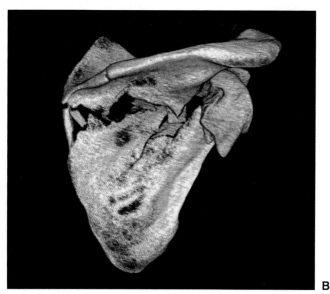

A   B

Figure 2.13. A. An intraoperative photo of the limited windows technique shows that the subcutaneous tissue is elevated with the deltoid muscle (behind the rake retractor) off the rotator cuff. The window depicted by the *upward yellow arrow* is the superomedial angle shown after the infraspinatus has been dissected from the posterior scapula; the procedure creates an axis for fracture reduction at this common location **(B)**. The other two retractors are in the interval between the infraspinatus and teres minor, and this interval is used to expose the lateral border. **B.** A 3D-CT scan shows a common fracture pattern, which lends itself to the exposure shown in **(A)**. The exposure allows for reduction and fixation at two key points: the glenoid neck and the superomedial angle. Both sites will be plated.

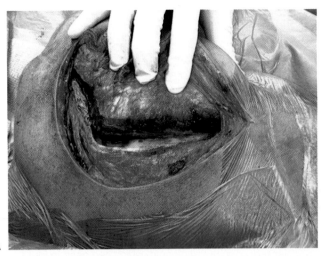
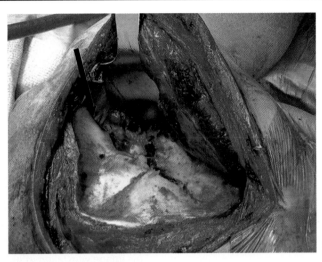

A **B**

Figure 2.14. **A.** The posterior Judet approach results in a flap from the acromial spine and vertebral borders. This extensile exposure will allow for visualization of the entire in-fraspinatus fossa (the posterior scapula) from the vertebral border to the lateral border as shown in **(B)**. The surgeon's fingers are reflecting the entire flap en mass, and a Cobb elevator is used to dissect the flap off the flat, posterior, scapular surface. This approach is best reserved for cases in which surgery has been delayed for more than 10 days from the time of injury or for cases in which severe comminution is present with several displaced-fracture lines exiting multiple scapular borders. It cannot be used when the surgeon desires intra-articular inspection. **B.** Image of same patient shown in **(A)** after flap elevation and retraction. This patient has a fracture variant that is characterized by a broken glenoid neck from the lateral border up into the supraglenoid notch. Extension of another fracture line into the body is apparent in this image, but the severe medialization and anteversion of the glenoid articular surface is not apparent. Note the threat of a retractor by virtue of traction on the suprascapular neurovascular bundle exiting from just below the acromion before it enters the infraspinatus muscle (*black arrow*).

border is between the trapezius and the deltoid, which lies at the inferior margin of the spine and is elevated to uncover the rotator cuff muscles. The deltoid should be dissected off the muscular origin of the infraspinatus and tagged through its fascial cuff for reattachment through bone tunnels later. A Key or Cobb elevator can be used to elevate the infraspina-tus and teres minor from the posterior fossa. At the vertebral border of the scapula, the intermuscular plane is between the infraspinatus–teres minor and the rhomboids.

The most important window in an intra-articular fracture is between the infraspinatus and teres minor because it allows access to the lateral border of the scapula and gleno-humeral joint. Identification of the correct interval is important to avoid denervation of the infraspinatus or injury to the axillary nerve and posterior humeral-circumflex artery in the quadrangular space. Once this important interval is developed, the lateral border of the scapula is exposed to allow reduction and correction of glenoid version or medialization. If the glenoid articular surface must be assessed directly, then a transverse capsulotomy can be made so a retractor can be placed on the anterior edge of the glenoid and the humeral head can be retracted (Fig. 2.15).

Aids for fracture reduction at the lateral border of the scapula are important because specific retractors and reduction tools have not been specifically designed for the scapula. At least two, small, pointed, bone reduction clamps and two, 4-mm, Schantz pins with a small external fixator set, as well as a pair of T-handle chucks, are helpful. Often a 2.7-mm, dynamic, compression plate straddling the lateral border fracture can be helpful for reduc-tion (as well as definitive fixation) because it can be applied perfectly straight on this border. Pointed reduction tenacula are frequently inadequate due to interference with the flap, so a Schantz pin in the proximal and distal segments can be placed in the proper orientation with a small external fixator to reduce the lateral border for subsequent plating. If the reduction is still not stable, a provisional 2.0-mm plate and screws placed slightly more medial can keep the lateral border aligned. Furthermore, a clamp can be placed at an

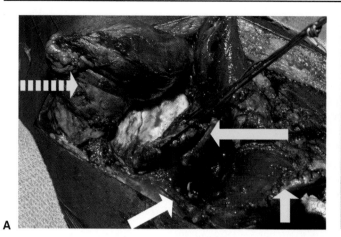
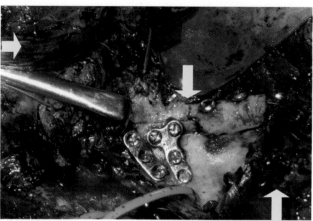

A   B

Figure 2.15. A. Intraoperative photo demonstrating the exposure after a capsulotomy. This image was taken after the articular reduction of the glenoid, which had been in four major fragments. The *rightward broken arrow* points to the deltoid muscle taken off the acromial spine. The sutures are tagging and retracting the joint capsule. The *leftward arrow* points to a fragment of displaced lateral border (glenoid neck). The *upward arrow* points to the infraspinatus, which has been tenotomized for better joint exposure and is on its neurovascular pedicle; the suprascapular artery and nerve are depicted by the *white arrow*. **B.** This image is of the same patient depicted in **(A)** after undergoing reconstruction of the lateral border and with the joint capsule retracted to the left over the joint. The *downward arrow* points to the lateral border; the *upward arrow* points to the infraspinatus; the vessel loop is on the suprascapular nerve and artery; the *rightward arrow* points to the deltoid.

associated fracture at the acromial or vertebral border to help off-load stresses on the lateral border while the reduction is maintained.

I favor 2.7-mm plates along the scapula borders, which are sufficiently strong and are not associated with breakage. In addition, they have a lower profile than 3.5 plates, are easier to contour, and allow for greater screw options. A 2.7-mm dynamic-compression plate is used on the lateral border where stresses are greatest, and 2.7-mm reconstruction plates are used for the acromial and vertebral borders of the scapula because they make contoured fitting, particularly around the superomedial angle, much easier (Fig. 2.16). I have found that two pedi-

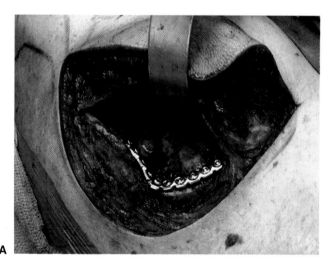
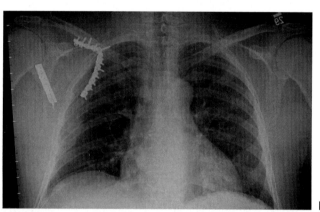

A   B

Figure 2.16. A. The superomedial angle postfixation with a 2.7-mm reconstruction plate. This implant is chosen for its malleability over a difficult contour. This is the same patient depicted in Figure 2.13. A 2.7-mm dynamic-compression plate was chosen for the lateral border because it is relatively strong and requires no contour to lay straight along the glenoid neck. **B.** An immediate postoperative AP chest x-ray that corresponds to the patient in Figure 2.16A. A chest x-ray is helpful to appreciate that the glenoid has been properly oriented relative to the opposite side.

atric Kocher clamps are useful for this maneuver. Longer plates with more screws should be used at the acromial and vertebral borders because each screw is typically 8 to 10 mm.

In the case of a posterior glenoid fracture or an intra-articular glenoid fracture with glenoid neck involvement and minimal displacement or involvement of the acromial spine and vertebral border, a direct posterior approach to the scapular neck or joint can be employed. In these cases, the pathology can be determined and the desired reduction and fixation can be accomplished through the interval between the teres minor and the infraspinatus muscles.

Occasionally, in patients with substantial articular comminution, greater exposure of the joint can be gained with an infraspinatus tenotomy where 1 cm of cuff insertion is left at the greater tuberosity for repair. This allows the slender musculotendinous portion of the infraspinatus to be retracted off the superior glenoid region for better access to the glenohumeral joint. It is repaired with two heavy-braided no. 2 sutures at closure. External rotation against resistance should be protected for 6 postoperative weeks in the case of this repair.

Before wound closure, the surgeon must insure that all extrinsic adhesions and shoulder stiffness are eliminated prior to waking the patient; this is especially important in cases where surgery has been delayed. This manipulation at the end of the procedure is one reason the entire extremity is preoperatively prepped. To insure that the repair is secure and early rehabilitation is possible, the wound is closed over a suction drain under the flap through use of braided no. 2 nonabsorbable sutures placed through several drill holes at the acromion spine and vertebral border. The rest of the musculofascial closure can be performed with a no. 1 absorbable, braided suture. For cosmesis, the skin is closed with a subcuticular absorbable stitch.

POSTOPERATIVE MANAGEMENT

Rehabilitation for the anterior and posterior approaches is based on an identical principle: stable fixation to withstand physiologic stresses of early motion to minimize shoulder stiffness. After surgery, full, passive range of motion should be instituted during the first week. Continuous passive motion (CPM) is not commonly used unless the patient cannot cooperate with rehabilitation adequately or also has an ipsilateral proximal humerus or elbow injury. For patients with profound brachial plexopathy, CPM may be used for extended periods.

The goal during the first 4 postoperative weeks is to regain and maintain shoulder motion. Activities of daily living are encouraged, but no lifting, pushing, pulling, or carrying is allowed for 4 weeks. The use of pulleys, push-pull sticks in the opposite extremity, and supine assisted motion is helpful. A regional anesthetic block with an indwelling interscalene catheter for the first 48 to 72 postoperative hours is an excellent adjunctive method to promote early shoulder motion. Ipsilateral elbow, wrist, and hand exercises including 3- to 5-lb weights (on a supported elbow) are encouraged. These exercises will prevent muscular atrophy and promote reduction of limb edema.

Patients are followed at 2, 6, and 12 week intervals postoperatively, and an AP, scapula Y, and axillary radiographs are obtained. Follow-up at 6 months and 1 year is appropriate to document return of maximum function. Patients with associated brachial plexopathy should be followed by an experienced specialist because some patients may benefit from brachial plexus exploration, tendon transfers, or neural grafting. For the patient with a dense or irrecoverable plexus lesion (flail shoulder) an arthrodesis should be strongly considered.

For anterior approaches to the shoulder, motion should be protected against external rotation past neutral. Likewise, motion against resistance should be avoided for a full 6 weeks to allow healing of the subscapularis, which had been repaired during exposure of the glenohumeral joint. After posterior approaches in which the infraspinatus and teres minor have been mobilized from their origins and in which the deltoid is taken off the acromial spine, these muscles must be protected for 6 weeks. At 6 weeks, patients begin a weight program, beginning with 3 to 5 lbs and increasing as the patient's symptoms allow.

On occasion, shoulder stiffness develops and does not improve with therapy. This is more common in patients with brachial plexus injuries, a head injury, halo-vest protection for spine injury, or complex associated fractures of the ipsilateral extremity. In these patients, a manipulation under anesthesia to jump-start shoulder motion can be helpful. At 3 months after surgery, restrictions can usually be lifted, and the patient can resume a strength and endurance program until fully conditioned.

COMPLICATIONS

Poor outcomes are often the result of associated injuries to the ipsilateral extremity, particularly when the brachial plexus is involved. Other complications include nonunion, malunion, degenerative glenohumeral joint disease, and instability. Shoulder instability and resultant pain and dysfunction can arise from severe angular deformity of the glenoid neck. These complications are far less likely to occur with anatomic restoration of the scapula and its articular surface.

Extensile, posterior, surgical approaches increase the risk of suprascapular nerve injury. This leads to wasting of the rotator cuff musculature, which may never recover. The surgeon must take intraoperative care to avoid excessive traction on the neurovascular bundle as the infraspinatus flap is retracted at the lateral border.

The most common complication is shoulder stiffness. Early aggressive rehabilitation, particularly in those patients with ipsilateral injuries, is recommended. If at the 6 week follow-up, motion is poor, manipulation of the patient's shoulder under anesthesia combined with shoulder arthroscopy is very useful in restoring shoulder motion.

ILLUSTRATIVE CASE FOR TECHNIQUE

A 42-year-old man had fallen 10 feet from a ladder while at work. He was evaluated at a hospital emergency room and subsequently admitted with severe left-shoulder pain and difficulty breathing. He was diagnosed with a broken scapula, clavicle, and multiple fractured left ribs (Fig. 2.17). After 2 days of pain control, the patient was sent home with a sling. He had been evaluated by an orthopedic surgeon in the hospital who explained to the patient that his broken bones would heal without additional treatment and that his prognosis for normal recovery was good.

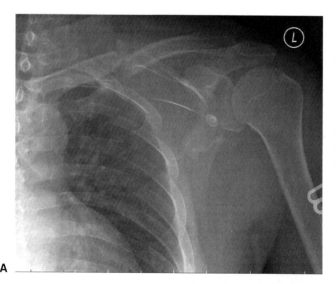
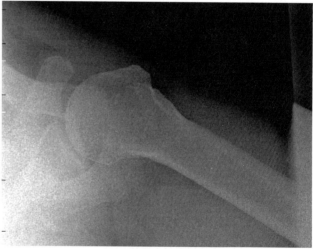

A

B

Figure 2.17. A. AP shoulder x-ray taken at the patient's first emergency room visit. This image reveals a minimally displaced clavicle fracture with a butterfly fragment, a scapula body fracture that exits the lateral border at the glenoid neck, and rib fractures of at least levels 2 through 5. Minimal glenoid medialization is found. **B.** An axillary view of the injured shoulder demonstrating no acromial nor coracoid process fractures, no intra-articular extension of the fracture, and no subluxation of the glenohumeral joint.

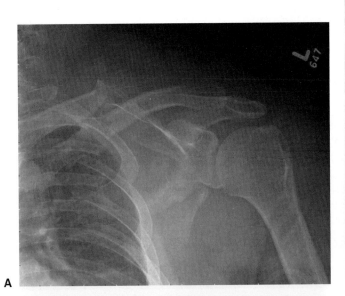

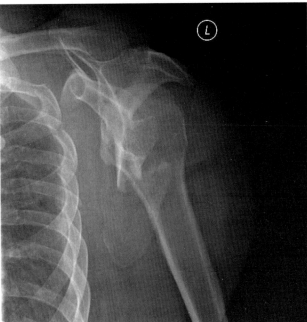

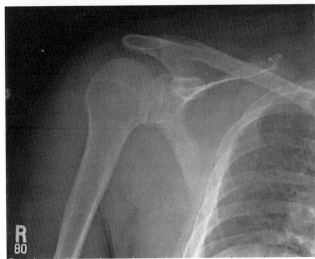

Figure 2.18. A. This AP x-ray image of the shoulder reveals substantial displacement of all fractured bones, which had not been evident in the initial films of the injury. The clavicle is medialized well over 1 cm; the glenoid has medialized markedly and has a caudad-facing attitude; perhaps most impressive, the marked displacement of all the rib fractures indicates that the entire forequarter has medialized en mass. **B.** This is a scapula Y radiograph taken 3 weeks after the injury showing substantial translation of the lateral border. This border is displaced by approximately 3 cm, and significant angular deformity is evident. **C.** A comparison view of the opposite shoulder was used as a template to evaluate the injured shoulder **(A)**. Side by side, these two images highlight the amount of scapular displacement, which is striking, as well as the coronal plane relationship to the chest wall.

After 3 weeks of significant pain and with no ability to move his shoulder, the patient presented in my office with a workers' compensation agent who had suggested that he obtain a second opinion. Physical examination revealed that the left shoulder was markedly depressed and medialized. The neurovascular exam at the level of the left hand revealed no abnormality. When the patient was asked to try and move his shoulder, the patient simply replied, "It won't move even when I want it to." Attempts at active range of motion were indeed futile; although he was taken passively to 30 degrees of forward flexion before stiffness could not be overcome. The pain was substantial. His neck was not tender, and his cervical motion was full, but he experienced spasms in the trapezius muscle.

New x-rays demonstrated significant displacement of the scapula (Fig. 2.18); this finding was different than that seen on the original film (Fig. 2.17). A CT scan was obtained (Fig. 2.19), and the patient learned the risks and benefits of surgery. Two days later the patient was taken to the operating room for surgical fixation of the scapula and clavicle. The relative indications for surgery were multiple and included medial displacement of more than 15 mm, angular deformity of greater than 25 degrees, grotesque clinical deformity, seven broken bones in the forequarter, and a floating shoulder (double lesion of the SSSC).

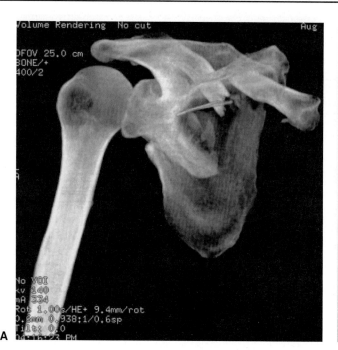
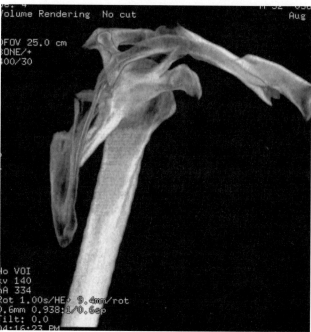

Figure 2.19. A. This is a 3D-CT reconstructed image of the scapula in the plane most perpendicular to the scapula body. This rotational image helps one to appreciate the medialization and angular deformity of the glenoid relative to the distal scapula-body fragment. The displacement of the scapula body at the superomedial angle can also be seen as a medialized, superior, scapula segment (attached to the glenoid). Comminution in the infraspinatus fossa is marked. The clavicular medialization is also confirmed in this image. **B.** A 3D-CT image representing the plane most parallel to the body of the scapula. In this view, semicoronal angular deformity can be measured off the proximal and distal scapula borders (35 degrees in this case). Also appreciated is the severe anteversion of the glenoid.

The patient was placed in the lateral decubitus position, flopping slightly forward, and a Judet posterior approach was used to mobilize the entire muscle flap. The callus was cleaned from the fracture lines so that the reduction could be visualized (Fig. 2.20). Schantz pin joysticks (with T-handled chucks) were used in the glenoid neck and lateral border to achieve the reduction. The lateral border was plated first followed by plating of the superomedial angle (Fig. 2.21).

The patient was re-prepped and draped after an intraoperative shoulder x-ray revealed marked clavicle-fracture displacement. The clavicle was subsequently fixed with a tension band plate along the superior border (Figs. 2.22 to 2.24).

Prior to awaking the patient from anesthesia, the surgeon manipulated the shoulder until full motion was restored. This manipulation also relieves the intrinsic and extrinsic contractures that form in a month. Formal postoperative x-rays were taken in the recovery room (Fig. 2.25). The patient worked with physical therapy immediately on full and aggressive, passive, range-of-motion exercises. He remarked (as most patients do) that his shoulder felt completely "different and restored" the day after surgery and that he was able to move it for the first time since his injury. At 1 month, he was advanced to full, active, range-of-motion activity with light weights (3 to 5 lb) beginning at 6 weeks. By 3 months after surgery, he had returned to work, had no pain, and stated that he had full motion.

Patients are followed in the office at 2, 6, 12, 24, and 48 postoperative weeks. This patient's 6 month x-ray is shown in Figure 2.26. At 6 months, his shoulder was asymptomatic. His motion was within at least 90% of the motion of opposite shoulder in all directions, and he complained of no deficit in strength. His Disabilities of the Arm, Shoulder, and Hand (DASH) exam score was 16 (scale 1–100; normative-scale functional score = 10.1).

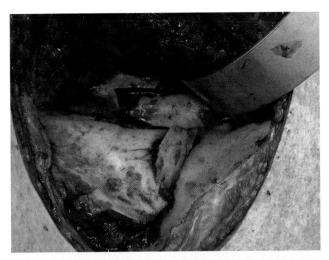

Figure 2.20. This intraoperative photograph was taken from the vantage point of the surgeon, who stood on the posterior side of the patient. Behind the retractor is the muscle flap containing the deltoid, infraspinatus, and teres minor. Fracture callus has been removed and saved to pack into fracture lines before wound closure. The open approach, in which the entire flap is elevated, was used because 3.5 weeks had passed since the time of this patient's injury; thus, this exposure was necessary to mobilize callus, and reduction aids were needed to overcome a static deformity.

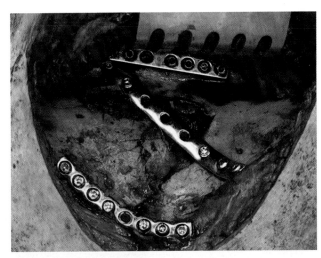

Figure 2.21. This intraoperative photograph shows the fixation construct using a nine-hole 2.7-mm dynamic compression plate (Synthes, Paoli, PA) for the lateral border, an eight-hole 2.7-mm reconstruction plate (Synthes) contoured around the superomedial angle of the scapula, and a seven-hole locking, one-third, tubular plate with locking screws (Synthes) deployed in the proximal and distal body fragments. The locking plate off-loads the other two nonlocking plates that have short screws: 8 to 10 mm on the vertebral border and 12 to 16 mm on the acromial and lateral borders. Directly behind and to the right of the Israel retractor is the suprascapular neurovascular bundle as it exits from beneath the acromion. Great care must be exercised in retracting this flap to preserve the functional integrity of these structures.

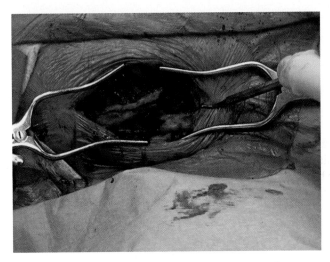

Figure 2.22. The surgical exposure of the clavicle fracture after it has been cleaned. The butterfly fragment is not in view; it had been reduced and fixed with 2.7-mm lag screws. The surgeon can access this site from either the anterior or posterior position. I have chosen to work from the posterior position (same as for the scapula) and thus the easiest access was to the superior border of the clavicle, which is more convenient in the patient who requires scapula surgery in the floppy lateral or forward position. The scapula and clavicle procedures can usually be done with a single prep and drape, but in this case, the procedures were done separately.

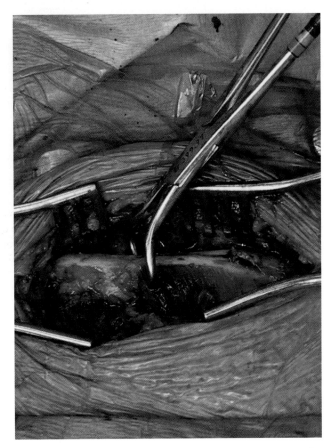

Figure 2.23. A pointed, bone, reduction forceps was used to reduce the fracture. The photograph is taken from the vantage point of the anesthesiologist.

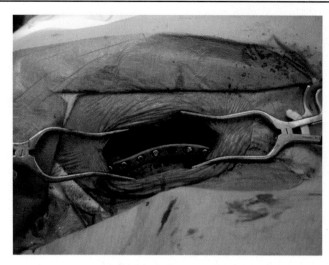

Figure 2.24. An eight-hole, precontoured, titanium, nonlocking plate (Acumed, Hillsboro, OR) was used for the clavicle stabilization.

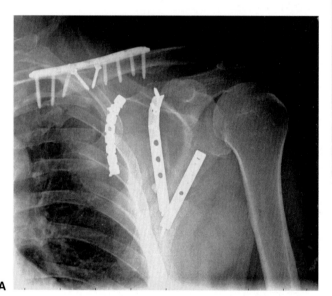

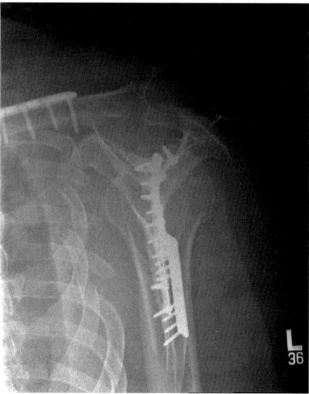

A   B

Figure 2.25. **A.** Postoperative AP x-ray showing the reconstructed scapula and clavicle in proper orientation. Note the gap at the lateral border, which is often difficult to define and reduce in the comminuted variants that undergo delayed surgery. **B.** A postoperative scapula-Y x-ray image demonstrating proper alignment and orientation of the lateral border. **C.** A postoperative, axillary, x-ray view can be used to insure that all screws are in extra-articular position. (*continues*)

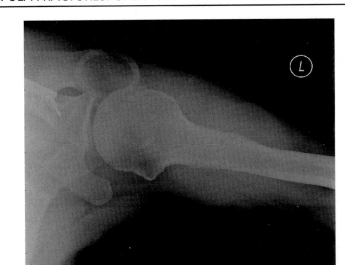

C

Figure 2.25. (*continued*)

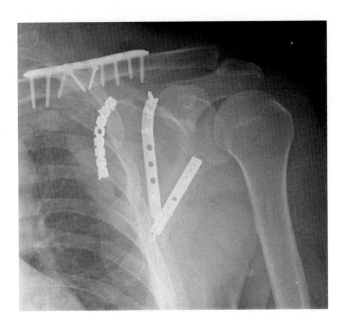

Figure 2.26. An x-ray image taken 6 months after the operation showing complete consolidation of fracture lines.

RECOMMENDED READING

Ada JR, Miller MD. Scapular fractures: analysis of 113 cases. *CORR* 1991;269:174–180.

Armstrong CP, Van Der Spuy J. The fractured scapula: importance and management based on a series of 62 patients. *Injury* 1984;15:324–329.

Bankart ASB. The pathology and treatment of recurrent dislocation of the shoulder joint. *Br J Surg* 1938;26:23.

Cole PA. Scapula fractures. *Orthop Clin North Am* 2002;33(1):1–18.

Goss TP. Fractures of the glenoid cavity. *J Bone Joint Surg Am* 1992;74:299–305.

Goss TP. Double disruptions of the superior shoulder suspensory complex. *J Orthop Trauma* 1993;7:99–106.

Goss TP. The scapula, coracoid, acromial and avulsion fractures. *Am J Orthop* 25:106–115, 1996.

Edwards SG, Whittle PA, Wood GW. Nonoperative treatment of ipsilateral fractures of the scapula and clavicle. *J Bone Joint Surg Am* 2000;82:774–780.

Hardegger FH, Simpson LA, Weber BG. The operative treatment of scapular fractures. *J Bone Joint Surg Br* 1984;66:725–731.

Ianotti JP, Gabriel JP, Schneck SL, et al. The normal glenohumeral relationships, an anatomical study of one hundred and forty shoulders. *J Bone Joint Surg Am* 1992;74:491–500.

Ideberg R, Grevsten S, Larsson S. Epidemiology of scapular fractures: incidence and classification of 338 fractures. *Acta Orthop Scand* 1995;66:395–397.

Imatani RJ. Fractures of the scapula: a review of 53 fractures. *J Trauma* 1975;15:473–478.

Lindblom A, Leven H. Prognosis in fractures of body and neck of scapula. *Acta Chir Scand* 1974;140:33–47.

Mayo KA, Benirschke SK, Mast JW. Displaced fractures of the glenoid fossa: results of open reduction and internal fixation. *CORR* 1998;347:122–130.

McGahan JP, Rab GT, Dublin A. Fractures of the scapula. *J Trauma* 1980;20:880–883.

McGinnis M, Denton J. Fractures of the scapula: a retrospective study of 40 fractured scapulae. *J Trauma* 1989;29:1488–1493.

Ogawa K, Naniwa T. Fractures of the acromion and the lateral scapular spine. *J Shoulder Elbow Surg* 1997;6:544–548.

Rowe CR. Fractures of the scapula. *Surg Clin North Am* 1963;43:1565–1571.

Van der Helm FC, Pronk GM. Three dimensional recording and description of motions of the shoulder mechanism. *J Biomech Eng* 1995;117:27–40.

Wilbur MC, Evans EB. Fractures of the scapula: an analysis of forty cases and review of the literature. *J Bone Joint Surg Am* 1977;59:358–362.

Williams GR Jr, Naranja J, Klimkiewicz J, et al. The floating shoulder: a biomechanical basis for classification and management. *J Bone Joint Surg Am* 2001;83A:1182–1187.

Wilson PD. *Experience of the management of fractures and dislocations (based on analysis of 4,390 cases) by staff of the Fracture Service MGH, Boston.* Philadelphia: JB Lippincott; 1938.

3

Proximal Humeral Fractures: Open Reduction Internal Fixation

Andrew H. Schmidt

INDICATIONS/CONTRAINDICATIONS

Proximal humeral fractures represent up to 5% of all fractures and occur most often as the result of a simple fall in an older patient with osteoporosis. The proximal humerus may also be fractured in younger patients as the result of high-energy trauma, and evaluation and management of associated injuries to the head, spine, chest, or other vital areas may take precedence over the shoulder fracture.

Even among experts, controversy exists regarding the indications for surgical versus non-operative management of many proximal humeral fractures. Furthermore, differences of opinion abound regarding whether internal fixation or arthroplasty provide better outcomes in selected fracture patterns. With the introduction of peri-articular locked plates in the past decade, the treatment of proximal humeral fractures has undergone a profound change.

The overriding goal in the treatment of proximal humeral fractures is the institution of early range of motion. Shoulder function depends on the complex interaction of the gleno-humeral and scapulothoracic motion, as well as the interplay of 7 or more muscle-tendon units. Soft-tissue scarring or loss of the gliding surfaces can leave the shoulder stiff and painful and results in poor outcomes. If a fracture of the proximal humerus is either unac-ceptably displaced or too unstable to allow early motion, then operative intervention should be considered to restore anatomy and useful shoulder function. Whether surgery is done by open reduction and fixation of the fracture or by prosthetic replacement depends on the patient's needs and expectations, fracture pattern, bone quality, available implants, and the experience of the surgeon.

The complex anatomy of the shoulder girdle must be understood to treat proximal humeral fractures successfully. Fractures of the proximal humerus occur in typical patterns that are influenced by muscular insertions that cause predictable displacement of the fracture frag-ments (Fig. 3.1). Although the Neer classification is often used for surgical decision making, multiple authors have shown that interobserver and intraobserver interpretations of plain ra-diographs vary widely. Fractures of the proximal humerus can involve the surgical neck and/or the tuberosities. Also, fracture displacement affects the biomechanical function of the

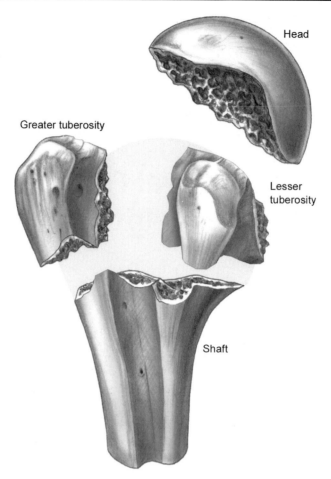

Figure 3.1. Drawing of the pathoanatomy of proximal humeral fractures.

shoulder and the vascularity of the fracture fragments. The inherent stability of the fracture is another factor affecting decision making. A fracture is considered stable if displacement is minimal and the patient will tolerate early functional motion. These fractures are usually treated nonoperatively. Surgery is indicated when fracture instability prevents early motion or when fracture displacement is sufficiently great that functional impairment is likely.

Isolated greater-tuberosity fractures are often associated with anterior shoulder dislocation, and displaced tuberosity fragments should be reduced and fixed. Tension-band techniques with heavy suture or wire can be utilized, or screw fixation may be considered when comminution is minimal and bone quality is good. Isolated lesser-tuberosity fractures are uncommon and may occur with posterior shoulder dislocations. Large lesser-tuberosity fragments may require open reduction and fixation if they are significantly displaced.

Fractures through the surgical neck of the humerus can be nondisplaced or displaced, simple or comminuted. Displaced surgical-neck fractures in physiologically young patients should be treated by reduction and fixation. A number of fixation techniques have been employed, including T-plate fixation, percutaneous pinning, tension-band wiring, and intramedullary nailing. With the advent of peri-articular locking plates, these methods of treatment have been rendered obsolete (Fig. 3.2). Locked plates dramatically increase angular stability, minimize screw toggle, and allow early range of motion in the shoulder. Therefore, locking plates are indicated for nearly every fracture of the proximal humerus for which surgical treatment is necessary.

Many fractures of the proximal humerus consist of various combinations of elementary fracture patterns. Three-part fractures generally represent the combination of surgical neck and greater-tuberosity fractures (Fig. 3.3). For these injuries, treatment should be based on the radiographic or computed tomography (CT) interpretation of the fracture, such as tuberosity or humeral-head displacement. Locking plates are ideal implants for these

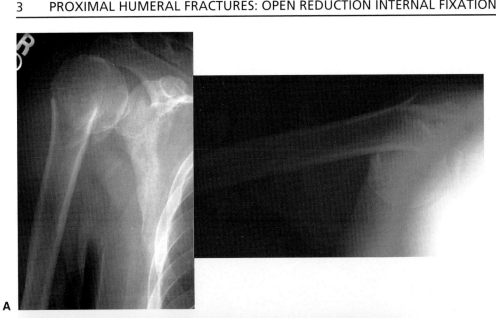

A

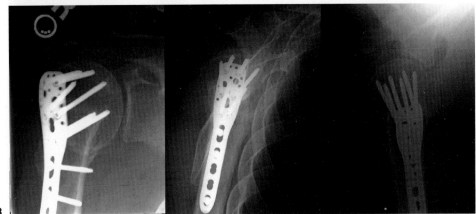

B

Figure 3.2. Example of a displaced surgical-neck fracture in a young patient treated with locking plate fixation. **A.** AP and axillary lateral views of a comminuted surgical-neck fracture. **B.** AP, Y, and axillary views 6 months after fixation with a locking proximal-humeral plate.

fractures because they provide stable fixation of the humeral head and a means to repair the greater or lesser tuberosities.

Several surgeons have reported successful results with open reduction and internal fixation for four-part fractures, and this treatment should be considered in relatively active, young patients. It is interesting that complications after operative repair of valgus-impacted four-part fractures seem to be less frequent than in other types of four-part fractures, and therefore, these valgus-impacted injuries may be a good indication for internal fixation. When a valgus-impacted fracture is identified, one must carefully look for evidence of lateral displacement of the humeral-head fragment (Fig. 3.4). If lateral displacement is found, the medial periosteal vessels that perfuse the articular segment may be ruptured, and avascular necrosis is more likely to result. In the absence of lateral displacement of the humeral-head fragment, the humeral head is likely to remain viable.

PREOPERATIVE PLANNING

Appropriate management of proximal humeral fractures begins with a thorough assessment of the functional needs and abilities of the patient, the presence of cognitive or physical impairments, the fracture pattern, bone density, the patient's expectations, and the ability of the patient to comply with a rehabilitation program. The goal of treatment is to

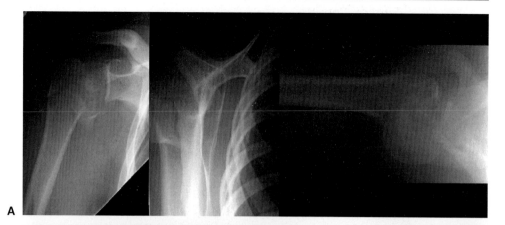

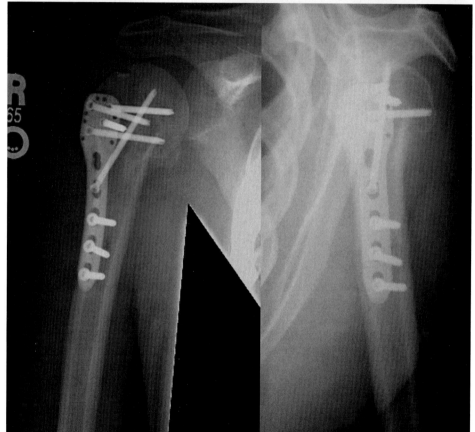

Figure 3.3. A three-part fracture dislocation of the shoulder following a seizure. **A.** AP, Y, and axillary lateral x-rays of the injury. Note the dislocation of the humeral head. **B.** AP and Y lateral views 4 months after open reduction and internal fixation with a locking plate.

obtain fracture union and maintain adequate function of the shoulder while avoiding complications. The skills of the surgeon and the resources available must also be considered.

In patients who require surgery, a thorough understanding of the fracture geometry and morphology is essential. Precise anteroposterior (AP) and axillary lateral radiographs of the shoulder should be scrutinized. Occasionally, oblique, Y views or arch views of the scapula can be helpful. If any doubt exists, a CT or magnetic resonance imaging (MRI) scan should be obtained in noncritically ill patients. In young patients with wide tuberosity displacement, an MRI scan often provides useful information about the rotator cuff. The fracture displacement should be carefully analyzed, so that reduction maneuvers can be planned. For example, in a valgus-impacted fracture, the greater tuberosity is displaced and the humeral head falls into the resultant void. In addition, an intact, medial, soft-tissue attach-

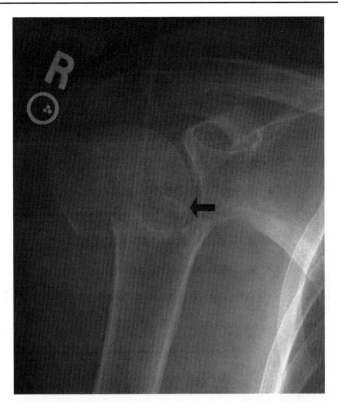

Figure 3.4. A valgus-impacted fracture with more than 5 mm of lateral displacement of the humeral head. This may signify disruption of all soft-tissue attachments to the articular segment.

ment is often found between the humeral head and shaft. Therefore, a valgus-impacted fracture is reduced by applying a medial force to the superior-lateral aspect of the humeral head and using the medial soft tissues as a hinge (Fig. 3.5). Once the humeral head is reduced, the greater tuberosity may be reduced into its bed, after which it serves to maintain reduction of the humeral head. In contrast, a humeral head that is displaced in varus will require the opposite maneuver to reduce the articular segment.

Open-reduction internal fixation of the proximal humerus is usually done through a classic deltopectoral approach. Although a deltoid-splitting approach is normally used for isolated greater-tuberosity fractures, the classic and splitting techniques may be combined if the greater tuberosity is displaced posteriorly such that reduction and fixation is difficult via the deltopectoral approach alone. This two-incision approach may also be helpful in patients with a large muscle envelope or significant soft-tissue swelling.

SURGERY

General Considerations

Surgery is done under general anesthesia with muscle paralysis to facilitate fracture reduction. Patients should receive prophylactic antibiotics within one hour of surgery. Multiply injured patients should have their cervical spines cleared because of issues with positioning of the head during surgery.

Patient Positioning

The patient is positioned in a beach-chair position on a standard operating table. The patient's torso should be at the edge of the table, and a soft bump should be placed behind the patient's chest to turn the individual slightly to the side opposite the injury. This

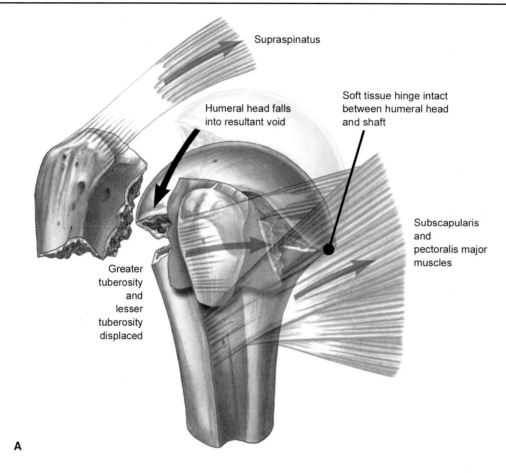

Supraspinatus

Humeral head falls
into resultant void

Soft tissue hinge intact
between humeral head
and shaft

Subscapularis
and
pectoralis major
muscles

Greater
tuberosity
and
lesser
tuberosity
displaced

A

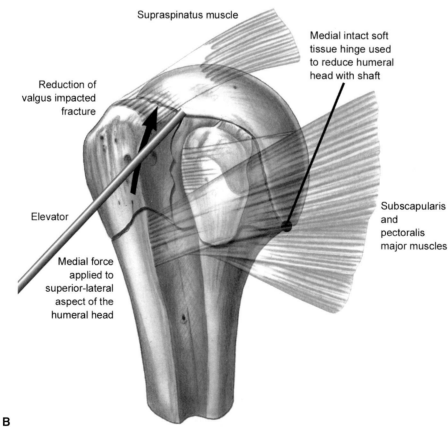

Supraspinatus muscle

Medial intact soft
tissue hinge used
to reduce humeral
head with shaft

Reduction of
valgus impacted
fracture

Subscapularis
and
pectoralis
major muscles

Elevator

Medial force
applied to
superior-lateral
aspect of the
humeral head

B

Figure 3.5. Drawings of reduction of a valgus-impacted fracture relying on a medial hinge.

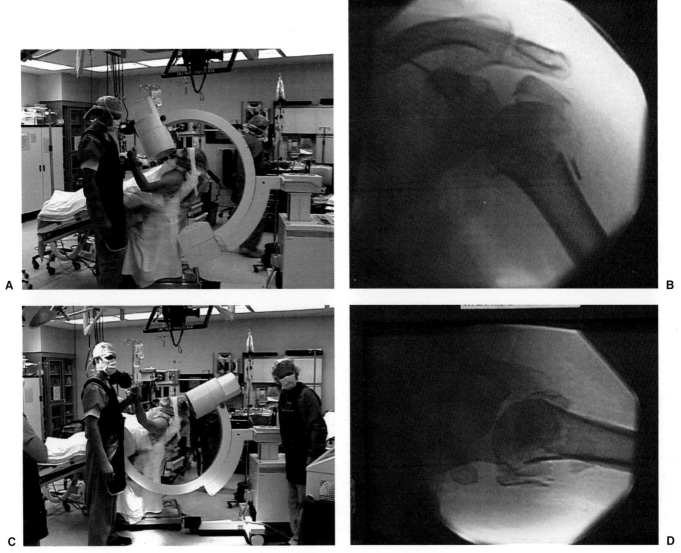

Figure 3.6. Positioning of the patient in a beach-chair position with the c-arm next to the patient's head. **A.** Positioning the c-arm for AP imaging of the shoulder. **B.** Example of the AP image obtained. **C.** Positioning the c-arm for axillary lateral imaging of the shoulder. **D.** Example of the axillary image obtained.

positioning facilitates imaging because the shoulder is slightly rotated away from the table. A radiolucent arm and/or shoulder rest is placed along the side of the bed. The entire upper extremity must be free to move or manipulate during surgery.

Complete visualization of the proximal humerus and glenoid must be possible with an image intensifier. The image intensifier is placed parallel to the table at the patient's head on the injured side (Fig. 3.6). With this arrangement, imaging in the AP and axillary planes is possible. Some surgeons prefer to bring the c-arm from the opposite side and obtain images in the AP and transscapular lateral planes, but this approach does not image the humeral head quite, as well as the axillary lateral view. In either position, trial images should be obtained prior to prepping.

Technique

The patient's shoulder, chest, neck, and arm are prepped and draped. A sticky prep solution, such as DuraPrep (3M Healthcare, St. Paul, MN), and an adherent, surgical, cover drape (Ioban, 3M Healthcare, St. Paul, MN) facilitate draping around the shoulder.

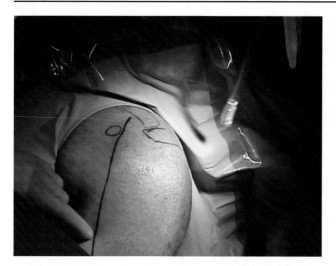

Figure 3.7. Bony landmarks outlined on the skin determine the proper placement of the skin incision.

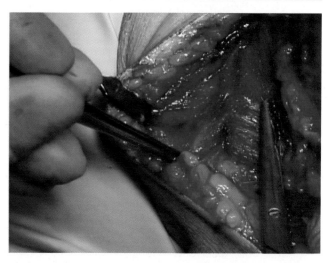

Figure 3.8. The deltopectoral interval is opened with sharp dissection. Note the cephalic vein visible just to the right of the scissors (left shoulder shown).

The bony landmarks of the clavicle, acromion, scapular spine, and coracoid process are outlined with a sterile marking pen (Fig. 3.7). The incision for the deltopectoral approach begins midway between the coracoid and clavicle, and it extends distally in an oblique manner to the deltoid insertion.

The skin may be infiltrated with local anesthetic and epinephrine if desired. The skin and subcutaneous tissues are divided, and the cephalic vein is identified. The vein marks the location of the deltopectoral interval (Fig. 3.8). The vein is most vulnerable to injury in the proximal part of the incision. The deltopectoral interval is deepened bluntly to the clavipectoral fascia. During deep dissection, an important landmark is the coracoid process and its associated strap muscles. The long head of the biceps tendon should be identified next because it defines the rotator cuff interval. The lesser tuberosity and subscapularis tendon lie medial to the biceps tendon, and the greater tuberosity and supraspinatus tendon insertion are lateral to the biceps. During the initial exposure and mobilization of the fracture, one should keep in mind that important vascular contributions to the articular segment are made by the ascending (arcuate) branch of the anterior, humeral, circumflex artery that is located along the bicipital groove. Likewise, the rotator cuff insertions will be exposed.

The deltopectoral interval is progressively developed. Shoulder abduction during the approach relaxes the deltoid and facilitates exposure. To facilitate exposure, reduction, and plate placement, the anterior one third of the deltoid insertion is released from the lateral humerus. Similarly, the upper portion of the pectoralis major insertion on the anteromedial aspect of the humerus may also be released. The surgeon must be cognizant of the potential for iatrogenic injury to the axillary or musculocutaneous nerve during surgery.

The fracture fragments are atraumatically identified and exposed. The long head of the biceps tendon is the key landmark for identifying the tuberosities. Heavy nonabsorbable sutures are placed in the subscapularis and supraspinatus tendons. The greater tuberosity is often displaced posteriorly and can be retrieved with the arm abducted. In patients with fractures more than 2 weeks old, a small, lateral, deltoid split can be performed to retrieve and repair the greater tuberosity; however, this type of dated injury is uncommon. Traction sutures should be placed in the tendinous insertions to hold and reduce fragments most securely (Fig. 3.9). Soft-tissue attachments should be maintained, but when needed, the rotator interval may be opened. The humeral head, as visualized via fluoroscopic imaging, is reduced with manipulation via blunt elevators or joysticks (Fig. 3.10). In the case of a displaced humeral head, a Kirschner (K) wire or Schantz pin may be used as a joystick to help reduce and/or stabilize the articular segment (Fig. 3.11).

A low-profile, precontoured, peri-articular, locking plate with angular stable screws is utilized (Locking Proximal Humeral Plate, Synthes USA, Westchester, PA) (Fig. 3.12). The plate is applied to the proximal lateral humerus just lateral to the biceps tendon and

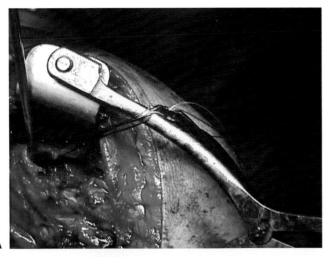

A

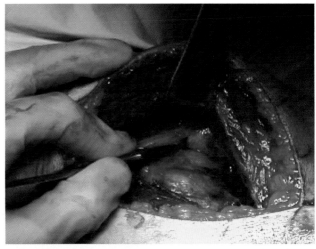

B

Figure 3.9. A. With the arm abducted, a blunt retractor is used to mobilize the greater tuberosity. Here, an elevator is shown beneath the coracoacromial ligament, allowing retrieval of the greater tuberosity from the subacromial space. **B.** Traction sutures are placed to the greater tuberosity in the rotator cuff insertion. These facilitate reduction of the tuberosity and are later used for its reattachment.

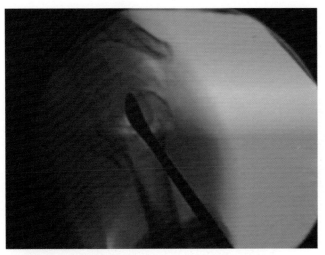

Figure 3.10. A blunt elevator is used to elevate the humeral head into anatomic position. A control image taken of the c-arm is shown.

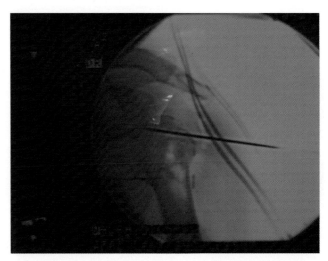

Figure 3.11. A K wire is shown maintaining the humeral head into a reduced position. The K wire can also be used to maneuver the humeral head.

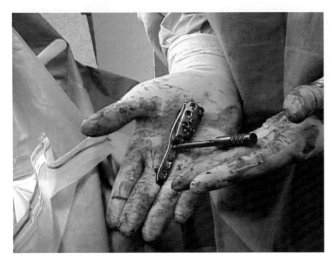

Figure 3.12. The locking plate and drill guide are assembled.

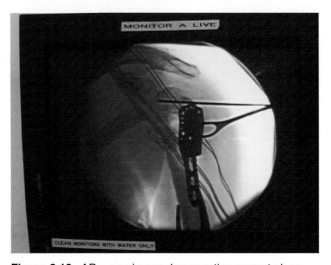

Figure 3.13. AP c-arm image documenting correct placement of the plate on the lateral humeral shaft. To avoid subacromial impingement, the plate should not be too high.

held with 1 or 2 K wires. The height of the plate is evaluated with the image intensifier to insure that the plate is not prominent superiorly (Fig. 3.13). A standard cortical screw is placed in the oval hole in the plate, lightly tightened and adjusted (as judged through fluoroscopy). To insert the locking screws into the head, a triple drill guide is threaded into the plate. A locking drill sleeve is threaded into the plate, and based on image intensification in two planes, a guide wire is advanced into the reduced humeral head (Fig. 3.14). The design of the locking plate ensures that the screws appropriately diverge within the humeral head. The screws are measured (Fig. 3.15) and inserted. The remaining screws are placed into the humeral head and shaft (Fig. 3.16). In a recent biomechanical study, Liew et al showed that the strength of screw fixation was related to screw position within the humeral head. Using paired cadaveric specimens, they found that the pull-out strength was greatest when the screws had subchondral fixation in the center of the humeral head.

The tuberosities are manipulated and reduced to the humeral shaft using traction sutures that were previously placed (Fig. 3.17). The sutures can be tied to the plate or to hole in the bone. It is desirable to have sutures placed between the tuberosity and the humeral shaft as well as in a horizontal cerclage fashion that incorporates the plate. The tuberosities must be repaired to their anatomic position and must be stable so that the musculotendinous unit of the rotator cuff is restored and can tolerate early motion. While directly observing the re-

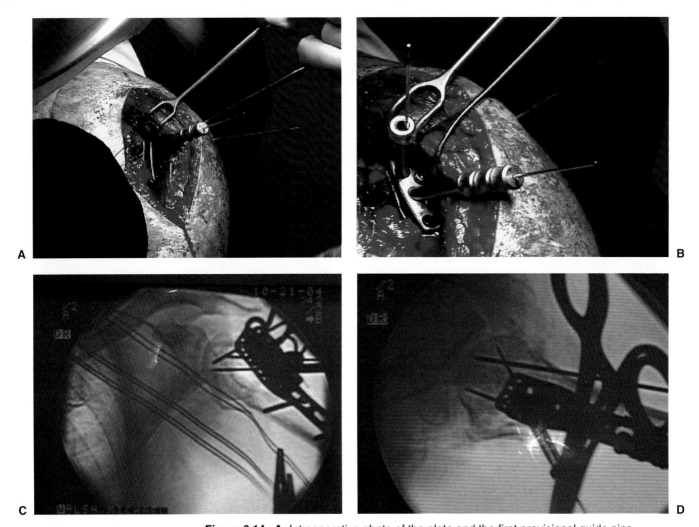

Figure 3.14. A. Intraoperative photo of the plate and the first provisional guide pins inserted into the humeral head. **B.** Intraoperative photo of the plate and 2 guide pins. **C.** Fluoroscopic AP and **D.** axillary lateral images documenting the correct position of the guide wires within the humeral head.

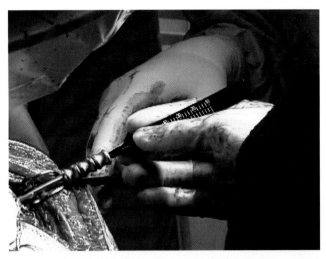

Figure 3.15. Measurement of screw length using the guide pin.

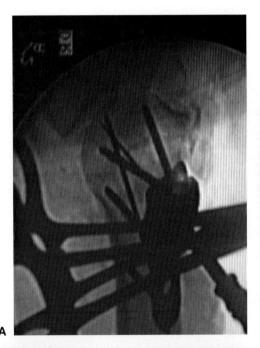

A

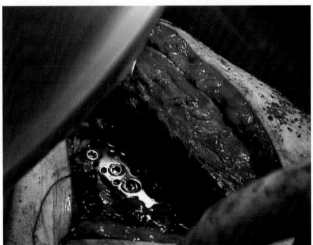

B

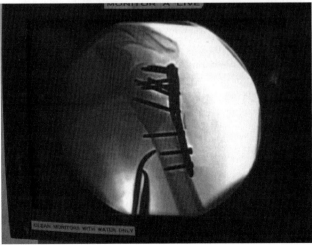

C

Figure 3.16. While using fluoroscopy, the surgeon inserts the remaining screws. **A.** C-arm axillary view showing several screws and the guide pin for another screw. All screws are divergent and contained within the humeral head. **B.** Photograph of the arm showing the plate beneath the deltoid. **C.** AP image of the shoulder showing the final construct.

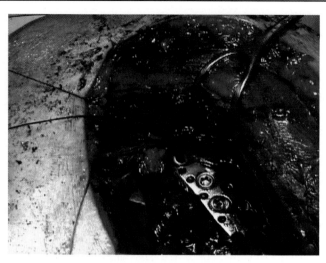

Figure 3.17. Utilizing multiple sutures in the rotator cuff insertions, the surgeon repairs the tuberosities to the plate and proximal humerus.

pair, the surgeon brings the shoulder through a range of motion so that limits of motion are determined for postoperative exercises.

After final repair of the tuberosities and confirmation, through imaging, of the reduction and fixation, the deltopectoral interval is closed. Drains are not typically used.

Tips and Tricks

- To confirm adequate visualization and reduction maneuvers, practice images with the c-arm should be taken before the patient is prepped and draped.
- Abduction of the shoulder relaxes the deltoid and facilitates exposure of the fracture.
- Sutures should be placed in the rotator cuff insertions to provide a means to reduce and then fix the tuberosities.
- The ubiquitous apex-anterior angulation of the surgical neck of the humerus is corrected by pushing toward the floor at the fracture site while lifting up on the distal arm.

POSTOPERATIVE MANAGEMENT

Rehabilitation after internal fixation of proximal humeral fractures is focused on early movement of the extremity within the limits of the soft-tissue repair determined at the time of surgery. Hodgson et al found that patients who started immediate physiotherapy had less pain and better motion compared to patients who were immobilized for 3 weeks. Pendulum exercises are usually begun immediately. Once the wound is healed, gentle active, assisted, range-of-motion exercises are initiated. When the greater-tuberosity fracture has been repaired, active abduction and external rotation should be delayed for soft-tissue healing. After lesser-tuberosity repair, the subscapularis must be protected from active internal rotation or passive external rotation. In general, active motion is begun within 4 to 6 weeks after surgery, and resistance exercises are started in 8 to 12 postoperative weeks.

COMPLICATIONS

Complications following open reduction and internal fixation of the proximal humerus fall into several broad categories that include shoulder stiffness, osteonecrosis, and malunion or nonunion. Complications that are unique to internal fixation of proximal humeral fractures include technical errors, such as inadequate reduction, incorrectly positioned implants, screw penetration into the joint, loss of fixation, tuberosity disruption, and nerve injury. The use of plates with angular stability, such as blade plates or plates with locking screws, and/or augmentation of the fracture with polymethylmethacrylate (PMMA) or calcium phosphate cement lessens this risk.

Osteonecrosis of the humeral head following fracture may be partial or complete; the significance of this complication on outcome remains controversial. Open reduction and internal fixation with plates requires a more invasive approach and may be associated with an increased risk of osteonecrosis. However, rigid fixation may promote better and more rapid revascularization by creeping substitution of the humeral head and may therefore lessen the risk of articular collapse when osteonecrosis occurs. Wijgman et al examined 60 patients with 3- or 4-part, proximal, humeral fractures that were managed with either plate or cerclage wire fixation at an average of 10 years after injury. Although 22 of the 60 patients (37%) had osteonecrosis, 17 of them (77% of those with osteonecrosis) had good or excellent functional outcomes. A correlation between the type of fixation and the development of osteonecrosis was not found.

RECOMMENDED READINGS

1. Chudik SC, Weinhold P, Dahners LE. Fixed-angle plate fixation in simulated fractures of the proximal humerus: a biomechanical study of a new device. *J Shoulder Elbow Surg* 2003;12:578–588.
2. Gerber C, Hersche O, Berberat C. The clinical significance of posttraumatic avascular necrosis of the humeral head. *J Shoulder Elbow Surg* 1998;7:586–590.
3. Hessmann MH, Blum J, Hofmann A, et al. Internal fixation of proximal humeral fractures: current concepts. *Europe J Trauma* 2003;5:253–261.
4. Hodgson SA, Mawson SJ, Stanley D. Rehabilitation after two-part fractures of the neck of the humerus. *J Bone Joint Surg Br* 2003;85:419–422.
5. Ko J-Y, Yamamoto R. Surgical treatment of complex fractures of the proximal humerus. *Clin Orthop* 1996;327:225–237.
6. Koval KJ, Blair B, Takei R, et al. Surgical neck fractures of the proximal humerus: a laboratory evaluation of ten fixation techniques. *J Trauma* 1996;40:778–783.
7. Kwon BK, Goertzen DJ, O'Brien PJ, et al. Biomechanical evaluation of proximal humeral fracture fixation supplemented with calcium phosphate cement. *J Bone Joint Surg Am* 2002;84: 951–961.
8. Liew ASL, Johnson JA, Patterson SD, et al. Effect of screw placement on fixation in the humeral head. *J Should Elbow Surg* 2000;9:423–426.
9. Misra A, Kapur R, Mafulli N. Complex proximal humeral fractures in adults—a systematic review of management. *Injury* 2001;32:363–372.
10. Schai P, Imhoff A, Preiss S. Comminuted humeral head fractures: a multicenter analysis. *J Shoulder Elbow Surg* 1995;4:319–330.
11. Wijgman AJ, Roolker W, Patt TW, et al. Open reduction and internal fixation of three and four-part fractures of the proximal part of the humerus. *J Bone Joint Surg Br* 2002;84A:1919–1925.
12. Zyto K, Kronberg M, Broström L-Å. Shoulder function after displaced fractures of the proximal humerus. *J Shoulder Elbow Surg* 1995;4:331–336.
13. Zyto K, Ahrengart L, Sperber A, et al. Treatment of displaced proximal humeral fractures in elderly patients. *J Bone Joint Surg Br* 1997;79:412–417.

4

Proximal Humeral Fractures: Arthroplasty

Louis U. Bigliani, Sean F. Bak, and Steven S. Goldberg

INDICATIONS/CONTRAINDICATIONS

Proximal humeral replacement is a useful surgical technique for acute displaced fractures of the proximal humerus (Fig. 4.1). The indications for placement of a prosthesis are (a) 4-part fractures and fracture dislocations, (b) head-splitting fractures, (c) impression fractures involving more than 40% of the articular surface, and (d) selected 3-part fractures in older patients with osteoporotic bone. The majority of severely displaced, proximal, humeral fractures occur in the older population, with predominance in women. Other methods of treatment, including closed reduction, open reduction-internal fixation, head excision, and fusion, have been reported to have a high percentage of unsatisfactory results.

The contraindications for proximal humeral replacement are active soft-tissue infection, chronic osteomyelitis, and paralysis of the rotator-cuff muscles. Deltoid paralysis is not a contraindication: Adequate yet compromised function can be achieved in such a shoulder.

PREOPERATIVE PLANNING

A detailed history and physical are essential, although an adequate clinical evaluation of the injured limb may be difficult because of pain and swelling. It is important to establish whether the patient has lost consciousness or has had a seizure. Neurovascular status should be assessed with a high index of suspicion for injuries to the axillary nerve and artery. Injuries to the axillary artery are limb threatening and should be evaluated with emergency arteriography and a vascular surgery consultation. Injuries to the brachial plexus or peripheral nerves are often overlooked initially. The vast majority of these are treated conservatively. Electromyographic analysis should be planned 3 to 4 weeks after injury to help clarify the extent of the injury. A neurologic deficiency should not delay definitive management of the fracture. Most injuries are neurapraxias and will resolve over time sufficiently to allow adequate function. If the neurologic status does not improve, any needed procedure to the axillary nerve can be done within 3 months of injury without compromise.

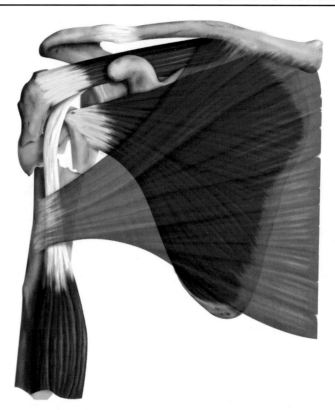

Figure 4.1. A four-part fracture of the proximal humerus. The humeral head is free floating and displaced from both tuberosities and the shaft. The lesser tuberosity fragment is pulled medially by the subscapularis; the greater-tuberosity fragment is pulled posteriorly and superiorly by the supraspinatus and infraspinatus; the shaft fragment is pulled medially by the pectoralis major.

To determine whether a humeral head replacement is the best treatment option for a displaced, proximal, humeral fracture, the fracture pattern must be clearly delineated. In the majority of cases, this can be achieved with a trauma series (Fig. 4.2). This includes a true anteroposterior (AP) view of the scapula (taken 30 to 40 degrees oblique to the coronal plane of the body), a transscapular lateral or Y view, and an axillary view. The axillary view is taken by abducting the arm 20 to 30 degrees and placing the tube in the axilla with the radiographic plate above the shoulder; there is no need to abduct the arm fully. Often the surgeon must position the arm because of pain. Alternately, a Velpeau axillary view can be obtained, with the patient remaining in the sling and leaning back over the plate and the tube directed downward. If displacement cannot be determined, or if the articular surfaces of the humeral head or glenoid are not clearly visualized, then a computed tomography (CT) scan also may be used to clarify the situation. Use of a preoperative scanogram of both the involved and the uninvolved arm often helps establish the proper length of the prosthesis relative to the remaining humeral shaft.

SURGERY

Patient Positioning

Proper patient positioning is the first step to a successful procedure, and its importance cannot be overemphasized. The goal is to have global access to the shoulder. This is achieved by having the involved shoulder elevated from the table and properly supported. We prefer a table with a cutaway section at the shoulder that allows greater access posteriorly and has an attached pneumatic arm positioner (Spider, Tenet Medical, Calgary,

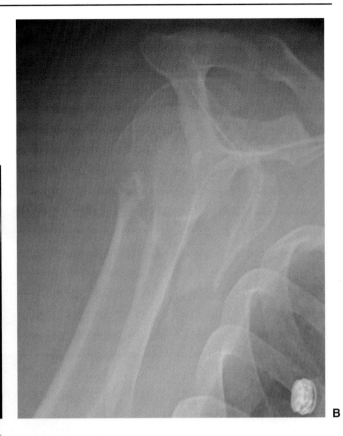

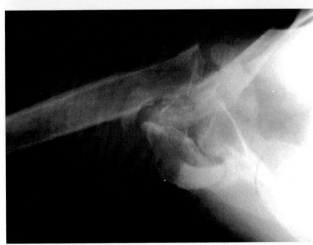

Figure 4.2. A. AP radiograph of a 4-part fracture.
B. Lateral view in the scapular plane. **C.** Axillary view.

Alberta, Canada) (Fig. 4.3). Our anesthetic of choice is an interscalene regional block because it provides excellent muscle relaxation, which facilitates exposure. Two small towels are placed under the medial border of the scapula to negate any retraction. The head is
secured in a positioner in neutral rotation and flexion with respect to the cervical spine. The
operating table should then be placed in a modified beach-chair position. The patient is first
flexed fully at the hips, and the foot of the table is lowered to slightly flex the knees. The
back of the operating table is then elevated so that the patient sits up at an angle of
approximately 45 to 50 degrees. Surgical drapes are used to isolate the operative field
superiorly to the midclavicle and inferiorly below the axilla so that the arm can be draped
free and is able to be moved throughout the surgery.

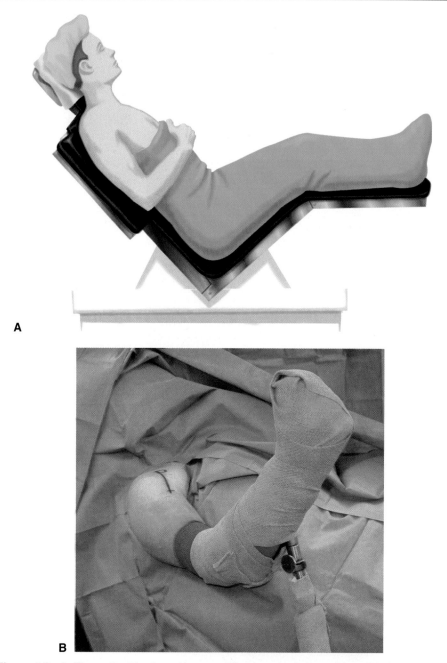

A

B

Figure 4.3. **A.** The patient is placed in a modified beach-chair position with the back flexed approximately 40 to 50 degrees, and the lateral border of the scapula is at the edge of the table. **B.** A pneumatic arm positioner can be used for hands-free universal positioning of the upper limb during the procedure.

Technique

Approach A long deltopectoral approach is performed, starting just below the clavicle and extending over the lateral aspect of the coracoid to the deltoid insertion on the humeral shaft (Fig. 4.4). Large Gelpi retractors can be placed in the skin to provide exposure. The cephalic vein is identified in the deltopectoral interval and is usually retracted laterally. There are fewer tributary veins on the medial side than on the lateral side, so retracting the vein laterally decreases bleeding. Often, however, there is a large crossover vein superiorly, which should be cauterized so that superior exposure is not compromised. It is important to preserve the deltoid origin on the clavicle and acromion. Rarely is the deltoid origin

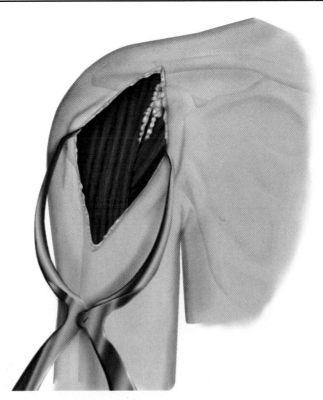

Figure 4.4. A long deltopectoral approach starts just below the clavicle and extends over the lateral aspect of the coracoid to the deltoid insertion on the humeral shaft.

removed. If more exposure is needed, the deltoid insertion may be partially elevated; however, the proximal third of the pectoralis insertion is usually detached from its humeral attachment (Fig. 4.5). This should be tagged with a suture and reattached during closure. At this stage, the coracoid and coracoid muscles should be identified. The coracoid is the lighthouse to the shoulder, and dissection should not be medial to this structure (Fig. 4.6). A

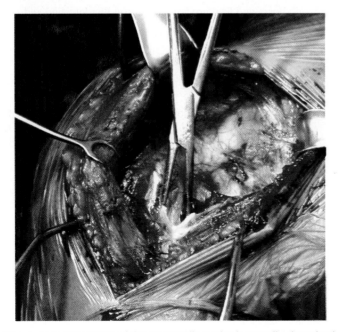

Figure 4.5. The superior insertion of the pectoralis major is usually detached and tagged to allow improved exposure.

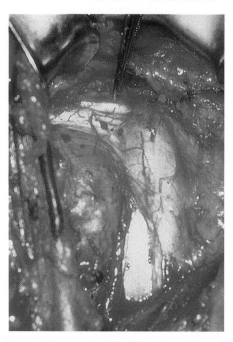

Figure 4.6. The coracoid should be readily identified (tip of clamp), and dissection should not proceed medial to it. The leading edge of the coracoacromial ligament may be resected to improve exposure of rotator cuff muscles.

broad retractor is placed beneath the lateral borders of the coracoid muscles. The coracoid muscles should not be cut nor the coracoid process osteotomized because they provide a barrier to protect the neurovascular bundle. The anterior portion of the leading edge of the coracoacromial ligament can be resected to facilitate exposure. The bulk of this ligament should remain intact to avoid any compromise in superior stability. Another retractor is placed underneath the deltoid and the muscle is retracted laterally. The long head of the biceps should be identified distally and followed proximally, as this is an important structure that will lead to the center of the shoulder at its glenoid insertion (Fig. 4.7).

Exposure of the Fracture Once the retractors have been placed in the appropriate position, hemorrhagic bursa and fracture hematoma can be identified and gently removed.

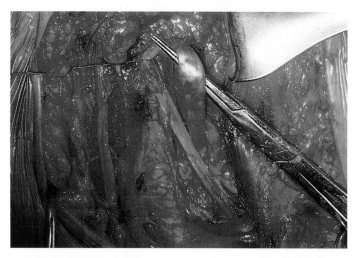

Figure 4.7. The tendon of the long head of the biceps should be identified and followed proximally because this will help to differentiate between the lesser and greater tuberosities and the area of the rotator interval. If possible, the long head of the biceps should be preserved to act as a head depressor.

It is important not to remove large pieces of bone that may be used later to support the prosthesis on the deficient proximal shaft. The key to recognizing the various components of the fracture is the long head of the biceps. As the biceps is followed proximally, the lesser tuberosity is on the medial side, and the greater tuberosity is usually on the lateral side (see Fig. 4.1).

As a rule, the rotator interval can be split in the area of the bicipital groove, as this is often fractured. This split can be carried proximally to help identify and mobilize the supraspinatus and subscapularis because they attach to the greater and lesser tuberosities, respectively. The interval is repaired later. The head usually lies between the tuberosities and is removed and used for sizing of the prosthetic head (Fig. 4.8).

If the head has been dislocated laterally, the greater and lesser tuberosities act almost as a hood and can be elevated intact. In this situation, the head can be extracted and the prosthesis can be placed without disturbing the rotator interval, greater-tuberosity, or lesser-tuberosity fragments. Generally, however, the interval must be opened in the area of the bicipital groove. Once again, it is important to preserve any loose fragments and pieces of bone to be used later in the procedure.

The biceps tendon should be preserved and tagged with a nonabsorbable suture. Both tuberosities are then mobilized and tagged with a no. 2, heavy, nonabsorbable suture. We prefer to use swedged-on needles and place them into the tendon at the tuberosity insertion. This preserves the integrity of the remaining bone attached to the tendon and avoids fragmentation of the tuberosity. Thorough mobilization superiorly and medially is important to allow secure fixation of the tuberosities, though this is often a tedious process as a significant amount of hemorrhagic subacromial bursa often obscures the tuberosities and rotator cuff. Often, superior exposure may be limited by the leading edge of the anterior fascicle of the coracoacromial ligament which, as mentioned previously, can be resected.

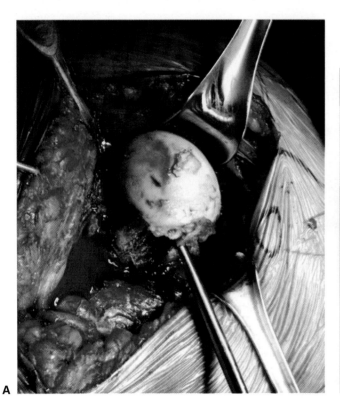
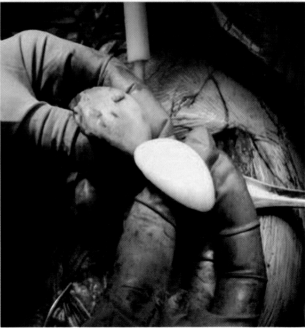

A   B

Figure 4.8. A. The humeral head is usually a free-floating fragment that can easily be removed by using a metal finger. It is important to evaluate the head for any soft-tissue insertion. **B.** A relatively intact head can be used to size the prosthetic head. The head may also be used as bone graft if needed or to support the prosthesis.

This is a good time to evaluate the patient for subacromial impingement. If there is a large subacromial spur in the ligament, or if the patient has an impingement configuration of the acromion, it may be worthwhile to perform an anterior acromioplasty. This is not a routine part of the procedure. Also at this stage, the rotator cuff should be examined for tears. Generally, the rotator cuff is intact in patients with subacromial impingement.

If there is an anterior dislocation of the humeral head below the coracoid and under the coracoid muscles, this should be slowly and carefully dissected, especially if there has been more than a week's delay in performing the procedure. Significant adhesions and scarring are invariably present and the sharp edges of the fractured head have the potential to injure the vital structures in this region if extraction is forceful or blind. In this instance, very gentle blunt dissection should be done from lateral to medial. Avoid placing any sharp instruments medial to the head without direct visualization. We prefer to use blunt retractors in this situation to avoid injuring the neurovascular bundle. If the head segment has been displaced posteriorly, the shaft and greater tuberosity are gently and laterally retracted so that the head can be removed. If the head is scarred posteriorly, it may need to be osteotomized into segments to facilitate removal.

Shaft Preparation and Prosthesis Placement   The proximal shaft of the humerus should be dealt with in a very gentle manner. The bone is often osteoporotic, and there may be a nondisplaced fracture of the shaft, which should not be disturbed. If a shaft component to the fracture is found, it is important to secure the shaft before prosthesis placement. This can usually be achieved with a cerclage wire and heavy nonabsorbable sutures. Canal preparation and stem implantation are carefully performed to avoid disrupting the repaired shaft. Successful placement of the humeral component supplements the shaft fixation and yields a solidly fixed construct.

Prior to preparation of the shaft, the arm is placed into extension and external rotation, delivering the shaft into the wound. The medullary canal is prepared with rasps and reamers (Fig. 4.9). In most general situations, there is not sufficient bone stock distally or support

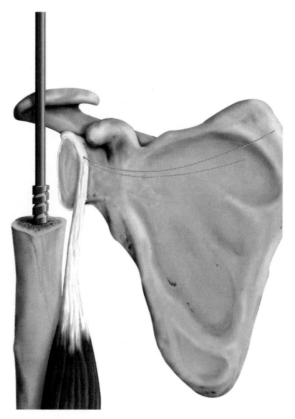

Figure 4.9. The medullary canal is prepared with rasps and reamers for cement fixation.

proximally to allow a press fit and cement is therefore necessary. In addition, with both tuberosities fractured, rotational stability of the implant is lost. The proximal part of the humerus should be prepared with drill holes to allow tuberosity fixation with heavy, non-absorbable sutures. Three or 4 holes should be placed in the area of the greater tuberosity (Fig. 4.10). We like to place no. 2 or no. 5 sutures with a swedged-on needle through the shaft. These sutures are then tagged with a clamp.

The next step is determination of proper prosthesis configuration. This involves three components: retroversion, height, and head size. Men tend to require a larger head size, and women, a smaller head size. We use the Bigliani/Flatow prosthesis (Zimmer, Inc., Warsaw, IN), which has multiple sizes with a choice of either standard or offset heads. We prefer the offset head because the humeral canal (and therefore the humeral implant) is offset from the center of the native head and better reproduces normal anatomy. Head size may be gauged by taking a radiograph of the contralateral shoulder or by using the head that was removed (if intact) for measurement. It is important, however, not to overstuff the joint as this may result in stiffness or subscapularis rupture.

The stem should not be seated so deeply that the head is placed against the remaining proximal shaft because such a placement will usually decrease the length of the humerus and effectively shorten the deltoid. In most general circumstances, the humeral head should be elevated above the proximal shaft to a position that will allow space for both the greater and the lesser tuberosities to be placed underneath the head. This is crucial. The system has sponges of different diameter that can be placed around the stem to support the shaft in the canal. Then a fin clamp is attached to the anterior fin of the prosthesis and securely holds it at the desired height and rotation on the shaft by way of metal pins or an outrigger that projects off the clamp (Fig. 4.11). This height is determined either by preoperative templating against the contralateral limb or by using intraoperative soft-tissue tension as a guide. The tension on the biceps tendon, if the tendon has been preserved, can act as a guide to the proper tension of the entire myofascial sleeve. If the prosthesis is inserted so deeply that the biceps is very slack in its anatomic position, then often the prosthesis has been placed too deeply into the medullary canal. A biceps tendon that is excessively taut usually indicates that the prosthesis is too proud. If the tuberosities are not placed below the head

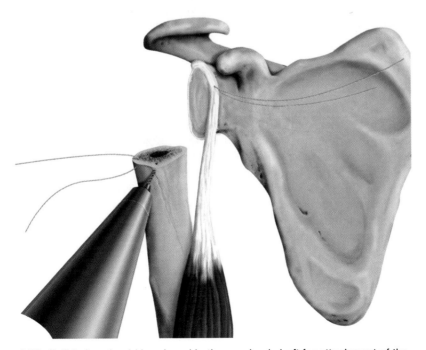

Figure 4.10. Drill holes should be placed in the proximal shaft for attachment of the tuberosities *before* cementing in the prosthesis. Three to 4 drill holes are placed in the greater tuberosity, and 1 to 2 holes in the lesser tuberosity.

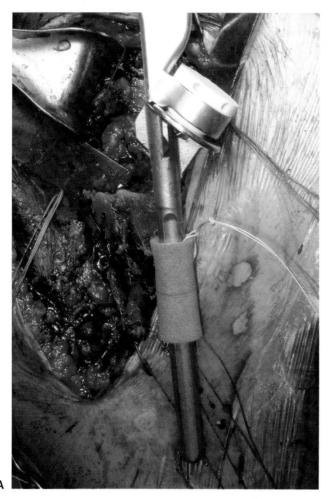

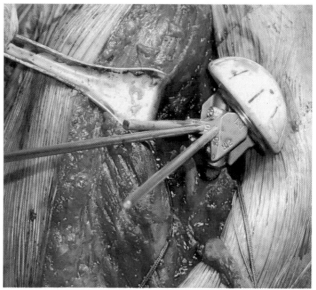

A   B

Figure 4.11. A. Sponge placed around the stem of the prosthesis will support the implant in the canal allowing for assessment of height and version. **B.** The fin clamp is attached to the prosthesis and the outrigger maintains the prosthesis at the desired height. The outrigger also can be attached by way of metal pins (not pictured).

of the prosthesis, impingement will occur. Also, these tuberosities must be attached to the proximal shaft. If extra bone has been saved, it should be used between the prosthesis and the shaft before cementing.

The third important component is the determination of the proper amount of retroversion. A rule of thumb is that the lateral fin of the prosthesis should be in the area of the bicipital groove. Often the majority of the bicipital groove is not present in fractures, but sometimes the distal part of the groove may be identified. Version rods can be attached to the humeral insertion tool or to the fin clamp (see Fig. 4.11). These can be used as reference for the forearm with the elbow flexed to 90 degrees, and in most patients, 30 degrees of retroversion is appropriate (Fig. 4.12). The fin clamp is used to hold the prosthesis at the desired height and rotation during the trial reduction. The head of the prosthesis is reduced on the glenoid to allow internal and external rotation to be assessed. If the prosthesis appears to be stable with 40 to 50 degrees of external rotation and internal rotation with the arm at the side, then the retroversion is adequate. If there has been a posterior-fracture dislocation, then the retroversion may be decreased by 5 to 10 degrees. If there is an anterior-fracture dislocation, then the retroversion may be increased by 5 to 10 degrees. Therefore, as a rule, the retroversion should never be less than 20 or more than 40 degrees. At this stage, the prosthesis can be cemented into place with the shaft properly supported (Fig. 4.13). It is important to make sure that the nonabsorbable sutures are through the holes in the proximal shaft prior to cementing.

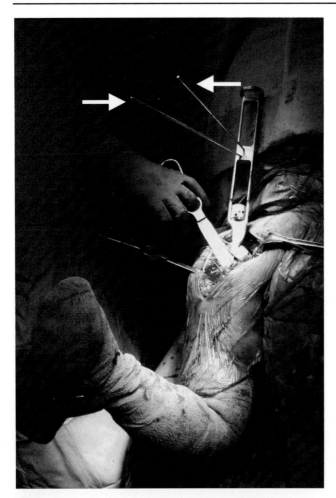

Figure 4.12. Version rods attach to the insertion device and reference off the forearm. One rod corresponds to 20 degrees of retroversion with the other at 40 degrees. Typically, the forearm should be oriented between these 2 rods to achieve 30 degrees of retroversion.

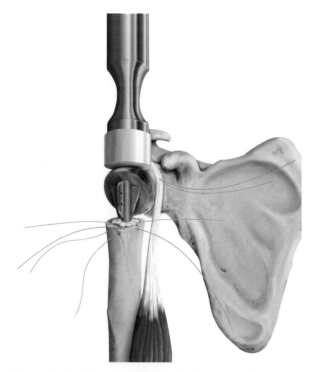

Figure 4.13. The stem is cemented into place to provide axial and rotational support.

Tuberosity Repair Tuberosity repair is the next important step. Tuberosity migration is one of the most common causes of failure of the procedure. The tuberosities must be attached to both the fin of the prosthesis and to the shaft of the proximal bone (Fig. 4.14). The nonabsorbable sutures that have been placed proximal to the tuberosities in the tendon can be used to mobilize the tendons and bring them forward. We generally reattach the greater tuberosity first, using 3 to 4 heavy nonabsorbable sutures. Next, the lesser tuberosity is fixed with two heavy sutures. The two sutures are placed through the fin of the prosthesis to both tuberosities and tightened. The arm should be supported in a slightly flexed and abducted position. The biceps tendon that has been preserved is now placed in its groove. The rotator interval that has been opened is now closed above the biceps tendon, so that the biceps tendon comes out at the distal aspect, which is now the bicipital groove (Fig. 4.15). At this point, the arm is gently internally and externally rotated and flexed to test the stability of the tuberosity repair. The proximal humerus and tuberosities should be moving as a single unit.

Closure A closed, suction drain should be used if there is any residual bleeding. These should exit laterally in the proximal deltoid to avoid injury to the axillary nerve. Drains are usually removed on the first postoperative day. The insertion of the pectoralis major should be repaired (Fig. 4.16). Multiple sutures should then be placed in the deltopectoral interval, and the skin is closed in a subcuticular fashion (Fig. 4.17). Steri-Strips are used to promote a cosmetic scar.

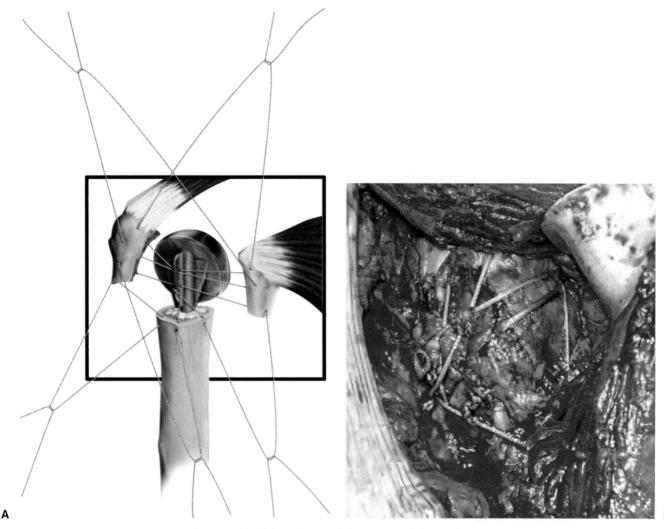

A   B

Figure 4.14. Tuberosity repair is an essential part of the procedure. **A.** Both tuberosities should be attached to the shaft and also to each other through the fin of the prosthesis. **B.** The tuberosities should move as a unit with the shaft after final repair.

POSTOPERATIVE MANAGEMENT

Proper postoperative rehabilitation is essential because adequate motion of the shoulder is required for optimal function. The patient's ability to participate in the physical therapy and to understand the restrictions on activity are crucial. In general, the goals are to perform early passive motion until the fracture has healed and then to begin strengthening exercises. Radiographs should be taken in the recovery room, at 1 week, 6 weeks, 3 months, and 1 year.

Passive motion is begun early, usually on the first postoperative day. Based on the intra-operative assessment of stability after the tuberosity reconstruction, the surgeon determines the limits of early motion. Consideration is given to the quality of bone, the status of the rotator cuff muscles and the deltoid, and the strength of the tuberosity fixation to the shaft and the prosthesis. On the first day, the surgeon usually passively elevates the arm in the scapular plane to approximately 80 to 90 degrees. On the second day, gravity-assisted pendulum exercises are done first to allow warm-up and obtain the patient's confidence. After this, passive forward elevation and supine external rotation with a stick are performed. The patient, after gaining some early motion with the help of a therapist, may lie supine and raise the arm by using the uninvolved contralateral arm. These 3 exercises are generally done for the first 6 weeks until adequate tuberosity healing has occurred. The

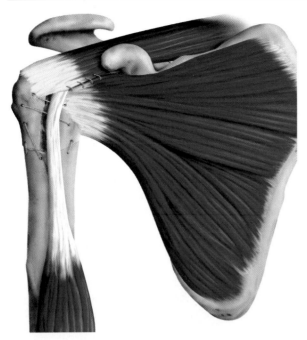

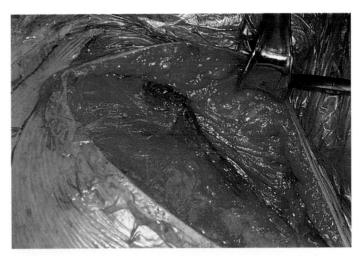

Figure 4.15. The biceps tendon should be preserved and placed in the rotator interval area.

Figure 4.16. A meticulous deltoid closure with repair of the pectoralis major insertion should be performed.

goal before discharge from the hospital should be 130 degrees of forward elevation in the scapular plane and 30 degrees of external rotation.

Radiographs should be taken before discharge to confirm that tuberosity displacement has not occurred. Furthermore, radiographs should be repeated at 6 weeks to assess tuberosity healing. When evidence of tuberosity healing is found at approximately 6 to 8 weeks, active assistive elevation with a pulley and isometric strengthening exercises for the rotator cuff and deltoid are initiated. Two to 3 weeks after this, progressive resistive and strengthening exercises are added. Activities of daily living such as personal hygiene and eating are allowed, and these help to build early muscle strength and endurance. Gentle strengthening is an important part of the prolonged physical therapy program. The patient is encouraged to perform the exercises on a daily basis for at least 6 months, preferably 1 year, to achieve optimal results.

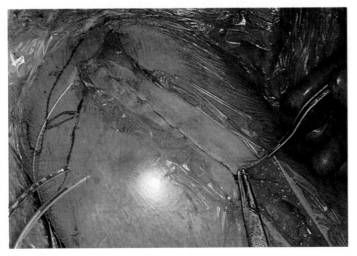

Figure 4.17. A subcuticular skin closure is performed.

The overall success of prosthetic replacement for humeral fractures depends on proper evaluation, surgical technique, and rehabilitation. If proper steps are followed, this procedure is highly successful, with a large percentage of satisfactory results. In a series of humeral head replacements performed at our hospital, 95% of patients had adequate pain relief, with 73% being essentially pain free. Overall, 82% of patients had a satisfactory result, and 18% had an unsatisfactory result. The impact on favorable or unfavorable results depends predominantly on the range of motion achieved by the patient rather than the degree of pain. The majority of failures reflected weakness and inability to raise the arm above horizontal. In addition, the single most important variable in a patient's ability to achieve a satisfactory result was found to be patient compliance in the postoperative rehabilitation program. Thus, that at the end of 1 year after prosthetic insertion for a 4-part fracture, most patients will be free of pain but will have variable range of motion and strength, often dependent on the adequacy of their rehabilitation.

COMPLICATIONS

Complications after proximal humeral replacement are not uncommon and in most instances can be directly related to failure of technique. Among the most common complications reported are tuberosity displacement, prosthesis problems, stiffness, and infection.

Tuberosity Displacement

The greater tuberosity is more likely to be displaced than is the lesser tuberosity, and it is most often found in older patient with osteopenic bone. Greater-tuberosity displacement is much more problematic because the attached supraspinatus, infraspinatus, and teres minor are critical for satisfactory motion and strength in the shoulder. In addition, with superior displacement of the greater tuberosity, motion may be mechanically blocked because the tuberosity occupies a portion of the subacromial space. If migration of the greater tuberosity happens postoperatively, then consideration should be given to early reattachment and regrafting. Although displacement of the lesser tuberosity occurs, it is not so problematic because other muscles can compensate for associated weakness of the subscapularis. Significant displacement can result in a mechanical block because the arm is internally rotated. In addition, wide displacement of the lesser tuberosity with the attached subscapularis may result in postoperative anterior instability.

The critical factor in eliminating tuberosity displacement is healing of the tuberosity to the shaft of the humerus. In patients adequately protected from postoperative active motion, secure fixation of the greater tuberosity to both the prosthesis and the shaft of the humerus, combined with bone graft between the tuberosity and shaft, will maximize the potential for tuberosity-shaft healing. We have recently used a trabecular metal (TM) proximal-humeral fracture prosthesis. The TM prosthesis features a metal surface designed for bony ingrowth in the proximal metaphysis including the sites of tuberosity attachment (Fig. 4.18). We have had excellent results using this in revisions for tuberosity nonunions and malunions, and we have also begun using it for primary proximal-humeral replacements in patients with marked osteopenia.

Whereas nonunion is often a far greater problem in terms of motion and strength, malunion of the greater tuberosity, either superiorly or posteriorly, frequently results in pain, either from impingement in the subacromial space or from the mechanical block caused by the displaced tuberosity. If the patient is symptomatic and malunion exists, strong consideration should be given to osteotomy and repositioning of the tuberosity.

Prosthetic Loosening

The bony support in the proximal humerus is often not ideal because of osteopenia. With loss of the rotational stability of the implant because of loosening, the version of the prosthesis may have changed and secondary pain, instability, or destruction of the

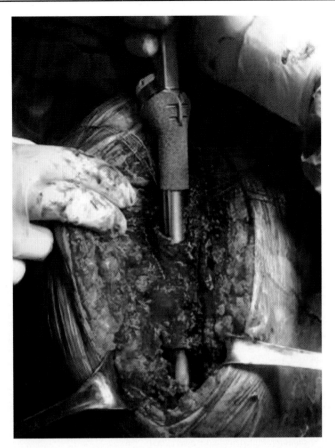

Figure 4.18. The TM humeral prosthesis has a proximal metal surface that promotes ingrowth of tuberosities.

previously normal glenoid. Whereas loosening caused by poor bone stock in an uncemented implant could have been avoided if cement had been used at implantation, loosening also may occur with a cemented implant. Because aseptic loosening of the humeral component is rare, the workup should include examination for infection. Revision of the prosthesis should be considered in the event of symptomatic loosening.

Malposition of the Prosthesis

Malposition may involve abnormal version, an abnormally proud prosthesis, or an abnormal depth of prosthesis. Mistakes made by cementing the implant in abnormal version are common because the landmark for correct version, the bicipital groove, is usually involved in the fracture. Three basic guides can be used to place the prosthesis in the proper amount of retroversion (20 to 40 degrees):

1. The prosthetic fin should be placed just lateral to the bicipital groove.
2. The prosthetic fin should be 20 to 40 degrees retroverted relative to the forearm, as judged by version rods on the prosthesis inserter corresponding to 20 and 40 degrees.
3. With the elbow bent 90 degrees and the arm at the side in 0 degrees of internal or external rotation, the implanted humeral head should face directly toward the glenoid fossa.

If the malpositioned prosthesis is too proud, impingement against the residual glenoid fossa may be found. If the humeral head is inserted too deeply into the intramedullary canal, instability of the humeral head may result because of inadequate tension of the deltoid. In addition, an overly deep insertion of the prosthesis makes the greater tuberosity relatively proud and may result in greater-tuberosity impingement on the acromion.

Postoperative Stiffness

Postoperative stiffness is an important complication because it is almost entirely preventable. Attention to the details of surgery, early, postoperative, passive motion, and patient cooperation with rehabilitation all play critical roles in avoiding postoperative stiffness. It must be emphasized to the patients that lack of compliance or understanding of the postoperative rehabilitation program is the single most common factor associated with rehabilitation failure and postoperative stiffness.

Infection

Infection is an uncommon complication, but it poses significant problems and a long treatment course before resolution. The final result after treatment of an infected prosthesis is frequently less than optimal.

RECOMMENDED READING

Bigliani LU. Proximal humerus fractures. In: Post M, Bigliani LU, Flatow EL, et al, eds. *The shoulder: operative technique.* Baltimore: Lipincott, Williams & Wilkins; 1998.

Bloom MH, Obata WG. Diagnosis of posterior dislocation of the shoulder with use of Velpeau axillary and angle-up roentgenographic views. *J Bone Joint Surg Am* 1967;49:943–949.

Hughes M, Neer CS. Glenohumeral joint replacement and post-operative rehabilitation. *Phys Ther* 1975; 55:850–858.

Lervick GN, Carroll RM, Levine WN. Complications after hemiarthroplasty for fractures of the proximal humerus. In: Ferlic DC. *Instructional course lectures.* Rosemont, IL: American Academy of Orthopaedic Surgeons; 2003.

Levine WN, Blaine TA, Bigliani LU. Fractures of the proximal humerus. In: Rockwood CA, Matsen FA, Wirth MA, et al, eds. *The shoulder.* Philadelphia: Elsevier; 2004.

Murthi AM, Bigliani LU. Humeral head replacement for four-part proximal humerus fractures. In: Levine WN, Marra G, Bigliani LU, eds. *Fractures of the shoulder girdle.* New York: Marcel Dekker; 2003.

Neer CS II. Articular replacement of the humeral head. *J Bone Joint Surg Am* 1955;37:215–228.

Neer CS II. Displaced proximal humerus fractures, Part I. *J Bone Joint Surg Am* 1970;52:1077–1089.

Neer CS II. Displaced proximal humerus fractures, Part II. *J Bone Joint Surg Am* 1970;52:1090–1103.

Neer CS II, McIlveen SJ. Remplacement de la tete humerale avec reconstruction des tuberosities et de la coiffe dans les fractures desplacees a 4 fragments. Resultats actuels et techniques. *Rev Chir Orthop* 1988;74(SII):31–40.

Tanner MW, Cofield RH. Prosthetic arthroplasty for fractures and fracture-dislocations of the proximal humerus. *Clin Orthop* 1983;179:116–128.

5

Humeral Shaft Fractures: Open Reduction Internal Fixation

Derek E. Robinson and Peter J. O'Brien

INDICATIONS/CONTRAINDICATIONS

Numerous studies have shown that the majority of humeral shaft fractures can be treated nonoperatively with high rates of union and excellent functional results. However, in specific clinical settings, open reduction and internal fixation (ORIF) are favored over closed functional methods. Good results can be expected (1–3) and outcomes are superior to comparable fractures treated with intramedullary nailing (4–6). Although there are no absolute indications for plate fixation, we favor its use in some patients and consider the fracture characteristics and the presence of concomitant injuries in our decision (Table 5.1).

Fracture Considerations

Internal fixation is indicated in patients with closed fractures in which a satisfactory reduction cannot be achieved or maintained. The most common cause of a poor reduction in an otherwise healthy individual is interposition of soft tissue. Failure to maintain an acceptable closed reduction sometimes occurs in obese patients or women with large breasts. Other indications include segmental and peri-articular fractures. The latter can be difficult to control, and the prolonged immobilization of the adjacent joint can lead to loss of motion.

Open fractures require surgical debridement and bony stabilization to allow optimal soft-tissue management. After thorough debridement, ORIF of the humerus is a good method of fracture stabilization for most grade I, II, and IIIA injuries with limited bony defects. It produces a stable limb, improving postoperative wound management. With extreme comminution or bone loss, acute shortening of up to 5 cm is usually well tolerated.

Experience has taught us that nonoperative treatment of pathologic humeral fractures frequently results in nonunion and persistent pain. There is widespread agreement that patients with a pathologic humeral fracture as a result of metastatic disease benefit from

Table 5.1. *Indications for Surgical Stabilization of Humeral Shaft Fractures*

Early	Late
Failure of closed treatment	Nonunion
Multiple injuries, patient	Malunion
Multiple injuries, limb	
Open fracture	
Pathologic fracture	
Associated arthrodesis	
Periprosthetic fracture	

surgical stabilization. Usually these fractures are best managed with a locked intramedullary nail, but occasionally, a fracture is not amenable to intramedullary nailing and is better managed with a long spanning plate (7).

Periprosthetic fractures around elbow or shoulder arthroplasty frequently require internal fixation. Fractures that occur around the stem of an implant occasionally require revision of the prosthesis.

Delayed unions and nonunions are additional indications for ORIF of a humeral fracture. Delayed union is generally accepted to mean that the fracture has failed to show progressive signs of healing within 3 to 4 months, whereas nonunion is defined when the healing is delayed or arrested beyond 6 months. Nonunions can occur because of fracture instability, poor bone vascularity, or marked displacement. Infection must be ruled out for nonunions of open fractures that have been surgically repaired. Union is usually obtained following revision ORIF and autogenous bone grafting (8), and in osteoporotic bone this may be done successfully with locking compression plates (9).

Malunion is rarely an indication for surgical intervention because angular deformity is often well tolerated after closed treatment. The amount of mal-alignment that can be accepted varies between patients and is influenced by level of activity and cosmesis. Most patients tolerate up to 20 degrees of varus, 15 degrees of anterior angulation, and 5 cm of shortening.

Concomitant Injuries

Internal fixation of humeral shaft fractures is also indicated in a variety of circumstances due to concomitant injuries. The patient with multiple injuries is the most common candidate for operative treatment of humeral shaft fractures (10–12). When patients sustain injuries to multiple body systems, early surgical stabilization of long bone fractures may be life-saving. Fixation should be undertaken early to reduce analgesic needs, allow early mobilization, and facilitate nursing care.

Patients with ipsilateral injuries to the shoulder, elbow, or forearm often require operative treatment of their humeral fracture. In bilateral humeral fractures or any contralateral upper-extremity injury, fixation may be necessary to allow activities of daily living and self-care. Humeral shaft fractures associated with a fracture of both forearm bones require fixation of both the forearm and the humerus to allow early range of motion. Finally, rehabilitation of injuries to the lower extremities can be accelerated by fixation of the humerus, which allows for the use of crutches through the stabilized humerus.

If an axillary or brachial artery injury is associated with a closed fracture, then this should be stabilized at the time of vascular repair. Internal fixation of the humerus through the vascular approach is recommended to protect the vascular repair, to facilitate ongoing assessment, and allow rehabilitation of the limb. Brachial plexus or peripheral nerve injuries in the ipsilateral limb are often an indication for internal fixation of a humeral fracture because concomitant brachial plexus injuries may be associated with high rates of delayed union, nonunion, and malunion of the humeral shaft when treated closed (13). To prevent these complications and to facilitate rehabilitation, operative treatment should be considered with this combination of injuries.

The management of humeral fractures with associated radial nerve injury remains controversial (14–16). The incidence of radial nerve injury in humeral fractures is approximately 10%, with a range reported between 2% and 26%. Humeral shaft fractures seen with a primary radial-nerve injury do not usually require nerve exploration. If the fracture reduction can be maintained, closed treatment will result in fracture healing and a good outcome with a greater than 80% chance of spontaneous nerve recovery. The majority of cases are neurapraxias, which should show signs of recovery by 3 to 4 months, with improvements in muscle grade up to 2 years after injury (11).

Some studies have shown that with modern microsurgical techniques and late exploration of radial nerve palsies, better than 90% recover (14,15). Therefore, we recommend initial observation and late exploration for nerve injuries that do not resolve. The injury should be documented clinically and electrophysiologically with electromyogram/nerve conduction studies (EMG/NCS) in the early stages. The hand should be splinted, and an intensive physiotherapy program should be initiated to maintain mobility at the elbow, wrist, and fingers. Patients are evaluated monthly and have a follow-up EMG/NCS at 6 and 12 weeks. If after 4 to 6 months there is no sign of radial nerve recovery, then we explore the nerve.

More controversial is the management of secondary radial-nerve palsy. Most commonly this occurs after closed reduction of a humeral fracture. Traditionally, a nerve palsy occurring in such a circumstance was considered an indication for nerve exploration and internal fixation. Although some have shown that the nerve can be trapped between the fracture fragments (17), and while it seems reasonable to explore the nerve and free it from any ongoing compression, there is no scientific evidence that the outcome is improved by early surgery. Secondary radial-nerve palsy, however, continues to be an accepted indication for early exploration.

Relative contraindications to plate fixation of humeral shaft fractures include grade IIIB open fractures with massive soft-tissue injury or extensive bone loss, soft-tissue or bone infection, as well as severe osteoporosis, that would preclude fixation.

PREOPERATIVE PLANNING

With all injured patients, a careful history and physical examination are mandatory. Associated injuries should be identified and carefully assessed. Physical examination should include the chest, neck, shoulder, arm, elbow, forearm, wrist, and hand. The physical signs of fracture are usually obvious after humeral shaft fractures with pain, swelling, crepitus, and motion at the fracture site. The neurologic examination of the limb must be meticulous. Radial nerve injury is the most commonly associated neurological injury, but any peripheral nerve, including the brachial plexus, can be injured in association with a humeral diaphyseal fracture. The vascular assessment includes palpation of the axillary, brachial, and radial pulses and an assessment of hand-tissue perfusion. The soft-tissue compartments of the arm and forearm should be evaluated for compartment syndrome.

Good quality radiographs of the humerus are essential. Anteroposterior (AP) and lateral views of the humerus should be obtained that include the shoulder and elbow joints. The anatomic location of the fracture, the fracture pattern, and the expected bone quality are critical when developing a preoperative plan.

Once a decision is made to operate on a humeral fracture, a surgical tactic should be developed that includes the patient position, the surgical approach, the steps necessary for fracture reduction, temporary fixation, and the implant to be used for final fixation.

There are four basic approaches to the shaft of the humerus: the anterolateral, straight lateral, posterior, and anteromedial. However, the anteromedial approach is rarely used in humeral-shaft fracture treatment and will not be discussed further. The decision about which surgical approach to use is based on the fracture level and configuration, the need for radial nerve exploration, and the patient's general condition. The most common approach is the anterolateral. Fractures located anywhere in the proximal two thirds of the humerus can be successfully managed through this approach, but it does not allow adequate exposure of the distal one third of the humerus; therefore, it cannot be used if the fixation must be extended into the distal third. In fractures involving the distal two thirds of the humerus, with an associated radial-nerve injury that requires surgery, we prefer the straight lateral approach. This approach can be extended into the anterolateral approach and thereby give access to the entire humerus if necessary. It may also be extended proximally by utilizing the same muscular interval but passing posteriorly to the deltoid, the proximal limit being the axillary nerve (18). The posterior approach can be used for fractures that involve the distal half of the humeral shaft.

The steps necessary for fracture reduction and temporary fixation before final fixation must be carefully considered. In most cases, direct reduction techniques are appropriate. The fracture hematoma is evacuated, and the fracture surfaces are anatomically reduced. For spiral or oblique fracture patterns, temporary fixation can usually be accomplished with Weber pointed reduction forceps. Transverse fractures can usually be stabilized temporarily with Kirschner (K) wires or by drilling a hole in each fragment and using pointed reduction forceps away from the site of anticipated plate application. Some comminuted fractures that still have cortical contact between the main proximal and distal pieces cannot be temporarily stabilized satisfactorily. In those cases, the appropriate plate is secured to one fragment, the fracture is then reduced under the plate, and fixation is completed.

Severely comminuted fractures may be amenable to indirect reduction techniques. The femoral distractor is used to secure the reduction, which is confirmed under image intensification. The appropriate plate is then secured to the main proximal and distal fragments. The soft-tissue attachments to the comminuted intercalary fragments are left intact. Bone grafting is not added when the indirect reduction technique is used.

When planning plate fixation in oblique or spiral fractures, surgeons strive to achieve interfragmentary compression, which can be done by using interfragmentary lag screws inserted either outside (Fig. 5.1) or through the plate (Fig. 5.2). Interfragmentary screws alone are insufficient fixation for humeral shaft fractures and must be supplemented with a neutralization plate. In transverse fracture patterns, interfragmentary compression is

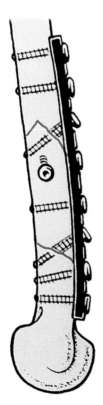

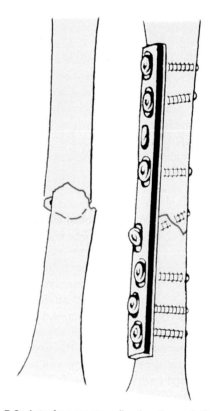

Figure 5.1. Initial fixation is accomplished with an interfragmentary screw. This is supplemented by a neutralization plate.

Figure 5.2. Interfragmentary fixation through the plate.

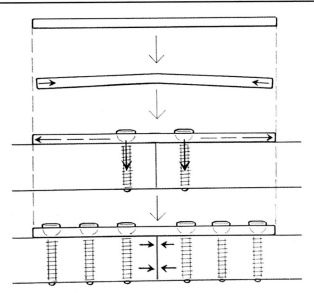

Figure 5.3. Transverse fracture pattern in which interfragmentary compression is achieved by using a prebent dynamic-compression plate.

achieved by using a limited-contact dynamic-compression (LCDC) plate, and the plate must be prestressed (prebent) to avoid a gap in the far cortex (Fig. 5.3). In general, the plate of choice is a broad 4.5-mm LCDC. This is a strong plate with a wide surface contact and offset screw holes to prevent longitudinal splitting of the shaft from collinear screws. In addressing acute fractures, we aim for at least six cortices of fixation above and below the fracture. When dealing with osteoporotic bone, we either use more cortices of fixation or locking compression plates. Bone grafting should be planned with comminuted fractures. If more than one third of the circumference of the humeral shaft is comminuted, we generally use an autogenous iliac-crest bone graft.

In many cases, the humerus is small, and the broad LCDC plate cannot be used. In such a situation, a narrow 4.5-mm LCDC plate can be used. Likewise, in the distal shaft, where extensive contouring of the plate is necessary, a 3.5-mm pelvic reconstruction plate is occasionally used for neutralization. However, this type of plate should be used only when there is excellent interfragmentary compression with multiple lag screws. It is important to avoid encroachment of the hardware in the olecranon or coronoid fossae when fixing the distal humerus.

SURGERY

All trauma patients are prescrubbed with a chlorhexidine nail brush: The area is washed off with saline and then chlorhexidine is poured over the limb prior to formal prepping and draping. However, for open fractures, iodine is preferred. A sterile tourniquet is used if the fracture is in the middle or distal one third. If it is used, the tourniquet is deflated prior to closure and hemostasis achieved; therefore, a drain is rarely necessary.

The anterolateral approach is performed with the patient supine and a pad beneath the scapula. The arm is free draped allowing access to the neck (subclavian vasculature) and placed on a radiolucent arm board. Surface landmarks, coracoid process, deltopectoral groove, lateral bicipital sulcus, and the lateral epicondyle, are marked with a sterile pen (Fig. 5.4). Depending on the fracture, the incision may extend from the coracoid process down to approximately 6 cm from the lateral epicondyle (Fig. 5.5). The deltopectoral groove is developed proximally. The belly of the biceps is identified and its lateral border mobilized, exposing the brachialis muscle (Fig. 5.6). Care is taken to avoid injury to the proximal cephalic vein and the lateral cutaneous nerve of the forearm in the medial aspect of the distal wound area. The biceps is retracted medially, and the brachialis is divided

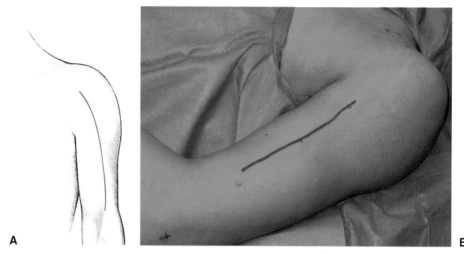

Figure 5.4. A,B. Incision for the anterolateral approach.

longitudinally, lateral to its midline and down to bone, aiming for the middle of the humeral shaft (Fig. 5.7). Through this approach, the radial nerve, which is lateral to the brachialis, is protected and the innervation of the lateral portion of the brachialis (radial nerve) is preserved. Flexion of the elbow, along with partial (anterior) detachment of the deltoid insertion and of the medial brachialis origin, is done to allow reduction and plating of the anterolateral surface of the humerus (Fig. 5.8).

The straight lateral approach requires careful dissection but allows excellent visualization of the radial nerve and adjacent structures. It is ideal for exploration of the radial nerve and fixation of the distal humerus in a multiply injured patient. With the patient supine, the arm is free draped and kept adducted along the patient's body. The surface landmarks are the lateral epicondyle, deltoid tuberosity, and the coracoid process as necessary (Fig. 5.9).

The incision extends longitudinally from the lateral epicondyle proximally to the deltoid tuberosity. After incision of the investing fascia of the arm, the intervals between the triceps and brachialis proximally and the brachioradialis and brachialis distally are identified. The distal interval is first developed bluntly as described by Henry (19): ". . . place well-gloved

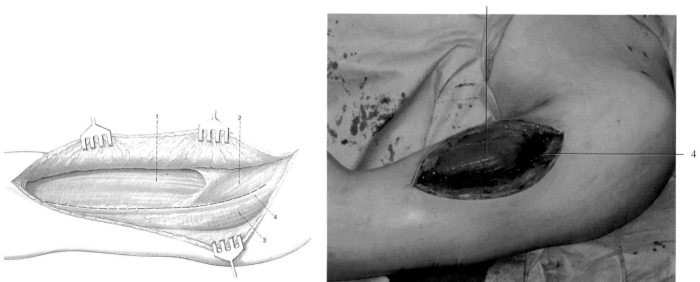

Figure 5.5. A,B. Initial muscular exposure: (1) biceps; (2) pectoralis major; (3) deltoid; and (4) cephalic vein.

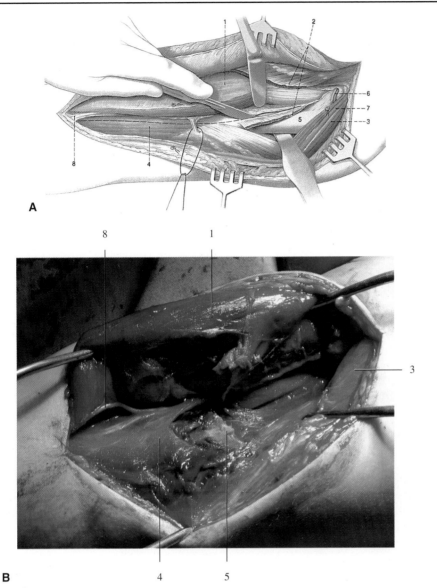

Figure 5.6. Splitting of the brachialis in the line of its fibers: (1) biceps; (2) pectoralis major; (3) deltoid; (4) brachialis; (5) humerus; (6) anterior, circumflex, humeral vessels; (7) cephalic vein; and (8) lateral cutaneous nerve of the forearm.

thumbs, lengthwise and parallel, on each belly (brachialis and brachioradialis), and open the plane like a book on your knee. The nerve marks the place" (Fig. 5.10). The radial nerve is isolated, looped with a rubber sling, and protected. The nerve is retracted laterally while the proximal dissection is completed. The periosteum anterior to the intermuscular septum is split longitudinally, and subperiosteal elevation progresses medially and proximally with direct visualization and protection of the nerve at all times. This can be gently elevated if further access is required. As the nerve courses posteriorly and proximally, one might need to incise the intermuscular septum to mobilize the nerve and visualize its relation to the fracture. The nerve is retracted anteriorly, and the distal dissection is completed. The distal plane between the brachioradialis and the triceps is identified (Fig. 5.11). This plane is incised sharply, and the brachioradialis is reflected anteriorly, protecting the distal portion of the nerve. The entire distal humerus is exposed laterally and anterolaterally (Fig. 5.12). A narrow, 4.5-mm LCDC plate positioned laterally is often the best implant with this exposure. The plate is often quite distal and screw placement in the coronoid/olecranon fossae must be avoided (Fig. 5.13).

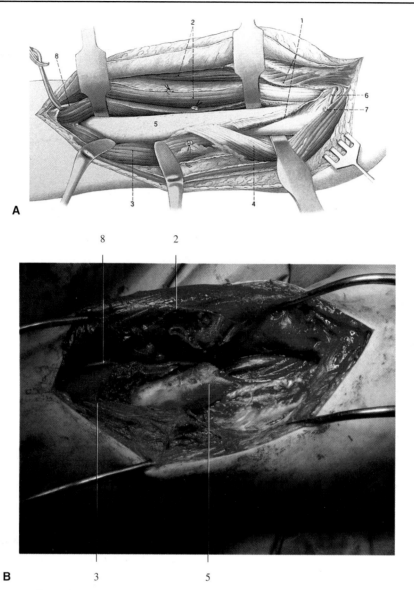

Figure 5.7. Completed exposure of the proximal two thirds of the humeral shaft: (1) pectoralis major; (2) biceps; (3) brachialis; (4) deltoid; (5) humerus; (6) anterior, circumflex, humeral vessels; (7) cephalic vein; and (8) lateral cutaneous nerve of the forearm.

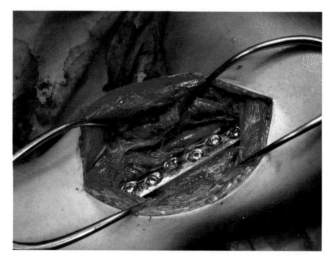

Figure 5.8. Prebent, broad, 4.5-mm, dynamic-compression plate applied to a transverse fracture via an anterolateral approach.

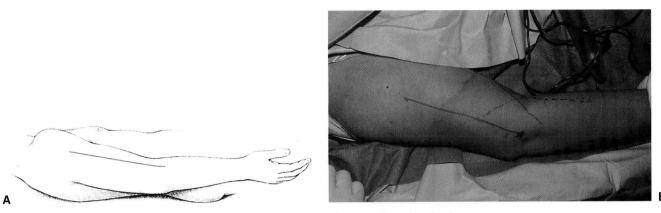

Figures 5.9. Positioning and skin incision for the straight lateral approach to the distal humerus.

The posterior approach is used in cases of isolated fractures in the distal half of the humerus. The patient is placed prone and brought to the edge of the operating table. The arm is free draped to allow access to the whole arm and the elbow. The shoulder is abducted 90 degrees in neutral flexion and supported distally at the elbow by a modified Mayo stand (Fig. 5.14). The stand can be altered by cutting a hole at the edge of the tray and padding the exposed rim of the stand. During the procedure, the forearm and hand are dropped into the hole, which is lined by a sterile c-arm pack protecting the forearm and hand from contamination that is possible due to their low-lying position. An additional advantage of using the Mayo stand is the ability to place instruments on it. An alternative is to place the patient in a lateral position with a bolster under the arm.

Surface markings are the posterolateral corner of the acromion and the olecranon. The straight incision extends from the distal border of the posterior deltoid, along the lateral edge of the long head of triceps, to the tip of the olecranon (Fig. 5.15). The long head can

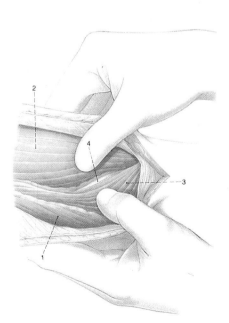

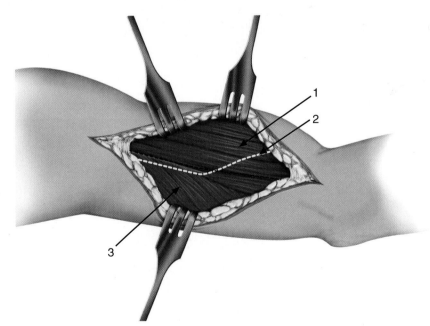

Figure 5.10. The radial nerve is identified in the interval between the brachialis and the brachioradialis: (1) triceps; (2) brachialis; (3) brachioradialis; and (4) radial nerve.

Figure 5.11. The intervals between brachialis and triceps proximally and between brachioradialis and triceps distally are developed: (1) biceps brachii muscle; (2) radial nerve; and (3) triceps brachii muscle.

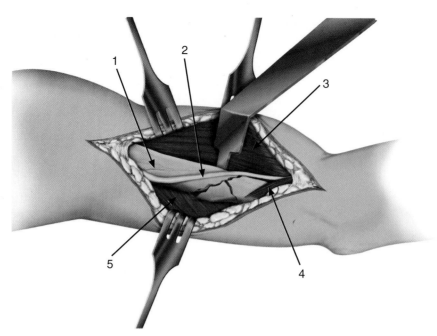

Figure 5.12. The brachialis and brachioradialis are retracted anteriorly and the triceps posteriorly exposing the distal humeral shaft: (1) humerus; (2) radial nerve; (3) brachialis muscle; (4) brachioradialis muscle; and (5) triceps brachii muscle.

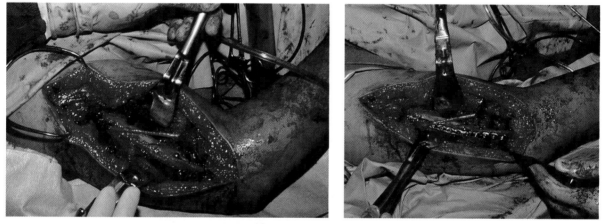

A   B

Figures 5.13. Reduction and internal fixation of a distal humeral fracture through the straight lateral approach.

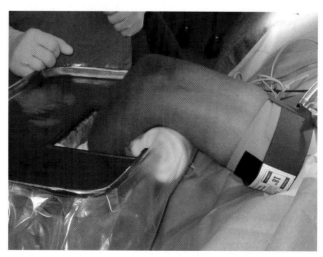

Figure 5.14. Positioning for the posterior approach with modified Mayo stand and sterile tourniquet.

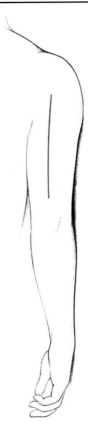

Figure 5.15. Skin incision for posterior approach.

be identified as a mobile mass on the posteromedial aspect of the arm. Skin, subcutaneous tissue, and fascia are incised and the distal, thick, white triceps tendon is identified. Proximally, the interval between the long and the lateral heads of the triceps is identified and dissected bluntly. Distally, these two superficial heads are sharply dissected by division of the triceps tendon (Fig. 5.16). Careful blunt dissection is carried out to identify the radial nerve on the proximal aspect of the deep head of triceps (Fig. 5.17). A rubber sling is placed around the radial nerve, which is protected throughout the case. The deep triceps is split longitudinally in its midline, and its medial and lateral portions are elevated, exposing the humerus (Fig. 5.18). Reduction and fixation can now proceed. The closure includes reapproximation of the triceps aponeurosis with absorbable suture and superficial layer closure.

POSTOPERATIVE MANAGEMENT

Postoperatively, a compression bandage is applied and patients are placed in a sling, which is removed to permit active range-of-motion exercises of the shoulder and elbow within 1 or 2 days of surgery. Full elbow and shoulder motion should be obtained within 6 weeks of surgery. Patients are seen on a monthly basis until the fracture is united and they have returned to normal activity. Radiographs are obtained at each visit. The patient is carefully assessed for shoulder, elbow, wrist, and hand function. The radiographs are studied for signs of fracture healing and any evidence of implant failure. With stable fixation, fracture union is often difficult to assess. If follow-up radiographs show maintenance of the reduction, light weights are usually allowed at 6 weeks and regular weights at 12 weeks. At 12 weeks, patients can begin returning to normal activities. Heavy work can be started at 16 weeks. Sporting activities, such as tennis and golf, can also be started about 4 months after surgery.

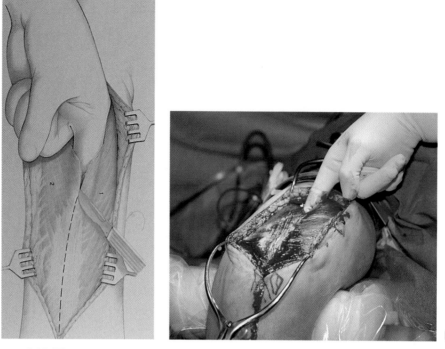

Figure 5.16. The posterior approach. Identification of the long and lateral heads of triceps: (1) long head of triceps and (2) lateral head of triceps.

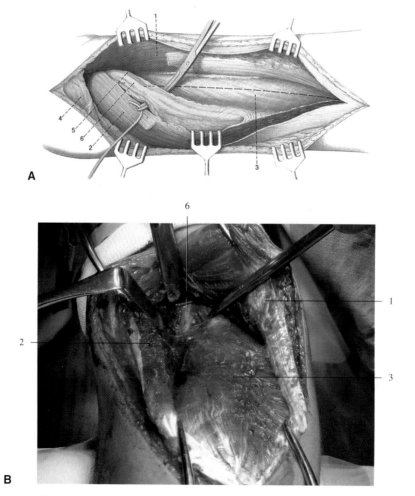

Figure 5.17. Exposure of the deep head of the triceps and radial nerve: (1) long head of triceps; (2) lateral head of triceps; (3) deep (medial) head of triceps; (4) deltoid; (5) deep brachial artery; and (6) radial nerve.

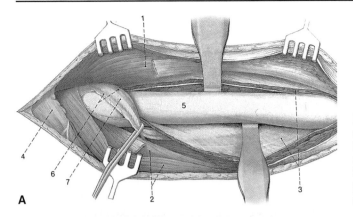

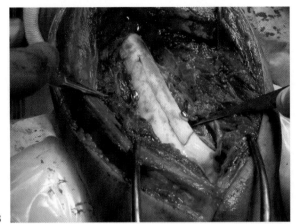

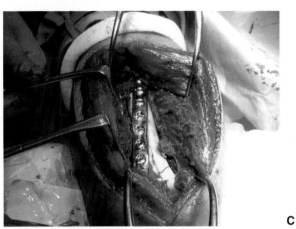

Figure 5.18. A. Exposure of the distal half of the humeral shaft: (1) long head of triceps; (2) lateral head; (3) medial head; (4) deltoid; (5) humerus; (6) deep brachial artery; and (7) radial nerve. **B.** By using the posterior approach, reduction and lag screw fixation is achieved. **C.** This is followed by placement of a neutralization plate positioned laterally to avoid encroachment on the olecranon fossa.

COMPLICATIONS

Most complications can be avoided by adhering to basic principles. Failure of fixation occurs in up to 4% of patients and can be avoided by careful preoperative planning and implant selection as well as limited soft-tissue dissection. When using a plate, interfragmentary compression, either with lag screws and a neutralization plate or with a compression plate alone, is essential. At least 6 points of cortical fixation on each side of the fracture must be obtained. If the fixation fails, revision ORIF is necessary, usually with a longer locking plate and bone graft because nonoperative management is rarely successful.

Nonunion after plate osteosynthesis occurs in 3% to 5% of cases. Factors thought to contribute to nonunion include open fractures, middle-third transverse fractures, pathologic fractures, patient alcohol abuse, or a technical error in the primary procedure. Factors that can be controlled by the surgeon include accurate fracture reduction, stability of fixation, and minimization of soft-tissue stripping and bone grafting. Nonunion is treated by revision ORIF and autogenous cancellous bone grafting. A longer plate must be used at the revision procedure. Nonunion after intramedullary nailing is also best treated by ORIF rather than exchange nailing (20).

With few studies assessing function in detail, loss of motion of the shoulder or elbow is probably underreported. Several studies report that 15% to 20% of patients have decreased shoulder and elbow motion after ORIF. Etiologic factors include fractures with extensive soft-tissue injuries or with ipsilateral bone or joint injury. Stable fixation and early motion are recommended. If significant stiffness is identified, a more vigorous physiotherapy program is initiated. We have not needed to use any surgical modalities to deal with joint stiffness after ORIF of humeral shaft fractures.

Infection is an uncommon complication of ORIF. The routine use of perioperative antibiotics, limited soft-tissue dissection, careful hemostasis, and thorough debridement of open fractures may reduce the rate of infection after ORIF. If infection develops, then the microorganism must be isolated. This is followed by assessing and correcting problems with stability, fragment approximation, vascularity, and soft-tissue coverage. The infected site should be incised, drained, and thoroughly debrided. The area is packed with antibiotic-loaded, acrylic, cement beads and systemic parenteral antibiotics are given. The choice of local and systemic antibiotic depends on the Gram stain findings and the final culture and sensitivities. Parenteral antibiotics are generally continued for 6 weeks. The local antibiotic depot is usually removed at 7 to 10 days during repeated debridement and irrigation. If the fixation is rigid, it is left in place, but if it is loose, it is revised and rigid fixation is obtained.

Radial nerve palsy most frequently occurs at the time of injury. Iatrogenic radial-nerve palsy occurs in about 5% of surgical cases. An intraoperative laceration should never occur, but if it does, it should be repaired immediately by a trained microsurgeon. A postoperative nerve palsy after identification and protection of the nerve should be observed, and full functional recovery anticipated.

RECOMMENDED READINGS

1. Meekers FS, Broos PL. Operative treatment of humeral shaft fractures: the Leuven experience. *Acta Orthop Belg* 2002;68:462–470.
2. Niall DM, O'Mahoney J, McElwain JP. Plating of humeral shaft fractures—has the pendulum swung back? *Injury* 2004;35:580–586.
3. Sarmiento A, Waddell JP, Latta LL. Diaphyseal humeral fractures: treatment options. *Instr Course Lect* 2002;51:257–269.
4. Chapman JR, Henley MB, Agel J, et al. Randomized prospective study of humeral shaft fracture fixation: intramedullary nails versus plates. *J Orthop Trauma* 2000;14:162–166.
5. McCormack RG, Brien D, Buckley RE, et al. Fixation of fractures of the shaft of the humerus by dynamic compression plate or intramedullary nail: a prospective, randomised trial. *J Bone Joint Surg Br* 2000;82:336–339.
6. Modabber MR, Jupiter JB. Operative management of diaphyseal fractures of the humerus: plate versus nail. *Clin Orthop* 1998;347:93–104.
7. Dijkstra S, Stapert J, Boxma H, et al. Treatment of pathological fractures of the humeral shaft due to bone metastases: a comparison of intramedullary locking nail and plate osteosynthesis with adjunctive bone cement. *Eur J Surg Oncol* 1996;22:621–626.
8. Marti RK, Verheyen CCPM, Besselaar PP. Humeral shaft nonunion: evaluation of uniform surgical repair in fifty-one patients. *J Orthop Trauma* 2002;16(2):108–115.
9. Ring D, Kloen P, Kadzielski J, et al. Locking compression plates for osteoporotic nonunions of the diaphyseal humerus. *Clin Orthop* 2004;425:50–54.
10. Bell MJ, Beauchamp CG, Kellam JK, et al. The results of plating humeral shaft fractures in patients with multiple injuries: the Sunnybrook experience. *J Bone Joint Surg Br* 1985;67:293–296.
11. Bleeker WA, Nisten MW, Duis H-J, et al. Treatment of humeral shaft fractures related to associated injuries: a retrospective study of 237 patients. *Acta Orthop Scand* 1991;62:148–153.
12. Heim D, Herkert F, Hess P, et al. Surgical treatment of humeral shaft fractures: the Basel experience. *J Trauma* 1993:35:226–232.
13. Brien WW, Gellman H, Becker V, et al. Management of fractures of the humerus in patients who have an injury of the ipsilateral brachial plexus. *J Bone Joint Surg Am* 1990;72:1208–1210.
14. Amillo S, Barrios RH, Martinez-Peric R, et al. Surgical treatment of the radial nerve lesions associated with fractures of the humerus. *J Orthop Trauma* 1993;7:211–215.
15. Samardzic M, Grujicic D, Milinkovic ZB. Radial nerve lesions associated with fractures of the humeral shaft. *Injury* 1990;21:220–222.
16. Sarmiento A, Horowitch A, Aboulafia A, et al. Functional bracing for comminuted extra-articular fractures of the distal third of the humerus. *J Bone Joint Surg Br* 1990;72:283–287.
17. Holstein A, Lewis GB. Fractures of the humerus with radial nerve paralysis. *J Bone Joint Surg Am* 1963;45:1382–1388.
18. Gerwin M, Hotchkiss RN, Weiland AJ. Alternative operative exposures of the posterior aspect of the humeral diaphysis. *J Bone Joint Surg Am* 1996;78:1690–1695.
19. Henry AK. *Extensile exposures.* 1st ed. Edinburgh: E. S. Livingstone; 1945.
20. McKee MD, Miranda MA, Reimer BL, et al. Management of humeral nonunion after the failure of locking intramedullary nails. *J Orthop Trauma* 1996;10:492–499.

6

Humeral Shaft Fractures: Intramedullary Nailing

Craig S. Roberts, Brent M. Walz, and
Jonathan G. Yerasimides

INDICATIONS/CONTRAINDICATIONS

The precise role for intramedullary nailing in the treatment of humeral shaft fractures is not defined (1). Although most humeral shaft fractures that require surgery are usually treated with plating, there remains a quiet optimism that newer approaches and implants for humeral nailing will lower the complication rate and thereby improve healing rates and patient outcomes.

Anatomic differences between the long bones of the lower extremity (tibia and femur) and the humerus narrow the indications for humeral nailing. The medullary canals of the femur and tibia extend distally into their respective metaphyses. In contrast, the humeral canal ends at the metaphysis. The isthmus of the femur is at the junction of the proximal and middle thirds, while the isthmus of the humerus is at the junction of the middle and distal thirds of the bone. The bone at the distal end of the medullary canals of the femur and the tibia is soft, metaphyseal bone, whereas the distal bone of the humeral canal is hard, diaphyseal bone. These anatomic differences highlight the need for newer design features and technologies for humeral nails that will differentiate them from tibial and femoral nails.

Besides anatomic differences, problems with classic antegrade (from the shoulder) nailing have limited its application. Shoulder pain following antegrade nailing may be unresolvable and has many similarities to anterior knee pain associated with tibial nailing. Nonunions associated with antegrade humeral nailing appear to be unique and more recalcitrant than those caused by other treatment methods (2). Furthermore, the humerus, unlike the tibia or femur, does not tolerate distraction at the fracture site. These formidable challenges with antegrade nailing are not resolved using standard approaches and available implant technology.

Humeral nailing is attractive because it is minimally invasive, can be done relatively quickly, and avoids the morbidity of extensive incisions. Because antegrade nailing has many potential complications, retrograde (from the elbow) nailing may be an attractive option for some patients. This chapter will review the techniques of both retrograde and antegrade nailing, detail possible complications, and provide a rationale for clinical application of these techniques.

Intramedullary nailing of the humerus can be performed either from the shoulder or the elbow. These two approaches enable the surgeon to nail diaphyseal fractures from the proximal fourth to the distal fourth of the humerus. The approach chosen should be based on Küntscher's principle of nailing from an insertion site as far from the fracture site as possible. Proximal shaft fractures should be nailed in a retrograde fashion; conversely, distal shaft fractures should be nailed in an antegrade fashion. Midshaft fractures may be approached from either end of the humerus. In adults, interlocking nailing is preferred over flexible nailing, which is occasionally used in pediatric fractures.

The surgeon should be familiar with both antegrade and retrograde approaches. The type of the fracture and its location, as well as overall condition of the patient, must be understood for selection of the correct approach and implant.

The indications for intramedullary nailing of the humerus are displaced transverse fractures of the diaphysis, segmental fractures, floating elbow injuries, pathologic fractures, fractures associated with thermal burns, and fractures in the polytrauma patient. A pathologic or impending pathological fracture may be the overall best indication for humeral nailing. Relative contraindications to intramedullary nailing include open fractures, fractures with associated radial-nerve palsy, long spiral fractures, open epiphyses, a narrow intramedullary canal, and prefracture deformity of the humeral shaft.

PREOPERATIVE PLANNING

Demographics, medical history, and information regarding the circumstances and mechanism of injury should be obtained. The arm should be carefully examined for neurovascular injuries. In general, intramedullary nailing should be avoided with open humeral fractures with or without obvious nerve palsy. Open humerus fractures are notorious for radial nerve interposition or laceration (3). Patients who are unable to cooperate with a neurological examination because of a head or spinal cord injury generally should undergo an open plating procedure with radial nerve exploration

Standard radiographs include anteroposterior (AP) and lateral views of the entire humerus. Because the arm should not be manually rotated through the fracture site in an attempt to obtain a lateral view, a transthoracic lateral is the preferred view. The diameter of the medullary canal size, canal length, and anterior deviation of the distal canal are measured on the lateral radiograph (4). Intramedullary canal sizes vary among patients, and therefore, these measurements provide an estimate for the dimensions of the nail. Measurements can be performed either manually or with a digital radiography system. The anterior deviation or distal humeral offset is visualized preoperatively to determine the relationship between the alignment of the humeral canal and the entry portal (Fig. 6.1) (4). With a small anterior deviation (distal humeral offset), the entry portal for retrograde nailing should be more distal and include the superior border of the olecranon fossa, which will require a longer bony defect. Conversely, if the anterior deviation (humeral offset) is large, the entry portal will need to be more proximal and will likely require a smaller length portal. The entry portal is usually 1.5 to 2.0 cm proximal to the olecranon fossa. Smaller canals require smaller nails and may be more susceptible to iatrogenic comminution. Multiplanar computed tomography (CT) can be helpful if there is any suspicion of fracture extension or a second fracture at a different level. Once adequate films are taken, the arm should be immobilized in a coaptation splint and sling (Fig. 6.2). The two most important preoperative decisions regard (a) whether a retrograde or an antegrade approach is indicated, and (b) if a retrograde approach is selected, the appropriate starting point as based on the patient's anatomy. The majority of displaced closed fractures can be surgically addressed in the first 10 days after injury.

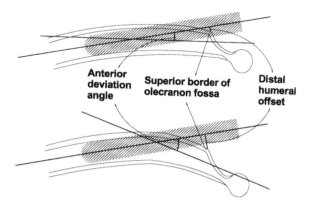

Figure 6.1. The anterior deviation or distal humeral offset must be appreciated to determine the linear relationship between the humeral canal and the distal, humeral, entry portal. The entry portal to the humeral canal can then be precisely placed in line with the humeral shaft. (From Lin J, Hou SM, Inoue N. Anatomic considerations of locked humeral nailing. *Clin Orthop Relat Res* 1999;368:247–254, with permission.)

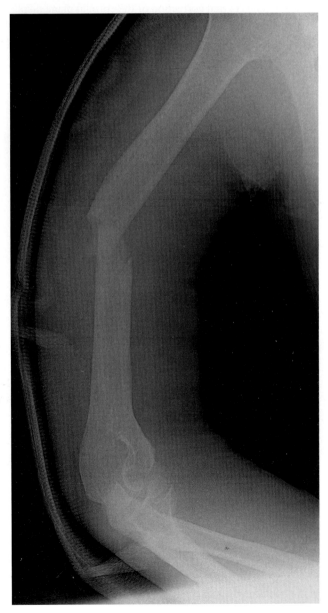

Figure 6.2. Preoperative radiograph of a diaphyseal fracture of the humerus.

Surgical Technique for Retrograde Interlocking Nailing

General endotracheal anesthesia is used, preoperative antibiotics are given, and the patient is positioned either in the lateral decubitus or prone position. We prefer the prone position (Fig. 6.3) and have found that an upper paint-roller type support is helpful in preventing traction injury to the brachial plexus, facilitating access to the olecranon fossa, and holding the arm in approximately 80 degrees of abduction. A 6-cm posterior incision, starting from the olecranon, is made in line with the humeral shaft (Fig. 6.4). The triceps tendon is split in line with its fibers and carried directly down to bone (Fig. 6.5). The olecranon fossa is identified and cleared of muscle with an elevator. The starting point for entry into the medullary canal must be individualized based on the anatomy of the distal humerus in the coronal plane and adjusted more proximally or distally, as previously described. The axis of the humerus is also in line with the lateral aspect of the olecranon fossa (Fig. 6.6). Using a drill guide, multiple, small, drill holes are made (Fig. 6.7) that outline the entry portal directly in line with the shaft of the humerus. These holes are then connected with a large drill bit and small rongeur to create an oval hole (Fig. 6.8). A router can also be used to enlarge the entry portal. Reduction of the fracture usually involves gentle traction on the distal humerus and correction of the coronal plane displacement (varus-valgus rotation). A ball-tip guide wire is inserted across the fracture site and confirmed fluoroscopically (Fig. 6.9A) and the canal is sequentially reamed up to an appropriate diameter, usually 1.0 to 1.5

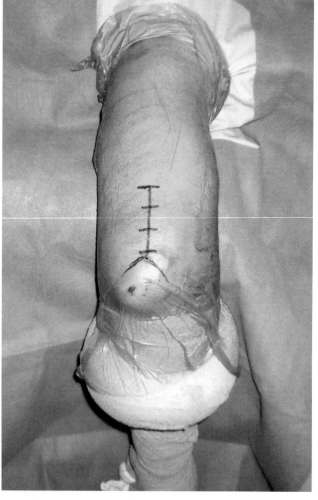

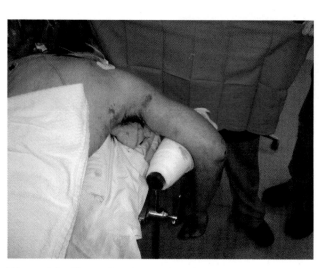

Figure 6.3. The patient is positioned in the prone position with the elbow flexed over the side of the table.

Figure 6.4. The skin incision is made for the entry portal from the tip of the olecranon to a point 6 cm proximal to the olecranon fossa.

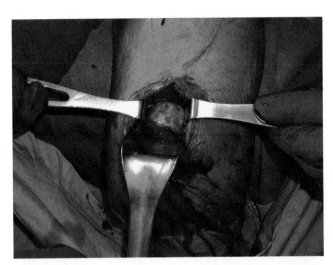

Figure 6.5. The exposure of the posterior humerus involves a triceps-splitting approach.

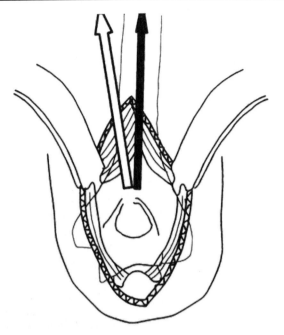

Figure 6.6. The axis of the humerus is usually in line with the lateral aspect of the olecranon fossa. This relationship should be used to place the entry portal in line with the humeral shaft. (From Lin J, Hou SM, Inoue N. Anatomic considerations of locked humeral nailing. *Clin Orthop Relat Res* 1999;368:247–254, with permission.)

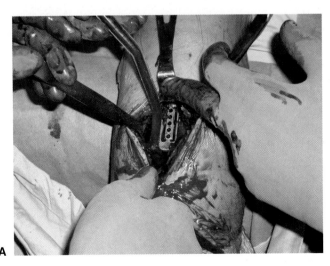

A

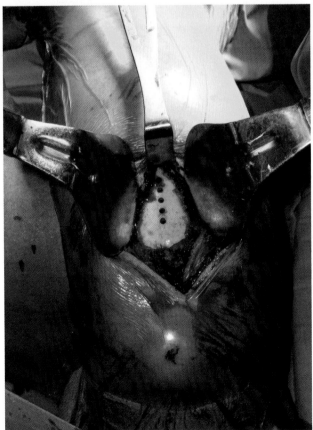

B

Figure 6.7. The entry portal is established using a **(A)** drill guide to drill **(B)** five collinear pilot holes.

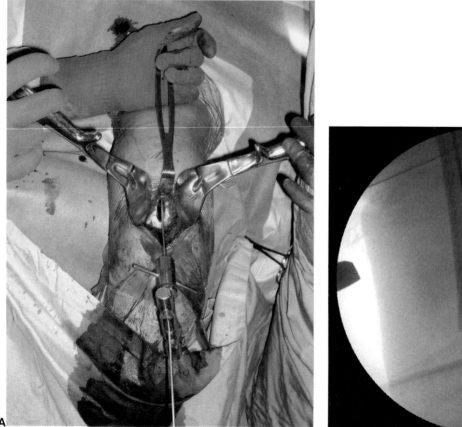

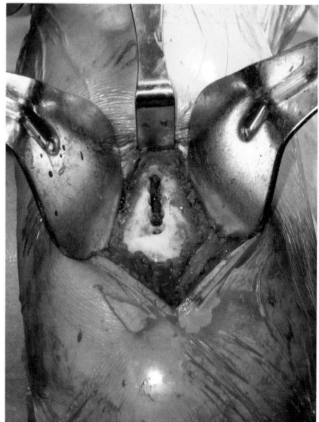

Figure 6.8. A. The collinear holes are enlarged and **(B)** connected using a large drill to establish a long, oval, entry portal.

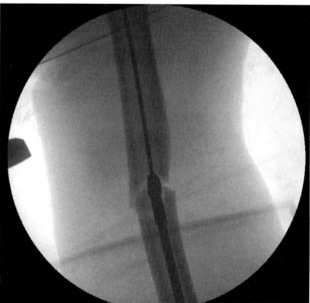

Figure 6.9. A. The guide wire is introduced by hand and **(B)** the fracture reduction is maintained while reaming.

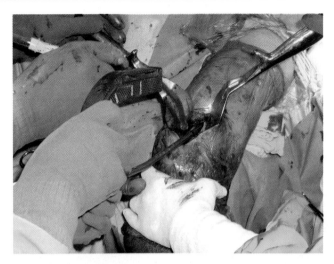

Figure 6.10. The nail is gently inserted by hand.

mm greater than the size of the nail (Fig. 6.9B). While reaming the canal, the surgeon must stay in line with the humeral shaft.

The nail is introduced gently by hand (Fig. 6.10). Forceful insertion may cause comminution of the fracture site or an iatrogenic supracondylar fracture. Distal locking is usually performed in a posterior-to-anterior direction (Fig. 6.11). After distal interlocking, the fracture should be compressed by gently tapping the insertion hand bolt with a mallet. Fracture distraction after nail insertion must be avoided. Proximal locking is performed from the posterior-to-anterior direction; a suture can be used as a safety line for retrieving a misplaced screw (Fig. 6.12). After the skin is incised over the screw hole, the soft tissues must be spread down to the bone with a hemostat to prevent injury to the axillary nerve. After radiographs are obtained in the operating room (Fig. 6.13), formal repair of the triceps tendon is performed and the skin is closed in a routine fashion.

An alternative to retrograde interlocked nailing is retrograde flexible nailing. This technique provides an option for exceptionally small intramedullary canals or resource-limited environments. This procedure may be performed from either a central portal above the olecranon fossa or through separate medial and lateral epicondylar portals. Multiple small-diameter nails are required to fill the canal. Postoperatively, fracture

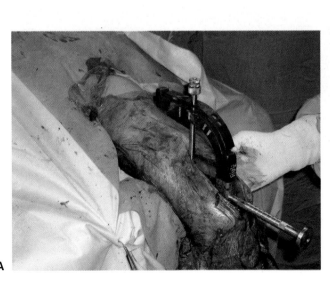

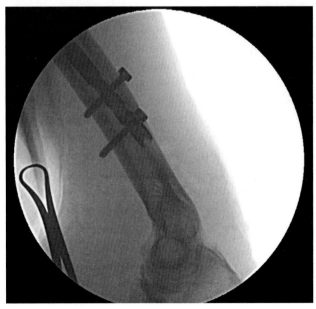

A   B

Figure 6.11. A. The nail is interlocked distally using the guide and **(B)** fluoroscopy.

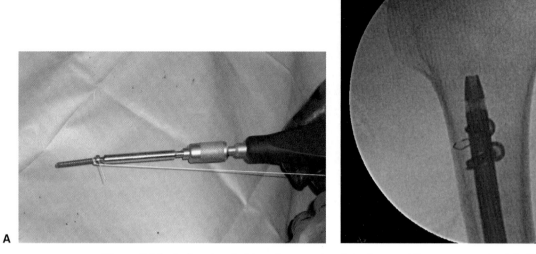

Figure 6.12. A. An absorbable suture can be placed around the screw as a safety line for **(B)** proximal interlocking.

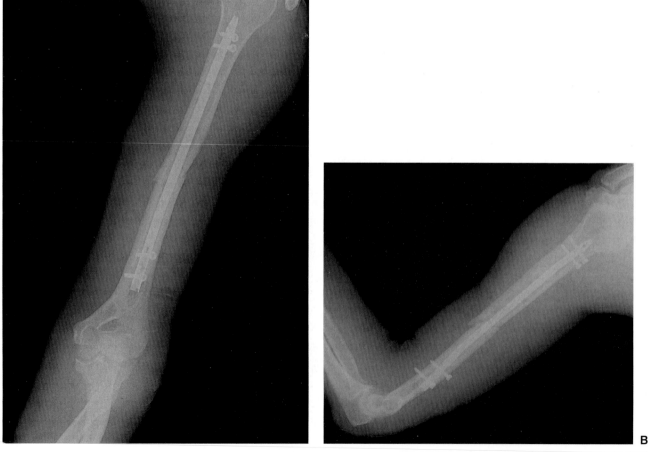

Figure 6.13. A. Postoperative AP and **(B)** lateral radiographs after retrograde nailing.

bracing is usually required to protect against rotational forces. A common complication with this procedure is flexible nail migration, which usually requires implant removal after fracture healing.

Surgical Technique for Antegrade Nailing

General endotracheal anesthesia is required with the endotracheal tube brought out toward the side opposite the humeral fracture. Preoperative antibiotics are given. Injury radiographs are available in the operating room (Fig. 6.14). The patient is positioned in a modified beach-chair position on a radiolucent operating table. A Mayfield headrest (Schaerer Mayfield USA, Inc., Cincinnati, OH) is invaluable because it facilitates the attainment of an intraoperative axillary view (Fig. 6.15). A small roll is placed between the scapulas, and the head is rotated toward the contralateral shoulder. The operative extremity should be draped free for reduction and imaging. The base of the c-arm is positioned at the foot of the bed, parallel to the operating table. This allows for AP and lateral imaging. Prior to prepping and draping, multiple fluoroscopic views should be obtained to confirm adequate visualization of the starting point as well as the fracture. The skin should be prepped sterilely from the hand to include the shoulder, chest, and neck.

The surface anatomy is palpated and outlined. The humeral head diameter is palpated from anterior to posterior to locate the midline. A 3-cm longitudinal incision is made from the edge of the acromion and carried distally (Figs. 6.16 and 6.17). The deltoid muscle is split in line with its fibers. The subacromial bursa is cleared bluntly with finger dissection. An incision is made in line with the fibers of the supraspinatus tendon, and the tendon edges are retracted. The correct starting point is critical. A curved awl is used to initiate the starting point just medial to the greater tuberosity and posterior to the bicipital tuberosity (see Fig. 6.17A). Adduction of the arm and extension of the shoulder will improve

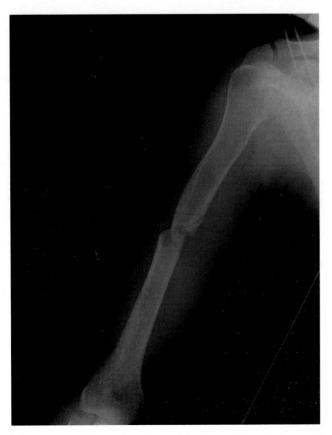

Figure 6.14. Preoperative AP radiograph before antegrade humeral nailing.

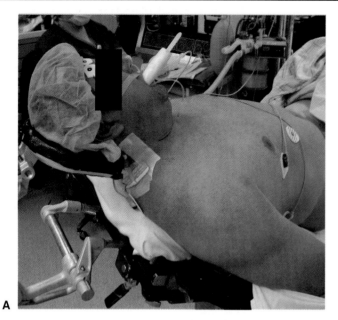

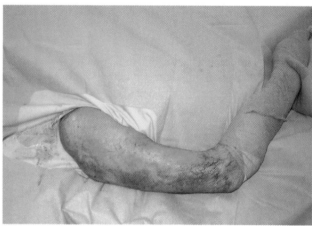

A   B

Figure 6.15. A. The patient is positioned supine eccentrically on the operating table, in a modified beach-chair position, with a Mayfield Headrest System table extension. **B.** The arm is draped free.

clearance of the acromion and facilitate awl access to the correct portal location. The awl is advanced into the intramedullary canal. Satisfactory position of the awl is confirmed fluoroscopically (see Fig. 6.17B).

Reduction of the fracture is usually achieved by a combination of adduction (arm against chest), neutral forearm rotation (forearm straight up toward ceiling), and traction. An assistant is necessary to maintain this reduction during reaming and nail insertion. A fracture gap should be avoided when nailing due to the potential of iatrogenic injury to the radial nerve. A ball-tipped guide wire, visualized via fluoroscopy, is inserted and passed down the medullary canal (Fig. 6.18). A small bend placed in the end of the guide wire allows for directional changes as the wire is advanced across the fracture site. Reaming is performed in 0.5-mm increments until 1.5 mm of cortical chatter is achieved. The nail is securely attached to the alignment and driving guide. An exchange tube may be used to replace the ball-tipped guide wire for a smaller, smooth wire with some nailing systems (Fig. 6.19). For solid nails, the reduction is

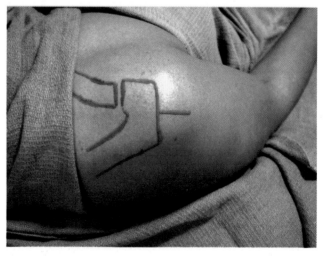

Figure 6.16. The skin incision is marked over the lateral aspect of the shoulder.

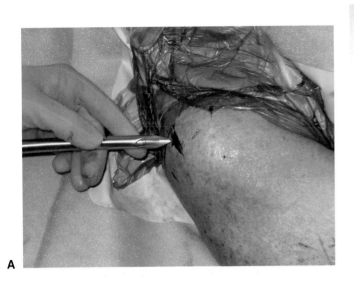

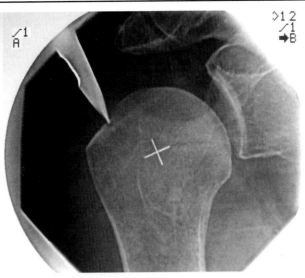

A   **B**

Figure 6.17. A. The entry site to the intramedullary canal is made with the cannulated awl. **B.** The entry site is verified fluoroscopically.

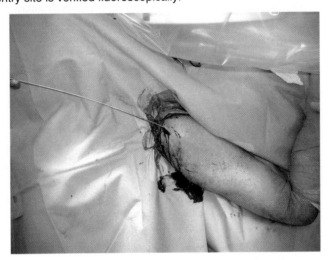

Figure 6.18. The guide wire is passed.

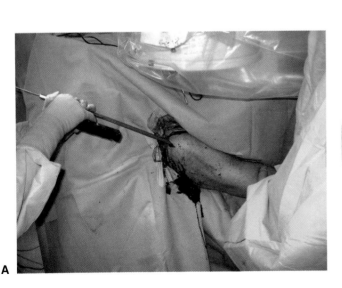

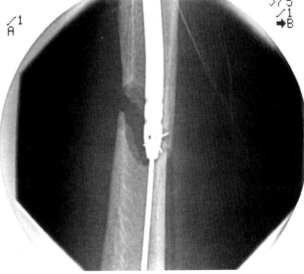

A   **B**

Figure 6.19. A. The nail is gently introduced by hand and **(B)** brought across under fluoroscopic control.

held firmly, the guide wire is removed, and the nail is carefully inserted by hand. The length of the nail should be carefully chosen. If measurements of the nail, made by the guide wire, show that the nails are in-between standard sizes, then the shorter size should be selected. The nail can bind in the distal canal and make countersinking difficult. The nail is driven below the cortical surface of the humeral head to prevent subacromial impingement and rotator cuff irritation. Multiple fluoroscopic images of the arm in various positions must be obtained to confirm that the nail is below the horizon of the humeral head and adequately countersunk. Fracture distraction after nail insertion should be avoided. The fracture can be compressed after proximal interlocking by tapping the insertion bolt with the mallet.

Drill guides are placed through the alignment guide to mark the skin for small stab incisions used to insert the proximal interlocking screws. The soft tissues are gently spread down to bone using a hemostat to ensure a safe screw path. The drill sleeve and trocar are inserted through the guide (Fig. 6.20) and advanced to bone with gentle taps from a mallet. Interlocking screws of the appropriate length are inserted after drilling and measuring. Oblique screws that course proximal-lateral to distal-medial are preferred because the insertion point is cephalad to the axillary nerve. Nonetheless, lateral screws that are very proximal can cause impingement when the arm is fully elevated.

Rotational alignment must be confirmed before static distal interlocking is performed. A freehand technique is used to target the distal interlocking screws. Distal interlocking screws inserted from an anterior-to-posterior direction are preferred because they avoid the radial nerve, which is more lateral. However, the surgeon must work only in the middle of the distal humerus in the coronal plane to avoid the brachial artery and vein. Adequate fluoroscopic images (perfect circles) of the distal, interlocking, screw holes are critical. Under fluoroscopy, a scalpel is placed over the skin to locate precisely the incision (Fig. 6.21A). An incision is made and a blunt hemostat is used to spread the brachialis muscle down to the bone. A short drill bit is useful to assist imaging under the c-arm, and based on an orthogonal view, the drill bit is centered in the locking hole. The drill bit is positioned perpendicular to the nail and the near cortex is drilled (Fig. 6.21B). The drill bit is detached from the drill and advanced through the nail up to the far cortex with gentle taps from a mallet, and satisfactory position of the drill bit is verified (Fig. 6.21C). The drill is then reattached to the drill bit and the far cortex is drilled. The bone at this level is fairly dense. The distal screws are usually 24 mm long. When placing these screws through a thick soft-tissue envelope, the surgeon should tie an absorbable suture to the screw so that if the screw becomes dislodged from the screwdriver it will not be displaced in the soft tissues. Final AP and lateral radiographs (Fig. 6.22) are taken in the operating room.

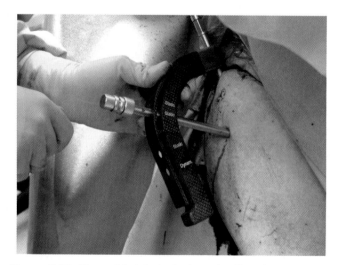

Figure 6.20. The nail is interlocked proximally using the guide.

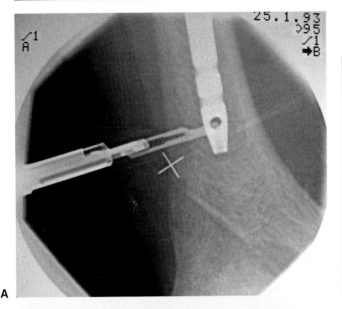

A

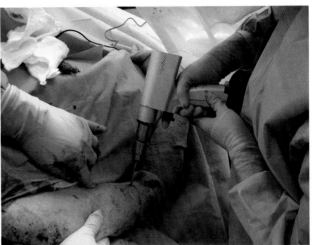

B

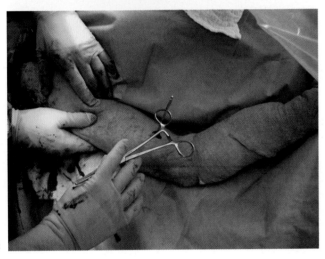

C

Figure 6.21. A. Distal interlocking is performed after the incisions are precisely placed under fluoroscopic control. **B.** A freehand technique is used, and **(C)** the position of the unchucked drill bit in the screw hole is verified.

A formal side-to-side rotator cuff repair is performed using nonabsorbable sutures. The deltoid raphe is also repaired. The skin and subcutaneous tissues are closed in a routine fashion.

POSTOPERATIVE MANAGEMENT

The arm is placed in a sling or shoulder immobilizer at the end of surgery. The postoperative dressing is removed after 2 days and gentle shoulder pendulum and elbow range-of-motion exercises are initiated. Postoperative rehabilitation is tailored to the method of nailing, fracture stability, and overall patient health. After antegrade nailing, patients commonly have shoulder symptoms; whereas after retrograde nailing, patients often have elbow symptoms. Patients are seen at 2 weeks for suture removal, with subsequent follow-up at 4- to 6-week intervals.

For retrograde nailing, initial elbow range of motion is limited to gentle passive motion by the patient. A sling is routinely used for the first 4 to 6 weeks after surgery. Formal physical therapy is not necessary, but the range-of-motion and shoulder pendulum exercises are required to prevent stiffness and loss of elbow extension. Large rotational stresses to the arm are avoided until radiographic evidence shows healing. Nail removal after healing is usually not required. However, if implant or soft-tissue irritation develops, the nail may be removed.

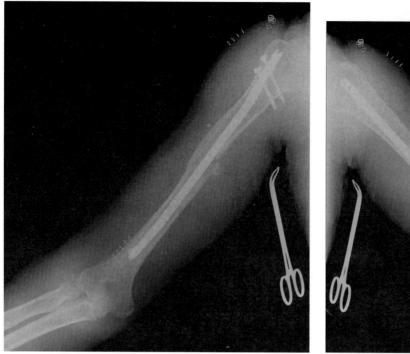
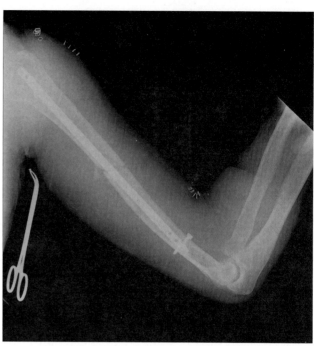

A   B

Figure 6.22. **A.** Final AP and **(B)** lateral radiographs after antegrade nailing.

COMPLICATIONS

Humeral nonunions associated with intramedullary nailing appear to be unique and more recalcitrant than humeral nonunions caused by other treatment methods. It is logical to assume that nonunion rates are similar for antegrade and retrograde nailing. However, in 2005, Court-Brown (5) reported nonunion rates of 11.6% for antegrade nailing and 4.5% rates for retrograde locked nailing. Nonunions after humeral nailing require nail removal followed by plate osteosynthesis with bone grafting. Unlike long bone nonunions in the femur or tibia, which respond well to exchange nailing, humeral diaphyseal nonunions rarely heal following renailing (2). When nails loosen or fatigue in conjunction with a nonunion, bone loss and cortical erosion are significant and complicate subsequent internal fixation. Most nonunions require exposure of the fracture site through an open approach, followed by debridement of the fracture site, osteosynthesis, and insertion of a bone graft.

Infection is rare after nailing, occurring in approximately 1% to 2% of cases. Infected humeral nails can be treated in a similar fashion to infected nails of the tibia and femur. Antibiotic-impregnated cement nails can be made with cement, powdered antibiotics, a chest tube, and an Ender nail. The cement is mixed with the antibiotics and injected into a small diameter (20–22 French) chest tube (approximately 6.7 to 7.3 mm), which is used as a mold. An Ender nail of appropriate length is then inserted in the middle of the cement. The eyelet of the Ender nail is left out of the end of the nail to allow for future removal of the antibiotic nail. After the cement hardens, the chest tube is incised in two areas over the length of the nail. The chest tube is then peeled off like a banana peel. These antibiotic nails can provide mechanical stability while delivering high local concentrations of antibiotics. To our knowledge, septic shoulders or septic elbows as a result of infected humeral nails have not been reported. Insertion site problems are the most common complication after intramedullary nailing.

Antegrade intramedullary nailing is associated with shoulder pain and loss of motion. If the nail is proud, subacromial impingement and rotator cuff irritation are universal. Even when the nail is buried beneath the cortical surface, shoulder pain can be a problem. Meticulous repair of the rotator cuff after nail insertion may decrease shoulder pain.

Iatrogenic fractures at the insertion site can also occur with antegrade nailing and occurs in 5.1% of cases (5).

Retrograde humeral nailing is associated with elbow pain and loss of elbow extension. Elbow pain appears to be caused by triceps tendon irritation or posterior elbow impingement. Iatrogenic comminution of the fracture site and/or supracondylar fracture at the insertion site reportedly occurred in 7.1% of retrograde nailing cases (5). These problems are not always of clinical significance.

Farragos et al (1) divided potential injury from humeral nailing to neurovascular structures into three areas: (a) risk to the radial nerve in the spiral groove from canal preparation and nail insertion; (b) risk to the axillary nerve from proximal interlocking; and (c) risk to the radial musculocutaneous and medial nerves, as well as brachial artery from distal interlocking. The potential for nerve injury in the spiral groove can be decreased by avoiding gap reductions and reaming in areas of comminution. The main trunk of the axillary nerve has been previously reported to be at risk with proximal screws placed in an anterior-to-posterior direction (6). In retrograde nailing, the axillary nerve is also at risk with proximal interlocking in a posterior-to-anterior direction. The axillary vessels are not at risk unless the drill penetrates several centimeters past the medial cortex (6). If a patient loses radial nerve function after humeral nailing, some surgeons advocate return to the operating room for exploration of the radial nerve. As an alternative, many surgeons favor observation for 3 to 4 months because many nerve palsies recover spontaneously.

Smaller axillary-nerve branches located 5 to 6 cm distal to the acromion at the lateral aspect of the humerus, where the axillary nerve arborizes, may also be injured from lateral-to-medial directed screws. Distal interlocking from a lateral-to-medial direction places the radial nerve at risk, while anterior-to-posterior or posterior-to-anterior interlocking places the medial and musculocutaneous nerves (especially the lateral antebrachial-cutaneous nerve) and brachial artery at risk. As a general rule, soft tissues should be spread down to the bone with a hemostat prior to drilling holes for any interlocking screws.

Iatrogenic comminution and distraction at the fracture site are also potential complications after intramedullary nailing of the humerus. The risk of fracture site distraction appears to be greater with antegrade nailing than with retrograde nailing. Comminution of the fracture after reaming is usually related to extension and propagation of radiographically occult secondary-fracture lines. Smaller humeral canals and larger diameter nails appear to increase the risk of iatrogenic comminution from nailing.

RECOMMENDED READINGS

1. Farragos AF, Schemitsch EH, McKee MD. Complications of intramedullary nailing for fractures of the humeral shaft: a review. *J Orthop Trauma* 1999;13(4):258–267.
2. McKee MD, Miranda MA, Riemer BL, et al. Management of humeral nonunion after the failure of locking intramedullary nails. *J Orthop Trauma* 1996;10(7):492–499.
3. Foster RJ, Swiontkowski MF, Bach AW, et al. Radial nerve palsy caused by open humeral shaft fractures. *J Hand Surg* 1993;18(1):121–124.
4. Lin J, Hou SM, Inoue N, et al. Anatomic considerations of locked humeral nailing. *Clin Orthop Relat Res* 1999;368:247–254.
5. Court-Brown C. Paper presented at: Orthopaedic Trauma Association Specialty Day Meeting; February 26, 2005; Washington, DC.
6. Riemer BL, D'Ambrosia R. The risk of injury to the axillary nerve, artery, and vein from proximal locking screws of humeral intramedullary nails. *Orthopedics* 1992;15(6):697–699.

7

Distal Humerus Intra-articular Fractures: Open Reduction Internal Fixation

Gary L. Zohman

INDICATIONS/CONTRAINDICATIONS

Intra-articular fractures of the distal humerus are uncommon injuries. Despite improved surgical techniques and implants, operative management does not guarantee an excellent clinical result. Indications for surgery include all displaced fractures in adults who are medically stable for surgery. Nonoperative management of displaced intra-articular fractures of the distal humerus are associated with unacceptably high rates of malunion, nonunion, and elbow joint stiffness, often leading to loss of independence and subsequent disability. The goal of surgery are identical to those of all intra-articular fractures: stable fixation to allow early joint motion in an anatomical position with healing of the fracture.

While early articular reconstruction is the treatment of choice for most fractures, some injuries in the osteoporotic elderly are probably best treated with primary elbow arthroplasty. Contraindications to surgery include selected grade-IIIB open fractures, active infection, extreme comminution such as found in gunshot wounds, lack of equipment, and surgeon inexperience.

PREOPERATIVE PLANNING

A thorough and meticulous examination of the upper extremity is performed. A detailed neurovascular examination as well as the status of the patient's compartments are documented. In multiply injured patients, evaluation of the head, chest, abdomen, and spine are essential. In many patients, concomitant injuries take precedence over the distal humeral fracture(s).

Initial radiographs of the elbow and distal humerus invariably show the fracture. However, a complete understanding of the fracture is difficult secondary to collapse of elbow anatomy caused by fracture displacement. In many cases, adequate radiographs may only be obtainable while patient is in traction and under intravenous sedation or anesthesia. Computed tomography (CT) is occasionally performed preoperatively. CT may reveal associated injuries of the radial head or neck that will alter the surgical plan. Coronal plane fractures of the anterior portion of the articular surface of the distal humerus are also identifiable by CT. As with plain radiographs, CT scans are most helpful when major fracture displacement has been corrected and the arm splinted. With the exception of open fractures, the vast majority of intra-articular fractures of the distal humerus are done semi-urgently.

The AO/ASIF has shown that with complex peri-articular fractures, results can be improved with the creation of a surgical plan. This involves a written step-by-step surgical tactic outlining each step of the operation, including the placement of screws, plates, bone grafts, and so forth. The creation of a preoperative plan ensures that needed implants can be ordered and will be available. In addition, when a preoperative plan is utilized, surgery and tourniquet times can be reduced and the need for bone graft clarified.

Available implants for internal fixation should include small diameter screws (1.5 through 2.4 mm) for comminuted peri-articular fragments as well as 3.5-mm compression and reconstruction plates and screws. Peri-articular and/or locking plates can be extremely useful. In some patients, 3.5-mm screws directed from medial to lateral in the supra-articular region will exceed the 50-mm maximum length available in the standard, small fragment instrument tray. Therefore, supplemental screw lengths should be readily available along with an accompanying extra-long 2.5-mm drill bit.

Two, large, pointed, reduction tenacula are invaluable in the articular reconstruction. A medium, serrated, reduction clamp is helpful during medial plate application. In patients with extensive comminution, the iliac crest should be prepped and draped or bank bone graft should be available.

SURGERY

Surgery is usually performed under general anesthesia, although regional anesthesia is occasionally employed. Prophylactic intravenous antibiotics are given before the procedure. Surgery can be done with the patient in the lateral or prone position. I prefer the lateral decubitus position. The arm is supported over a padded small-diameter post that will allow intraoperative flexion of the elbow to 110 degrees (Fig. 7.1). The entire upper extremity, flank, and iliac crest are prepped in the same field through the utilization of pairs of U-shaped split drapes. The arm is exsanguinated and a sterile tourniquet applied.

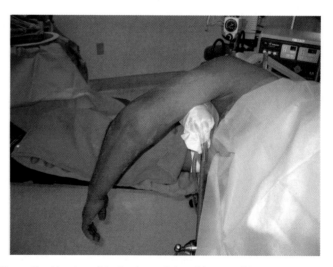

Figure 7.1. The patient is placed in the lateral decubitus position with the arm draped over a padded roll; this position allows for intraoperative flexion of the ulna to 110 degrees.

The tourniquet is later removed after the articular reconstruction is complete. A c-arm image intensifier must be available so fracture reduction and screw placement can be assessed.

A posterior longitudinal incision is made beginning at the midpoint of the arm and extending over the dorsal surface of the ulna onto the proximal forearm. The incision is placed slightly medial or lateral to the tip of the olecranon (Fig. 7.2.). The ulnar nerve is identified and followed proximally to where it emerges from the medial intermuscular septum and distally to where it enters the flexor carpi ulnaris. The nerve is protected with a moistened Penrose drain (Fig. 7.3).

Exposure of the articular fracture fragments is done with either a formal olecranon osteotomy or a triceps slide. For most patients, I prefer a modified Morrey triceps-splitting approach; the split is extended longitudinally down the fascial sleeve of the proximal

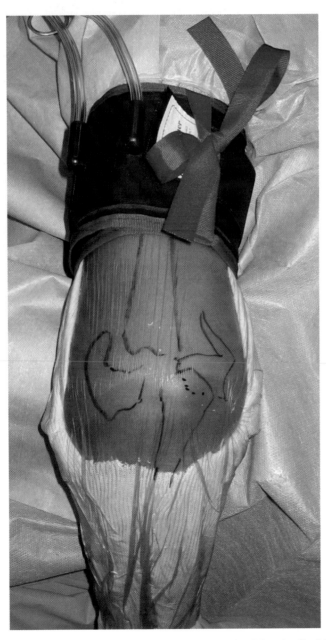

Figure 7.2. The anatomy is marked with ink pen on the skin. A longitudinal incision is made slightly lateral to the tip of the olecranon.

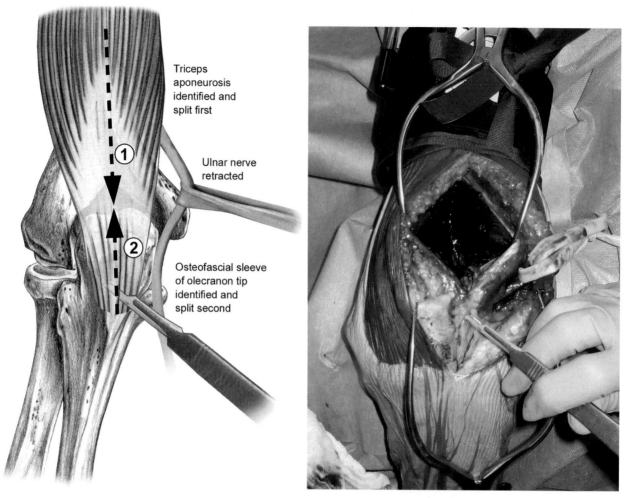

Triceps
aponeurosis
identified and
split first

Ulnar nerve
retracted

Osteofascial sleeve
of olecranon tip
identified and
split second

Figure 7.3. The ulnar nerve is protected with a Penrose drain. The split in the triceps tendon is connected to the split in the forearm fascia by sharp elevation of the olecranon medially and laterally.

forearm. This approach provides excellent access to the distal humerus and decreases some of the complications associated with an olecranon osteotomy. The extended triceps-splitting approach may be desirable when there is transverse disruption of the extensor mechanism (which often occurs in open fractures) and the distal humeral-shaft-fracture fragment protrudes posteriorly through the triceps tendon.

The triceps-tendon split is begun just proximal to the olecranon fossa and is carried down to the bone. The split is extended through the posterior fat pad of the elbow joint down to the tip of the olecranon. To expose the humeral shaft, the triceps muscle mass is split proximally using medial and lateral countertraction and a vertically oriented, sharp, half-inch periosteal elevator. Proximal extension is dictated by the extent of the fracture into the diaphysis. If the distal humerus must be exposed through the lower diaphysis, the radial nerve must be identified and protected.

Tendinous attachments to the olecranon are temporarily left intact while attention is turned to the most distal portion of the incision. The interval between the flexor carpi ulnaris and extensor carpi ulnaris is split down to the ulnar shaft. Sharp subperiosteal dissection from distal to proximal exposes both sides of the ulna. The depth of dissection should be to the ulnohumeral joint line medially and to the proximal radioulnar joint laterally; the dissection should be maintained proximal to the annular ligament of the radius.

The dissection is completed by meticulously peeling away the dense tendinous attachments remaining at the tip of the olecranon with several, fresh, knife blades. This is most successfully performed by proceeding toward the olecranon both proximally and distally.

In this way, the entire extensor mechanism is opened longitudinally and is later repaired side to side (Fig. 7.4). Small rents in the extensor mechanism, exposing a portion of the olecranon, will not impede healing or eventual extensor function.

The cord of a laparotomy sponge (or Mersilene tape) is then passed around the trochlear notch of the ulna and is used to apply longitudinal distraction to the ulna (along the axis of the humeral shaft) as the forearm is flexed approximately 110 degrees. The entire articular surface of the distal humerus is now exposed and the fracture may be addressed (Fig. 7.5).

If an olecranon osteotomy is to be used, the periosteum over the proximal ulna is incised and elevated 15 mm distal to the olecranon tip. A shallow Chevron osteotomy is planned. A 2.0-mm Kirschner (K) wire is used to drill multiple holes along the plane of the planned osteotomy, which is completed with an osteotome. The olecranon and the entire triceps muscle can then be reflected proximally, exposing the entire posterior aspect of the distal humerus. At the conclusion of the case, the osteotomy is stabilized with a 6.5-mm screw or tension band wire technique.

Every effort is made to preserve the soft-tissue attachments to fracture fragments as they are cleansed of adherent clot using a dental pick and forceps. Fracture reconstruction then proceeds from distal to proximal. The articular fragments are pieced together and provisionally held with multiple K wires. A large, pointed, tenaculum clamp often facilitates reduction. Two screws are placed transversely from medial to lateral through the ulnar sulcus (Fig. 7.6). These screws are countersunk to avoid ulnar nerve irritation. Safe sites for screw entry are limited, and many surgeons prefer to use 4.0-mm cannulated screws.

If central articular comminution is present, compression may distort the trochlear fragments leading to ulnotrochlear incongruence. In this case, it is important to fix the trochlea

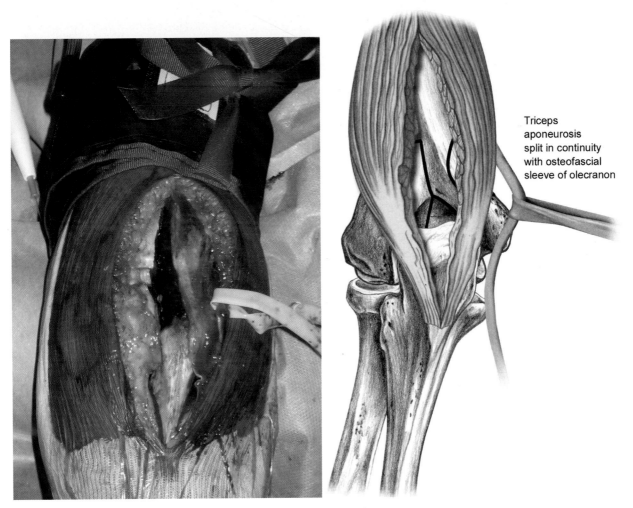

Triceps
aponeurosis
split in continuity
with osteofascial
sleeve of olecranon

Figure 7.4. The triceps-splitting approach is complete.

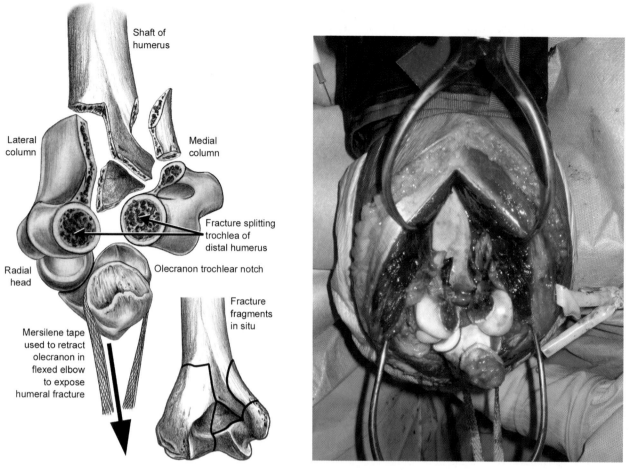

Shaft of humerus

Lateral column

Medial column

Fracture splitting trochlea of distal humerus

Radial head

Olecranon trochlear notch

Mersilene tape used to retract olecranon in flexed elbow to expose humeral fracture

Fracture fragments in situ

Figure 7.5. The fracture is exposed by flexing the ulna 110 degrees and applying longitudinal traction through the trochlear notch with the cord of a laparotomy sponge.

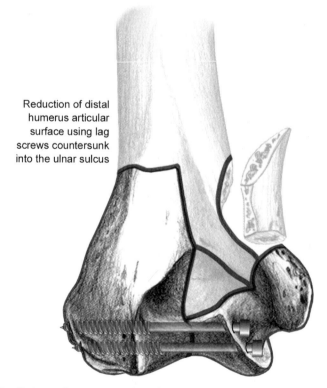

Reduction of distal humerus articular surface using lag screws countersunk into the ulnar sulcus

Figure 7.6. The first step in reconstruction: the articular surface is reduced and stabilized with lag screws countersunk medially into the ulnar sulcus.

at the appropriate width using interposition bone graft and fully threaded positioning screws rather than lag screws. In typical instances, at least one of the trochlear fracture fragments will also remain attached to its respective epicondyle. This side should be used to fasten the articular surface to its respective humeral column.

The tourniquet is now released and removed from the arm. The next step in the reconstruction is realigning and reattaching the articular surface to the distal humeral metaphysis. Plates on both the lateral and medial column are recommended. Plates are contoured to lie posterior on the lateral column and medial on the medial column. Whenever possible, compression plates are used at both sites to increase stability. However, a reconstruction plate placed medially is often necessary. Locking plates are advantageous especially on the lateral column where distal fixation is otherwise limited to short, unicortical, cancellous screws with conventional low-compression dynamic-compression (LCDC) plates.

K wires may be passed retrograde up the medial and lateral columns into the humeral shaft to reduce and stabilize the metadiaphyseal component of the injury. Often definitive reduction and compression to the shaft can only be performed after one of the plates has been applied distally.

The lateral plate requires a short curve only at the site of the two most distal holes. The proximal portion of the lateral plate is usually left straight. (Fig. 7.7) The lateral plate is placed as distal as possible to the edge of the capitulum without impinging on the radial head when the elbow is fully extended. Placing the lateral plate posteriorly provides a stable construct and avoids the additional soft-tissue stripping required to place the plate on the lateral aspect of the distal humerus. In severely comminuted or osteoporotic fractures, however, the addition of a third plate along the lateral aspect of the lateral column may improve stability.

The medial plate requires a relatively large curvature radius over most of the plate. The distal tip of the plate will lie superior to the most prominent portion of the medial epicondyle. Stable fixation can be compromised if the medial epicondyle is separated from the articular fragments by fracture. In this case, specially designed, anatomically congruent plates that curve around the medial epicondyle may have an advantage over standard or

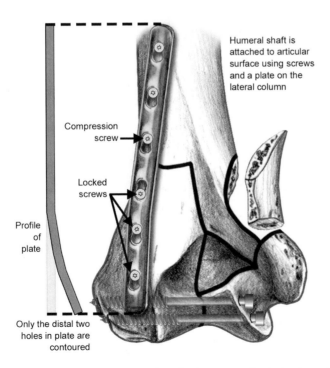

Figure 7.7. The second step in reconstruction: the less comminuted column (in this case, lateral) is used to attach the articular surface to the shaft. Only the distal two holes in the lateral plate should be contoured; the proximal portion should be straight.

reconstruction compression plates. It is very difficult to contour a compression plate around the medial epicondyle and is not recommended.

In cases where the fracture line lies below the medial epicondyle, an alternative fixation construct may be used. Purchase in the small distal fragment may be improved via a contoured 3.5-mm reconstruction plate that curves around the posterior aspect of the medial column occupying the ulnar sulcus. If the curve in the plate is sufficient, the two distal screws may be inserted orthogonally to each other and can interlock within the bone.

When permitted by the fracture pattern, stability is increased by fixing the reconstructed articular surface to the shaft under compression. This can be performed by using the offset drill guide in the oblique holes of the compression plate. In another alternative, a unicortical push-pull screw may be inserted temporarily proximal to the plate. A Verbrugge clamp is then used to pull the plate toward the screw, achieving considerable compressive stability (Fig. 7.8).

During fixation, attempts are made to place as many screws as possible through plates and into the distal fragments. In ideal situations, screws placed from medial to lateral through the medial plate are anchored into a fragment on the lateral side that is fixed by the lateral plate. To maximize distal screw length, two screws are passed through the medial plate straddling the olecranon fossa (Fig. 7.9).

An extra-long, calibrated, 2.5-mm drill bit is helpful during placement of hardware from the medial to lateral direction. The extra length facilitates protection of the bulky soft-tissue envelope traversed by the drill. Calibrations on the drill bit and self-tapping screws may eliminate the need to measure and tap.

The number of screws used for proximal fixation in each plate should roughly equal the number of screws achieved distally for a balanced fixation construct. The elbow joint is reduced and taken through a normal range of motion while the fixation is observed.

A suction drain is placed in the wound and brought out through the proximal triceps split. The extensor mechanism is repaired with resorbable suture, and the ulnar nerve is allowed to resume its normal anatomic position (Fig. 7.10). If the demands of fixation require screw heads or tips protruding into the ulnar sulcus beneath the medial epicondyle, then an anterior subcutaneous transposition of the ulnar nerve is performed.

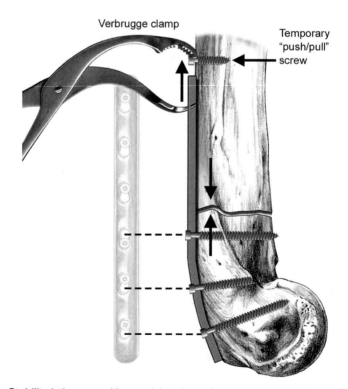

Figure 7.8. Stability is increased by applying the columnar plates under compression. Laterally, a Verbrugge clamp and push-pull screw may be used.

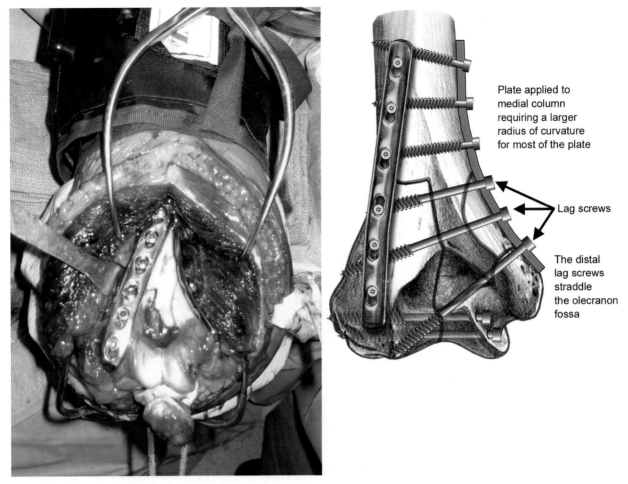

Plate applied to
medial column
requiring a larger
radius of curvature
for most of the plate

Lag screws

The distal
lag screws
straddle
the olecranon
fossa

Figure 7.9. The final step in reconstruction: a medially applied medial column plate.

Fluoroscopic images or plain radiographs are performed in the operating room. The arm is immobilized in a plaster splint with the elbow flexed 90 degrees and supinated.

POSTOPERATIVE MANAGEMENT

Prophylactic intravenous antibiotics are continued for 24 hours. The suction drain is removed the day following surgery, and the patient is encouraged to begin active finger exercises. The splint is removed on the third postoperative day, and the wound is recovered with sterile dressings and a padded elbow sleeve. A sling is used for comfort and is removed at least three times daily so the patient can begin active and assisted range of motion in the elbow. Skin sutures are removed in 7 to 10 postoperative days, and formal physical therapy may begin.

Therapy is aimed chiefly at regaining range of motion. Resistive strengthening is avoided until the fracture has healed and functional range of motion has been achieved, typically at 12 weeks. Dynamic splinting is sometimes helpful in regaining terminal extension of the elbow. Postoperative radiographs are checked at 3, 6, 12, and 24 weeks after surgery.

COMPLICATIONS

Early failure of internal fixation will be accompanied by pain and inability to mobilize the patient. Late failure of fixation may be associated with delayed union or nonunion. The

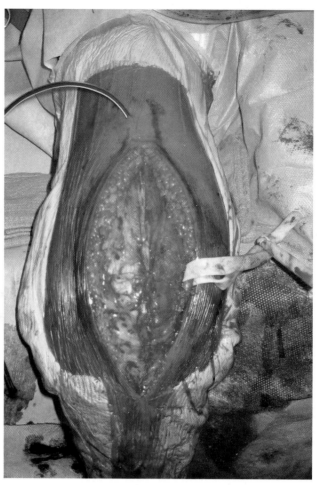

Figure 7.10. The triceps split has been repaired in continuity with the forearm fascial sleeve. A suction drain is in place.

use of compression plates rather than reconstruction plates may enhance the longevity of the fixation construct and reduce the risk of fixation failure.

Iatrogenic complications associated with olecranon osteotomy, such as nonunion, may be reduced by using the extended triceps-splitting exposure described.

Infection can prove to be catastrophic. If suspected, extensive wound debridement, lavage, and intravenous antibiotics are required. Stable internal fixation should be retained if possible until union occurs. If the infection cannot be eradicated in the presence of the hardware, then after the fracture heals, the implants may need to be removed.

RECOMMENDED READING

Helfet DL, Kloen P, Anand N, et al. ORIF of delayed unions and nonunions of distal humeral fractures: surgical technique. *J Bone Joint Surg Am* March 2004;86:18–29.

Jupiter JB, Morrey BF. Fractures of the distal humerus in the adult. In: Morrey BF, ed. *The elbow and its disorders.* Philadelphia: W.B. Saunders; 1993:328–366.

Korner J, Diederichs G, Arzdorf M, et al. A biomechanical evaluation of methods of distal humerus fracture fixation using locking compression plates versus conventional reconstruction plates. *J Orthop Trauma* May-June 2004;18:286–293.

Morrey BF, ed. *The elbow and its disorders.* Philadelphia: W.B. Saunders; 1993:139–166.

O'Driscoll SW, Sanchez-Sotelo J, Torchia ME. Management of the smashed distal humerus. *Orthop Clin North Am* January 2002;33:19–33.

Ring D, Gulotta L, Chin K, et al. Olecranon osteotomy for exposure of fractures and nonunions of the distal humerus. *J Orthop Trauma* 2004;18:446–449.

8

Olecranon Fractures: Open Reduction Internal Fixation

Gregory J. Schmeling and Lawrence J. Maciolek

INDICATIONS/CONTRAINDICATIONS

Olecranon fractures are a result of direct or indirect forces, or a combination of both (1). Direct forces drive the olecranon into the distal humerus, often producing comminuted fractures with depressed joint fragments, similar to a tibial plateau fracture. Olecranon fractures, which occur indirectly through the contraction of the triceps muscle, generally produce transverse or short oblique fracture patterns.

Minimally displaced olecranon fractures are defined as less than 2 mm of joint gap or step-off, intact, active-elbow extension, and no significant fragment motion with elbow flexion. Fractures are displaced if they do not meet these criteria (1).

The treatment objectives for olecranon fractures are reconstruction of the articular surface, restoration of the elbow extensor mechanism, preservation of elbow motion and function, and prevention or avoidance of complications (2). The indications for operative treatment include displaced fractures, injuries with elbow extensor-mechanism disruption, and open fractures. Indications for conservative treatment include nondisplaced fractures, injuries where the elbow extensor mechanism is intact, and poor overall medical condition of the patient.

Operative treatment options include open reduction and internal fixation (ORIF) and fragment excision with elbow extensor-mechanism reconstruction (2–4). For displaced fractures, the treatment goals are met most often with internal fixation techniques. These techniques consist primarily of tension band wiring or plate osteosynthesis.

Olecranon fractures usually occur as isolated injuries, but they are occasionally found in the polytrauma patient. With isolated fractures, a history of a fall with elbow pain is the most common presenting complaint. Physical examination reveals a painful, swollen elbow, and in displaced fractures, a palpable defect is often identified. Crepitus with elbow motion may also be present. The inability to extend the elbow against gravity suggests loss of the integrity of the elbow extensor mechanism. Neurovascular evaluation should include particular attention to the ulnar nerve. The proximity of the ulnar nerve places it at risk for injury, especially when direct forces are involved in the accident.

Essential radiographs include an anteroposterior (AP) view and a true lateral view. When the olecranon fracture is part of an elbow fracture dislocation, traction radiographs are used to evaluate the injury as well. The lateral radiograph reveals the extent of the fracture and the presence of comminution or joint depression. The integrity of the radial head–capitulum articulation is examined, and subluxation or dislocation of the semilunar notch from the trochlea is noted. The AP radiograph is examined for sagittal fracture lines that are not well visualized on the lateral view. Comparison radiographs can be helpful in complex fracture patterns.

PREOPERATIVE PLANNING

To optimize outcomes, a preoperative plan is drawn and a surgical tactic developed. The preoperative plan begins with a tracing of the fracture fragments. The fragments are then reduced on paper. The need for bone graft to support depressed intra-articular fragments is determined. The proposed fixation is added. The method of fixation chosen is dependent on the fracture geometry and the experience of the surgeon. The surgical tactic is a sequential outline of the planned procedure and is added to the drawing (Fig. 8.1).

Although there are many classification schemes for olecranon fractures, we prefer that of the Orthopaedic Trauma Association (5). The location of the fracture is in the proximal segment of the radius and ulna (6). The fractures are divided into three types: extra-articular (21-A), articular and involving the surface of one bone (21-B), and articular and involving the surface of both bones (21-C). Extra-articular avulsion fractures are type 21-A

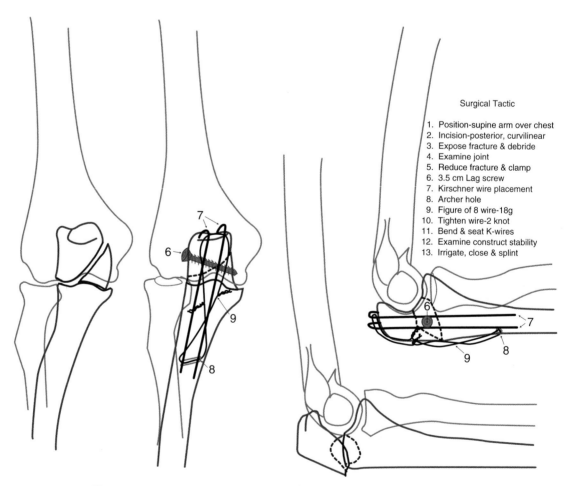

Surgical Tactic

1. Position-supine arm over chest
2. Incision-posterior, curvilinear
3. Expose fracture & debride
4. Examine joint
5. Reduce fracture & clamp
6. 3.5 cm Lag screw
7. Kirschner wire placement
8. Archer hole
9. Figure of 8 wire-18g
10. Tighten wire-2 knot
11. Bend & seat K-wires
12. Examine construct stability
13. Irrigate, close & splint

Figure 8.1. Preoperative plan. This is a tracing from the radiographs: ulna (blue); fixation (red); and humerus/radius (black).

while intra-articular fractures are type 21-B. A more detailed description of this classification is found in the Orthopaedic Trauma Association's *Fractures and Dislocation Compendium* (5).

It is easier to conceptualize olecranon fractures as transverse, oblique, comminuted, or elbow fracture dislocations (Fig. 8.2). Transverse and oblique fractures may have a depressed joint segment similar to that seen in tibial plateau fractures. Depressed segments are elevated and may require bone graft or other support to maintain elevation. Oblique fractures can be oriented proximally or distally. Lag screws are frequently used with oblique fractures. Comminuted fracture patterns usually occur in isolation, but the radiographs must be scrutinized to rule out a fracture dislocation of the elbow.

The two most common methods of fixation are either tension band wiring or plate osteosynthesis with or without a lag screw (3,6,7–26). A tension band construct may consist of two Kirschner (K) wires with a figure-of-eight wire or cable, or it may be made of an intramedullary screw with a figure-of-eight wire. Alternatively, a lag screw and dorsal plate (3.5-mm semitubular or reconstruction) can be used (Fig. 8.3A–C). The cable is easier to place and has a low-profile crimp rather than two prominent wire knots. A figure-of-eight wire alone does not provide sufficient stability to resist physiologic loading (21). Advocates of the lag screw–dorsal plate technique cite less operative time, better reductions, fewer

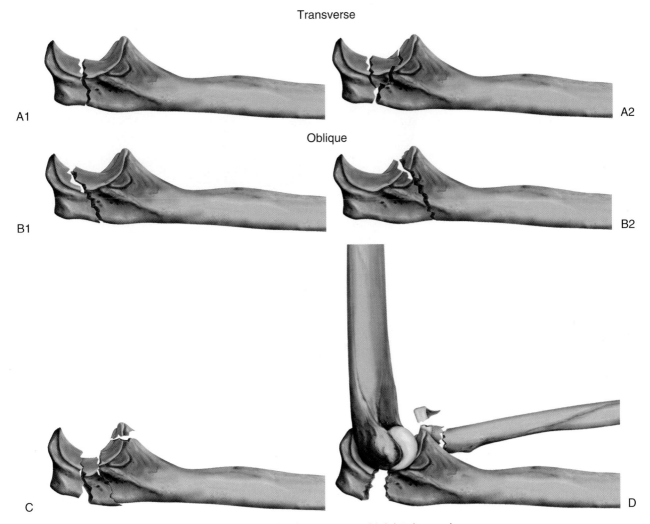

Transverse

A1   A2

Oblique

B1   B2

C   D

Figure 8.2. Olecranon fractures: **(A1)** transverse, **(A2)** transverse with joint depression, **(B1)** proximal oblique, **(B2)** distal oblique, **(C)** comminuted, **(D)** fracture-dislocation. (From McKee MD, Jupiter JB. Trauma to the adult elbow and fractures of the distal humerus. In: Browner BD, Jupiter JB, Levine AM, et al, eds. *Skeletal trauma.* Philadelphia: W.B. Saunders; 1992:1455–1522; Fig. 41-16.)

hardware symptoms, less postoperative loss of reduction, and lower incidence of infection (7,10,20,26). The lag screw–neutralization plate construct consists of a lag screw across the fracture and a radial, ulnar, or dorsal neutralization plate. Two K wires with a figure-of-eight wire will also neutralize the lag screw (Fig. 8.3D).

Based on the injury pattern, patient profile, and clinical experience, the surgeon must determine which fixation technique to employ for a given fracture. In the absence of complications, outcomes for each of the fixation techniques are comparable (12,21). However, biomechanical and clinical evidence suggests that certain techniques may be advantageous when applied to specific fracture patterns.

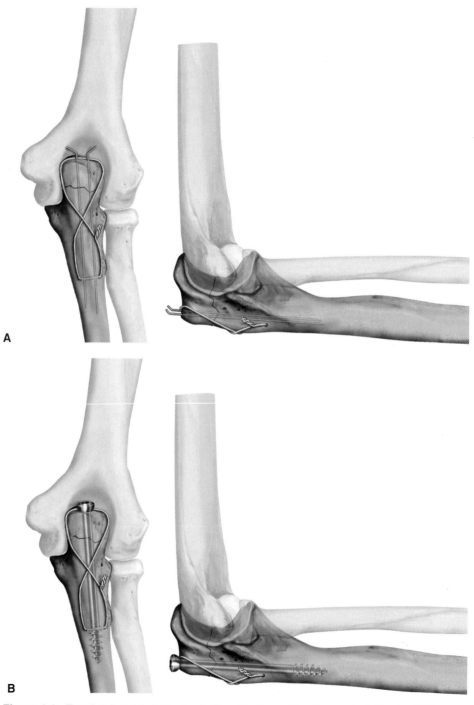

Figure 8.3. Tension-band constructs. **A.** Two K wires with a figure-of-eight wire (33). **B.** Medullary screw with a figure-of-eight wire (33). (*continues*)

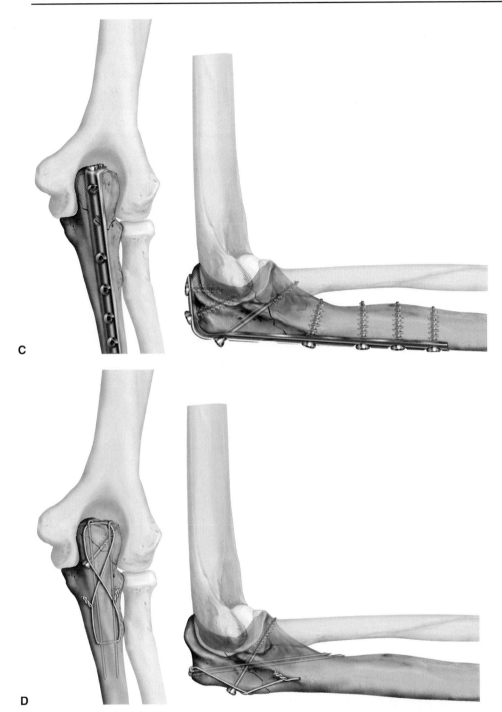

C

D

Figure 8.3. (*continued*) **C.** Dorsal plate with lag screw. **D.** Two K wires that engage the anterior cortex plus lag screw. (**A** and **B** from Macko D, Szabo RM. Complications of tension-band wiring of olecranon fractures. *J Bone Joint Surg* 1985;67A: 1396–1401; **C** and **D** from Helm U. Forearm and hand/mini-implants. In: Muller ME, Allgower M, Schneider R, et al, eds. *Manual of internal fixation.* Berlin: Springer-Verlag; 1991: 453–484, Fig. 8.6.)

Tension band wiring techniques are the mainstay of treatment for transverse, noncomminuted, olecranon fractures, but they may also be used in some comminuted fracture patterns. In commonly used constructs, intramedullary K wires or an intramedullary screw, combined with either braided cable or monofilament wire, are used. In terms of biomechanics, tension band techniques are thought to convert the force generated by the elbow extensor mechanism into a dynamic compressive force along the articular surface of the semilunar notch during active elbow motion (7). Although the validity of this biomechanical principle has been recently challenged, the clinical efficacy of tension band techniques is well documented (15,18,22).

Plate fixation is particularly effective when used to bridge areas of fracture comminution (7). A plate, often in conjunction with a lag screw, can also be used in oblique fractures. Whereas proximal oblique fractures are effectively treated with either tension band wiring or interfragmentary lag screws with a neutralization plate, the interfragmentary lag-screw fixation-neutralization plate construct has been demonstrated to possess a biomechanical advantage in treating more distal oblique fractures (14). Because of the subcutaneous location of the olecranon, mini and small fragment plates are indicated (Fig. 8.4D). Recently, olecranon- specific peri-articular plates have been developed as have standard locking plates.

Fractures with depressed osteo-articular fragments require joint elevation and bone grafting. Larger joint depressions may require adjunctive fixation with miniscrews or

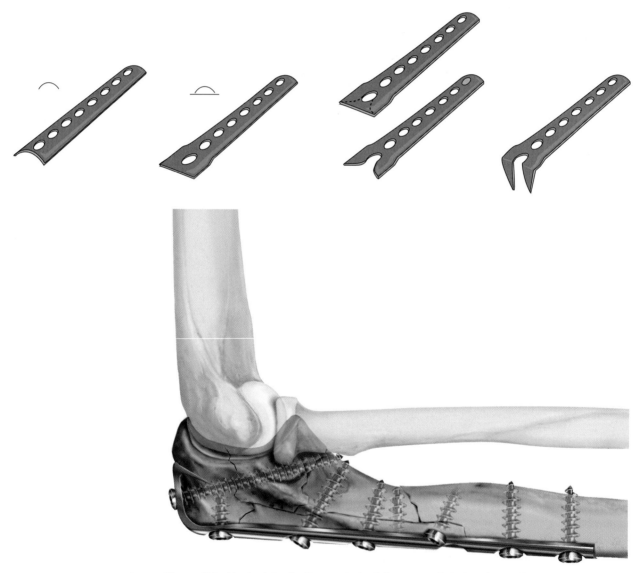

Figure 8.4. Hook plate. **A.** One end of a 3.5-mm semitubular plate is **B.** flattened with a mallet and bending irons. **C.** A wire cutter is used to cut away a portion of the distal plate hole. **D.** The two cut ends are then bent to 90 degrees. The plate is then contoured to the olecranon. Two holes are placed in the proximal olecranon to ease insertion of the hooks into the fragment. **E.** Cut portions of the plate are bent 90 degrees. (From Mast JW, Jakob R, Ganz R. *Planning and reduction techniques in fracture surgery.* Berlin: Springer-Verlag; 1989; Figs. 3.17 and 4.37.)

plates, K wires, and absorbable pins. A lag screw and a 3.5-mm plate or two K wires with a figure-of-eight wire are indicated for proximal and distal oblique fractures. Bone graft, lag screws, and a dorsal-neutralization 3.5-mm semitubular hook (see Fig. 8.4D), reconstruction, or compression plate all are required for comminuted fractures. Repair or reconstruction of the associated injuries in comminuted olecranon fractures is also required.

Excision and triceps advancement is indicated for a small, comminuted, olecranon fracture or in cases of severe osteopenia (27–30). Although some authors have demonstrated maintenance of elbow stability with excision of up to 80% of the trochlear notch, others have demonstrated a linear decline in elbow stability with increasing amounts of bone excision. Furthermore, several investigators have shown that fragment excision results in relatively elevated joint pressures in comparison to those found after internal fixation (7,18,28). Whenever possible, the amount of resected bone should be minimized.

Although discussions of transolecranon fracture dislocations of the elbow are beyond the scope of this chapter, we implore the surgeon to be vigilant in the identification of associated radial-head fractures, coronoid fractures, and Monteggia fracture-dislocations. When treating olecranon fractures, these additional injuries must be addressed because they may compromise the elbow function if left untreated.

SURGERY

The patient is placed supine on the operating table and either regional (Bier or axillary block) or general anesthesia is administered. A tourniquet is applied, and the arm is placed in an arm holder across the patient's chest (Fig. 8.5). Antibiotic prophylaxis consists of a cephalosporin for closed injuries, and for open injury, an aminoglycoside or penicillin (or both) are added to cefazolin. A c-arm image intensifier is positioned at either the head or foot of the table on the side of injury.

The arm is then prepped and draped (Fig. 8.6). A sterile Kerlex dressing (Kendall Healthcare Products, Mansfield, MA) is wrapped around the wrist, and a weighted speculum attached to the end of the Kerlex is passed off the table (Fig. 8.7). The weighted speculum provides enough traction to maintain the arm on the arm holder with the dorsal surface exposed. This eliminates the need for an assistant to hold the arm. As an alternate, the patient may be placed in a lateral decubitus position with the arm over a post. The elbow rests in flexion. The elbow is then extended to aid in the reduction. An iliac crest is also prepped and draped if the preoperative plan specifies the need for a bone graft.

The limb is exsanguinated, and the tourniquet inflated. The incision is begun distally on the subcutaneous border of the ulna (Fig. 8.8). It is continued proximally in line with the

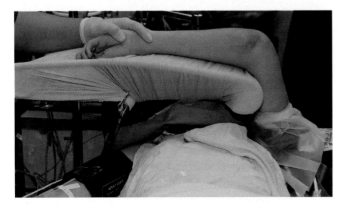

Figure 8.5. The patient's arm is placed across the chest on an arm holder. A tourniquet is applied.

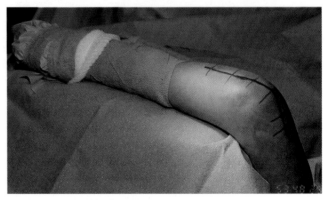

Figure 8.6. The patient's arm is prepped and draped for surgery and placed on the arm holder.

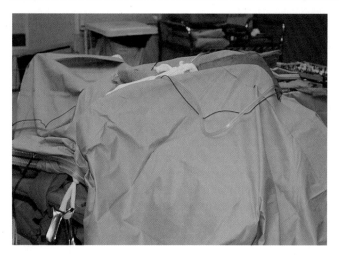

Figure 8.7. A sterile Kerlex is wrapped around the patient's forearm. A weighted vaginal speculum is attached to the Kerlex. The traction holds the arm on the arm holder.

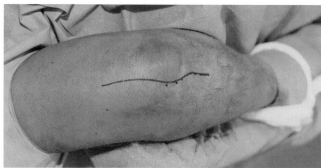

Figure 8.8. The skin incision is begun distally along the ulnar subcutaneous border and is curved radially around the tip of the olecranon and extended proximally in the midline.

subcutaneous border of the ulna to the olecranon area, where it is curved radially around the tip of the olecranon and then extended proximally in the midline 3 to 5 cm.

The incision is developed down to the fascia. A subcutaneous flap is elevated over the tip of the olecranon from radial to ulnar. The dorsal component of the fracture line is now usually visible (Fig. 8.9). Two millimeters of periosteum is reflected from either side of the fracture lines to simplify visualization and fracture reduction. Distally, muscle origins are reflected extraperiosteally as needed. The fracture lines are cleaned of clot and debris. The joint is visualized by retracting the proximal fragment. The joint is cleaned of clot and debris.

Fracture reduction begins with elevation of any depressed articular component, if present. Bank or autogenous bone graft is used if necessary to support the depressed fragments. Small-screw fixation can be added if necessary. The fracture is then reduced and temporarily held in place with K wires or pointed reduction clamps. Additional lag screws are used if needed (Fig. 8.10). The fixation construct is determined by the preoperative plan.

With tension band wiring, two 1.6-mm K wires are placed by use of a parallel drill

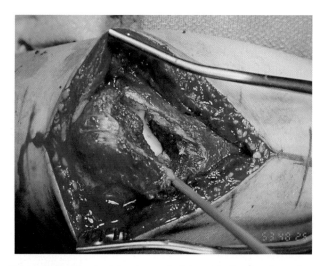

Figure 8.9. The incision is carried down to the fascia and periosteum. A subcutaneous flap is developed radially with the skin over the tip of the olecranon. The dorsal component of the fracture line is now visible.

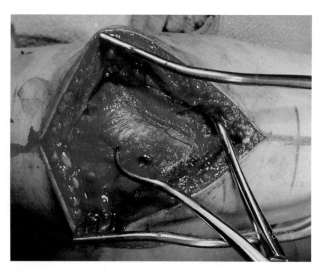

Figure 8.10. The fracture is reduced and held in place with a pointed reduction clamp. In this case, one lag screw is placed across the fracture.

guide (Fig. 8.11). The K wires are over-inserted 1.0 to 1.5 cm and then are backed out to ease seating to the final depth. The K wires are placed down the intramedullary canal of the ulna. Alternately, the K wires can engage the anterior cortex of the ulna (see Fig. 8.3D), which may diminish pin migration. Intraoperative radiographs are obtained to verify the reduction and fixation position. We have abandoned the technique of anterior cortical engagement because precisely estimating the K wire length is technically difficult but necessary for preventing forearm rotational impingement or neurovascular injury should the K wire excessively protrude through the anterior cortex.

A 2-mm hole is drilled perpendicular to the long axis of the ulna approximately 3 to 4 cm distal to the fracture (distal anchor hole). This drill hole is approximately halfway between the volar and dorsal surfaces of the ulna. Anterior placement of this drill hole has been advocated based on a mathematical analysis (24). The anchor hole may be drilled before or after fracture reduction and K wire placement. Drilling the distal anchor hole before K wire placement avoids the potential complication of the drill hitting the K wires but does not eliminate the possibility that the K wires will prevent tension-band-wire placement in the distal anchor hole.

An 18-gauge figure-of-eight wire is passed through this distal drill hole. This wire is then crossed over the dorsal surface of the olecranon. A small loop is added to the wire proximal to the point where the wire crosses the dorsal olecranon surface on the radial side (Fig. 8.12). A 14-gauge angiocatheter is then passed from ulnar to radial side between the triceps tendon and the tip of the olecranon to help avoid injury to the ulnar nerve. The needle is removed. The radial limb of the figure-of-eight wire is inserted into the angiocatheter (see Fig. 8.12), and the angiocatheter is gently pulled back out (Fig. 8.13). The figure-of-eight wire is now located anterior to the triceps insertion, which has been shown to be the optimal position (8). This portion of the wire is twisted to the other end of itself. Two knots are now present in the wire, one knot on each side of the ulna.

The wire knots are then tightened simultaneously. This provides more uniform tension to the bone-implant construct. The knots are cut to a length of 3 to 4 mm, bent down, and buried in the soft tissues (Fig. 8.14). The K wires are bent dorsally just past 90 degrees with a metal suction tip (Fig. 8.15) and cut, leaving 3 to 4 mm of wire remaining past the bend. By using a wire pliers, the K wires are bent over to 180 degrees (Fig. 8.16) and rotated un-

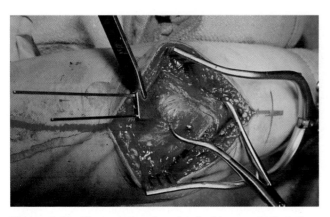

Figure 8.11. The preoperative plan in this case included a tension band construct with K wires and a figure-of-eight wire. Two 1.6-mm K wires are placed across the fracture site with a parallel drill guide.

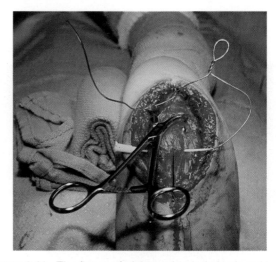

Figure 8.12. The figure-of-eight anchor hole is placed in the distal fragment. A wire is passed through the hole and crossed over the dorsal cortex of the ulna. A twist with a loop is placed into the limb of the wire that is now radial. A 14-gauge angiocatheter is passed from ulnar to radial side anterior to the triceps tendon along the tip of the olecranon. The needle is removed. The radial limb of the wire is put into the angiocatheter.

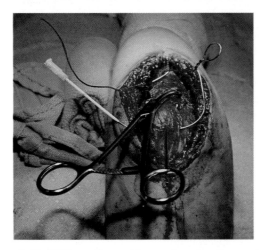

Figure 8.13. With gentle pushing on the wire, the angio-catheter is removed. The figure-of-eight wire now lies anterior to the triceps tendon on the tip of the olecranon. This end of the wire is twisted to itself.

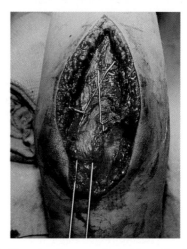

Figure 8.14. By using two needle holders, the figure-of-eight wire is tightened by twisting the loop on the radial side and the knot on the ulnar side. The twists are cut to a length of 3 to 4 mm.

til the short portion of the bent wire is anterior. The K wires are then seated with a mallet and nail set (Fig. 8.17).

We prefer to use a 1.3-mm stainless-steel cable with a small crimp instead of figure-of-eight wire. The cable sleeve is placed along the ulna so that the soft tissues can easily cover it, making it less prominent. In theory, the cable has the ability to achieve greater tension in a more symmetric fashion than the figure-of-eight wire. Care must be exercised to avoid applying too much tension on the cable, resulting in fragment crushing and loss of reduction.

The tourniquet is released. Final radiographs are obtained. The fracture is examined through a full range of elbow motion to verify stability (Fig. 8.18). The wound is irrigated and closed in layers. A drain is not used if adequate hemostasis is obtained after tourniquet release. The arm is placed into a posterior plaster splint. Antibiotics are continued for 24 hours.

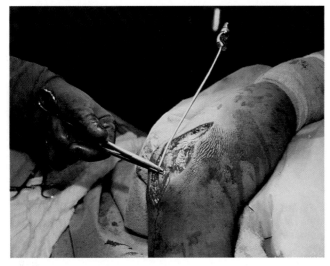

Figure 8.15. The two K wires are bent dorsally to 90 degrees with a metal suction tip and a heavy needle holder.

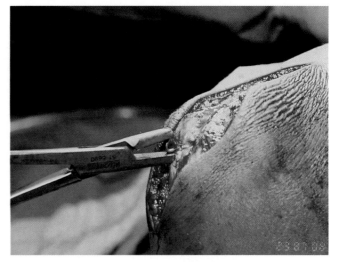

Figure 8.16. The K wires are then cut, leaving 3 to 4 mm past the bend. A heavy needle holder is used to bend the K wires to 180 degrees.

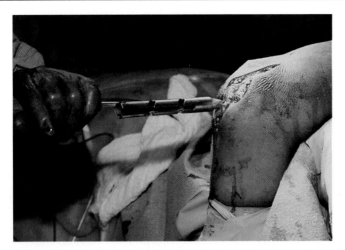

Figure 8.17. The bent K wires are rotated 180 degrees so that the short end of the bend is now anterior. The K wires are seated with a nail set.

Alternative Constructs

Medullary Screw with a Figure-of-Eight Wire. A medullary screw can substitute for the K wires in the previously described technique (see Fig. 8.3B). Advocates of this technique point out that static and dynamic compression are applied, that the screw is less likely to back out, and that this fixation is the strongest biomechanical construct (12,16,21). Disadvantages include prominent hardware and loss of reduction as the screw engages the distal ulnar canal, causing fragment translation.

The medullary screw is placed after fracture reduction. A 6.5-mm cancellous (32-mm thread length) or 4.5-mm malleolar screw is used. A washer is used to help anchor the figure-of-eight wire proximally. The triceps tendon is split in line with its fibers. The pilot hole is drilled, starting at the tip of the olecranon, and subsequently tapped. An alternative method is to leave the fracture displaced and to drill the pilot hole retrograde into the proximal fragment. The fracture is then reduced and held in place with clamps. The pilot hole is identified in the proximal fragment and the drill bit is inserted through it into the distal fragment.

As the screw engages the distal ulna, translation of the proximal fragment can occur. Before final seating of the screw, the figure-of-eight wire is inserted as described. The wire is passed around the screw below the triceps tendon. After the wire is tightened, the screw is

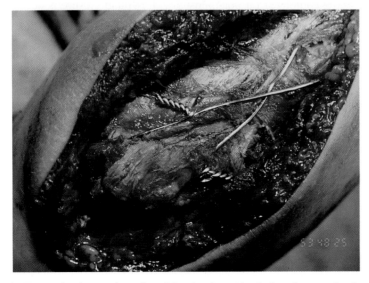

Figure 8.18. The reduction and quality of fixation is evaluated as the arm is placed through a range of motion.

seated. The washer is located on the bone deep to the triceps tendon. This technique avoids injury to the triceps tendon during final seating of the screw. The procedure continues as described.

Lag Screw and Tension Band Plate. This technique involves placing a lag screw, usually through the plate, across the fracture, and placing a plate on the dorsal surface of the olecranon (see Fig. 8.3C). It is especially useful with oblique fractures in the sagittal plane. The lag screw is usually inclined from just distal to the tip of the olecranon to the coronoid process. The plate is bent around the tip of the olecranon, and two screws are placed proximally. The plate is tensioned by first placing a screw distal to the end of the plate. One limb of a Verbrugge clamp is then placed around the screw head, and the other hooks the last hole in the plate (Fig. 8.19). Closing the clamp applies tension to the plate. As an alternative, an articulated tensioning device can be used to tension the plate. Three to four screws are then added distally. The procedure continues as described previously. The use of a peri-articular plate with or without locking screws can be very helpful.

Comminuted Fractures. The surgical exposure described previously is used for comminuted fractures. Care is taken to avoid devascularization of bone fragments. Reduction proceeds in a step-wise fashion. Temporary fixation is achieved with K wires. The quality of the reduction, proposed final fixation, and bone is now assessed. If the fracture cannot be reduced, a spanning or bridging plate can be considered, or the fragments excised, and the triceps tendon advanced.

If adequate fixation can be achieved with an anatomic reduction, then final fixation is applied. K wires are replaced with lag screws. Bone graft is used to support osteochondral fragments. A dorsal plate is then applied to neutralize the lag screws. Several custom-designed plates are currently available. In addition, locking plates now offer other alternatives for fixation. While their role needs to be better defined biomechanically before advocating routine use, we have found locking plates very useful when the fracture is comminuted or is in osteopenic bone. A pelvic reconstruction plate can also be shaped to fit dorsally to the tip of the olecranon. In another alternative, a 3.5-mm semitubular plate is fashioned into a hook plate (see Fig. 8.4A–C) and shaped to fit dorsally to the tip of the olecranon (Fig. 8.4E). The hooks engage the olecranon at the most proximal point. This supplies additional points of fixation. The quality of fixation is assessed by moving the elbow neutral to 120 degrees. Closure continues as previously described.

Open Fractures. Patients with open fractures are taken to the operating room immediately, where irrigation and debridement of the injury are completed. The open wounds are extended as needed. Fixation proceeds as previously described. Part of the wound is left open, but the joint may be closed over a suction drain. The patient is returned to the operating room on postinjury days 2 and 4 for wound and fracture irrigation and debridement. Wound closure is completed on postinjury day 4. Wound closure is accomplished by

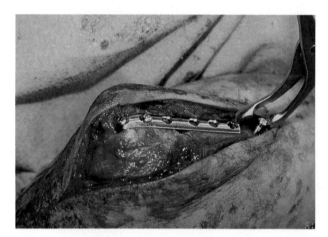

Figure 8.19. The fracture is reduced and a plate applied. A screw is placed into the ulna. A Verbrugge clamp is applied to the screw and the plate. Closing the clamp puts tension on the plate. This is unmeasured tension and care must be taken so the fracture is not displaced.

delayed primary closure, skin graft, local rotational flap, or free-tissue transfer as needed. Antibiotics are used for 24 hours after each wound manipulation.

POSTOPERATIVE MANAGEMENT

The postoperative rehabilitation is divided into three phases: initial, motion, and strengthening. Initially, the limb is splinted at 90 degrees for 3 to 5 days to promote soft-tissue healing. The second phase (motion) depends on the fixation used. Patients with fractures fixed with the tension band principle begin early active motion on day 5. A cast brace is used as needed; the decision is based on fixation quality and patient reliability. Fractures fixed with the lag screw–neutralization principle are placed in a long arm cast for a total of 2 to 3 weeks. A cast brace is used for an additional 3 to 4 weeks. Active and active-assisted motion exercises continue until the patient enters phase three. Isometric and isotonic exercises are started early as dictated by patient tolerance.

Phase three consists of strengthening. The prerequisites for entering this phase are radiographic evidence of progression to union, clinical evidence of union (no pain with physiologic stress), and an active range of motion of at least 75% of the contralateral elbow (75% of normal with bilateral injuries). The patient begins a progressive-resistance program designed to strengthen the entire upper extremity. Functional capacity evaluations are used for return to work for manual laborers.

The rehabilitation protocol is tempered by the quality of fixation and the intraoperative stability achieved. If stable fixation is achieved, even in comminuted fractures, then the protocol continues as described. If the quality of fixation will not withstand early motion, then the arm is splinted for 3 weeks. The rehabilitation protocol then continues as described and is adjusted if needed.

COMPLICATIONS

The most frequent complications of internal fixation of olecranon fractures are related to the hardware. Hardware symptoms are present in 22% to 80% of cases (7,10,13,26,29, 31–33). K wire migration occurs in up to 15% of the cases. Hardware removal is required in 20% to 66% of fractures. Hardware failure occurs in 1% to 5% of cases.

When a K wire and figure-of-eight wire construct is used, several steps may help avoid symptoms related to the implants. K wires are over-inserted 1 cm and then backed up to ease deep final seating. The K wires are bent 180 degrees before final seating so that the bent portion of the wire penetrates the tip of the olecranon, making the wires less prominent. K wires that engage the anterior cortex may prevent the wires from backing out (23). The figure-of-eight wire knots should be buried in the surrounding muscle to avoid their prominence. The use of plate fixation may decrease the incidence of hardware-related complaints and the need for subsequent hardware removal (25,34). However, hardware prominence, symptoms, and removal may be unavoidable in this very superficial area. The preoperative discussion should include a description of the hardware-related symptoms and the frequent necessity for hardware removal.

Infection occurs in 0% to 6% of cases. The risk of infection is reduced with the use of perioperative antibiotics and in open fractures with attention to the soft tissues and wound closure. Acute infection is managed with irrigation and debridement as needed, antibiotics, and wound closure or soft-tissue reconstruction (tissue transfer).

Ulnar neuritis is present postoperatively in 2% to 12% of the cases. The ulnar nerve is not routinely exposed during ORIF, but the surgeon's constant awareness of its location minimizes the possibility of injury. Observation is usually all that is required as symptoms either quickly resolve or improve with time. Late neurolysis may reduce symptoms in some patients.

Heterotopic ossification occurs in 2% to 13% of fractures. Indomethacin is recommended to help prevent heterotopic ossification in fractures at risk (associated, severe, soft-tissue injury, or elbow dislocation). Significant heterotopic ossification is treated with delayed resection and prophylactic irradiation.

RECOMMENDED READINGS

1. Hotchkiss RN, Green DP. Fractures and dislocations of the elbow. In: Rockwood CA Jr, Green DP, Bucholz RW, eds. *Rockwood and Green's fractures in adults*. Philadelphia: J.B. Lippincott; 1991:795–805.
2. Jupiter JB, Mehne DK. Trauma to the adult elbow and fractures of the distal humerus. In: Browner BD, Jupiter JB, Levine AM, et al, eds. *Skeletal trauma: fractures, dislocations, ligamentous injuries*. Philadelphia: W. B. Saunders; 1992:1125–1176.
3. Hak DJ, Golladay GJ. Olecranon fractures: treatment options. *J Am Acad Orthop Surg* 2000;8:266–275.
4. Schatzker J. Fractures of the olecranon. In: Schatzker J, Tile M, eds. *The rationale of operative fracture care*. Berlin: Springer-Verlag; 1987:89–95.
5. Orthopaedic Trauma Association Committee for Coding and Classification. Fracture and dislocation compendium. *J Orthop Trauma* 1996;10:S1–S155.
6. McKee MD, Seiler JG, Jupiter JB. The application of the limited contact dynamic compression plate in the upper extremity: an analysis of 114 consecutive cases. *Injury* 1995;26:661–666.
7. Bailey CS, MacDermid J, Patterson SD, et al. Outcome of plate fixation of olecranon fractures. *J Orthop Trauma* 2001;15:542–548.
8. Coleman NP, Warren PJ. Tension-band fixation of olecranon fractures: A cadaver study of elbow extension. *Acta Orthop Scand* 1990;62:58–59.
9. Colton CL. Fractures of the olecranon in adults: classification and management. *Injury* 1973;5:121–129.
10. Danziger M, Whitelaw GP, Cimino W, et al. Postoperative complications of tension band wiring of olecranon fractures. Paper presented at: The Eighth Annual Orthopaedic Trauma Association Meeting; October, 1992; Minneapolis, Minnesota.
11. Finsen V, Lingaas PS, Storro S. AO tension-band osteosynthesis of displaced olecranon fractures. *Orthopedics* 2000;23:1069–1072.
12. Fyfe IS, Mossad MM, Holdsworth BJ. Methods of fixation of olecranon fractures: an experimental mechanical study. *J Bone Joint Surg* 1985;67B:367–372.
13. Horne JG, Tanzer TL. Olecranon fractures: a review of 100 cases. *J Trauma* 1981;21:469–472.
14. Horner SR, Sadasivan KK, Lipka JM. Analysis of mechanical factors affecting fixation of olecranon fractures. *Orthopedics* 1989;12:1469–1472.
15. Hutchinson DT, Horwitz DS, Ha G, et al. Cyclic loading of olecranon fracture fixation constructs. *J Bone Joint Surg* 2003;85A:831–837.
16. Johnson RP, Roetker A, Schwab JP. Olecranon fractures treated with AO screw and tension bands. *Orthopedics* 1986;9:66–68.
17. Kozin SH, Berglund LJ, Cooney WP, et al. Biomechanical analysis of tension band fixation for olecranon fracture treatment. *J Shoulder Elbow Surg* 1996;5:442–448.
18. Moed BR, Ede DE, Brown TD. Fractures of the olecranon: an in vitro study of the elbow joint stresses after tension-band wire fixation versus proximal fracture fragment excision. *J Trauma* 2002;53:1088–1093.
19. Montgomery RJ. A secure method of olecranon fixation: a modification of tension band wiring technique. *J R Coll Surg Edinb* 1986;31:179–182.
20. Morrey BF. Current concepts in the treatment of fractures of the radial head, the olecranon, and the coronoid. *Instr Course Lect* 1995;44:175–185.
21. Murphy DF, Greene WB, Gilbert JA, et al. Displaced olecranon fractures in adults: biomechanical analysis of fixation methods. *Clin Orthop* 1987;224:210–214.
22. Paremain GP, Novak VP, Jinnah RH, et al. Biomechanical evaluation of tension band placement for the repair of olecranon fractures. *Clin Orthop* 1997;335:325–330.
23. Prayson MJ, Williams JL, Marshall MP, et al. Biomechanical comparison of fixation methods in transverse olecranon fractures: a cadaveric study. *J Orthop Trauma* 1997;11:565–572.
24. Rowland SA, Burkhart SS. Tension band wiring of olecranon fractures: a modification of the AO technique. *Clin Orthop* 1992;277:238–242.
25. Tejwani NC, Garnham IR, Wolinsky PR, et al. Posterior olecranon plating: biomechanical and clinical evaluation of a new operative technique. *Bull Hosp Joint Dis* 2002;61:27–31.
26. Wolfgang G, Burke F, Bush D, et al. Surgical treatment of displaced olecranon fractures by the tension band wiring technique. *Clin Orthop* 1987;224:192–204.
27. Fern ED, Brown JN. Olecranon advancement osteotomy in the management of severely comminuted olecranon fractures. *Injury* 1993;24:267–269.
28. Gartsman GM, Sculco TP, Otis JC. Operative treatment of olecranon fractures: excision or open reduction with internal fixation. *J Bone Joint Surg* 1981;63A:718–721.
29. Murphy DF, Greene WB, Dameron TB. Displaced olecranon fractures in adults: clinical evaluation. *Clin Orthop* 1987;224:215–223.
30. Teasdall R, Savoie FH, Hughes JL. Comminuted fractures of the proximal radius and ulna. *Clin Orthop* 1993;292:37–47.
31. Helm RH, Miller SWM. The complications of surgical treatment of displaced fractures of the olecranon. *Injury* 1987;18:48–50.
32. Holdsworth BJ, Mossad MM. Elbow function following tension band fixation of displaced fractures of the olecranon. *Injury*. 1984;16:182–187.
33. Macko D, Szabo RM. Complications of tension-band wiring of olecranon fractures. *J Bone Joint Surg* 1985;67A:1396–1401.
34. Hume MC, Wiss DA. Olecranon fractures: a clinical and radiographic comparison of tension band wiring and plate fixation. *Clin Orthop* 1992;285:229–235.

9

Radial Head Fractures: Open Reduction Internal Fixation

David Ring

The advent of techniques and implants for internal fixation of small fractures (1) coincided with an increasing appreciation of the important contributions of the radial head to the stability of the elbow and forearm (2–5). As a result, and also due to the inadequacy and problems associated with the silicone rubber radial-head prostheses (2,6–8), it became popular to attempt to save even the most complex fracture of the radial head by operative fixation (9). Early reports of open reduction and internal fixation (ORIF) of radial head fractures were very positive, perhaps due to the prevalence of isolated, partial, radial-head fractures for which good results would be expected (10–15). Some subsequent reports have stated that complex fractures of the radial head are prone to early failure, nonunion, and poor forearm rotation after operative fixation (9,16–18). Combined with increased availability and use of more-predictable metal radial-head prosthesis for complex fractures of the radial head (19,20), the role of ORIF is being redefined.

INDICATIONS/CONTRAINDICATIONS

Historical Background

For most of the last century, excision of the radial head was the only commonly used treatment for fractures of the radial head (21,22), and decision making was simple: excise or do not excise. If excision was elected, the entire head was resected because the results of partial head excision were usually poor (23–26). In the 1980s, with the advent of techniques and implants for the fixation of small fractures and articular fracture fragments, ORIF became a more viable option (1).

On one hand, the incidence, severity, and consequences of proximal migration of the radius after excision of isolated radial-head fractures have long been a source of debate (24).

On the other hand, there is agreement on the value of retaining the fractured radial head amidst complex combined injury with instability of the forearm or elbow, such as an Essex-Lopresti injury (22,27) (radial head fracture and rupture of the interosseous ligament of the forearm) or a terrible triad injury (posterior dislocation of the elbow with fractures of the radial head and coronoid process) (28–31). The radial head is increasingly recognized as an important stabilizer of the forearm and elbow (2–5,22,28–33). Some authors even suggest that ulnohumeral arthrosis after elbow fracture-dislocation is accelerated in the absence of a radial head (34).

The initial reports of ORIF on radial-head fractures focused primarily on isolated fractures involving only part of the radial head (10–15). The good results in these series, the popularity of the new techniques for internal fixation of small fractures, and the increasing recognition of the importance of the radial head led many to emphasize the importance of preserving the native radial head. Unfortunately, subsequent papers have reported unpredictable results after internal fixation of more complex radial-head fractures (9,16–18), particularly very comminuted fractures with greater than three articular fragments (9).

Due to recent improvements in prostheses, surgeons are focused on deciding whether to use fixation or prosthetic replacement for radial head fractures associated with forearm and/or elbow instability. Problems related to the articulation of a metal radial-head implant with native capitular cartilage have been reported, but the majority of these problems are related to an oversized prosthesis (35). In general, results of prosthetic replacement of the radial head have been quite favorable (19,20), making it a useful alternative to ORIF.

Goals of Treatment

Fracture of the radial head can restrict forearm rotation, compromise the stability of the forearm or elbow, and in relatively rare cases, cause radiocapitellar arthrosis. The primary goal of treatment is to ensure forearm rotation. Incongruity of the radial head in the proximal radioulnar joint causes loss of rotation. Painful arthrosis of the proximal radioulnar joint is not usually observed. Although some studies dispute these observations, my training and experience lead me to conclude that partial fractures of the radial head that do not restrict forearm rotation are usually consistent with excellent elbow and forearm function no matter the radiographic appearance (13).

Operative fixation can restrict forearm rotation either via implant prominence, scarring, or heterotopic bone formation. Some patients with healed and apparently well-aligned fractures of the radial head after operative fixation have substantial loss of motion that is not attributable to implant prominence (9). This result may be due to articular incongruities, but based on observations of my own patients and similar observations noted in the literature (36), I suspect that many fractures of the radial head are impacted in a way that expands the diameter of the radial head. Healing of the radial head with this deformity might contribute to loss of forearm motion. Loss of ulnohumeral motion is usually related to capsular contracture and only rarely related to interference from displaced fracture fragments.

When the interosseous ligament of the forearm has been torn [the so-called Essex-Lopresti lesion (27) and variants (37,38)], the initial treatment must include restoration of contact between the radial head and capitulum to prevent marked proximal migration of the radius. Although restoration of the radial head does not guarantee good function in this complex injury, failure to restore the radial head will result in chronic forearm instability that currently has no good solution (39). Attempts to save the radial head at all costs might be unwise in this setting. For instance, many chronic Essex-Lopresti lesions result from failure of attempted operative fixation of the radial head. In this circumstance, where the radial head is essential, tenuous fixation of a complex radial-head fracture may be inadequate and prosthetic replacement might be preferable.

The circumstance is similar for elbow fracture-dislocations. Particularly for unstable elbow injuries, such as the terrible triad pattern of elbow fracture-dislocation (29), secure reconstruction of the radial head is requisite. If the fracture is too complex to achieve reconstruction, then radial head replacement may be preferable. Many partial radial-head fractures are difficult or impossible to repair securely and should also be considered for prosthetic replacement.

Although radiographic criteria for acceptable alignment of the radial-head articular surface are frequently offered (24,31,40, 41), little data support them. The oft-repeated 2-mm limit for acceptable articular alignment, derived from Knirk and Jupiter's study of intra-articular distal radius fractures (42), may not apply to the radiocapitellar joint. Although displaced fractures of the radial head are extremely common, radiocapitellar arthritis is an uncommon presenting complaint about which very little has been published (43).

Treatment Rationale According to Injury Pattern

Isolated Partial Radial-Head Fractures. Slightly displaced fractures involving part of the radial head do relatively well with nonoperative treatment (41,44). They rarely block motion, cause pain, or lead to arthrosis. Although radiographic criteria for operative treatment have been suggested, they lack scientific support.

One generally accepted indication for operative treatment of an isolated partial fracture of the radial head is a fracture that blocks forearm rotation. Because it can be difficult to assess forearm rotation in the setting of an acute, painful, elbow hemarthrosis, it can be useful to aspirate the hemarthrosis and place a local anesthetic in the elbow joint. Alternatively (perhaps preferably) if the patient is evaluated in the office at least 4 or 5 days after injury, the pain is sufficiently relieved to allow a reliable examination. Without block to motion, crepitation with forearm rotation does not seem predictive of problems, but this phenomenon deserves further study.

Because few problems arise with nonoperative treatment [a minimum of 75% good results in long-term follow-up as measured according to a very strict rating scale (45)], the surgeon should not take too much credit for good elbow function after operative treatment of isolated partial fractures of the radial head. In addition, operative treatment provides an opportunity for several complications and so should be undertaken with care.

Isolated fractures of the radial head that are more than slightly displaced are very uncommon (approximately 4% of all radial-head fractures in an unpublished review of over 300 patients treated at Massachusetts General Hospital). Among this small group of patients, blocks to forearm rotation were uncommon. The surgeon should therefore approach the management of the patient with an isolated partial fracture of the radial head with the understanding that these fractures rarely benefit from operative treatment.

Partial Radial-Head Fracture as Part of a Complex Injury. The treatment rationale for partial radial-head fractures that are part of a complex injury pattern is entirely different than in other cases. Such fractures are usually displaced and unstable with little or no soft-tissue attachments; occasionally some fragments are lost. Even a relatively small fracture can make an important contribution to the stability of the elbow and forearm. Usually, the anterolateral aspect of the radial head is fractured with resultant loss of the anterior buttress of the ulnohumeral joint.

While such fractures would seem to be obvious candidates for ORIF because the majority of the head remains intact, they can be very challenging to treat due to fragmentation, the small size of the fragments, lost fragments, poor bone quality, limited subchondral bone on the fracture fragments, and metaphyseal comminution and bone loss. Early failure of fixation of these fractures is potentially problematic, particularly in an Essex-Lopresti injury or a terrible triad fracture-dislocation of the elbow. Therefore, many partial-head fractures associated with complex injuries may be best treated with prosthetic replacement even though this means removing a substantial amount of uninjured radial head. ORIF is indicated when stable, reliable fixation can be achieved.

Displaced, partial radial-head fractures are common among patients with posterior olecranon fracture dislocations; the majority of these candidates are older, osteoporotic women. Some authors believe that radial head excision is acceptable in these cases as long as the ulnohumeral joint is stable (46). In some cases, I have neglected or excised a small, partial, radial-head fracture in these patients, with good results, but favor retaining the stability and support of radiocapitellar contact in most cases. I believe that a low-energy injury in an older patient is a relatively favorable situation in which to consider neglecting or resecting the radial head; however, retention of the radial head, either with operative fixation or prosthetic replacement, would be preferable in healthy, active patients injured in high-energy activities.

Fractures Involving the Entire Head of the Radius. Fractures involving the entire head of the radius [type 3 according to the Mason system (21)] are almost always part of a more complex injury. Some older, low-demand patients are best treated with resection of the radial head without prosthetic replacement but only if the elbow and forearm are stable. The rare young patient with an isolated injury involving the entire radial head can also be considered for excision without prosthetic replacement, but retention of the radial head may improve the function and durability of the elbow, particularly with forceful use.

When treating a fracture-dislocation of the forearm or elbow with associated fracture involving the entire head of the radius, ORIF should only be considered a viable option if stable, reliable fixation can be achieved. There is a definite risk of both early failure and later nonunion, both of which can contribute to recurrent instability. Other factors, such as loss of fragments, metaphyseal bone loss, impaction and deformity of fragments (36), and the size and quality of the fracture fragments may make ORIF a less predictable choice. In particular, if more than three articular fragments are presented, the rates of early failure, nonunion, and poor forearm rotation may be unacceptable (9). The optimal fracture for ORIF will have three or fewer articular fragments without impaction or deformity, each of sufficient size and bone quality to accept screw fixation, and little or no metaphyseal bone loss.

PREOPERATIVE PLANNING

Plain radiographs are useful for determining the overall pattern of injury. In my experience in both patient care and research, fractures of the radial head can occur either in isolation or in association with one of several discrete injury patterns, including (a) fracture of the radial head and rupture of the interosseous ligament of the forearm (Essex-Lopresti and variants) (Fig. 9.1A) (27,37,38); (b) fracture of the radial head and rupture of the medial collateral-ligament complex and/or fracture of the capitulum (see Fig. 9.1B); (c) fracture of the radial head and posterior dislocation of the elbow (47,48); (d) posterior dislocation of the elbow with fractures of the radial head and coronoid process (18,29,48) [the so-called terrible triad (49)] (Fig. 9.1C); and (e) posterior olecranon fracture-dislocations (posterior Monteggia pattern injuries) (see Fig. 9.1D) (28,50–52). As has been emphasized by Davidson et al (36), complex fractures of the radial head are nearly always associated with a complex injury. Intraoperative evidence of ligament injury should always be sought (53), particularly if simple excision is being considered (22).

Plain radiographs frequently underestimate the complexity of a radial head fracture (Fig. 9.2). Computed tomography (CT), particularly three-dimensional reconstructions with the distal humerus removed (see Fig. 9.2B), are very useful for characterizing the fracture and planning surgery. When facing a complex injury pattern, the surgeon should always be prepared for prosthetic replacement of the radial head in case operative fixation proves unfeasible or unwise (see Fig. 9.2C,D).

SURGERY

Patient Positioning

The majority of radial head fractures are treated with the patient supine on the operating table, under general or regional anesthesia, with the arm supported on a hand table. To improve access to the elbow, a sterile tourniquet is preferred to a nonsterile one. Posterior olecranon fracture-dislocations are often best treated in a lateral decubitus position with the arm supported over a bolster.

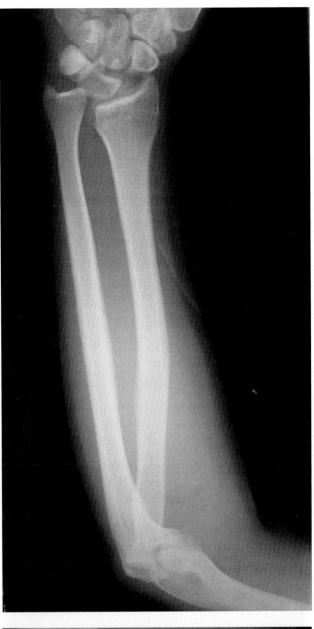

Figure 9.1. When evaluating a fracture of the radial head, one should consider the possibility of one of the following complex injury patterns: **(A)** an Essex-Lopresti lesion or variant; **(B)** fracture of the radial head and medial collateral-ligament injury; **(C)** an elbow fracture-dislocation; and **(D)** an olecranon fracture-dislocation. (Copyright © David Ring, MD.)

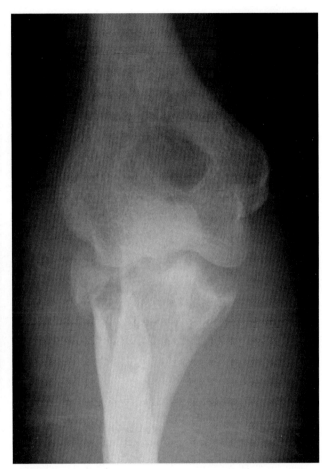

A

B

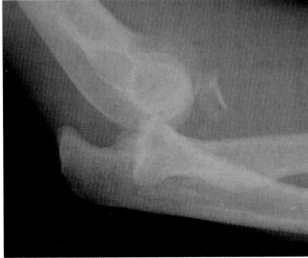

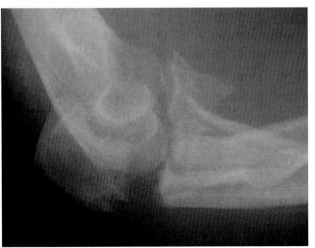

C

D

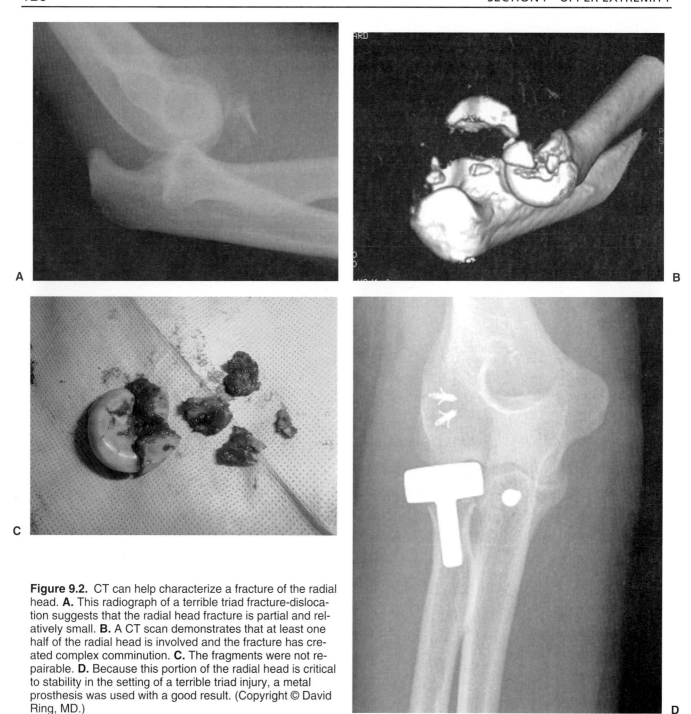

Figure 9.2. CT can help characterize a fracture of the radial head. **A.** This radiograph of a terrible triad fracture-dislocation suggests that the radial head fracture is partial and relatively small. **B.** A CT scan demonstrates that at least one half of the radial head is involved and the fracture has created complex comminution. **C.** The fragments were not repairable. **D.** Because this portion of the radial head is critical to stability in the setting of a terrible triad injury, a metal prosthesis was used with a good result. (Copyright © David Ring, MD.)

Techniques

Operative Exposures. The most popular interval for the exposure of fractures of the radial head is between the anconeus and extensor carpi ulnaris (Kocher exposure) (Fig. 9.3) (54,55). This interval is fairly easy to define intraoperatively. It represents the most posterior interval and provides good access to fragments of the radial head that displace posteriorly. It also provides greater protection to the posterior interosseous nerve. However, attention must be paid to protecting the lateral collateral-ligament complex. The anconeus should not be elevated posteriorly, and the elbow capsule and annular ligament should be incised diagonally, in line with the posterior margin of the extensor carpi ulnaris (56).

A more anterior interval protects the lateral collateral-ligament complex but places the posterior interosseous nerve at greater risk (22). Some authors recommend identifying the nerve if dissection onto the radial neck is required (22). Kaplan described an interval between the extensor carpi radialis brevis and the extensor digitorum communis (54), whereas Hotchkiss recommends going directly through the extensor digitorum-communis muscle (see Fig. 9.3) (22). I find these intervals difficult to define precisely based upon intraoperative observations. A useful technique for choosing a good interval and protecting the lateral collateral-ligament complex was described by Hotchkiss (22): Starting at the supracondylar ridge of the distal humerus, if one incises the origin of the extensor carpi radialis, elevates it, and incises the underlying elbow capsule, it is then possible to see the capitulum and radial head. The interval for more distal dissection should be just anterior to a line bisecting the radial head in the anteroposterior (AP) plane.

In my practice, the vast majority of radial head fractures that merit operative treatment are associated with fracture-dislocations of the elbow. In this context, exposure is greatly facilitated by the associated capsuloligamentous and muscle injury (9,28,57). When the elbow has dislocated, the lateral collateral ligament has ruptured and the injury always occurs [or, according to some authors (57), nearly always occurs] as an avulsion from the lateral epicondyle. Along with a variable amount of muscle avulsion from the lateral epicondyle (57–61), these injuries leave a relatively bare epicondyle (Fig. 9.4). A frequently found split in the common extensor muscle can be developed more distally.

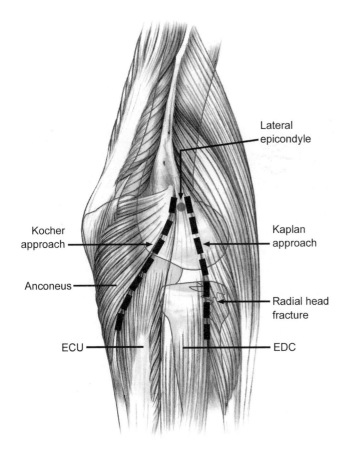

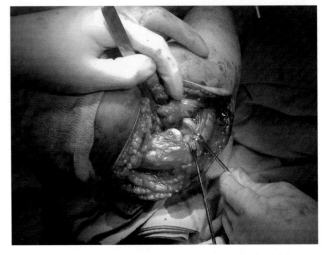

Figure 9.3. Several, lateral, muscle intervals have been described. The most commonly used interval is that of Kocher (between the anconeus and extensor carpi ulnaris). This interval is particularly good for retrieving posterior fracture fragments. The relatively anterior Kaplan interval places the lateral collateral ligament at less risk and provides good exposure to the more anterolateral aspects of the radial head that are typically fractured, but it puts the posterior interosseous nerve at greater risk.

Figure 9.4. The vast majority of complex radial-head fractures are associated with an elbow dislocation. Elbow dislocation results in avulsion of the lateral collateral-ligament origin and a variable amount of the common extensor musculature from the lateral epicondyle resulting in a relatively bare epicondyle. This damage should be used to enhance exposure to the radial head. (Copyright © David Ring, MD.)

In the setting of a posterior olecranon fracture-dislocation (posterior Monteggia pattern injury) the radial head often displaces posteriorly through capsule and muscle. In such cases, the surgeon will usually extend this posterior injury to mobilize the olecranon fracture proximally to expose and manipulate the coronoid fracture through the elbow articulation. This usually provides adequate access to the radial head as well (Fig. 9.5). Slight additional dissection between the radius and the ulna is acceptable because of the usually extensive injury in this region, but extensive new dissection in this area may increase the risk of proximal radioulnar synostosis.

When treating a complex fracture of the radial head with the lateral collateral-ligament complex intact (for instance an Essex-Lopresti injury), it may be difficult to gain adequate exposure without releasing the lateral collateral-ligament complex from the lateral epicondyle. This can be done either by directly incising the origin of the lateral collateral-ligament complex from bone or by performing an osteotomy of the lateral epicondyle (Fig.9.6) (1,11,17,62,63). In either case, a secure repair and avoidance of varus stress (shoulder abduction) in the early postoperative period are important.

The posterior interosseous nerve wraps around the radial neck, directly adjacent to the neck in some patients and separated by some muscle fibers in others. It is at risk during ORIF. It can be protected by pronating the forearm, by dissecting the supinator bluntly with or without identifying the nerve, and by avoiding the use of retractors placed over the radial neck (22). A recent study showed that, with pronation, the posterior interosseous nerve is an average of 3.8 cm distal to the articular surface of the radius (64).

Implants and Implant Placement   Small (1.0 to 2.4 mm) headed or headless screws (such as the Herbert screw) can be used. Standard screws placed in the articular area of the radial head should be countersunk below the articular surface. Some small fragments can only be repaired with small K wires. Threaded wires are usually used because of the tendency for smooth wires to migrate and potentially travel to various parts

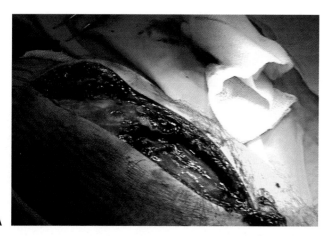

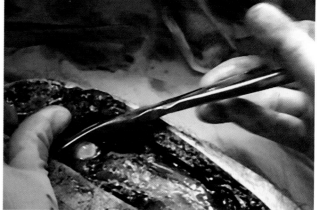

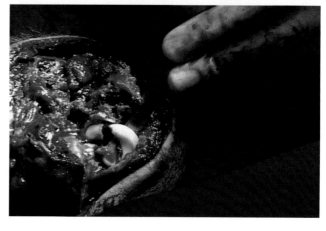

Figure 9.5. A. Posterior olecranon fracture-dislocations (very proximal, posterior, Monteggia injuries) create posterior muscle injury that can be used to expose a fracture of the radial head. **B.** Mobilizing the olecranon fracture fragment proximally as one would do for an olecranon osteotomy exposure of the distal humerus provides access to the joint. **C.** Recreating the posterior subluxation of the radial head that occurred at the time of injury provides good exposure to the radial head. (Copyright © David Ring, MD.)

A

B

C

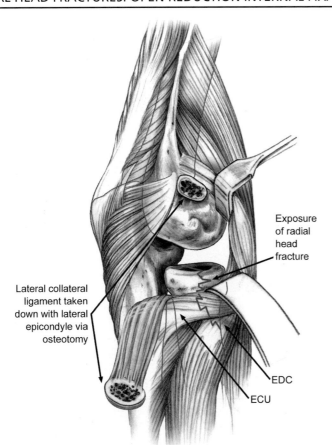

Exposure
of radial
head
fracture

Lateral collateral
ligament taken
down with lateral
epicondyle via
osteotomy

EDC

ECU

Figure 9.6. In the uncommon circumstance that a complex fracture of the radial head is not associated with injury to the lateral collateral ligament (e.g., Essex-Lopresti injury), it may be necessary to take down the origin of the ligament to obtain satisfactory exposure of the radial head. This can be done by releasing the soft-tissue attachment or via an osteotomy of the lateral epicondyle.

of the body (65). Absorbable pins and screws are being developed for similar uses (66,67) but are still somewhat brittle and associated with an inflammatory response.

Small plates are available for fractures that involve the entire head. Plate types include T-shaped and L-shaped plates with standard screws, small (condylar) blade plates, and new plates designed specifically for the radial head (many of which incorporate angular stable screws that thread directly into the plate). The use of plates that are placed within the radial head or countersunk into the articular surface has also been described (62).

The majority of the radial head articulates with either the proximal ulna or the distal humerus. Implants can be placed on the small nonarticular area without impinging during motion, but implants placed in other areas must be countersunk below the articular surface. By simple visual inspection, the articular surface of the radial head with the proximal ulna can be difficult to distinguish from the nonarticular surface, particularly when the radial head is fractured. Smith and Hotchkiss (68) characterized the nonarticular portion of the radial head based upon reference points made in the operative wound. If the radial head is bisected in the anterior-posterior plane with the elbow in neutral, full pronation, and full supination, the safe zone can be defined as half the distance between the middle and posterior marks and half the distance plus a few millimeters (roughly two thirds the distance) between the middle and anterior marks (68). Caputo et al (69) have approximated this zone according to landmarks on the distal radius as lying between the radial styloid and Lister's tubercle. In one study, small plates were applied to the radial head with the forearm in neutral rotation, and the results show that the procedure did not result in impingement (70).

Operative Techniques for Specific Fracture Types

Isolated, Partial Radial-Head Fractures. For isolated, partial, radial-head fractures, a Kocher or Kaplan exposure is used, with the surgeon taking care to protect the uninjured, lateral collateral-ligament complex. In these isolated injuries, the anterolateral aspect of the radial head is usually fractured, and the process to expose through these intervals is straightforward (Fig. 9.7A,B). The fracture is usually only slightly displaced. In fact, it is usually impacted into a stable position (see Fig. 9.7D). The periosteum is

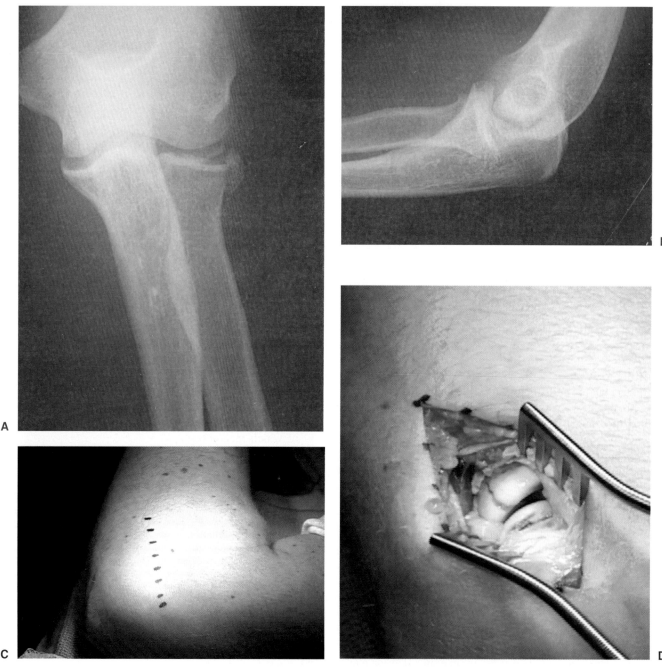

Figure 9.7. ORIF of a isolated fracture of the radial head. **A.** This impacted partial-head fracture blocked forearm rotation. **B.** There were no other apparent injuries. **C.** A lateral skin incision in line with the muscle interval is used. **D.** In this case, the interval between the anconeus and the extensor carpi ulnaris was used, and the elbow capsule and annular ligament were incised anterior to the lateral collateral ligament. (*continues*)

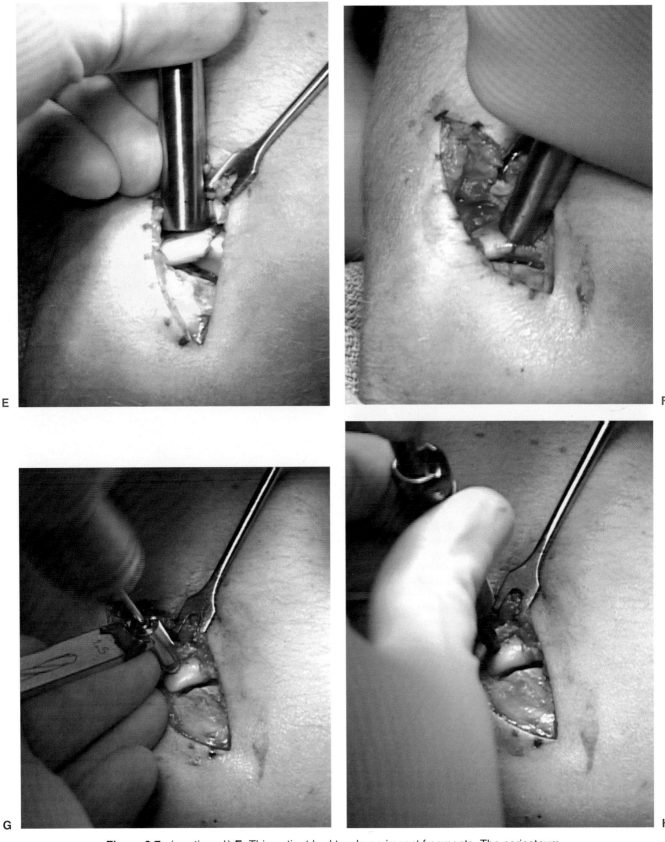

Figure 9.7. (*continued*) **E.** This patient had two large impact fragments. The periosteum was intact and the position of the fragments was quite stable. **F.** A bone tamp was used to realign the fragments without disrupting soft-tissue attachment and to attempt to preserve some of the inherent stability of this impacted fracture. **G.** A 1.5-mm drill was used initially. **H.** Careful screw-size measurement with a depth gauge is important. (*continues*)

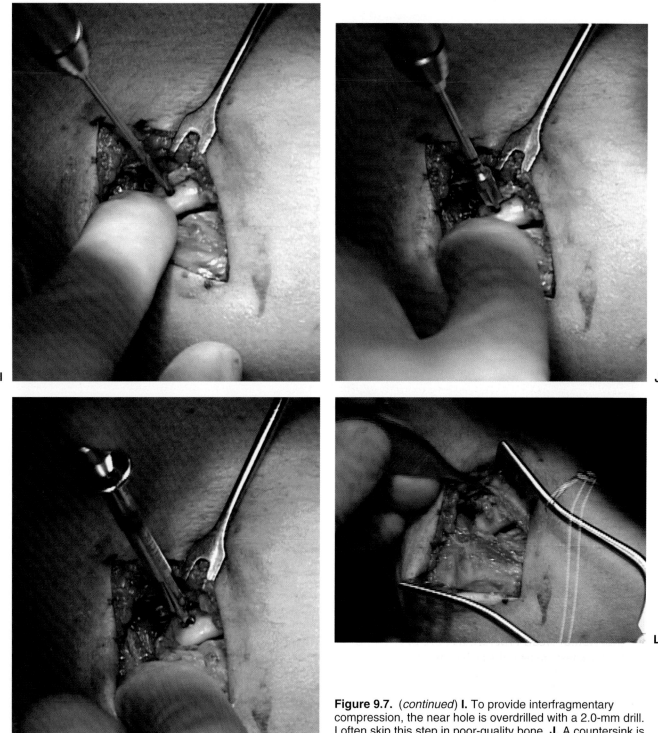

Figure 9.7. (*continued*) **I.** To provide interfragmentary compression, the near hole is overdrilled with a 2.0-mm drill. I often skip this step in poor-quality bone. **J.** A countersink is used to diminish screw prominence. **K.** It is particularly important to place the screw below the articular surface when it is within the area that articulates with the proximal ulna. **L.** The annular-ligament elbow capsule is sutured.

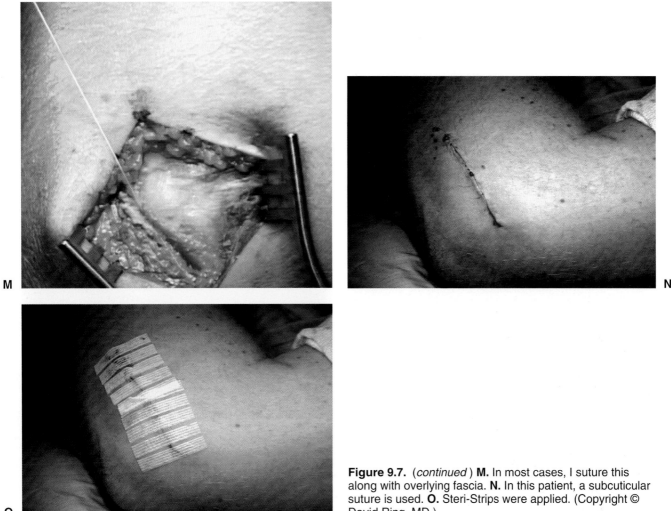

Figure 9.7. (*continued*) **M.** In most cases, I suture this along with overlying fascia. **N.** In this patient, a subcuticular suture is used. **O.** Steri-Strips were applied. (Copyright © David Ring, MD.)

usually intact over the metaphyseal fracture line. Every attempt is made to preserve this inherent stability by using a bone tamp to reposition the fragment (see Fig. 9.7E,F). After the fragments have been realigned, one or two small screws are used to secure each fragment.

Partial Radial-Head Fracture as Part of a Complex Injury. Exposure of radial-head fractures that are part of an elbow fracture-dislocation is straightforward because of associated capsuloligamentous and muscle injury. In the absence of this soft-tissue injury, most partial radial-head fractures can be treated through a Kocher or Kaplan exposure. Reduction and screw fixation is usually used, but if any metaphyseal bone loss or comminution is found, a plate may be preferable (Fig. 9.8).

Fractures Involving the Entire Head of the Radius. To correct fractures to the entire radial head, excellent exposure is requisite, and the surgeon should not hesitate to release the origin of the lateral collateral-ligament complex to improve exposure in the unusual situation where it is not injured (Fig. 9.9). In many cases, the surgeon will remove the fracture fragments from the wound and reassemble them outside the body (on the "back table"). The sacrifice of any small, residual, capsular attachments made in this type of reassembly seems an acceptable trade-off to achieve the goal of stable, anatomical fixation. This reconstructed radial head is then secured to the radial neck with a plate. Consideration should be given to applying bone graft to metaphyseal defects; sufficient bone can often be obtained from the lateral epicondyle or olecranon.

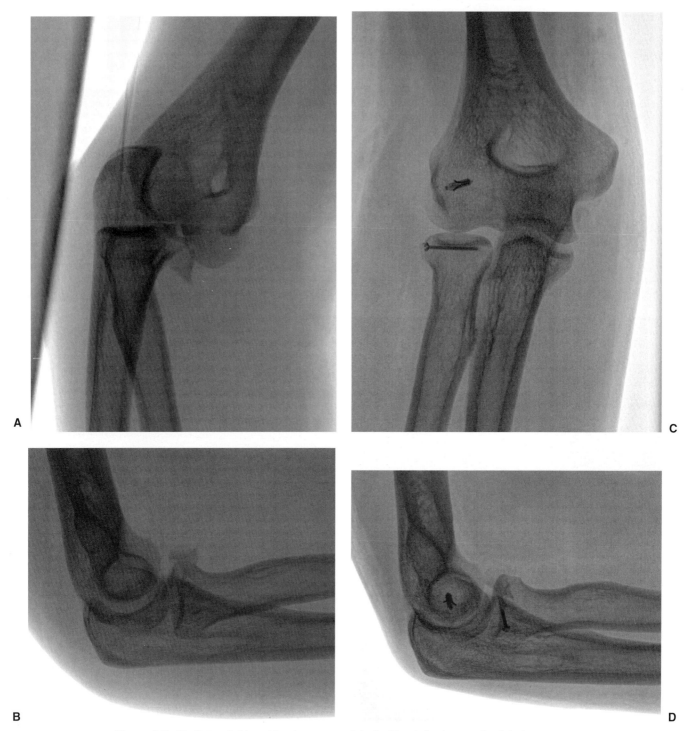

A

B

C

D

Figure 9.8. Partial radial-head fractures associated with relatively complex injuries are usually displaced and instable. **A.** This is a terrible triad injury with the coronoid fragment visible anterior to the coronoid. **B.** A lateral radiograph after manipulative reduction shows both coronoid and radial head fragments. **C.** The radial head fracture was a single small fragment that was repairable with a screw. **D.** The coronoid was repaired with sutures through drill holes, and the lateral collateral ligament was reattached to the lateral epicondyle. (Copyright © David Ring, MD.)

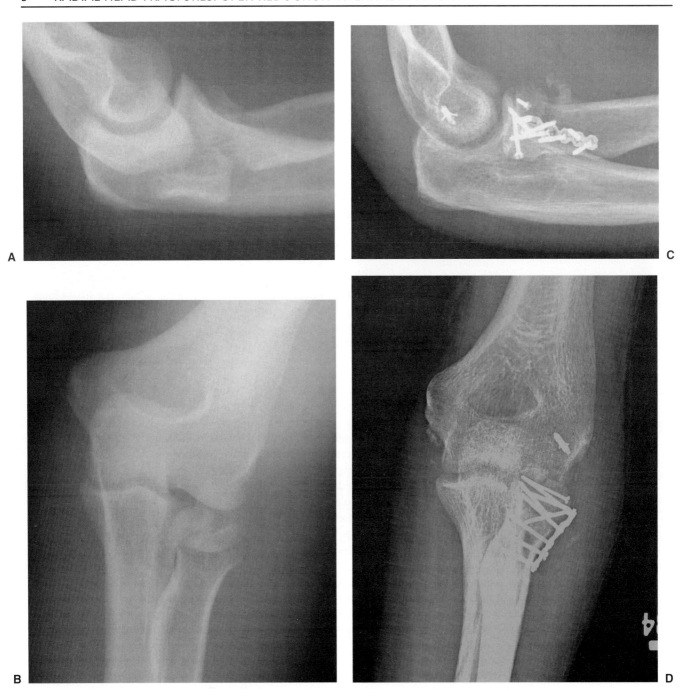

Figure 9.9. Complex fractures of the entire head are very challenging to repair. **A.** This patient received a fracture-dislocation while playing hockey. The majority of the radial head is dislocated posteriorly. **B.** The complexity of the fracture is apparent on the AP radiograph. **C.** A 2.0-mm blade plate and screws were used to repair the fracture, which consisted of two large head fragments and substantial metaphyseal comminution. **D.** The lateral collateral ligament was also repaired. (Copyright © David Ring, MD.)

RESULTS

Along with my colleagues, Quintero and Juniper (9), I recently reviewed the results of ORIF of a fracture of the radial head in 56 patients. The 15 patients with isolated partial fractures of the radial head experienced excellent results. Among the 15 patients with displaced fractures of the radial head as part of a complex injury, 4 (27%) recovered fewer than 100 degrees of forearm rotation, and the results were considered unsatisfactory.

Thirteen of the 14 (93%) patients with Mason type 3, comminuted, radial-head fractures comprised of more than three articular fragments had unsatisfactory results. Three had early failure of fixation, and so required radial head excision; six had painful nonunions treated with excision; four had 70 or fewer degrees of forearm rotation. In the 12 patients with a type 3 fracture in which the radial head was split into two or three simple fragments, no one experienced early failures, two had nonunion, and all achieved an arc of forearm rotation of 100 or more degrees.

POSTOPERATIVE MANAGEMENT

The elbow is prone to stiffness and is best managed with active exercises as soon as possible after injury and surgery. Furthermore, elbow stability is enhanced by early, active, elbow motion. For these reasons, the goal of surgery should be to create a situation stable enough to allow active motion after a very short period of comfortable immobilization.

If the lateral collateral ligament has been repaired, shoulder abduction should be avoided for approximately 6 weeks (so-called varus stress precautions). I have not found hinged braces nor continuous passive motion useful or worth the added expense, and no data are available to support their use.

COMPLICATIONS

Laceration or permanent injury to the posterior interosseous nerve during ORIF of a radial head fracture is unusual. This complication is most commonly experienced as a palsy related to retraction or exposure and resolves over weeks to months. To limit the potential for this complication, retractors should not be placed around the radial neck, the forearm should be pronated during exposure of the radial neck, and when relatively distal dissection and internal fixation are needed, particularly when a more anterior muscle interval is used for exposure, the nerve should be identified and protected.

Injury to the lateral collateral-ligament complex, leading to posterolateral, rotatory, elbow instability, is an uncommon complication related to injury or inadequate repair of the lateral collateral-ligament complex. Awareness of this potential complication and the anatomic landmarks used to prevent it should help limit its occurrence. This complication is treated by reconstruction of the lateral collateral-ligament complex (71).

Stiffness after radial head fracture is usually related to the hemarthrosis and perhaps inadequate early movement of the elbow. This could be exacerbated by the trauma of the operative dissection, particularly if the fixation achieved was tenuous and the surgeon opted to immobilize the elbow and forearm. Heterotopic ossification, usually in the form of anterior heterotopic bone that blocks flexion or a proximal radioulnar synostosis that blocks forearm rotation, is also a risk of operative treatment. Stiffness, with or without heterotopic bone, is treated with exercises, dynamic or static-progressive splinting, or operative release (72).

Early failure of fixation is somewhat frequent, particularly with complex fractures (Fig. 9.10). In a recent series, 3 of 14 fractures involving the entire radial head and more than three articular fragments had fixation failure within the first month (9). Because it can contribute to instability of the forearm or elbow, unstable or unpredictable fixation is undesirable, and such fractures should probably be treated with prosthetic replacement.

Radial head fractures are also associated with nonunion (Fig. 9.11). Nonunions of partial head fractures are usually asymptomatic, and therefore, the number of incidences is unknown (Fig. 9.12). Among fractures of the entire radial head, 6 of 11 in one series (17) and 8 of 26 fractures in another series (9) (including 2 of 12 fractures with three or fewer fragments and 6 of 14 fractures with more than three articular fragments) were classified as nonunions.

Delayed resection of the radial head has usually been performed to improve forearm rotation and not for painful arthrosis of the radiocapitellar joint (73, 74). Incongruity of the

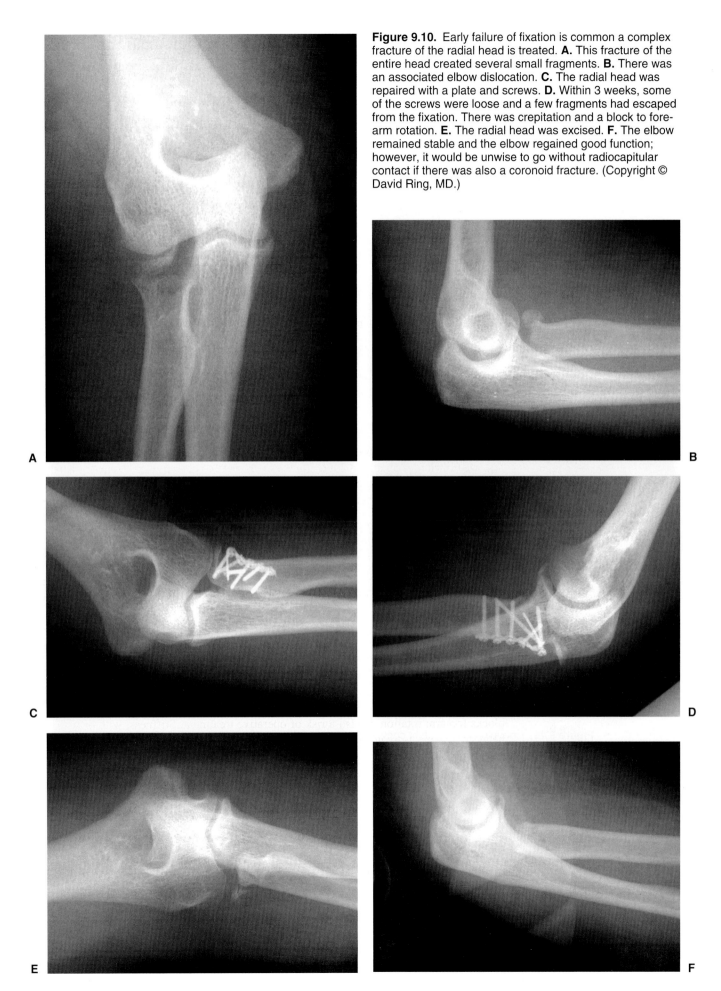

Figure 9.10. Early failure of fixation is common a complex fracture of the radial head is treated. **A.** This fracture of the entire head created several small fragments. **B.** There was an associated elbow dislocation. **C.** The radial head was repaired with a plate and screws. **D.** Within 3 weeks, some of the screws were loose and a few fragments had escaped from the fixation. There was crepitation and a block to forearm rotation. **E.** The radial head was excised. **F.** The elbow remained stable and the elbow regained good function; however, it would be unwise to go without radiocapitular contact if there was also a coronoid fracture. (Copyright © David Ring, MD.)

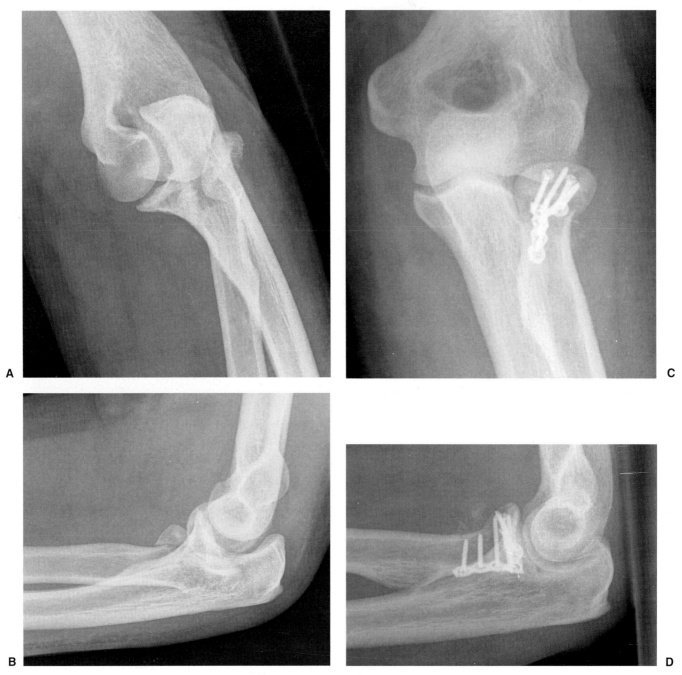

Figure 9.11. Nonunion is a frequent complication of complex fractures of the entire head of the radius. **A.** After reduction of fracture-dislocation of the elbow, a fracture of the entire head of the radius is apparent. **B.** The elbow remains well aligned. **C.** Operative fixation with a plate and screws was performed. **D.** The lateral collateral ligament was reattached to the epicondyle with sutures through drill holes. (*continues*)

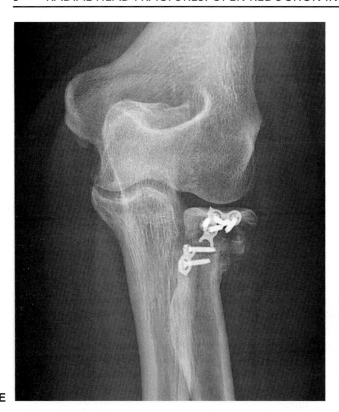

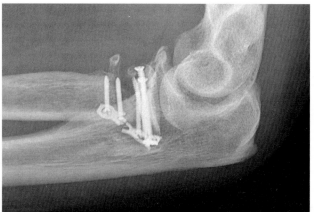

Figure 9.11. (*continued*) **E.** Six months later, the plate is broken and the fracture remains a nonunion. **F.** The patient has nearly full forearm rotation with crepitation and some pain. (Copyright © David Ring, MD.)

E

F

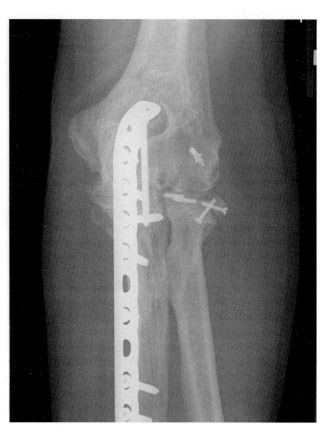

Figure 9.12. Partial radial-head fractures can also fail to heal. This seems to be more common in association with complex injury patterns and metaphyseal bone loss. (Copyright © David Ring, MD.)

proximal radioulnar joint presents as stiffness rather than pain or arthrosis, and incongruity of the radiocapitellar joint inconsistently and unpredictably leads to radiocapitellar arthrosis, which seems to be an uncommon problem.

RECOMMENDED READINGS

1. Heim U, Pfeiffer KM. *Internal Fixation of Small Fractures*. 3rd ed. Berlin, Germany: Springer-Verlag; 1988.
2. Hotchkiss RN, Weiland AJ. Valgus stability of the elbow. *J Orthop Res* 1987;15:327–333.
3. Morrey BF, An KN. Articular and ligamentous contributions to the stability of the elbow joint. *Am J Sports Med* 1983;11:315–320.
4. Morrey BF, An KN, Stormont TJ. Force transmission through the radial head. *J Bone Joint Surg* 1988;70A:250–256.
5. Morrey BF, Chao EY, Hui FC. Biomechanical study of the elbow following excision of the radial head. *J Bone Joint Surg* 1979;61A:63–68.
6. Gordon M, Bullough PG. Synovial and osseous inflammation in failed silicone-rubber prosthesis. *J Bone Joint Surg* 1982;64A:574–580.
7. Vanderwilde RS, Morrey BF, Melberg MW, et al. Inflammatory arthritis after failure of silicone rubber replacement of the radial head. *J Bone Joint Surg* 1994;76B:78–81.
8. Carn RM, Medige J, Curtain D, et al. Silicone rubber replacement of the severely fractured radial head. *Clin Orthop* 1986;209:259–269.
9. Ring D, Quintero J, Jupiter JB. Open reduction and internal fixation of fractures of the radial head. *J Bone Joint Surg* 2002;84A:1811–1815.
10. Bunker TD, Newman LH. The Herbert differential pitch bone screw in displaced radial head fractures. *Injury* 1987;16:621–624.
11. Geel CW, Palmer AK, Rüedi T, et al. Internal fixation of proximal radial head fractures. *J Orthop Trauma* 1990;4:270–274.
12. Kelberine F, Basseres B, Curvale G, et al. Fractures of the radial head: an analysis of 62 surgically treated cases. *Rev Chir Orthop* 1991;77:322–328.
13. Khalfayan EE, Culp RW, Alexander AH. Mason type II radial head fractures: operative versus nonoperative treatment. *J Orthop Trauma* 1992;6:283–289.
14. Pearce MS, Gallannaugh SC. Mason type II radial head fractures fixed with Herbert bone screws. *J R Soc Med* 1996;89:340–344.
15. Odenheimer K, Harvey JP. Internal fixation of fracture of the radial head: two case reports. *J Bone Joint Surg* 1979;61A:785–787.
16. King GJW, Evans DC, Kellam JF. Open reduction and internal fixation of radial head fractures. *J Orthop Trauma* 1991;5:21–28.
17. Heim U. Surgical treatment of radial head fracture. *Z Unfallchir Versicherungsmed* 1992;85:3–11.
18. Heim U. Combined fractures of the upper end of the ulna and the radius in adults: a series of 120 cases. *Rev Chir Orthop* 1998;84:142–153.
19. Knight DJ, Rymaszewski LA, Amis AA, et al. Primary replacement of the fractured radial head with a metal prosthesis. *J Bone Joint Surg* 1993;75B:572–576.
20. Moro JK, Werier J, MacDermid JC, et al. Arthroplasty with a metal radial head for unreconstructable fractures of the radial head. *J Bone Joint Surg* 2001;83:1201–1211.
21. Mason ML. Some observations on fractures of the head of the radius with a review of one hundred cases. *Br J Surg* 1959;42:123–132.
22. Hotchkiss RN. Displaced fractures of the radial head: internal fixation or excision. *J Am Acad Orthop Surg* 1997;5:1–10.
23. Wagner CJ. Fractures of the head of the radius. *Am J Surg* 1955;89:911–913.
24. Radin EL, Riseborough EJ. Fractures of the radial head. *J Bone Joint Surg* 1966;48A:1055–1065.
25. Murray RC. Fractures of the head and neck of the radius. *Brit J Surg* 1940;28:106–118.
26. Carstam N. Operative treatment of fractures of the upper end of the radius. *Acta Orthop Scan* 1950;19:502–526.
27. Essex-Lopresti P. Fractures of the radial head with distal radioulnar dislocation. *J Bone Joint Surg* 1951;33B:244–247.
28. Ring D, Jupiter JB. Fracture-dislocation of the elbow. *J Bone Joint Surg* 1998;80A:566–580.
29. Ring D, Jupiter JB, Zilberfarb J. Posterior dislocation of the elbow with fractures of the coronoid and radial head. *J Bone Joint Surg* 2002;84A:547–551.
30. Morrey BF. Complex instability of the elbow. *J Bone Joint Surg* 1997;79A:460–469.
31. Morrey BF. Current concepts in the treatment of fractures of the radial head, the olecranon, and the coronoid. *J Bone Joint Surg* 1995;77A:316–327.
32. Sojberg JO, Ovesen J, Gundorf CE. The stability of the elbow following excision of the radial head and transection of the annular ligament. *Arch Orthop Trauma Surg* 1987;106:248–250.
33. Morrey BF, Tanaka S, An KN. Valgus stability of the elbow: a definition of primary and secondary constraints. *Clin Orthop* 1991;265:187–195.
34. Sanchez-Sotelo J, Romanillos O, Garay EG. Results of acute excision of the radial head in elbow radial head fracture-dislocations. *J Orthop Trauma* 2000;14:354–358.
35. van Riet RP, Glabbeek FV, Verborgt O, et al. Capitellar erosion caused by a metal radial head prosthesis: a case report. *J Bone Joint Surg* 2004;86A:1061–1064.
36. Davidson PA, Moseley JB, Tullos HS. Radial head fracture: a potentially complex injury. *Clin Orthop* 1993;297:224–130.
37. Jupiter JB, Kour AK, Richards RR. The floating radius in bipolar fracture-dislocations of the forearm. *J Orthop Trauma* 1994;8:99–106.
38. Odena IC. Bipolar fracture-dislocation of the forearm. *J Bone Joint Surg* 1952;34A:968–976.

39. Szabo RM, Hotchkiss RN, Slater RR. The use of frozen-allograft radial head replacement for treatment of established symptomatic proximal translation of the radius: preliminary experience in five cases. *J Hand Surg* 1997;22A:269–278.
40. Bennett JB. Radial head fractures: diagnosis and management. *J Should Elbow Surg* 1993;2:264–273.
41. Weseley MS, Barenfeld PA, Eisenstein AL. Closed treatment of isolated radial head fractures. *J Trauma* 1983;23:36–39.
42. Knirk JL, Jupiter JB. Intraarticular fractures of the distal end of the radius in young adults. *J Bone Joint Surg* 1986;68A:647–659.
43. Morrey BF, Schneeberger AG. Anconeus arthroplasty: a new technique for reconstruction of the radiocapitellar and/or proximal radioulnar joint. *J Bone Joint Surg* 2002;84A:1960–1969.
44. Miller GK, Drennan DB, Maylahn DJ. Treatment of displaced segmental radial head fractures: long-term follow-up. *J Bone Joint Surg* 1981;63A:712–717.
45. Herbertsson P, Josefsson PO, Hasserius R, et al. Uncomplicated Mason type II and III fractures of the radial head and neck in adults: a long-term follow-up study. *J Bone Joint Surg* 2004;86A:569–574.
46. O'Driscoll SW, Jupiter JB, King GJ, et al. The unstable elbow. *Instr Course Lect* 2001;50:89–102.
47. Broberg MA, Morrey BF. Results of treatment of fracture-dislocations of the elbow. *Clin Orthop* 1987;216:109–119.
48. Josefsson PO, Gentz CF, Johnell O, et al. Dislocations of the elbow and intraarticular fractures. *Clin Orthop* 1989;246:126–130.
49. Hotchkiss RN. Fractures and dislocations of the elbow. In: Rockwood CA, Green DP, Bucholz RW, et al, eds. *Rockwood and Green's fractures in adults*. 4th ed. Philadelphia: Lippincott-Raven; 1996:929–1024.
50. Penrose JH. The Monteggia fracture with posterior dislocation of the radial head. *J Bone Joint Surg* 1951;33B:65–73.
51. Pavel A, Pittman JM, Lance EM, et al. The posterior Monteggia fracture: a clinical study. *J Trauma* 1965;5:185–199.
52. Ring D, Jupiter JB, Simpson NS. Monteggia fractures in adults. *J Bone Joint Surg* 1998;80:1733–1744.
53. Smith AM, Urbanosky LR, Castle JA, et al. Radius pull test: predictor of longitudinal forearm instability. *J Bone Joint Surg Am* 2002;84:1970–1976.
54. Morrey BF. Surgical exposures of the elbow. In: Morrey BF, ed. *The elbow and its disorders*. 2nd ed. Philadelphia: W.B. Saunders; 1993:139–166.
55. Kocher T. *Textbook of operative surgery*, 3rd ed. London: Adam and Charles Black; 1911.
56. Cohen MS, Hastings H. Rotatory instability of the elbow: the anatomy and role of the lateral stabilizers. *J Bone Joint Surg* 1997;79:225–233.
57. McKee MD, Schemitsch EH, Sala MJ, et al. The pathoanatomy of lateral ligamentous disruption in complex elbow instability. *J Shoulder Elbow Surg* 2003;12:391–396.
58. Ring D, Jupiter JB. Surgical exposure of coronoid fractures. *Tech Should Elbow Surg* 2002;3:48–56.
59. Dürig M, Müller W, Rüedi TP, et al. The operative treatment of elbow dislocation in the adult. *J Bone Joint Surg* 1979;61:239–244.
60. Josefsson PO, Gentz CF, Johnell O, et al. Surgical versus non-surgical treatment of ligamentous injuries following dislocation of the elbow joint. *J Bone Joint Surg* 1987;69:605–608.
61. Josefsson PO, Johnell O, Wendeberg B. Ligamentous injuries in dislocations of the elbow joint. *Clin Orthop* 1987;221:221–225.
62. Geel C. Fractures of the radial head. In: McQueen MM, Jupiter JB, eds. *Radius and ulna*. Oxford: Butterworth-Heinemann; 1999:159–168.
63. Patterson SD, Bain GI, Mehta JA. Surgical approaches to the elbow. *Clin Orthop* 2000;370:19–33.
64. Diliberti T, Botte MJ, Abrams RA. Anatomical considerations regarding the posterior interosseous nerve during posterolateral approaches to the proximal part of the radius. *J Bone Joint Surg* 2000;82:809–813.
65. Lyons FA, Rockwood CA. Migration of pins used in operations on the shoulder. *J Bone Joint Surg* 1990;72:1262–1267.
66. Hirvensalo E, Böstman O, Rokkanen P. Absorbable polyglycolide pins in fixation of displaced fractures of the radial head. *Arch Orthop Trauma Surg* 1990;109:258–261.
67. Pelto K, Hirvensalo E, Bostman O, et al. Treatment of radial head fractures with absorbable polyglycolide pins: a study on the security of fixation in 38 cases. *J Orthop Trauma* 1994;8:94–98.
68. Smith GR, Hotchkiss RN. Radial head and neck fractures: anatomic guidelines for proper placement of internal fixation. *J Shoulder Elbow Surg* 1996;5:113–117.
69. Caputo AE, Mazzocca AD, Santoro VM. The nonarticulating portion of the radial head: anatomic and clinical correlations for internal fixation. *J Hand Surg* 1998;23:1082–1090.
70. Soyer AD, Nowotarski PJ, Kelso TB, et al. Optimal position for plate fixation of complex fractures of the proximal radius: a cadaver study. *J Orthop Trauma* 1998;12:291–293.
71. Nestor BJ, O'Driscoll SW, Morrey BF. Ligamentous reconstruction for posterolateral rotatory instability of the elbow. *J Bone Joint Surg* 1992;74:1235–1241.
72. Hastings HI. Elbow contractures and ossification. In: Peimer CA, ed. *Surgery of the hand and upper extremity*. New York: McGraw-Hill; 1997:507–534.
73. Goldberg I, Peylan J, Yosipovitch Z, et al. Late results of excision of the radial head for an isolated closed fracture. *J Bone Joint Surg* 1986;68:675–679.
74. Broberg MA, Morrey BF. Results of delayed excision of the radial head after fracture. *J Bone Joint Surg* 1986;68:669–674.

10

Forearm Fractures: Open Reduction Internal Fixation

Steven J. Morgan

INDICATIONS

The radius and the ulna form a complex articulation that permits elbow, forearm, and wrist motion. Loss of normal angular alignment results in loss of forearm supination and pronation (1,2). Angular deformity in single bone fractures of the forearm with associated soft-tissue injury result in dislocation. Isolated ulna fractures are often referred to as Monteggia fractures and are recognized as having an associated injury or dislocation of the proximal radioulnar joint. Isolated fractures of the radius are accompanied by a distal radioulnar joint (DRUJ) dislocation and are often called a Galeazzi fracture. Open reduction and internal fixation (ORIF) of displaced forearm fractures in the skeletally mature patient remains the standard treatment for displaced forearm fractures. Internal fixation allows for maintenance of fracture alignment during healing while the patient performs functional range of motion with the arm. Outcomes following internal fixation provide better results than nonoperative treatment (3–8).

Isolated ulna fractures resulting from a direct blow remain the exception to this general rule. The "night stick" fracture, as it is commonly called, does not have the degree of soft-tissue injury recognized in other fractures of the forearm, and the likelihood of acute instability of the distal or proximal radioulnar articulations is absent. Fractures involving the distal third of the ulna should be evaluated closely and observed carefully over time as angular deformity can result in significant functional impairment at the DRUJ. Operative fixation of isolated ulna fractures, regardless of injury mechanism, is recommended in open fractures, fractures angulated greater then 10 degrees in any plane, and in fractures with greater than 50% comminution (9).

INITIAL EVALUATION, MANAGEMENT, AND SURGICAL PLANNING

Initial evaluation of the patient and the radiographs is necessary for developing a treatment plan. A detailed history related to mechanism of injury, hand dominance, occupation, previous injury, and associated medical problems is required. The entire extremity needs to be carefully examined for associated injuries. Circumferential inspection of the extremity should be performed to identify the presence of an open fracture as well as to assess the extent and severity of the soft-tissue injury. Any violation of the skin in reasonable proximity to the fracture should be enough to consider the injury an open fracture. Ecchymosis, fracture blisters, and edema suggest that the soft tissue absorbed significant energy and the index of suspicion for compartment syndrome should be high. Palpation for tenderness and instability should be performed from the shoulder to the hand. The elbow, wrist, and carpal bones should receive special attention.

Injuries to the DRUJ or proximal radioulnar joint, scaphoid fractures, and carpal instability are common. Neurological examination should be focused and include the motor and sensory status of the radial (posterior interosseous, superficial radial), ulnar, and median nerves. Vascular examination should focus on the perfusion of the extremity and should include palpation of the brachial radial and ulnar pulses.

Initial radiographic evaluation, prior to the application of splinting material, should consist of orthogonal radiographs (AP and lateral) that include both the wrist and the elbow. In situations when the physical examination indicates additional injury or radiographs are inadequate or inspire suspicion that associated injuries exist, joint specific views of the wrist and elbow should be obtained. Radiographic evaluation should never inhibit the overall care of the patient. In the patient with multiple injuries as well as in the patient with soft-tissue injury or neurological or vascular compromise, a provisional reduction and splint should be applied prior to obtaining radiographs. Traction radiographs often facilitate evaluation of comminuted fractures. Difficult to obtain without proper sedation, these radiographs are best obtained following induction of anesthesia prior to surgery. Stress radiographs of the joints for associated instability can also be obtained at this time, and fluoroscopy is often helpful in this regard.

Initial management of the forearm fracture following the physical examination consists of basic open-fracture wound management (if present) and gross realignment and splint immobilization of the forearm to limit pain and further soft-tissue injury while definitive fracture fixation is pending. In cases of marked angulation or vascular compromise, realignment should be performed immediately. In a Monteggia fracture with a dislocated radial head, gentle traction and supination with conscious sedation or regional anesthesia (Bier block) is necessary to reduce the dislocation. In most other situations, adequate analgesia will permit gross realignment and splint application of the forearm. A long-arm posterior splint is preferred. A sugar tong splint, while adequate in many patients, can result in unnecessary skin breakdown in the supracondylar area. Following any manipulation, the neurological and vascular status of the extremity should be reevaluated and documented.

The timing of surgery is largely dependent on the condition of the soft tissues and the general condition of the patient. Internal fixation is warranted on an emergent basis for open fractures, impending or frank compartment syndrome, and irreducible dislocation with impending skin breakdown or neurological deficit. In other situations, the surgery can be performed in a more elective setting. The reduction, however, becomes more difficult with time, and additional soft-tissue dissection may be required to achieve reduction when fracture fixation is delayed beyond 72 hours. Several studies on open fractures have shown no increased morbidity with immediate plate fixation (6,10). Repeat irrigation and debridement are dictated by the severity of the soft-tissue injury and viability following initial plate fixation. In the patient with multisystem trauma and an open forearm fracture, external fixation following irrigation and debridement may be used as a temporizing measure until the patient's general condition is allowed to improve.

The implant of choice for forearm fracture fixation is a 3.5-mm plate that allows for dynamic compression and application of lag screws through the plate. These implants are available in full contact and limited contact designs. They are available in either titanium or stainless steel from a variety of manufacturers. In theory, low-contact plates limit devitalization of the underlying bone, and titanium decreases the likelihood of stress shielding. Excellent results can be achieved with any of these implant choices. Recently, locked compression plates have been introduced as a fixation option. Their role in diaphyseal fractures of the forearm remains undefined and to a large extent appears to be unnecessary except in cases of significant osteoporosis (11). In adults, reconstruction and one-third tubular plates are contraindicated.

Implant selection and size, with reasonable variations, should be determined following full evaluation of radiographs and characterization of the fracture pattern. Implant templates are available to aid in this process and should be used liberally. Traditional technique has called for the use of plates that can obtain a minimum of 6 cortices of fixation on either side of the fracture. The use of long plates with spaced screws is also an option. More important, a well thought-out surgical plan should be developed to achieve reduction and fixation. This is paramount when utilizing indirect reduction aids to restore length and alignment.

General Surgical Technique

While regional anesthesia can be utilized in these cases, general anesthesia is preferred so that accurate postoperative assessment of neurological function and evaluation for compartment syndrome can be ensured. The patient is positioned supine and the arm is placed on a radiolucent arm board. Following the induction of anesthesia, a nonsterile tourniquet is applied, and in the case of comminuted fractures, traction radiographs are obtained by applying longitudinal traction to the hand while an assistant or the surgeon applies counter traction in the upper arm.

The extremity is prepped and draped in a standard fashion. In the case of open fractures, the tourniquet is not utilized so that further anoxic injury to the traumatized soft tissue can be avoided. In closed fractures, the limb is exsanguinated and the tourniquet is inflated to 250 psi. Surgical incisions are then drawn on the extremity, and the fracture site is localized with the C-arm and marked. In general, the least comminuted fracture is approached first to aid in the indirect reduction of the other fracture(s). In noncomminuted fractures, the radius is generally approached first. Loop magnification may be utilized for volar forearm dissections to better recognize and control bleeding vessels. Bipolar cautery is utilized when the surgeon is working in close proximity to the nerves, and small ligature clips are utilized liberally during the dissection.

Surgical Approaches

Flexor Carpi Radialis Approach For fractures involving the distal third of the radius, a volar approach based on the flexor carpi radialis (FCR) is utilized. The surgical incision is located just radial to the FCR tendon (Fig. 10.1). Following the skin incision, the FCR tendon sheath is split longitudinally and the FCR tendon is retracted ulnarly. The floor of the tendon sheath is then incised. The flexor pollicis longus (FPL) is then encountered and

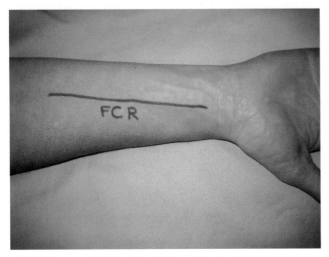

Figure 10.1. The surgical incision is based just radial to the FCR tendon.

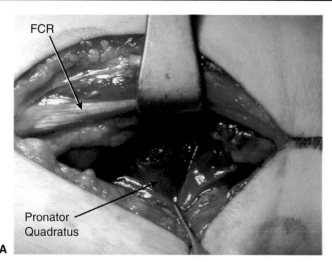

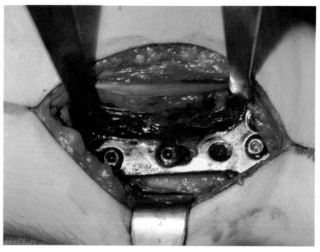

A

B

Figure 10.2. A. The floor of the tendon sheath is incised. The FPL is encountered and re-tracted ulnarly. **B.** The pronator quadratus is elevated from the periosteum and retracted ulnarly.

retracted ulnarly; this action adds further protection to the median nerve. The pronator quadratus is then incised, elevated from the periosteum, and retracted ulnarly to expose the distal third of the radius (Fig. 10.2). This exposure offers the benefit of avoiding direct dissection of the radial artery, which the FCR sheath protects.

Volar Approach of Henry The extensile volar approach of Henry is utilized for most fractures of the proximal radius (12). Adequate exposure can be obtained from the biceps tuberosity to the distal-radial articular surface. The surgical skin incision extends from the biceps tendon to the radial styloid, generally following the lateral aspect of the FCR (Fig. 10.3). In the distal aspect of the incision, the radial artery is in close proximity to the volar fascia, and careful scissor dissection initiated proximally and proceeding distally will keep the surgeon from injuring this structure. The proximal plane between the brachioradialis and the FCR should be developed (Fig. 10.4).

The radial artery is mobilized and retracted in the direction dictated by associated soft-tissue conditions. Loop dissection is tremendously helpful when dissecting the radial artery because it allows for recognition of the small vascular branches that are associated with the artery and their subsequent clip ligature or cautery.

The superficial radial nerve should be protected. The nerve is found on the under surface of the proximal brachioradialis. It pierces the fascia and emerges on the superficial surface of the brachioradialis. Deep dissection distally includes incising the pronator quadratus

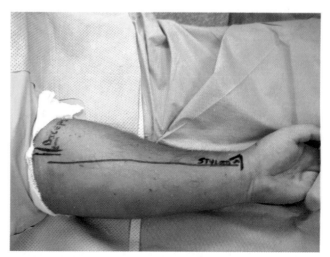

Figure 10.3. The surgical incision is based just radial to the FCR tendon.

Radial Artery

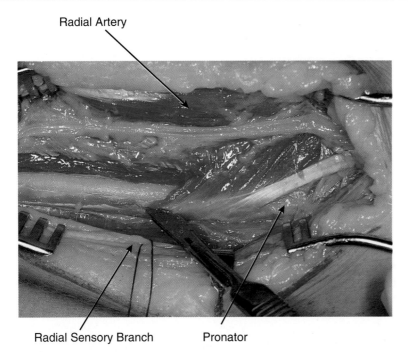

Radial Sensory Branch   Pronator

Figure 10.4. The volar fascia is opened to expose the brachioradialis and the FCR muscles. The interval between these muscles is developed bluntly. The sensory branch of the radial nerve courses beneath the brachioradialis and pierces the volar fascia in the distal third.

from its radial attachment such that it is dissected off the underlying periosteum and retracted ulnarly along with the FPL (Fig. 10.5).

The proximal pronator teres can be detached by pronating the forearm and releasing the tendinous attachment from the radius (Fig. 10.6). In an alternative, the pronator teres attachment can be preserved and the tendon can be elevated from the volar surface of the radius to accommodate a submuscular/tendinous plate (Fig. 10.7).

The supinator is elevated from the periosteum with an elevator and retracted radially while the flexor digitorum superficialis is elevated and retracted ulnarly to expose the

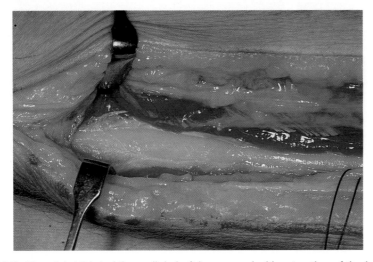

Figure 10.5. The distal third of the radial shaft is exposed with retraction of the brachioradialis radially and FCR ulnarly. The radius is relatively flat in this zone, and the plate generally needs minimal contouring.

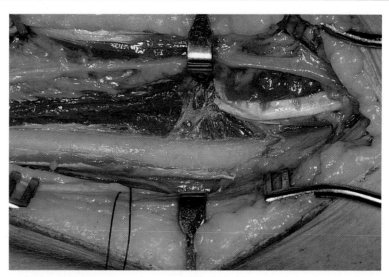

Figure 10.6. The pronator teres has been elevated sharply to expose the middle third of the radius.

biceps tuberosity (Fig. 10.8). In this area, bipolar cautery should be utilized secondary to the proximity of the posterior interosseous nerve.

Dorsal or Thompson Approach   The Thompson approach is an extensile exposure to the radius that offers complete access from the radial head to the distal articular surface (13). Secondary to the risk to the posterior interosseous nerve and irritation caused by dorsal plate fixation of the overlying tendons, this approach is used less frequently than the FCR or Henry approaches. The dorsal approach is reserved for open fractures with a dorsal-based soft-tissue lesion, fractures that require exploration of the posterior interosseous nerve, and select proximal-third radial fractures. The skin excision extends from the lateral epicondyle to the ulnar aspect of Lister's tubercle (Fig. 10.9).

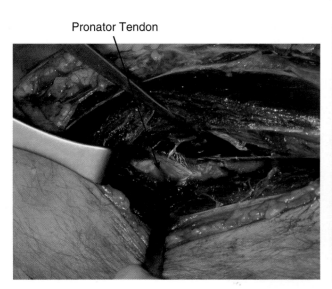

Pronator Tendon

Figure 10.7. The pronator attachment can be preserved and the tendon can be elevated from the volar surface of the radius allowing submuscular/tendinous placement of a plate.

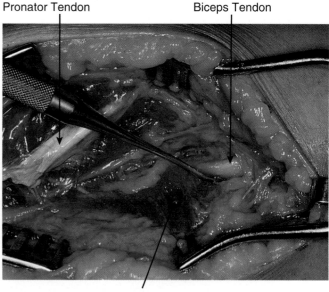

Pronator Tendon   Biceps Tendon

Supinator

Figure 10.8. The Henry approach can be extended to the proximal third of the radius if needed. The probe shows the insertion of the bicipital tendon.

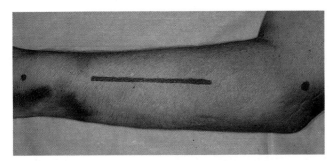

Figure 10.9. The dorsal approach to the radius is marked along a line from the lateral humeral epicondyle to the ulnar side of Lister's tubercle.

The interval between the extensor carpi radialis brevis (ECRB) and the extensor digitorum comminus (EDC) is developed proximally. The interval between the muscles is more easily recognized in the distal forearm (Fig. 10.10). Once this interval is developed, the posterior interosseous nerve (PIN) is localized as it emerges from the mid substance of the supinator muscle. The nerve must be dissected out of the supinator while care is taken to protect the branches of the nerve to the supinator muscle (Fig. 10.11).

As in the volar approaches, loop magnification can be beneficial. The arm is supinated to expose the attachment of the supinator and the pronator teres, both of which are detached and subperiosteally elevated toward their origins. As the approach is developed distally, the abductor pollicis longus (APL) and the extensor pollicis brevis are obliquely crossing the radius (Fig. 10.12). The muscles are elevated from the underlying periosteum and retracted either radially or ulnarly to facilitate exposure. In the most distal aspect of the approach, the interval between the ECRB and the extensor pollicis longus (EPL) is developed. As with all approaches to the forearm, the extent of dissection is based on the fracture location and the length of the plate to be utilized.

Dorsal Approach to the Ulna The subcutaneous nature of the ulna facilitates a direct dorsal approach to the entire ulna. The arm is flexed on the table to provide access to the subcutaneous border and needs to be supported during dissection (Fig. 10.13). The interval is between the extensor carpi ulnaris (ECU) and the flexor carpi ulnaris. To avoid subcutaneous placement of internal fixation, the ECU is retracted and the dorsal aspect of the ulna is exposed (Fig. 10.14).

The subcutaneous nature of the ulna also facilitates percutaneous plate placement, particularly in comminuted fractures. Following indirect reduction of the ulna by either plate fixation of the radius or provisional reduction utilizing an external fixator, 2-cm incisions

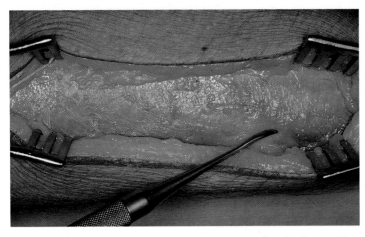

Figure 10.10. The dorsal investing fascia is examined to define the interval between the ECRB and the EDC.

PIN (nerve)

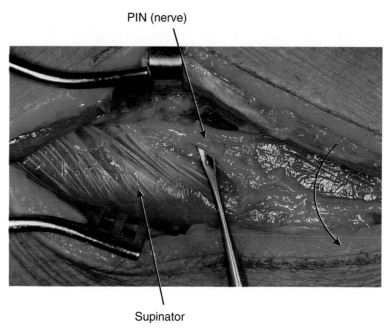

Supinator

Figure 10.11. The forearm is pronated, which brings the PIN closer to the operative field and may increase the risk for injury.

are made along the subcutaneous border of the ulna, and the overlying skin is mobilized from the deep tissue with an elevator directed toward the fracture. The plate is then inserted along the bone until it is exposed in the opposite incision. The process is visualized with an image intensifier. The plate is then secured to the bone with screws via the two small incisions and strategically placed stab incisions along the subcutaneous border of the ulna (Fig. 10.15). When placed percutaneously in this manner, plates lie along the subcutaneous border and thus increase the likelihood of symptoms related to the internal fixation.

Reduction and Plate Fixation Techniques

The fracture pattern dictates the technique utilized for reduction and internal fixation. Soft tissues are retracted with right angle retractors or strategically placed (extraperiosteally when possible) small Homan retractors. Broad retractors should be avoided to eliminate unnecessary soft-tissue stripping (Fig. 10.16). In transverse and short, oblique

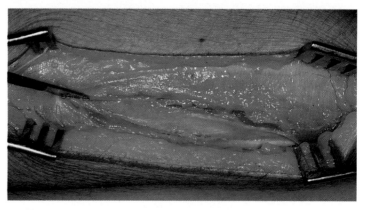

Figure 10.12. The dorsal fascia is incised along this interval. The APL crosses the dorsal surface of the radius obliquely in the distal portion of the exposure.

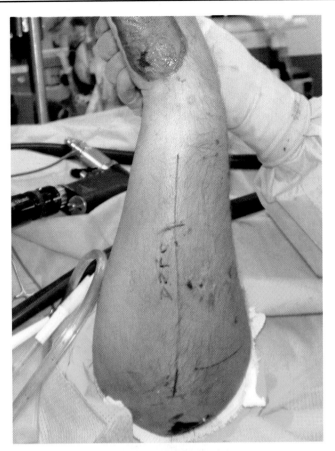

Figure 10.13. The subcutaneous approach to the ulna is marked with the elbow flexed and the forearm in neutral rotation. The fracture site should be palpated to determine the midpoint of the incision.

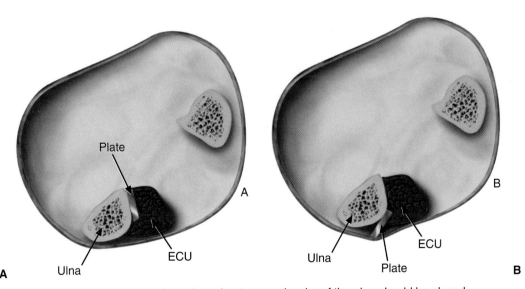

Figure 10.14. A. The plate along the subcutaneous border of the ulna should be placed so that it lies beneath the ECU and is recessed dorsal to the subcutaneous border of the ulna. **B.** This reduces painful symptoms related to a prominent plate that most frequently occurs when the forearm is placed on a rigid surface.

fracture patterns, direct reduction followed by lag screw and compression plating techniques are recommended. Pointed reduction forceps or serrated reduction forceps are used to grasp the bone and draw it out to length; the fracture is then reduced under direct visualization (Fig. 10.17).

Oblique fracture patterns are temporarily maintained in a reduced position by placing the pointed reduction forceps perpendicular to the fracture line. Compression across the fracture should then be obtained with a lag screw. When the fracture orientation permits, lag screw fixation through the plate (after compression of the fracture with the plate) will enhance the stability of the construct. In transverse fractures, a contoured plate is secured to the bone with a bicortical screw in the most distal aspect of the plate after the surgeon ensures it is centered on the bone. Opposite the fracture, an additional bicortical screw is

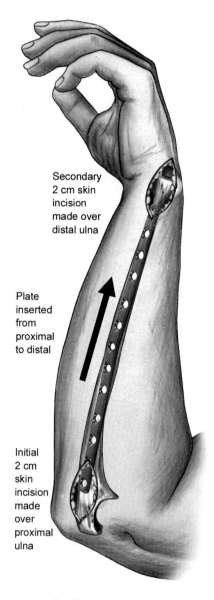

Secondary
2 cm skin
incision
made over
distal ulna

Plate
inserted
from
proximal
to distal

Initial
2 cm
skin
incision
made
over
proximal
ulna

Figure 10.15. An incision measuring 2 cm is made over the subcutaneous proximal ulna and carried down to the periosteum. The subcutaneous tissue is elevated from the periosteum by pushing a plate along the subcutaneous border of the ulna. With the plate inserted, a separate 2-cm incision is made over the plate at the distal ulna. The plate is then centered on the bone at both ends and screws are placed. If additional screws are required closer to the fracture, stab wounds are made over the plate and screws are inserted percutaneously.

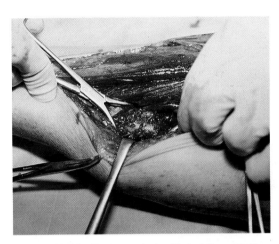

Figure 10.16. Exposure is facilitated through the use of right-angle retractors and small Weber clamps. Extensive dissection of soft tissue with wide exposure of the fracture site is avoided.

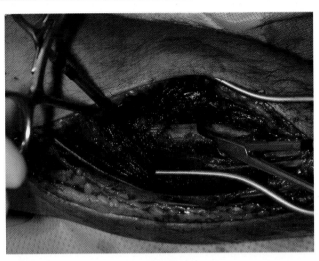

Figure 10.17. Pointed reduction forceps or serrated reduction forceps are used to grasp the bone and draw it out to length. The fracture is reduced under direct visualization.

placed in an eccentrically drilled hole to compress effectively the fracture as it is tightened. Prior to final tightening, the clamps anchoring the plate to the bone should be loosened or removed to allow the plate to slide in relationship to the compressing screw. The clamps are then removed and two additional screws are placed in the neutral position on either side of and in close proximity to the fracture. Additional screw fixation is unnecessary in bone of regular quality. In poor quality bone, a minimum of six to eight cortices of fixation should be obtained on either side of the fracture or use of a locked plate device should be considered.

Comminuted fractures are fixed utilizing indirect reduction techniques and the application of a bridge plate. In this situation, individual reductions of the comminuted fragments are avoided and dissection in the area of the main fracture should be limited. Restoration of length and alignment can be obtained by several methods. The fracture can be brought out to length by the surgeon grasping the bone with pointed reduction forceps or serrated reduction forceps on opposite sides of the fracture, drawing it out to length, and then clamping the plate to the bone to maintain length while screw fixation is obtained.

More reliable methods for restoring and maintaining length and alignment include application of the plate to the distal aspect of the bone with one or two screws placed in the neutral position, then the application of a push-pull screw in the proximal aspect of the plate. A tension distraction device or a lamina spreader is then utilized to push the fracture out to length. During this process, two loosely applied clamps placed perpendicular to one another around the plate will control alignment during the distraction process (Figs. 10.18 and 10.19). When the bone is appropriately brought out to the correct length, two screws are placed in the neutral position; one in close proximity to the fracture and one in the most proximal aspect of the plate. With good indirect technique, bone grafting is not required even in comminuted fractures (Fig. 10.20) (14).

Following plate fixation of both bones of the forearm, the range of motion and the stability of both the proximal and distal radial and ulnar articulations should be checked. In Galeazzi fractures, if the DRUJ is stable through a full range of motion no immobilization is required. If it is only stable in supination, the extremity should be initially splinted and then casted in supination for 6 weeks. If the DRUJ is unstable in all positions, the joint should be reduced and pinned with a 2.0-mm Kirschner (K) wire, and ulnar styloid fractures should be repaired. The extremity should then be immobilized in a cast in the reduced position for 6 weeks.

In Monteggia fractures, if the radial head is not reduced, the fracture reduction needs to be carefully checked to ensure that anatomic length of the ulna has been restored. If

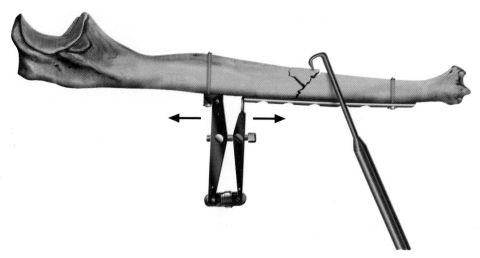

Figure 10.18. Indirect reduction of the ulna is depicted. A laminar spreader and screw are used for distraction of the fracture. The dental pick is used to tease the wedge fragment into position. The laminar spreader is then gradually released, and the fracture is compressed with an eccentrically placed screw.

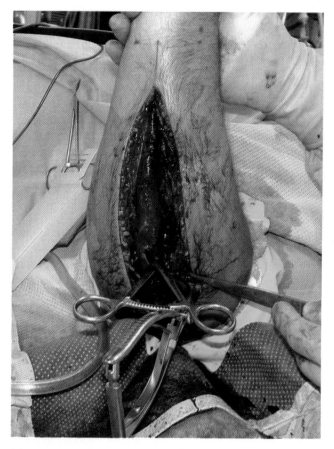

Figure 10.19. A lamina spreader is utilized to push the fracture out to length. During this process, two loosely applied clamps placed perpendicular to one another around the plate will control alignment.

the radial head remains dislocated and the ulna has been correctly reduced, then the proximal radioulnar joint should be explored and the annular ligament reconstructed. If the joint is reduced and stable, then no additional immobilization is required, but if it is unstable, then it should be reduced in a stable position, usually supination, for 6 weeks.

In both-bone forearm fractures, failure to achieve full range of motion under anesthesia suggests residual mal-alignment of the fracture. In all cases, full length radiographs should be obtained in the operating room to ensure accurate fracture reduction. The tourniquet, if utilized, should be deflated prior to closure and hemostasis obtained. The

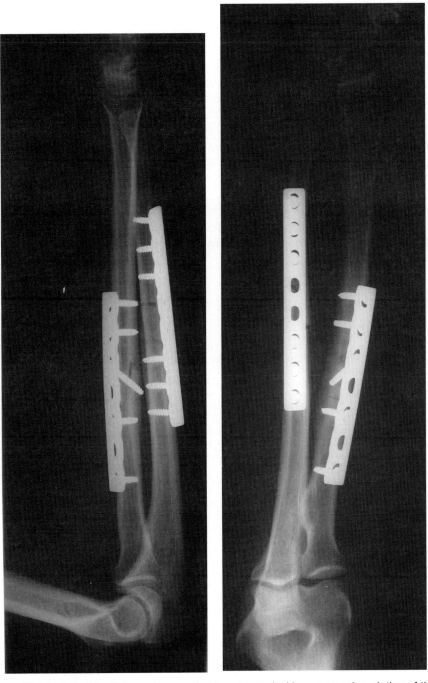

A   B

Figure 10.20. A,B. A both-bone forearm fracture treated with compression plating of the radius and bridge plate fixation of the ulna is shown. A long plate with minimal screw insertion was utilized to minimize bone devitalization.

deep structures, such as the pronator teres, supinator, and pronator quadratus, are placed back in their anatomic locations but do not require repair. The fasciae on both the volar and dorsal exposures are not closed to decrease the likelihood of a compartment syndrome following closure. The skin is then closed with an interrupted no. 2-0 absorbable suture in the subcuticular layer and either a running subcuticular stitch or interrupted nonabsorbable suture.

POSTOPERATIVE CARE

If instability is not found in the proximal or distal radioulnar joint, the surgical incision sites are dressed, and with the wrist in neutral or slight dorsiflexion, a light, volar, wrist splint is applied. This postoperative immobilization is provided to rest the soft tissues and increase the comfort of the patient in the immediate postoperative period. The splint is discontinued on the first postoperative visit, and active-assisted range of motion of the upper extremity is initiated at that time as tolerated. The patient is encouraged to begin using the extremity for activities of daily living, with restrictions against lifting objects greater than 10 to 15 pounds. The lifting restriction is eased at 6 to 10 weeks depending on clinical and radiographic signs of fracture union, and typically all restrictions are removed at approximately 3 to 4 months. Return to work is encouraged with restrictions in the first 7 to 10 days following surgery, and return to sport is allowed 4 to 6 months following injury. Radiographs are obtained on the second postoperative visit, typically 6 weeks following injury, then on a 4 to 6 week basis thereafter until union.

Patients are instructed that the hardware will be retained indefinitely unless complications arise related to internal fixation. Hardware removal before 1 year should be avoided. When it is performed, the patient should be carefully counseled regarding the inherent risk of nerve injury and refracture (15,16).

RECOMMENDED READINGS

1. Dumont CE, Thalmann R, Macy JC. The effect of rotational malunion of the radius and the ulna on supination and pronation. *J Bone Joint Surg Br* 2002;84(7):1070–1074.
2. Schemitsch EH, Richards RR. The effect of malunion on functional outcome after plate fixation of both bones of the forearm in adults. *J Bone Joint Surg Am* 1992;74:1068–1078.
3. Anderson LD, Sisk TD, Tooms RE, et al. Compression-plate fixation in acute diaphyseal fractures of the radius and ulna. *J Bone Joint Surg Am* 1975;57:287–297.
4. Burwell HN, Charnley AD. Treatment of forearm fractures in adults with particular reference to plate fixation. *J Bone Joint Surg Br* 1964;46:404–425.
5. Chapman MW, Gordon JE, Zissimos AG. Compression-plate fixation in acute diaphyseal fractures of the radius and ulna. *J Bone Joint Surg Am* 1989;71:159–169.
6. Duncan R, Geissler W, Freeland AE, et al. Immediate internal fixation of open fractures of the diaphysis of the forearm. *J Orthop Trauma* 1992;6:25–31.
7. Mih AD, Cooney WP, Idler RS, et al. Long-term follow-up of forearm bone diaphyseal plating. *Clin Orthop* 1994;299:256–258.
8. Moed BR, Kellam JF, Foster JR, et al. Immediate internal fixation of open fractures of the diaphysis of the forearm. *J Bone Joint Surg Am* 1986;68:1008–1017.
9. Mackay D, Wood L, Rangan A. The treatment of isolated ulnar fractures in adults: a systematic review. *Injury* 2000;31(8):565–570.
10. Jones JA. Immediate internal fixation of high-energy open forearm fractures. *J Orthop Trauma* 1991;5(3):272–279.
11. Leung F, Chow SP. A prospective, randomized trial comparing the limited contact dynamic compression plate with the point contact fixator for forearm fractures. *J Bone Joint Surg Am* 2003;85(12):2343–2348.
12. Henry WA. *Extensile exposures*. 2nd ed. New York: Churchill Livingstone; 1973:100.
13. Thompson JE. Anatomical methods of approach in operations on the long bones of the extremities. *Ann Surg* 1918;68:309.
14. Wright RR, Schmeling GJ, Schwab JP. The necessity of acute bone grafting in diaphyseal forearm fractures: a retrospective review. *J Orthop Trauma* 1997;11(4):288–294.
15. Beaupre GS, Csongradi JJ. Refracture risk after plate removal in the forearm. *J Orthop Trauma* 1996;10:87–92.
16. Langkamer VG, Ackroyd CE. Removal of forearm plates: a review of complications. *Bone Joint Surg Br* 1990;72:601–604.

11

Forearm Fractures: Intramedullary Nailing

Daniel M. Zinar

INDICATIONS/CONTRAINDICATIONS

Diaphyseal fractures of the forearm in adults are relatively common injuries that usually occur after intermediate or high-energy trauma. With widespread dissemination of the methods of fixation advocated by the AO/ASIF, plate fixation of these injuries has become the gold standard. Numerous authors have shown high rates of union and excellent functional outcomes after plate osteosynthesis of these fractures. The chief drawbacks with this fixation method are the long incisions and wide exposure necessary to reduce and fix the fractures. Radial nerve palsies are common after open reduction and internal fixation (ORIF), and refracture rates of the forearm vary from 1% to 20% and are most common in the proximal one third. Furthermore, the resultant scar can be a significant cosmetic deformity, particularly in female patients.

Intramedullary nailing of forearm fractures is not meant to replace conventional plate fixation. Rather, it is indicated in a small subgroup of patients in whom nailing may be more advantageous than plate osteosynthesis. The indications for intramedullary nailing of the radius and ulna include segmental fractures, gunshot fractures with severe comminution, refracture of the forearm after plate removal, fracture occurring above or below an existing plate, unstable fractures in children or adolescents, and fractures in athletes who participate in contact sports.

Forearm nailing is contraindicated in adults whose intramedullary canal measures less than 3 mm at the narrowest point. Fractures less than 3 cm from the proximal or distal end of the bone should not be nailed because of inadequate fixation of the short segment of bone (Fig. 11.1). Nailing should be avoided in patients with preexisting deformity of the forearm that would preclude nailing without an osteotomy. Finally, nailing is not the fixation method of first choice to stabilize corrective osteotomies or treat nonunions.

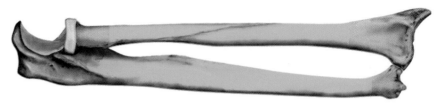

Figure 11.1. Portion of radius and ulna that can be treated with an interlocking forearm nail. At least 3 cm of intact bone on either end must be present.

PREOPERATIVE PLANNING

Forearm fractures may occur as an isolated injury or after multiple trauma. In the severely injured patient, basic and advanced trauma life support (ATLS) and a full trauma evaluation and resuscitation are mandatory. Once life-threatening and limb-threatening injuries have been addressed, the injured arm is carefully evaluated. The entire upper extremity is inspected for open wounds, ecchymosis, abrasion, deformity, and other injury. The limb is palpated from shoulder to fingers by the surgeon looking for areas of tenderness or fracture crepitus. Ipsilateral injuries to the shoulder, upper arm, elbow, wrist, and hand commonly occur after high-energy trauma. The arm is critically examined to ensure that a compartment syndrome does not exist. If the surgeon has any doubt, the compartment pressure should be measured. After the lower leg, the forearm is the second most common site for a compartment syndrome. The axillary, brachial, radial, and ulnar pulses should be palpated and compared with those of the opposite side. The sensory and motor components of the radial, medial, and ulnar nerves must be documented. In patients with proximal injuries, the function of the brachial plexus requires evaluation. If the fracture is open, the wounds should be sterilely dressed, the limb splinted, and intravenous antibiotics administered. The patient should be brought to the operating room as soon as possible for irrigation and debridement.

Anteroposterior (AP) and lateral radiographs of the entire injured and uninjured forearm are obtained to determine proper nail length, diameter, and radial bow. Three methods of determining correct nail length are used: First, the patient's uninjured arm is measured with a tape measure from the tip of the olecranon to the ulnar styloid, and 1 cm is subtracted from the measurement; second, a nail of known length is intraoperatively placed against the affected bone while traction is used to keep the bone to the appropriate length, and the fit of the nail is checked fluoroscopically; or third, the fit is checked preoperatively through the use of radiographic templates with known magnification parameters. Because the radial head is often difficult to palpate, the radial length can be determined by subtracting 2 cm from the ulnar length.

Special projections, such as oblique radiographs, computed tomography (CT) scanning, or other imaging modalities, are not helpful in preoperative planning.

SURGERY

General anesthesia is preferred over regional anesthesia because the relaxation obtained improves the chances of achieving a closed reduction. Closed nailing is more successful if surgery is done within 72 hours of injury. The patient is placed supine on an operating table, and a radiolucent arm table is used to support the extremity (Fig. 11.2). A mobile, C-arm, image intensifier is brought in from the head of the table. The surgeon sits at the axilla while the assistant is positioned at the end of the hand table. For ulnar nailing, the shoulder is abducted and internally rotated, and the elbow is flexed to 90 degrees. The elbow is "bumped" with a stack of towels for easier access to the olecranon (Fig. 11.3).

Fracture reduction can be accomplished by a closed or open method. Closed nailing is preferable because it preserves blood supply and enhances fracture healing. Closed reduction is achieved by longitudinal traction or direct pressure at the fracture site. Traction

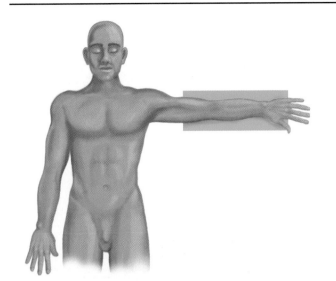

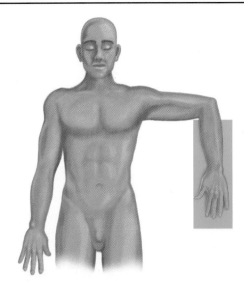

Figure 11.2. The patient is positioned supine with a radiolucent arm board. The surgeon sits facing the axilla, while the image intensifier comes in from the head of the table. A stack of towels is placed under the wrist.

Figure 11.3. With nailing of the ulna, the elbow is bent 90 degrees for access to olecranon, where the surgeon will place the entry portal. A stack of towels is placed under the elbow.

devices with finger traps have not been successful. The surgical assistant should wear sterile lead gloves to minimize radiation exposure to his/her hands. When the fracture fragments are locked in bayonet apposition, a mini–open technique through a 2- to 4-cm incision may be used to reduce the fragments (Fig. 11.4).

Entry Portal

A tourniquet is used whenever possible to minimize blood loss. If both bones are fractured, the radius is approached first. However, both bones are prepared for nailing before nailing is initiated in either bone. A 1.5-cm incision is made just lateral to Lister's tubercle at the distal radius (Fig. 11.5). The extensor pollicis longus (EPL) tendon is identified and

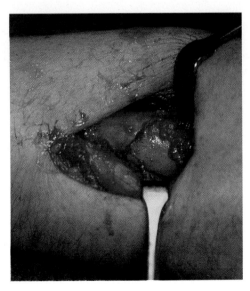

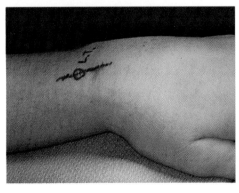

Figure 11.4. A 4-cm mini–open incision is used to reduce a completely displaced fracture of the radius.

Figure 11.5. A 2-cm incision is centered over Lister's tubercle for creation of an entry portal into the radius.

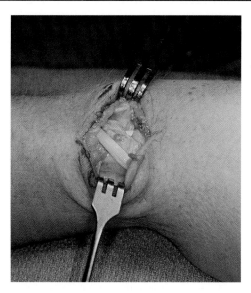

Figure 11.6. The extensor retinaculum is divided to expose the EPL tendon. The EPL tendon is then released from its surrounding sheath.

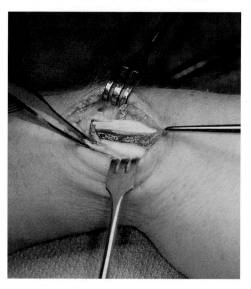

Figure 11.7. The interval between the extensor carpi radialis longus (ECRL) is developed. The EPL is retracted radially with the ECRL.

released from its sheath around Lister's tubercle (Fig.11.6). The interval between the short and long wrist extensors is identified (Fig. 11.7). The surgeon must identify the distal edge of the radius to avoid inadvertent insertion through the scaphoid. The medullary canal is entered obliquely through a 2.0-mm pilot drill hole at the dorsal margin of the radius (Fig. 11.8). The wrist is flexed and placed over a stack of towels to prevent inadvertent perforation of the volar cortex (Fig. 11.9). The entry portal is enlarged with a cannulated 6.0-mm reamer (Fig. 11.10).

Because the ulna bows toward the radius in the proximal third, the point of insertion for the ulna is toward the radial side of the olecranon, and is made approximately 5 mm from the lateral cortex. A 1-cm incision is made with the 2.0-mm drill to access the medullary canal, and then a 6-mm cannulated reamer is used.

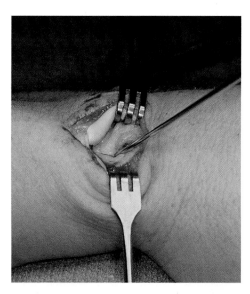

Figure 11.8. The 2.0-mm guide pin is introduced at a point 5 mm from the distal edge of the radius. The pin is started vertically so entry into the bone can be gained.

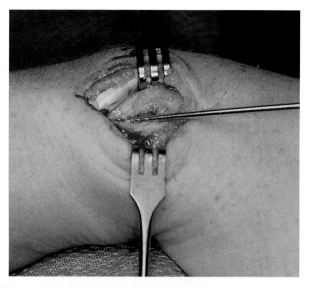

Figure 11.9. The wrist is flexed, and the pin is brought into a more horizontal direction to avoid penetration of the volar cortex.

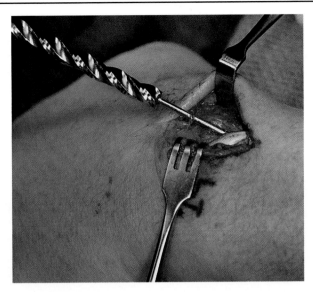

Figure 11.10. To enlarge the entry portal, the surgeon introduces a 6-mm cannulated reamer over the 2.0-mm trocar wire.

Canal Preparation

Proper-sized reamers are essential for successful nailing because they help the surgeon avoid nail incarceration. Both hand and power reamers are available (Fig. 11.11). Small end-cutting and side-cutting reamers are manufactured by Smith & Nephew Richards (Memphis, TN). The narrowest portion of the intramedullary canal may range from 3 to 7 mm. Preoperative canal sizing is used to determine whether reaming is necessary before nail insertion. The medullary canal should be overreamed by 0.5 to 1.0 mm to prevent nail incarceration, fracture comminution, or distraction at the fracture site.

Whether open or closed nailing is performed, both fractures should be reduced and prepared before either bone can be nailed; otherwise, the stability of the nailed bone may make reduction of the other fracture difficult. When closed nailing is performed, the rotational control obtained by the interference fit of the nail is less important than it is with open nailing. If open nailing is performed, the canal may be reamed from the fracture site (Fig. 11.12). After the last reamer is used, it is replaced with a 2.4-mm, straight, guide rod. The

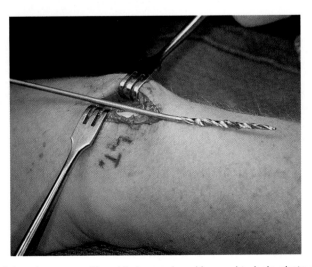

Figure 11.11. A hand reamer with a 15-degree bend is used to help skate off the volar cortex. Reamers are available in sizes from 3.0 to 5.5 mm in 5-mm increments.

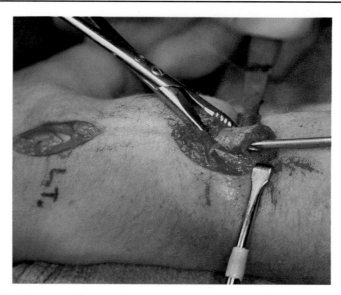

Figure 11.12. To prepare the canal at the fracture site, the surgeon uses a power reamer during an open nailing.

radius is reduced and temporarily stabilized with a guide rod. The ulna is prepared in a fashion similar to that of the radius.

Forearm nails are manufactured in several different materials and shapes. Some are made of stainless steel, and others are comprised of titanium. Some are prebent to conform to the normal dorsoradial bow of the radius and lateral ulna bow. Other nails are straight and must be contoured with a nail bender before insertion. The radial nail should be contoured with respect to the normal dorsoradial bow. The angle to which the nail should be bent can be determined through radiographs of the uninjured forearm. This process is similar to that used to bend reconstruction plates before implantation (Fig. 11.13). After proper nail contouring (Fig. 11.14), orientation of the implant with respect to anatomy is most important. After assembly of the nail on the driver and drill guide (Fig. 11.15), the nail is inserted with hand pressure or light hammering. Proper rotational alignment is confirmed by the use of the image intensifier. Orientation of the bicipital tuberosity and the radial styloid is helpful in confirming correct rotation of the radius. In addition, at the completion of the procedure, an intraoperative check of the arc of forearm rotation is essential to prevent malreduction. The nail is seated so that the driving end is countersunk just below the cortex (Fig. 11.16).

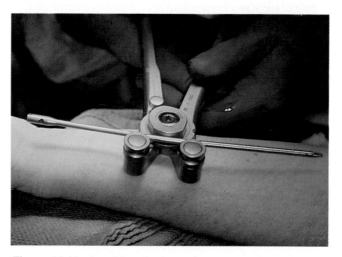

Figure 11.13. A nail bender is used to contour the radial nail.

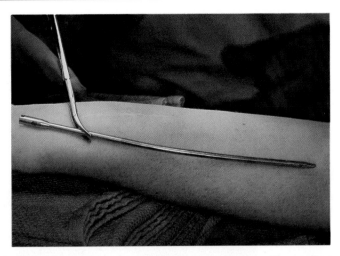

Figure 11.14. The nail is bent to re-create the dorsoradial bow. The amount of bow can be determined by preoperatively measuring the radiographs of the uninjured radius.

Interlocking Screw Insertion

The nail can be locked statically (screws at both ends) or dynamically (screws at only one end). Fracture stability, expected patient compliance, and appropriate level of postoperative immobilization all must be considered. For unstable fracture patterns, possible noncompliant patients, and patients who desire to be free of any postoperative immobilization, static locking should be performed for optimal rotational control and length maintenance. If the surgeon has any doubt about the length or rotational stability of the fracture, static interlocking should be done.

A 2.0-mm drill is used to prepare both the distal and proximal interlocking screws (Fig. 11.17). One, 2.7-mm, fully threaded, locking screw is placed through a targeting guide on the driving end of the nail. In the radius, this screw is placed from radial to ulnar through a 1-cm incision (Fig. 11.18). The soft tissues are spread to make sure the drill guide is firmly on bone to avoid injury to the superficial branch of the radial nerve. To avoid injury to the ulnar nerve, the driving end screw is placed from ulnar to radial through a l-cm incision of the ulna.

Interlocking the far end of the nail is difficult. It is done with the aid of an image intensifier in magnification mode. A perfect circle view of the hole is obtained. To avoid injury to the posterior interosseous nerve, the surgeon makes an incision to expose the bone in the proximal radius. To decrease the possibility of injury to the posterior interosseous nerve, the arm should be kept in neutral position with the hole no more than 3 cm from the end of the radius. The length of the screw is measured from a calibrated drill, and a unicortical 2.7-mm screw is inserted.

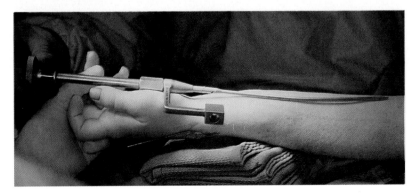

Figure 11.15. The nail driver and proximal targeting guide are assembled. Orientation of the nail in relation to the normal, dorsal, radial bow is shown.

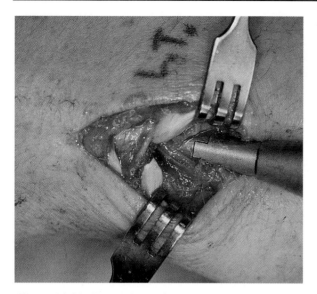

Figure 11.16. The nail is seated so that the female end is countersunk just below the cortex to avoid irritation of the extensor tendons.

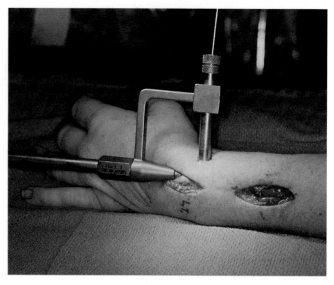

Figure 11.17. A 1.5-cm incision is made to insert the driving-end interlocking screw. Drill and screw guides must be placed onto bone to avoid injury to the superficial branch of the radial nerve.

After placement of the screws, the range of motion of the arm is checked, and the arc of rotation is recorded. Both screw holes are checked via image intensification to ensure proper position of the nail and screws.

Bone Grafting

With closed nailing, bone grafting is not usually necessary. If nailing is done as an open procedure, a primary bone graft should be done, especially if comminution, a bone defect, or any distraction or gap at the fracture site is present. When small amounts are needed, bone from the reamed area at the entry portal may be sufficient (Fig. 11.19). Cancellous

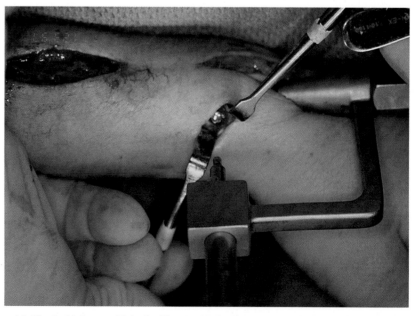

Figure 11.18. A driving-end interlocking screw is shown seated on bone. Image intensification is used to verify that the screw has engaged the hole in the nail.

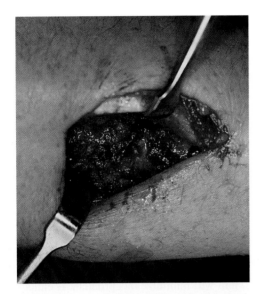

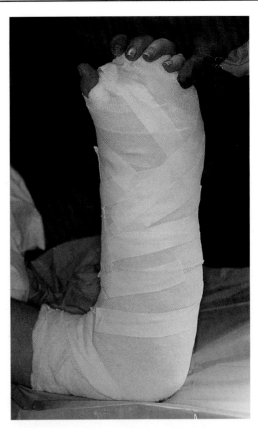

Figure 11.19. Bone graft obtained from the reamed entry portal is used to pack around the fracture site through the mini–open incision.

Figure 11.20. To reduce swelling and control pain, a bulky hand dressing is postoperatively incorporated via use of a sugar-tong splint that provides even compression. The dressing is removed at 2 postoperative weeks for suture removal.

bone from the distal radius or proximal ulna can also be used. If larger amounts of bone are needed, an iliac-crest bone graft should be obtained. We have no experience with the use of bone-bank grafts or synthetic bone in conjunction with forearm nailing.

POSTOPERATIVE MANAGEMENT

If secure fixation is achieved in a compliant patient, then a long-arm posterior splint or sugar-tong splint is applied for 2 weeks (Fig. 11.20). In noncompliant patients or in patients whose nailing was done as an open procedure or was dynamically locked, the arm is immobilized for 4 to 6 weeks. Heavy lifting and twisting should be avoided for 3 months. Patients are followed up at monthly intervals to determine clinical outcomes and assess radiographic evidence of healing. Recreational activities such as golf or tennis are permitted at approximately 6 months. Hardware removal is not recommended unless the patient is severely symptomatic.

At Los Angeles County, Harbor-University of California at the Los Angeles Medical Center, both retrospective and prospective reviews have been completed to evaluate forearm nailing by Langkamer and Ackroyd; Marek; and Rush and Rush. Union rates of 97% have been reported with good and excellent results in 25 patients. This compares favorably with results of other series of forearm fractures treated with plating. All studies emphasized the need for proper patient selection and careful surgical technique with attention to detail. Ulna nailing was described successfully by De Pedro et al.

Marek reported that neither nonunions nor infections were found in his series of patients treated with intramedullary nailing. Street et al reported a 93% union rate in their series of patients treated with a square forearm nail. Studies by DePedro et al have correlated accuracy of reduction and the restoration of radial bow in forearm fractures with return of function.

COMPLICATIONS

The most common complications of forearm nailing include nail incarceration, iatrogenic comminution of the fracture, fracture distraction, nonunion, and cortical perforation during reaming or nail insertion. Successful nailing eliminates the problem of refracture after implant removal, which has been reported with plating of forearm fractures. The major complication of nonunion can be minimized if (a) closed nailing is done whenever possible, (b) distraction at the fracture site is avoided, and (c) bone grafting is done when open nailing is necessary in comminuted fractures. Radiographic evidence of consolidation at the fracture can be slow and should not limit restoration of function. Technical problems such as nail incarceration, fracture distraction, iatrogenic comminution, and cortical perforation are preventable with careful attention to surgical technique and preoperative planning.

Nail incarceration is the most common complication. The surgeon can avoid it by making sure that the nail advances with each blow of the hammer. A change in pitch should alert the surgeon that the nail may be too tight. Removal of the nail with a vise grip or splitting of the cortex may be necessary to remove an incarcerated nail. This correction is followed by overreaming of the canal by 1 mm and reinsertion of the nail with static locking.

Fracture distraction and iatrogenic comminution also can be prevented by proper canal preparation. Overreaming by 0.5 to 1.0 mm will minimize this problem. If either of these occurs during open nailing, then bone grafting is recommended.

Nonunion is best managed by compression-plate osteosynthesis. Hypertrophic nonunion does not require bone grafting. Atrophic nonunions should be treated with plating and supplemental, cancellous, bone grafts.

Cortical perforation usually occurs during creation of the entry portal into the radius. Flexion of the wrist to 90 degrees over a stack of towels will prevent the drill or reamer (or both) from exiting through the volar cortex.

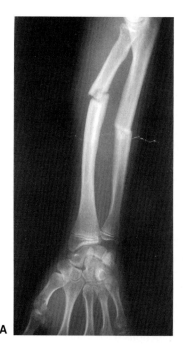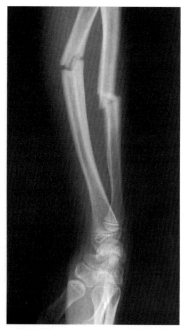

Figure 11.21. AP **(A)** and lateral **(B)** radiograph of preoperative radius and ulna.

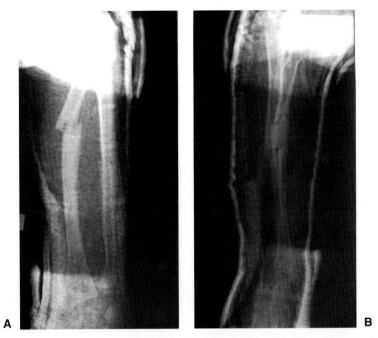

Figure 11.22. Preoperative AP **(A)** and lateral **(B)** radiograph after closed reduction.

ILLUSTRATIVE CASE FOR TECHNIQUE

A 16-year-old male presented with a radius and an ulna fracture after having sustained a forearm fracture 6 months before (Fig. 11.21). Closed reduction had been performed with an unsatisfactory result (Fig. 11.22). In the second treatment, closed nailing was performed (Fig. 11.23). The fracture had healed at 8 postoperative weeks operatively and patient enjoyed full restoration of function.

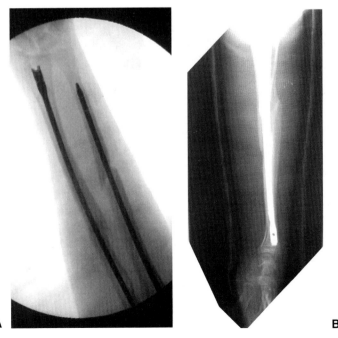

Figure 11.23. Postoperative AP **(A)** and lateral **(B)** radiographs after closed nailing.

RECOMMENDED READING

Amit Y, Salai M, Checkik A, et al. Closing intramedullary nailing for the treatment of diaphyseal fore-arm fractures in adolescence: a preliminary report. *J Pediatr Orthop* 1985;5:143–146.

Anderson LD, Sisk TD, Tooms RE, et al. Compression-plate fixation in acute diaphyseal fractures of the radius and ulna. *J Bone Joint Surg Am* 1975;57:287.

Chapman MW, Gordon JE, Zissimos AG. Compression-plate fixation of acute fractures of the diaphyses of the radius and ulna. *J Bone Joint Surg Am* 1989;71:159.

De Pedro JA, Garcia-Navarette F, DeLucas FG, et al. Internal fixation of ulnar fractures by locking nail. *Clin Orthop* 1992;283:81.

Hidaka S, Gustilo RB. Refracture of bones of the forearm after plate removal. *J Bone Joint Surg Am* 1984;66:1241.

Langkamer VG, Ackroyd CE. Safe forearm plate removal: fact or fallacy? *J Bone Joint Surg Br* 1989;71:875.

Marek FM. Axial fixation of forearm fractures. *J Bone Joint Surg Am* 1961;41:1099.

Rush LV, Rush HL. Technique for longitudinal pin fixation of certain fractures of the ulna and of the femur. *J Bone Joint Surg* 21:619, 1939.

Schemitsch E, Richards R. The effect of malunion on functional outcome of fractures of both bones of the forearm in adults. *J Bone Joint Surg Am* 1992;74:1068.

Smith H, Sage FP. Medullary fixation of forearm fractures. *J Bone Joint Surg Am.* 1957;39:91.

Street, D. Intramedullary forearm nailing. *Clin Orthop* 1986;212:219.

Street D, Plut J, Wood W. Intramedullary forearm nailing. Paper presented at: American Academy of Orthopaedic Surgeons Exhibit, 1979.

Street DM. Medullary nailing of forearm fractures. *J Bone Joint Surg Am* 1957; 39:715.

Wolgin M, Zinar DM: Intramedullary fixation of forearm fractures using the Street square forearm nail. Paper presented at: American Academy of Orthopaedic Surgeons meeting; 1990; New Orleans, LA.

Zinar DM, Wolgin M, et al. Prospective evaluation of forearm i.m. nailing. Paper presented at: American Academy of Orthopaedic Surgeons Meeting; 1992; Washington, DC.

12

Distal Radius Fractures: External Fixation

Michael W. Grafe, Paul D. Kim, and
Melvin P. Rosenwasser

Distal radius fractures are one of the most common injuries in clinical practice. They tend to occur in a bimodal fashion with a peak associated in children and adolescents as well as elderly patients. Nonarticular fractures of the distal radius and most epiphyseal fractures in children are typically treated, with predictable success, by cast immobilization. With increasing age, osteoporosis and falls lead to fragility fractures of the distal radius, particularly in women. These fractures often have significant fracture comminution with instability, making closed treatment less successful. In young patients with normal bone stock, these fractures are often caused by motor vehicle accidents or a fall from a height, and they often result in highly comminuted fracture patterns. While many of these fractures can be reduced by closed means, comminution and instability lead to loss of reduction and malunion.

The inability to maintain fracture alignment by closed reduction and casting defines fracture instability. Many authors have proposed criteria to predict which fracture patterns are inherently unstable and may benefit from surgical treatment. Lafontaine et al (1) proposed five factors that indicated fracture instability: (a) initial dorsal angulation greater than 20 degrees, (b) dorsal comminution, (c) radiocarpal intra-articular involvement, (d) associated ulnar fractures, and (e) age greater than 60 years. In their experience, patients with three or more of these factors had a high incidence of reduction loss with cast treatment. Nesbitt et al (2) used the criteria of Lafontaine et al and determined that age was the only significant risk factor in predicting instability. In patients over the age of 58 years, there was a 50% risk for secondary displacement, while patients over 80 years had a 77% increased risk. In addition to the Lafontaine factors, carpal malalignment and postreduction incongruity (the combination of articular step-off and fracture gap) have been shown to have a negative impact on functional outcome (3,4).

In the past decade, new implants for fixation of unstable distal-radius fractures have become available, especially the use of anatomically designed plates for the volar, radial, and dorsal aspects of the radius. In the past, external fixation had been the workhorse for unstable distal-radius fractures which had been judged to be too unstable for cast treatment. With advances in internal fixation, external fixation is used more commonly as an adjunctive procedure to other fixation techniques. These techniques include Kirschner (K) wire fixation, Kapandji pin technique, arthroscopically assisted articular-surface reduction (5) and the placement of fragment-specific miniplates. These techniques are frequently augmented with metaphyseal bone fillers such as cancellous allograft chips and hydroxyapatite cement. Thus, external fixation devices that span the fracture can be used to neutralize the forces around the wrist and to protect the fracture reduction obtained by other direct or indirect means.

In some cases a non–joint-spanning external fixator can be used as both the reduction tool and the neutralization device. This is accomplished through the use of dorsally applied half pins which can directly manipulate and reduce displaced fragments. This construct combines the principle of Kapandji, dorsal, and blocking pins with the security of half pins locked to the frame. It also improves restoration of palmar tilt, which is difficult to accomplish with spanning frames (6).

CLINICAL EVALUATION

A careful history and physical examination, including information gathering on hand dominance, occupational requirements, medical co-morbidities, and patient expectations, are important factors in crafting a treatment strategy. The mechanism of injury and a careful examination of the limb allow the surgeon to assess soft-tissue integrity. Any signs or symptoms of increased compartment pressure or evolving neurological deficits mandate that any splints or cast be removed for more precise evaluation and treatment. Furthermore, it is necessary to check the forearm and elbow for instability and the possibility of combined fracture-dislocation patterns such as Galeazzi, Monteggia, or Essex-Lopresti injuries. The carpus should be carefully palpated to determine if any focal sources of pain or deformity can be found in carpal injuries or dislocations. The hand should also be carefully evaluated for signs and symptoms of injuries to the metacarpals and phalanges.

Careful, systematic examination of the hand for sensation and motor integrity should be documented and the results assessed. The encompassing, and often incorrect assumption of "neurovascularly intact," should not be used when evaluating patients with a distal radius fracture.

Unrelated, but often present, osteoarthritis of the digits, especially the basal joint of the thumb, should be noted. Often joints with preexistent stiffness are adversely affected by the postfracture swelling, pain, and immobilization, and as a result hand function is compromised.

Acute, concomitant tendon injuries are rare following closed distal-radius fractures. However, the surgeon should caution patients about the small risk of late, extensor pollicis longus (EPL) tendon ruptures.

Extrinsic motor function can be simply assessed by asking the patient to grasp, and to confirm anterior interosseous nerve integrity, by paying particular attention to the flexor pollicis longus (FPL) and flexor digitorum profundus (FDP) to the index finger. Abducting and adducting the second ray will confirm ulnar-nerve intrinsic function. Tip pinch will confirm median nerve thenar function.

IMAGING

Following falls or injuries to the wrist, anteroposterior (AP) (7), lateral, and oblique radiographs should be obtained. True lateral x-rays of the wrist are more difficult to obtain when the wrist is immobilized in flexion and ulnar deviation. Contralateral films can be helpful in assessing the normal radial and ulnar lengths as well as radial inclination of the wrist.

A critical review of the initial injury films can be useful in predicting the magnitude of the forces involved as well as the displacement and comminution. Traction films obtained in the emergency room or operating room will allow assessment of articular incongruities such as scaphoid or lunate die-punch injuries. Traction films can also reveal subtle, combined, carpal bone and or ligamentous injury (i.e., transradial styloid-perilunate instability).

Ulnar styloid fractures occur in more than one half of all distal-radius fractures. Although most ulnar styloid fractures heal uneventfully with a fibrous union, some ulnar-styloid fractures are associated with distal radioulnar joint (DRUJ) instability. Ulnar styloid fractures that occur through the base and those displaced greater than 2 mm have highest likelihood of associated DRUJ instability (8). However, DRUJ stability is assessed following stabilization of the radial fracture.

Parameters of acceptable reduction are restoration of radial length to within 2 to 3 mm of uninjured wrist. Radial inclination is approximately 21 degrees and radiocarpal congruence is within 1 mm. The lateral view should demonstrate a collinear relationship with the radial shaft and lunocapitate axis: There should be no more than 5 to 10 degrees of articular dorsal tilt and preferably neutral or inclined toward the normal 10-degree palmar tilt.

Carpal alignment will generally follow the gross reduction of the distal radius. Residual angular or rotational instability, such as dorsal, intercalated, segment instability (DISI), is usually a sign of laxity of the extrinsic capsular ligaments, which can occur secondary to a loss of axial length or from rupture. The peri-articular shear fractures, either dorsal or palmar, are essentially ligamentous injuries that require secure repositioning of the fracture to effect stable reduction. Assessment of the break in the carpal arcs, as described by Sarmiento et al (9), should be recognized; these breaks may be unmasked by traction films taken in the emergency or operating room.

Computerized tomography (CT) scans are not routinely necessary for preoperative planning. In fact, standard two dimensional CT scans done prior to reduction may create more confusion in interpreting the position of unstable, unreduced fragments. We prefer a traction film taken in the operating room for its simplicity in preoperative planning.

TREATMENT PARADIGM

Based on a careful history and physical examination, as well as a thorough review of the radiographs, surgical or nonsurgical treatment is recommended. Based on criteria elaborated previously, we attempt to identify stable and unstable fracture patterns. The ultimate treatment plan is based upon the patient's expectations, functional requirements, and medical conditions; each plays a role in the indication for surgery. With regard to marked loss of radial length, radial inclination, and reversal of palmar tilt, numerous studies have shown measurable deficits in the objective and subjective outcomes following cast treatment. These differences in outcomes are magnified when loss of articular congruence and carpal subluxation are found (3,4). Treatment decisions should be made in the context of the entire person and not on the radiographic findings alone.

Most patients with displaced distal-radius fractures seen in the emergency room undergo a closed reduction and application of a sugar tong splint with application of a Bier block or a fracture hematoma injection. If a hematoma block is used, one must remember to also inject the ulnocarpal joint to achieve complete anesthesia of the injury. The ulnar side of the wrist joint is almost always involved in a distal radius fracture through an ulnar styloid fracture or peripheral triangular, fibrocartilage complex (TFCC) tear.

Nonsurgical treatment can be considered if postreduction radiographs show restoration of radial length, minimal loss of palmar tilt, and most important, good cortical apposition and minimal fracture comminution. The wrist is held in slight flexion, ulnar deviation, and neutral forearm rotation. Weekly follow-up x-rays for the first 3 weeks are necessary to guard against loss of reduction. The palmar extent of the cast must always be contoured to allow for full metacarpal-phalangeal joint flexion. Casting usually continues for 6 weeks followed by transitional splinting with a removal prefabricated splint. If finger motion can be maintained, then little formal occupational therapy is required. If stiffness or swelling in the immediate postreduction period is significant, then supervised occupation therapy is recommended.

If the fracture is deemed unstable by the criteria of Lafontaine (1), then surgical management is indicated in all but the most elderly or infirm. In most cases, it is better to perform primary osteosynthesis rather than late three-dimensional osteotomy and grafting.

Although most unstable distal-radius fractures can be treated with external fixation, few should be treated with a spanning construct alone. The fracture morphology usually will dictate if additional or augmented fixation is necessary (10). This may include Kapandji dorsal intrafracture K wire pinning, transradial styloid-interosseous pinning, and metaphyseal-bone filler support with allograft or hydroxyapatite-based bone cements (11). In minimally comminuted fractures, with sufficient distal-fragment bone stock, a non–joint-spanning external fixation may be a superior technique for restoring the radial length, inclination, and palmar tilt (6). Dorsal volar-shearing type fractures, such as Smith and volar Barton, should be treated with a buttress plate. Scaphoid or lunate die-punch injuries should be treated with elevation of fragments and subchondral support which can often be performed with arthroscopic assistance (12).

SURGICAL TECHNIQUES

Surgery is performed under general or regional anesthesia with either an infraclavicular or axillary block. This is performed with nerve stimulation assistance to avoid transaxillary arterial puncture. Regional anesthesia allows full muscle relaxation and postsurgical pain relief for 8 to 12 hours.

The patient is placed supine on the operative table, and the arm is abducted and placed on a radiolucent arm board. A C-arm image intensifier must be available. A first generation cephalosporin is given intravenously prior to the inflation of the arm tourniquet, which is used in all cases. If a penicillin allergy exists, vancomycin is substituted.

The arm is prepped and draped, and the tourniquet pressure is set at 250 mm Hg in the adult, but for very large or small circumference limbs, it may be adjusted to within 70 mm Hg of mean systolic pressure. Tourniquet times should be limited to less than 120 minutes to limit muscle weakness from prolonged tissue ischemia.

We routinely utilize a sterile, horizontally applied, traction apparatus attached to the arm board to assist in preliminary fracture reduction. The traction apparatus can also be used to facilitate intraoperative traction radiographs. It can also help with the application of adjunctive K wire fixation prior to the distraction through the completed external-fixation construct.

When arthroscopy is used, the equipment is positioned near the foot of the bed. The overhead traction tower may also be used to facilitate the arthroscopic examination.

K Wire Fixation

In most patients with dorsal comminution and angulation of the distal fragment, we employ a combination of K wire insertion techniques following fracture reduction. The Kapandji technique is useful in providing a prop or support to prevent gradual fracture resettling that is secondary to dorsal cortex incompetence. We use two or three dorsal, intrafocal 0.625 K wires. The K wires are introduced by hand directly into the fracture site and up to but not through the palmar cortex. Respecting the dorsal extensor tendon, we place one wire radial to the fourth dorsal compartment and another ulnar to the fourth compartment. The power wire driver is used to assist this process if the bone is particularly dense. The pin is then directed distally to affect a clockwise rotatory force to correct the dorsal displacement and reversal of palmar tilt. Once this is accomplished, the K wire is then driven in a retrograde fashion to engage the palmar cortex and is thus stabilized against migration. The force and direction of the Kapandji pins tends to translate the distal radius fragment in a palmar direction. This tendency is accentuated when the palmar cortex is comminuted. To prevent this secondary deformity of overreduction, one must place a transradial, styloid, intramedullary pin. Following placement of the K wires, we favor a neutralizing, spanning, external-fixation frame until fracture union. We prefer to leave K wires percutaneous to allow for ease of removal in the outpatient. The K wires are cut, with 2 to 3 cm protruding from the skin, and then pin caps are applied (Figs. 12.1 and 12.2).

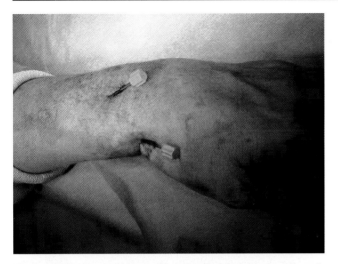

Figure 12.1. Dorsal Kapandji and radial styloid pins placed.

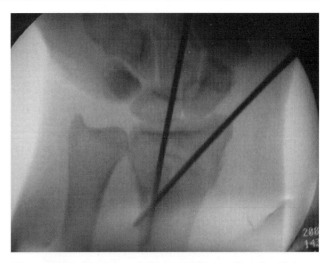

Figure 12.2. Fluoroscopic image of Kapandji and radial styloid pins.

If the reduction is deemed satisfactory, a decision is made regarding the presence and magnitude of residual, metaphyseal, bone loss. Many patients with severe osteopenia will have significant bony defects that can lead to late settling and reduction loss despite proper placement of K wires (11). Placing a bone filler or substitute is effective and avoids the morbidity of an iliac-crest bone graft. We use freeze-dried, allograft, cancellous-bone chips, which can be crushed and placed into the void with an impaction grafting technique. This will supplement the fixation with rapid incorporation and remodeling (7). This technique also decreases the stress on the K wire and external fixation construct, and therefore, it can prevent late settling and loss of radial length even after the external fixation frame is removed. One can also use hydroxyapatite cements, which provide similar mechanical support, but with some reduction in bone remodeling that is secondary to slow, and perhaps, incomplete resorption (10).

A 2-cm longitudinal incision is made between the third and fourth dorsal compartments just ulnar to Lister's tubercle. The proximal extensor retinaculum is divided. The EPL is retracted radially and the extensor digiti communis (EDC) is retracted ulnarly. The fracture site is visualized and used as the window for bone grafting. A cavity is then created within the fracture site. This is done by compacting and compressing the cancellous bone within the metaphysis of the distal radius. The crushed cancellous bone chips are then place into the void. They are then impacted with an elevator against the subchondral surface until the entire void is filled with the allograft chips (Figs. 12.3 and 12.4).

Arthroscopically Assisted Articular Reduction

Wrist arthroscopy can be helpful for reduction of selected articular-fracture fragments. These injuries can be reduced from the metaphyseal side with elevators as a prelude to bone or bone substitute grafting. However, certain fractures will not reduce this way and arthroscopy is less invasive than a formal arthrotomy. Arthroscopy is performed with vertically applied traction. This setup allows for intraoperative fluoroscopy and extra-articular K wire elevators can be used to fine tune the reduction (Fig. 12.5).

Traction is applied through sterile finger traps to the index and long fingers and is generally set at 4.5 kg. Care is taken to pad and protect the ulnar nerve. Arthroscopy portals are outlined with a skin marker and follow the dorsal compartment intervals. The workhorse portals are the 3–4 and 4–5, but all may be used. Dorsal veins are noted so that they are avoided during portal creation.

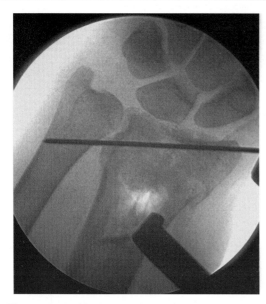

Figure 12.3. Metaphyseal void under fluoroscopy.

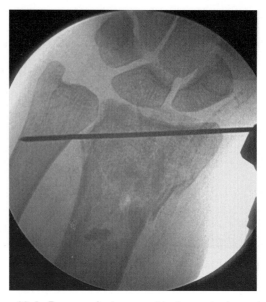

Figure 12.4. Bone graft placement in the metaphyseal void under fluoroscopy.

Prior to arthroscopy, the tourniquet is inflated. The joint is then distended with 3 to 5 cc of normal saline injected through the 3–4 portal. Joint triangulation is tested with an 18-gauge needle. The portals are then created with a nick-and-spread method to protect the articular cartilage from iatrogenic injury. A 2 to 3 mm incision is made with a no. 11 blade and then a small, curved hemostat is used to penetrate the dorsal joint capsule. A hemostat is spread wide enough to allow a 2.7-mm blunt trochar and cannula to be inserted into the 3–4 portal. Visualization is usually obscured with clotted blood in the joint. This is rapidly cleared with pressurized joint lavage set at a maximum of 25 mm Hg. A synovial shaver can also help clear joint debris quickly. In many patients, there is an articular defect on the carpal side of the injury from axial load and impaction. One major additional benefit of arthroscopy is the ability to evaluate intercarpal ligament injuries, as well as TFCC tears, which are common and often unrecognized (13). Extra-articular placement of joystick K wires and bone elevators allows reduction and elevation of fragments, which can then be secured by subchondral wires and supported by a spanning, external, fixation frame and a bone graft or filler as indicated (Fig. 12.6).

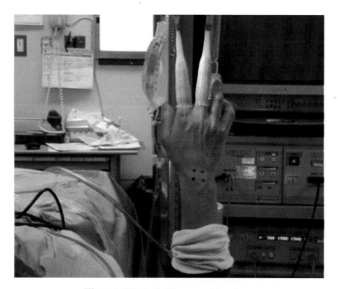

Figure 12.5. Arthroscopic setup.

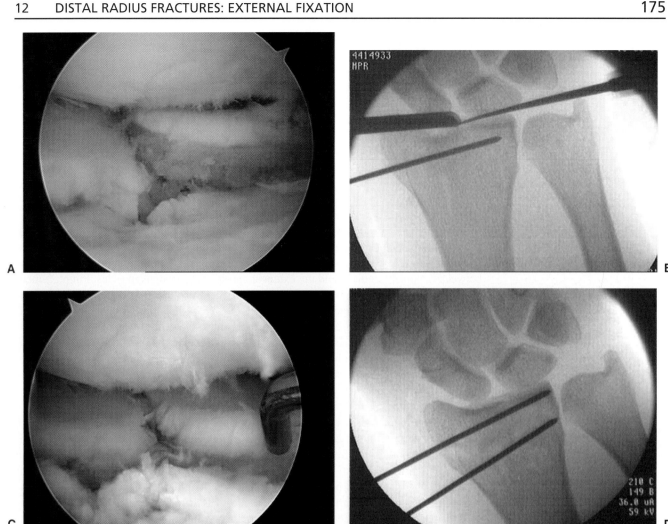

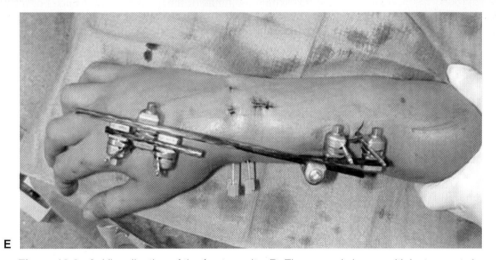

Figure 12.6. A. Visualization of the fracture site. **B.** Fluoroscopic image with instruments in place. **C.** After arthroscopically assisted articular reduction of the fracture site. **D.** K wires used to hold together the reduction. **E.** After arthroscopically assisted reduction, an external fixator is placed. Note the midline dorsal incision where the metaphyseal bone graft was placed.

External Fixation Technique

Once the percutaneous or limited open reduction of the fracture has been accomplished, a decision to proceed with either non–joint-spanning or joint-spanning external fixation is made. If the distal fracture fragment is large enough, we always prefer to use a non–joint-spanning external fixator. However, if the fracture fragment is too small or if there is too much comminution, then we will use a spanning external fixator.

Several studies support the use of non–joint-spanning external fixation as the best way to control radial length, inclination, and most of all, the restoration of palmar tilt (6). The studies of Bartosh and Saldana (14) clearly demonstrate the difficulty of attaining full correction of palmar tilt with a spanning device: the palmar capsule is symmetrically tensioned and thus limits the correction to neutral tilt.

The proximal pins are always placed first because they can be used with the spanning and the nonspanning external fixators. The proximal pins are placed about 10 cm proximal to the tip of the radial styloid. They are positioned in the bare interval of the midradius between the brachioradialis and the extensor carpi-radialis longus muscles. Pin placement is done through a limited open approach to insure identification and protection of the radial sensory and lateral antebrachial-cutaneous nerves (15). The limited open approach also insures that the pilot holes and half pins are placed in the central axis of the radial shaft. To minimize the risk of heterotopic ossification, one must be careful not to violate the interosseous membrane with the drill or half pins. We prefer self-tapping pins that engage the distal cortex. Prestressing the pins during the assembly of the external fixator is unnecessary and may lead to resorption of the bone around the pins and subsequent premature loosening.

Once the proximal screws are placed, the distal pin placement is finalized. Most fractures that have at least 6 mm of cortex proximal to the subchondral plate can accept the 3 mm threaded half pins. If the fracture is amenable to a non–joint-spanning external fixator, a longitudinal, transradial, styloid, K wire is placed to prevent overtranslation of the distal fragment. The pins should be inserted through 2-cm longitudinal incisions that are placed between the dorsal compartments. Because most distal-radius fractures include a radial styloid and/or scaphoid facet fragment and an ulnar or lunate facet fragment, the two distal half pins must stay within the limits of those fracture fragments. For the protection of all soft tissues, including cutaneous nerves and tendons, we prefer to use small incisions instead of percutaneous placement of the half pins. Pilot holes (1.5 mm) are drilled for the self-tapping 3-mm half pins. It is important to use the designated soft tissue sleeves to facilitate pin placement, and to be secure, the half pins must engage the palmar cortex (Fig. 12.7).

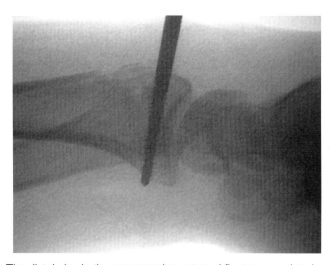

Figure 12.7. The distal pins in the nonspanning external fixator engaging the palmar cortex.

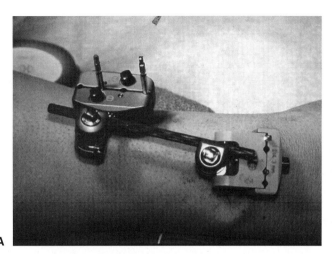
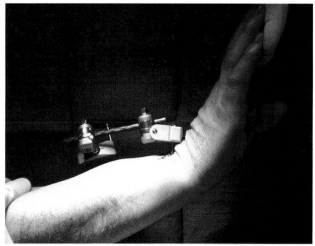

Figure 12.8. A,B. Final construct of non–joint-spanning external fixator.

Once the proximal and distal pins are placed, the frame is applied with pin-to-rod connectors. A moderate amount of traction is applied to unload the previously placed adjunctive K wires and/or metaphyseal bone filler. We use graphite rods because they are light and radiolucent (Fig. 12.8).

If a non–joint-spanning external fixator cannot be employed, then a joint-spanning external fixator is created. The metacarpal pin placement should also be done through a limited open approach (Fig. 12.9). The incision is positioned over the proximal third of the second metacarpal and is centered in the bare area between the first dorsal interosseous muscle and the extensor tendon to the index finger. To avoid the possibility of a stress fracture, the pilot holes for the 3-mm half pins must be placed in the center of the cylindrical metacarpal shaft. The more proximal pin of the pair can be oriented to cross the bases of the 2nd and 3rd metacarpals. This enables four cortices to be captured because the bases of these two are in close proximity, and there is no violation of the interossei muscles. The metacarpal pins must be kept in the proximal third of the second metacarpal. This pin placement prevents encroachment upon the metacarpal-phalangeal joint capsule or interference with the smooth gliding of the lateral bands. The orientation of these pins should be 45 degrees to the long axis to permit full abduction and extension of the thumb (15). As noted previously, to have maximal purchase for the duration of the frame application, one must ensure that the terminal threads of the self-tapping half pins engage the far cortex fully (Fig. 12.10).

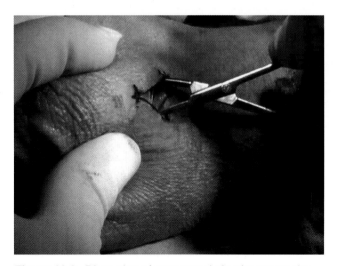

Figure 12.9. Dissection of metacarpal pin-placement site using a limited open incision.

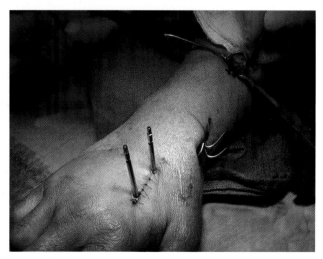

Figure 12.10. Location of proximal and distal screw site placement.

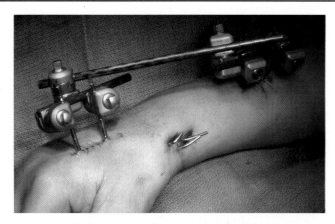

Figure 12.11. Final frame assembly.

Limited open incisions should be closed in layers with the muscle interval closed over both the proximal and distal pin groupings. The skin should be closed by the orientation that provides the least skin tethering because most of the pin-skin interface problems are due to excessive traction on the skin. Poor closures can cause wound necrosis, which ultimately leads to local pin-tract infection and early pin loosening.

Once the wounds are closed, the frame assembly is finalized (Fig. 12.11). The pin clamps and connecting bars are placed close to the skin to minimize the profile and to make it easy to wear shirts and coats. The final wrist position need not be in the classic Cotton-Loder ulnar deviation and wrist flexion as the ligamentotaxis effect is not required for maintenance of reduction. The distal fragment must not be overpronated in the spanning frame. Overpronation of the distal fragment will restrict restoration of supination. A few degrees of volar flexion and ulnar deviation are all that usually are necessary. Tighten all remaining pins and bar clamps.

At this stage, it is important to examine the stability of the distal radioulnar joint. If dorsopalmar translation is greater than on the contralateral wrist, arthroscopic evaluation and repair of the TFCC ligaments may be indicated. Alternatively, the position of the forearm in the fixator may be adjusted to increase stability. Occasionally, K wire fixation of the distal radioulnar joint may be necessary.

The incisions are dressed with Xeroform gauze about the pins, and early motion of the fingers and thumb is encouraged. Index MP flexion or thumb abduction and extension should not be discouraged. Final intraoperative x-rays should not demonstrate any carpal distraction at either the proximal or midcarpal articulations. Surgical incisions are infiltrated with 0.5% Marcaine as a postoperative analgesic. Palmar plaster splints may be used to control wrist motion if a non–joint-spanning fixation frame is employed.

POSTOPERATIVE CARE

Most patients stay in the hospital overnight for comfort and pain management. In the morning of the first postoperative day, patients are seen by an occupational therapist to review finger, elbow, and shoulder range of motion exercises. They are encouraged to use their fingers, elbow, and shoulder for activities of daily living. The use of a sling is used intermittently for comfort and to control swelling. Pin sites are cleaned with hydrogen peroxide and cotton tip applicators.

Patients are seen 10 to 14 days after surgery for suture removal and x-rays. They can now shower and have water run over their fixator. If patients have limited finger mobility or are reluctant to use their hands, formal, supervised, hand therapy is begun.

Six weeks to 8 weeks after surgery, the external fixator and pins are removed under local anesthesia. Hand therapy is intensified with emphasis on functional tasks and the return to previous activities. Most patients can transition to a home program at 2 to 4 months after surgery, but gains in strength can continue for up to 1 year.

COMPLICATIONS

The most common complication with external fixation is pin track infection. Most can be managed by pin care and oral antibiotics. If the pins loosen, they must be replaced if the frame is still required. Modern frames have excellent articulations and usually will not loosen. It is important to check for frame tightness at each postoperative visit.

Some patients present with extreme swelling and stiffness early in the postoperative period. They should be aggressively treated to avoid arthrofibrosis. This is not a complex regional pain syndrome (CRPS) as is often suggested. If a CRPS is present, a multimodal and interdisciplinary approach is used and may include regional blocks, pain management, and even manipulation under anesthesia prior to the onset of unyielding capsular contractures.

RECOMMENDED READINGS

1. Lafontaine M, Hardy D, Delince P. Stability assessment of distal radius fractures. *Injury* 1989;20(4):208–210.
2. Nesbitt KS, Failla JM, Les C. Assessment of instability factors in adult distal radius fractures. *J Hand Surg [Am]* 2004;29(6):1128–1138.
3. McQueen MM, Hajducka C, Court-Brown CM. Redisplaced unstable fractures of the distal radius: a prospective randomised comparison of four methods of treatment. *J Bone Joint Surg Br* 1996;78(3):404–409.
4. Trumble TE, Schmitt SR, Vedder NB. Factors affecting functional outcome of displaced intra-articular distal radius fractures. *J Hand Surg [Am]* 1994;19(2):325–340.
5. Doi K, Hattori Y, Otsuka K, et al. Intra-articular fractures of the distal aspect of the radius: arthroscopically assisted reduction compared with open reduction and internal fixation. *J Bone Joint Surg Am* 1999;81(8):1093–1110.
6. McQueen MM. Redisplaced unstable fractures of the distal radius. A randomised, prospective study of bridging versus non-bridging external fixation. *J Bone Joint Surg Br* 1998;80(4):665–669.
7. Herrera M, Chapman CB, Roh M, et al. Treatment of unstable distal radius fractures with cancellous allograft and external fixation. *J Hand Surg [Am]* 1999;24(6):1269–1278.
8. May MM, Lawton JN, Blazar PE. Ulnar styloid fractures associated with distal radius fractures: incidence and implications for distal radioulnar joint instability. *J Hand Surg [Am]* 2002;27(6):965–971.
9. Sarmiento A, Pratt GW, Berry NC, et al. Colles' fractures. Functional bracing in supination. *J Bone Joint Surg [Am]* 1975;57(3):311–317.
10. Wolfe SW, Austin G, Lorenze M, et al. A biomechanical comparison of different wrist external fixators with and without K-wire augmentation. *J Hand Surg [Am]* 1999;24(3):516–524.
11. Trumble TE, Wagner W, Hanel DP, et al. Intrafocal (Kapandji) pinning of distal radius fractures with and without external fixation. *J Hand Surg [Am]* 1998;23(3):381–394.
12. Wolfe SW, Easterling, KJ, Yoo HH. Arthroscopic-assisted reduction of distal radius fractures. *Arthroscopy* 1995;11(6):706–714.
13. Geissler WB, Fernandez DL, Lamey DM. Distal radioulnar joint injuries associated with fractures of the distal radius. *Clin Orthop Relat Res* 1996;327:135–346.
14. Bartosh RA, Saldana, MJ. Intraarticular fractures of the distal radius: a cadaveric study to determine if ligamentotaxis restores radiopalmar tilt. *J Hand Surg [Am]* 1990;15(1):18–21.
15. Seitz WH, Putnam MD, Dick HM. Limited open surgical approach for external fixation of distal radius fractures. *J Hand Surg [Am]* 1990;15(2):288–293.

13

Distal Radius Fractures: Open Reduction Internal Fixation

George S.M. Dyer and Jesse B. Jupiter

The past decade has witnessed widespread enthusiasm for operative treatment of distal radial fractures (1–17). A number of factors have contributed to this changing perspective. Among these include a greater recognition of the wide variation in fracture patterns (18–20). The availability of computed tomography (CT) has permitted a three-dimensional projection of the fracture morphology (Fig. 13.1) (5,21). In fact, distal radial fractures differ to the extent that only the distal nature of the injury is in common among them (Fig. 13.2). Fractures that involve a shearing mechanism displacing part of the articular surface along with the carpus (Barton's and reverse Barton's fracture) (22–25), radiocarpal fracture-dislocations, displaced articular fractures associated with high-energy trauma and metaphyseal-diaphyseal comminution, articular compression fractures involving rotation of a volar lunate facet component, and some unstable extra-articular fractures are all amenable to open reduction and internal fixation.

Along with a greater understanding of the variety of fracture patterns has been an expanded appreciation for the structural anatomy of the distal radius. Rikli and Regazzoni (26) divided the distal radius into a strong, cortical radial "column"; an intermediate column, which contains the articular surfaces of both the lunate facet as well as the sigmoid notch; and the distal ulna column with its firm attachment to the radius through the triangular fibrocartilage complex (Fig 13.3). Recognition of this unique anatomical orientation and patterns of articular injury has led to the development of a method of operative treatment coined "fragment-specific fixation," through which small strategically-placed implants are used to support the critical structural components of the fracture (Fig. 13.4).

A third factor that has led to the operative treatment of certain fractures involves those injuries associated with intercarpal injury (27,28). Fracture patterns involving compression or shearing of the radial styloid and/or scaphoid facet of the distal radius are recognized to have the potential of accompanying injuries to the scapholunate ligament as well as the lunate facet and the lunotriquetral ligament (Fig 13.5).

Associated instability of the distal radioulnar joint (DRUJ) has also stimulated more operative intervention. DRUJ instability following stabilization of the radius fracture,

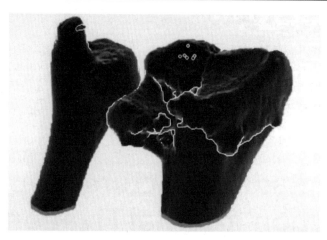

Figure 13.1. A three-dimensional CT image clearly shows the components of the articular injury.

especially in the presence of a large ulnar-styloid fracture, is best treated by operative fixation of the ulnar styloid.

Interest in operative intervention has been further generated by the development of a variety of technologically advanced implants that are specific to the distal radius. These new pieces have features, such as locking screws that enhance fixation in osteopenic bone, that have led to interest in the volar approach to internal fixation of dorsally displaced fractures. A volar approach would limit the potential for problems involving the overlying extensor tendons on the dorsal surface.

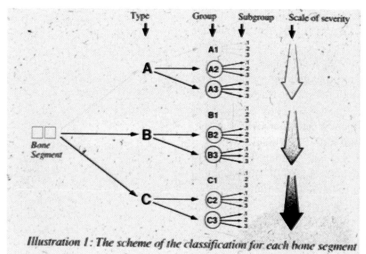

Illustration 1: The scheme of the classification for each bone segment

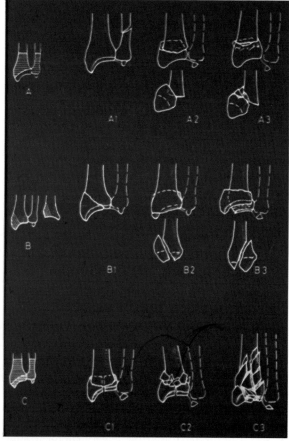

Figure 13.2. The comprehensive classification of the AO/ASIF demonstrates three major types, nine groups, and twenty-seven subgroups reflecting the enormous variation of fracture patterns.

Column Theory

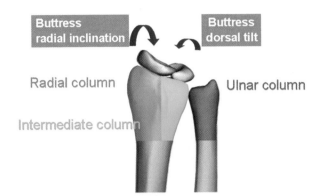

Figure 13.3. The column concept, developed by Rikli and Regazzoni (26), includes the radial, intermediate, and ulnar columns.

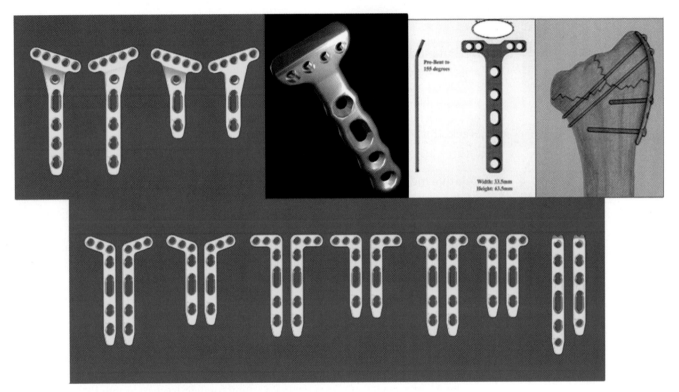

Figure 13.4. Implants constructed specifically for the anatomy of the distal radius have allowed limited fixation of fracture components and minimization of prior problems associated with larger nonspecific implants.

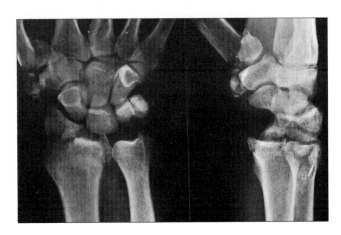

Figure 13.5. Fractures involving compression or shearing of the articular surface may be accompanied by intercarpal ligament injury.

Table 13.1. *Definite Indications for Open Reduction and Internal Fixation*

- Volar or dorsal radiocarpal subluxation/dislocations
- Displaced radial-styloid fractures
- Rotated, volar, lunate-facet fracture
- Displaced articular fractures seen late (after 3 weeks)

INDICATIONS/CONTRAINDICATIONS

A number of factors are considered when surgeons decide on operative fixation of distal radius fractures: specific aspects of the fracture itself, the presence of associated soft-tissue injury such as median nerve dysfunction; associated ipsilateral limb injury, and the overall physical and medical condition of the patient. With the advent of fixed-angle locking screw-plate constructs, underlying osteopenia is no longer a contraindication to internal fixation.

Definite Indications for ORIF

Fracture patterns including volar or dorsal radiocarpal subluxations or dislocations, displaced radial-styloid fractures, articular fractures involving a displaced and rotated volar lunate-facet component, and those displaced fractures presented 3 weeks after the injury (Table 13.1).

Relative Indications

Relative indications for ORIF include a host of different fractures. These include bilateral displaced fractures, fractures associated with ipsilateral limb trauma, some fractures with associated progressive swelling or nerve dysfunction, open fractures, fractures associated with DRUJ instability, or unstable extra or intra-articular fractures that were not reduced after closed reduction and cast immobilization (Table 13.2).

Relative Contraindications

Patients with medical conditions that prohibit the use of anesthesia, with poor compliance, or with local soft-tissue conditions, such as active infection or complex regional pain syndrome, may not benefit from internal fixation for their fracture (Table 13.3).

PREOPERATIVE PLANNING

As with any musculoskeletal injury, a careful evaluation of the patient's overall condition, as well as that of the involved limb and hand, must be made before a decision is rendered to proceed with operative intervention. The fracture characteristics are not always easily appreciated before the fracture is reduced and repeat x-rays are taken. Furthermore,

Table 13.2. *Relative Indications for ORIF*

- Bilateral, displaced, articular fractures
- Fractures associated with ipsilateral limb trauma
- Fractures associated with excessive swelling or nerve dysfunction
- Open fractures
- Fractures associated with DRUJ instability
- Unstable extra-articular fractures that failed cast immobilization

Table 13.3. *Relative Contraindications to ORIF*

- Patients with medical conditions that prohibit anesthesia use
- Poor patient compliance
- Poor local soft-tissue conditions or complex regional-pain syndrome

additional x-ray views, including oblique views to focus on the articular surface, or CT studies may further influence the decision about intervening operatively.

When the fracture involves impacted articular fragments and/or extensive metaphyseal comminution, the potential for autogenous, allograft, bone-substitute grafts should be noted in the preoperative plan. The patient should also be informed that bone grafting may be necessary.

OPERATIVE TECHNIQUES

We prefer to use regional anesthesia, pneumatic tourniquet control, and have the involved limb extended on a hand table. The advent of relatively small, versatile, mini c-arms has greatly facilitated intraoperative imaging. Because distal radius fractures may be operatively approached through different exposures, we will highlight several approaches with emphasis on the pitfalls and pearls for each.

Anterior Approach

The uncomplicated volar shearing as well as the extra-articular, volar, displaced Smith's and many dorsally displaced fractures may be approached through the standard distal limb of the Henry exposure. The interval is created between the radial artery and flexor carpi radialis tendon. (Fig. 13.6).

Relatively complex fractures associated with high-energy trauma or those involving a small, displaced, volar, lunate-facet fragment are better exposed through an extended ulnar-based incision that creates an interval between the ulnar nerve and artery and flexor tendons. Extending this incision distally to release the transverse carpal ligament will further facilitate exposure (Fig. 13.7).

Orbay (29) has developed an additional, extensile, volar, radial approach. By extending the Henry approach more distally, the surgeon releases the fibrous septum overlying the flexor carpi radialis and step cuts the insertion of the brachioradialis tendon, which will permit further displacement of the distal fragment and thus allow for exposure of the dorsal surface of the distal fragment (Fig. 13.8).

When approaching the radius from the volar surface, the surgeon must take care to retract the muscle belly of the flexor pollicis longus exposing the pronator quadratus. The pronator is necessarily and sharply elevated in L fashion either from the radial aspect of the radius or from its ulnar attachment. Whenever possible, the proximal pedicle of the anterior interosseous artery should be preserved to maintain muscle viability and limit the potential for a pronation contracture that develops due to ischemia of the pronator quadratus (Fig. 13.9).

The vast majority of fractures can be manipulated into reduction using longitudinal traction and direct digital manipulation of the distal fracture fragment(s). Another advantage of the anterior approach is the surgeon's ability to judge rotational alignment as well as length by reducing the volar, cortical fracture lines; this area is less likely to be comminuted even in impacted, dorsally displaced fractures (see Fig. 13.9C).

The locked-screw application of implants contoured to the specific anatomy of the volar surface increase stability of fixation. The distal screws, if placed in the subchondral position further enhance the stability of fixation, especially in osteopenic bone (see Fig 13.9D–K).

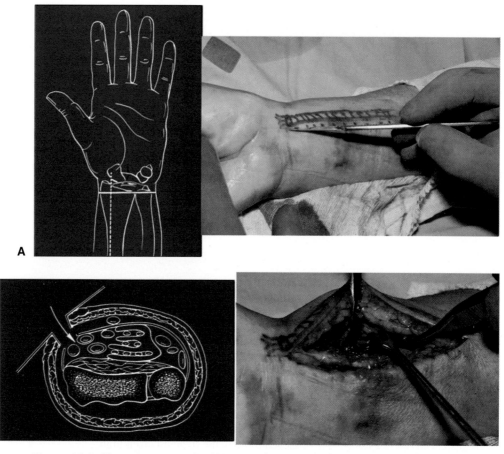

Figure 13.6. The volar approach of Henry creates an interval between the flexor carpi radialis and radial artery.

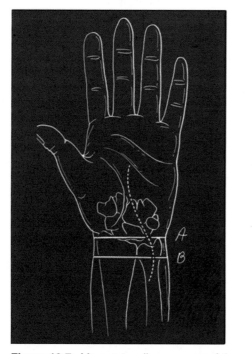
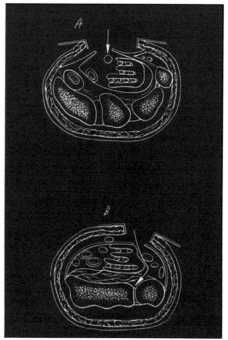

Figure 13.7. More extensile exposure of the volar aspect of the distal radius is achieved through a volar ulnar incision that creates an interval between the ulnar artery and nerve and flexor tendons.

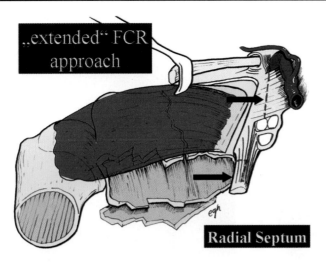

Figure 13.8. The extensile flexor carpi-radialis exposure developed by Orbay involves distal release of the flexor carpi radialis septum, which permits wide exposure of the anterior surface as well as the ability to gain access to the dorsal surface of the distal fragment. (Courtesy of Jorge Orbay, MD.)

Following internal fixation, x-rays should be taken with the beam 20 degrees inclined from distal to proximal to ascertain both the articular reduction. X-rays also ensure that distal screws have not penetrated into the radiocarpal joint (Fig 13.10).

If possible, we prefer to reapproximate the pronator quadratus to serve as a covering over the implant. The postoperative wrist is kept in a splint for 7 to 10 days after which sutures are removed and active wrist motion is initiated.

Anterior Approach

Several specific fractures patterns have potential pitfalls that may lead to loss of reduction or problems with internal fixation:

1. When approaching the displaced volar fracture in the older patient, one must suspect an element of dorsal cortical comminution even if it is not apparent on the lateral x-ray. An implant applied as a buttress pushing up the displaced, volar, distal fragment has the potential of dorsally translating the fragment. This will cause loss of the normal volar tilt of the distal articular surface (Fig. 13.11).

2. The volar, shearing, radiocarpal fracture-subluxation (Barton's fracture) most often will have two or more distal-radius fragments. In some, the volar ulnar component may be relatively small. Failure to support this fragment can result in postoperative volar subluxation of both the small fragment as well as the carpus (Fig 13.12). The very distal, articular rim of the radius dips anteriorly both at the radial styloid as well as at its most ulnar aspect. Therefore, one implant may be unable to support the entire, distal, articular rim adequately (30).

3. When stabilizing a three- or four-part articular fracture through an anterior approach, the radial styloid (column) component may not be protected against displacing shearing forces when a single volar implant is used. In these instances, an additional, small, contoured radial implant can be applied through the same exposure by step-cutting the brachioradialis insertion (Fig. 13.13). In addition, the volar lunate-articular facet fragment may be found to be rotated with minimal subchondral bony support (31). We loop a wire through the volar capsular attachments to the fragment and through a hole drilled transversely in the distal radius metaphysis (Fig. 13.14) (32).

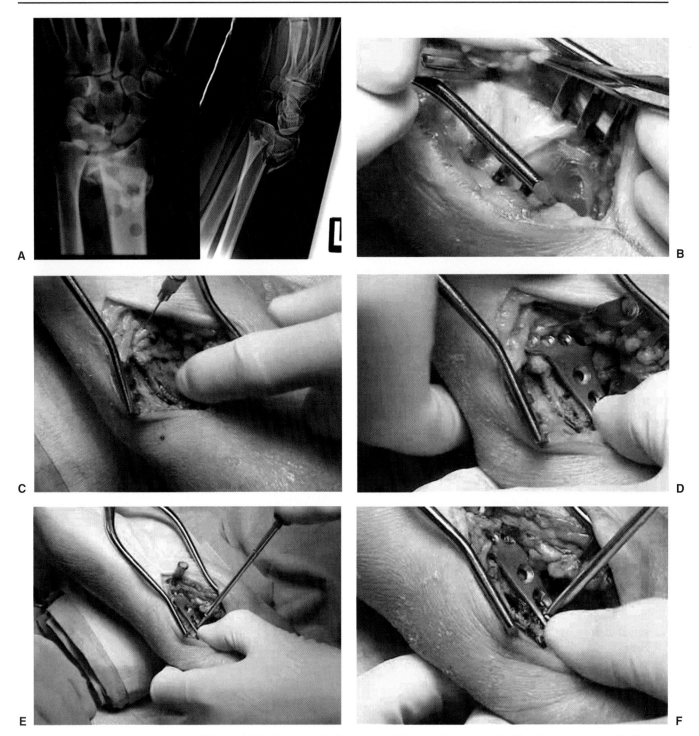

Figure 13.9. An unstable fracture in 56-year-old woman. **A.** The fracture x-rays. **B.** Exposure of the pronator quadratus. **C.** Following elevation of the pronator quadratus, a needle is placed into the radiocarpal joint marking the distal volar cortical rim. The fracture is reduced. **D.** The 2.4-mm plate is placed and checked using intraoperative fluoroscopy. **E,F.** The initial screw is placed in a proximal oval hole that will allow additional stability. (*continues*)

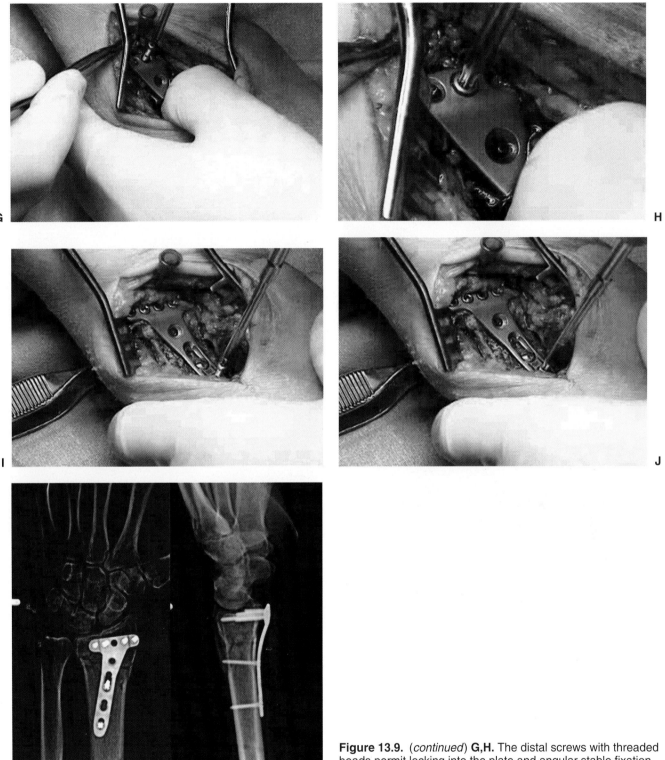

Figure 13.9. (*continued*) **G,H.** The distal screws with threaded heads permit locking into the plate and angular stable fixation. **I,J.** Final screw insertion. **K.** Postoperative x-rays.

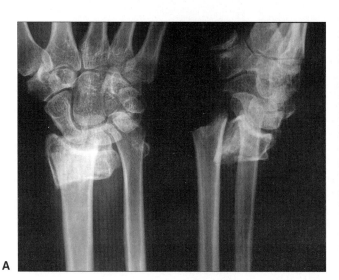

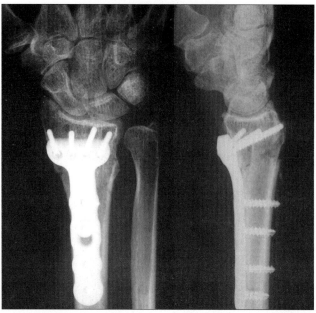

Figure 13.10. Volar implants with locked head screws provide angular stability even in osteoporotic patients. Stability is enhanced by placing the distal screws in a subchondral position especially when stabilizing a dorsally displaced fracture from a volar approach.

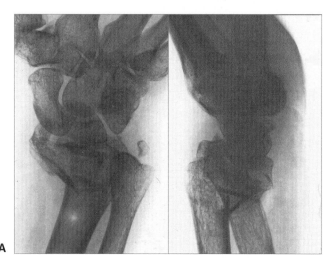

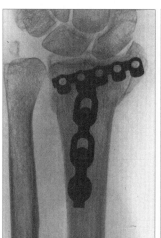

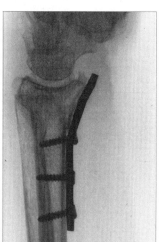

Figure 13.11. Dorsal translation of the distal fragment is a potential fixation problem of an unstable extra-articular fracture from a volar approach. The result is loss of normal volar angulation of the distal articular fragment.

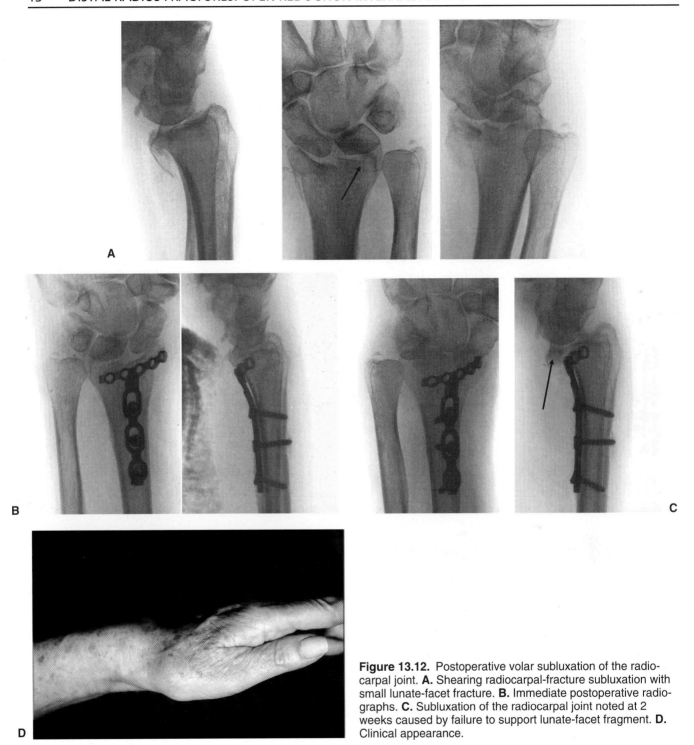

Figure 13.12. Postoperative volar subluxation of the radio-carpal joint. **A.** Shearing radiocarpal-fracture subluxation with small lunate-facet fracture. **B.** Immediate postoperative radiographs. **C.** Subluxation of the radiocarpal joint noted at 2 weeks caused by failure to support lunate-facet fragment. **D.** Clinical appearance.

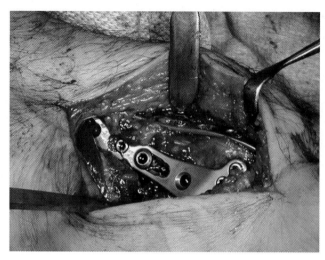

Figure 13.13. Complex articular fractures involving both the radial column and intermediate column can be stabilized from the volar approach using a radial column plate and volar surface plate.

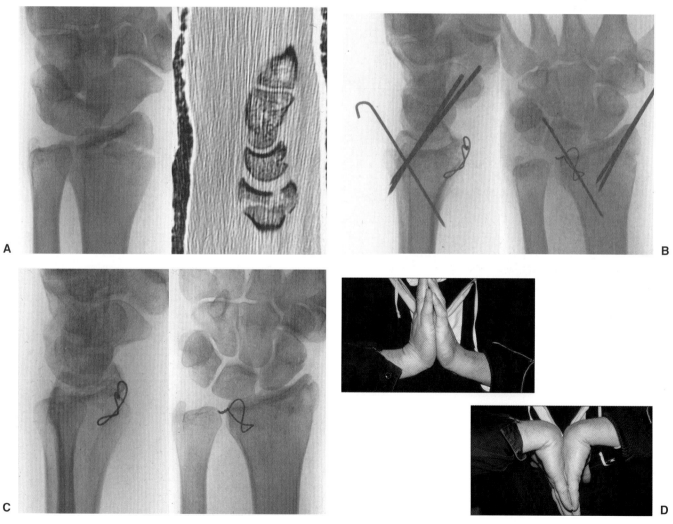

Figure 13.14. Fixation of a displaced, rotated, volar, ulnar, lunate-facet fragment can be done using a small gauge wire looped through the volar capsule and radius in a figure-of-eight fashion. **A.** Preoperative x-ray and CT scan reveal a displaced, volar, lunate facet. **B.** The radial styloid and dorsal lunate facet could be reduced and held with K wires, but the volar lunate facet required open reduction and wire loop fixation. **C.** Healed fracture at 1 year. **D.** Clinical wrist motion.

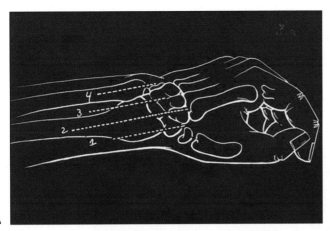
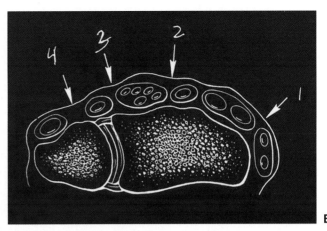

A   B

Figure 13.15. The surgical approach to the dorsal aspect of the radial styloid is through the first and second dorsal extensor compartment.

Dorsal Approach

A number of fracture patterns represent acceptable indications for a dorsal approach to the reduction and internal fixation of the distal radius fracture. These include radial, styloid, shearing fractures with associated impaction of the articular surface; some complex four-part articular fractures in which the dorsal, lunate, facet component cannot be reduced from a volar approach; complex fractures associated with intercarpal ligament descriptions; and some dorsally displaced fractures seen 3 weeks or more postinjury.

Several surgical approaches can be used to access the dorsal aspect of the distal radius. When approaching a radial styloid fracture, the surgeon can make the incision on the dorsal radial aspect, creating exposure between the first and second extensor compartments. Care is always taken to avoid traction injuries to the branches of the radial sensory nerve (Fig. 13.15).

In an alternative approach, the surgeon places the incision more dorsally and has several options for exposure of the distal radius. The extensor retinaculum can be opened between the third and fourth extensor compartments and the fourth extensor compartment can be elevated subperiosteally toward the ulnar fragment. The second extensor compartment can also be elevated subperiosteally (Fig. 13.16).

The exposure to the dorsoradial and intermediate columns can also be made through two exposures through the extensor retinaculum. One is between the first and second compartments, and another is between the fourth and fifth compartments (Fig. 13.17A–E).

Dorsal Approach

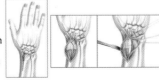

1   Straight dorsal incision

2   Incise the extensor retinaculum and open third extensor compartment (extensor pollicis longus)

3   Incision third compartment/ Preparation

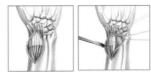

Figure 13.16. An extensile approach to the dorsal aspect of the distal radius is between the third and fourth extensor compartments. The fourth compartment and second extensor compartments are elevated subperiosteally.

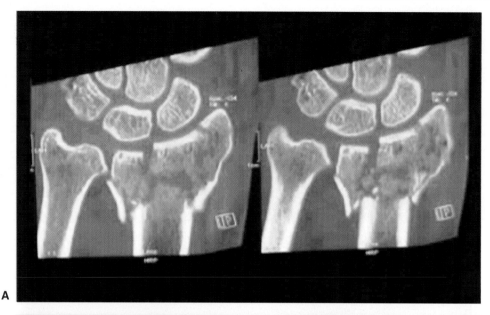

A

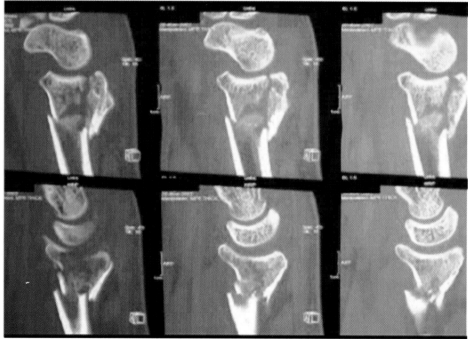

B

Figure 13.17. A complex intra-articular fracture treated with a fragment-specific plate through a dorsal approach. **A,B.** Anterior and lateral CT scans demonstrate clearly the articular and metaphyseal injury. (*continues*)

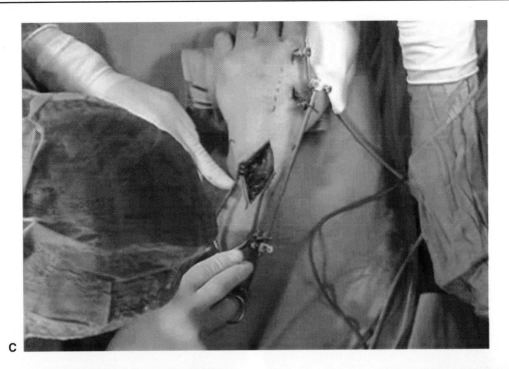

C

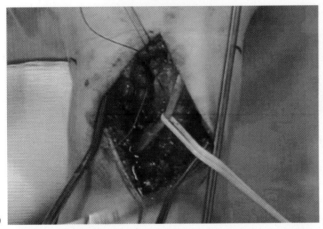

D

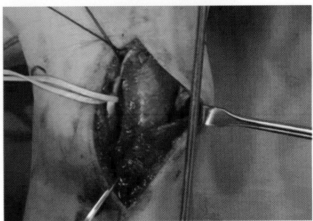

E

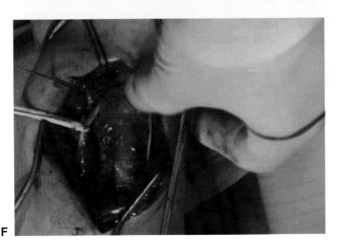

F

Figure 13.17. (*continued*) **C.** A dorsal radial incision with a temporary external fixator on the limb. **D.** The extensor pollicis longus is elevated from its third extensor retinacular compartment. **E.** Exposure of the radial column can be made through the first and second extensor retinacular compartments. **F.** The radial column plate is placed in this interval. (*continues*)

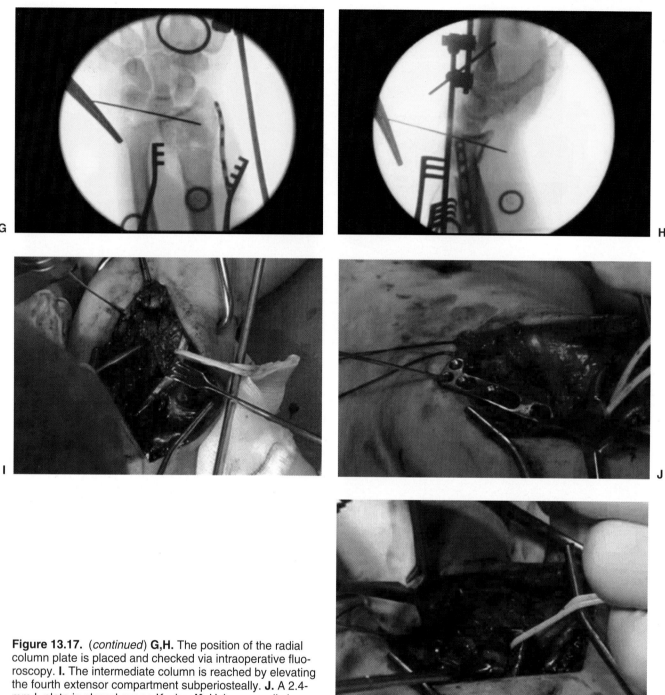

Figure 13.17. (*continued*) **G,H.** The position of the radial column plate is placed and checked via intraoperative fluoroscopy. **I.** The intermediate column is reached by elevating the fourth extensor compartment subperiosteally. **J.** A 2.4-mm L plate is placed over a K wire. **K.** Using a small clamp to hold both plates, the initial proximal screw is placed. (*continues*)

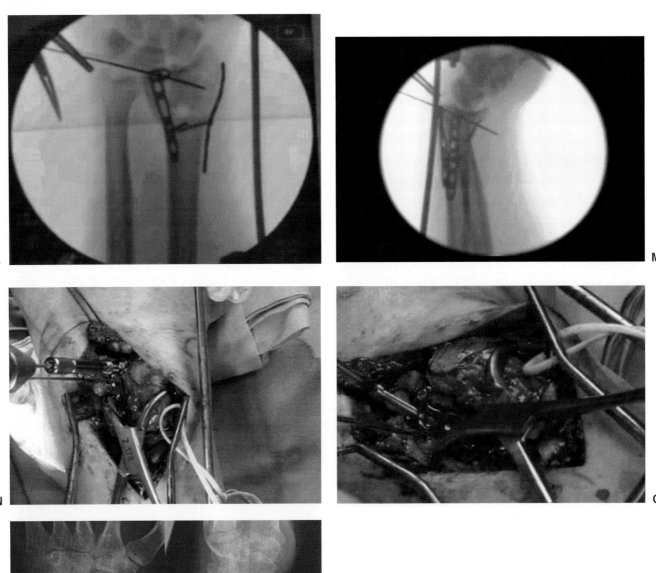

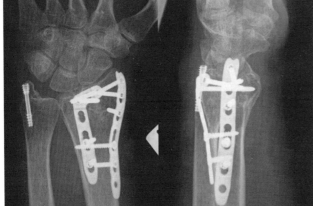

Figure 13.17. (*continued*) **L,M.** The position of both plates and fracture reduction is controlled through use of intraoperative fluoroscopy. **N.** A special drill guide permits the locking head screws to be placed directly in the center of the hole.
O. The distal screws are placed and locked into the plate.
P. Postoperative radiographs of the internal fixation.

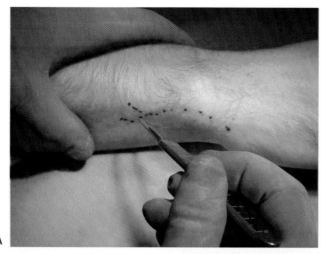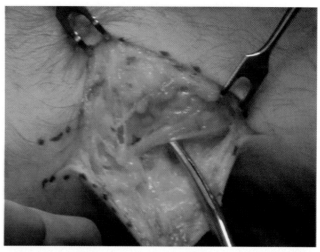

Figure 13.18. A dorsoulnar approach to the distal ulna and ulna styloid. **A.** The incision is marked out. **B.** Identification and protection of the branches of the dorsal ulnar sensory nerve.

For the most part, fracture reduction can be accomplished by longitudinal traction and direct manipulation of the fracture fragments (see Fig. 13.17F–O). A central articular impaction, which may be ineffectively reduced with traction alone, will require direct elevation through the fracture site and control of the articular reduction that is judged after an arthrotomy of the radiocarpal joint. Direct evaluation is also advisable when concern exists regarding intercarpal ligament injury.

The use of either external fixator or finger trap traction can be considered. It is especially useful for fractures seen late or associated with soft-tissue swelling.

Provisional fixation with smooth Kirschner (K) wires is of importance with unstable articular fractures. It will help control the reduction when using intraoperative image intensification.

An additional exposure is necessary primarily for problems involving the distal ulna. A longitudinal incision is created along the diaphysis. The surgeon notes that the ulnar styloid lies relatively anterior to the ulnar diaphysis (Fig. 13.18).

Stable Internal Fixation

A number of options regarding internal fixation are dependent upon the fracture pattern and available implants. The concept of "fracture-specific fixation" espoused independently by Medoff as well as Rikli and Regazzoni (26) has led to the use of small strategically placed implants to support the specific fracture fragments. These include anatomically shaped plates, pins, and wire forms (Figs. 13.19 and 13.20).

The indications for additional support, either with autogenous bone graft, bone substitute, or allograft, will be based upon whether a defect exists under an articular fragment and/or the stability of the internal fixation. The development of implants with locked screw heads, which creates angular stable fixation, has substantially decreased the requirement for bone graft.

We usually prefer to close the extensor retinaculum. This leaves the extensor pollicis longus outside of the retinacular closure.

Fixation of Distal Radioulnar-Joint Instability

A distal radius fracture is commonly associated with an injury to the distal radioulnar joint. While most do not result in instability, they are best recognized and treated concomitantly with the radius fracture.

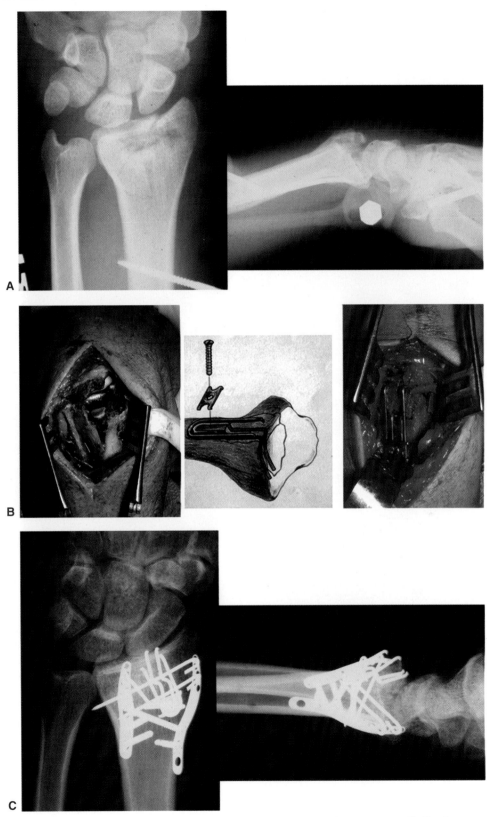

Figure 13.19. A complex intra-articular fracture treated with fragment specific fixation using wire forms and pin plate. **A.** The x-rays of the fracture. **B.** The use of the wire form to support the impacted articular fracture. **C.** X-rays of the healed fracture. (Case courtesy of Dr. Robert Medoff).

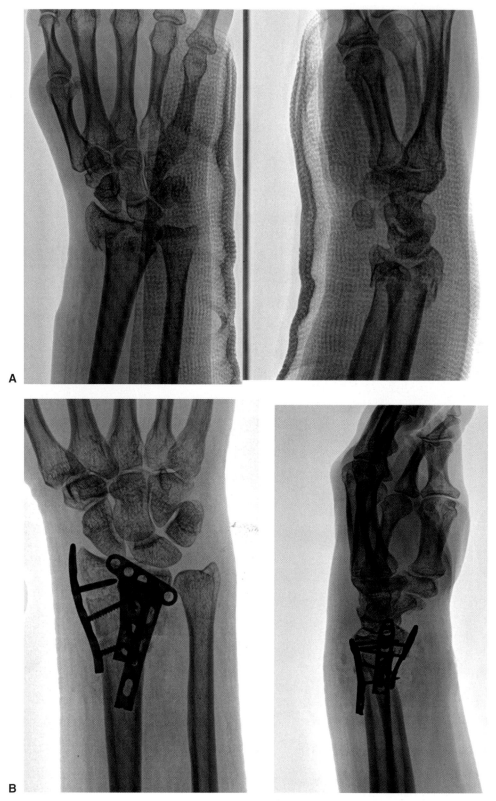

Figure 13.20. A complex intra-articular fracture treated with fragment-specific volar and dorsal plates. **A.** The initial fracture x-rays. **B.** X-ray of the three plates at 3 months post-surgery.

Following internal fixation of the radius fracture, the stability of the distal radioulnar joint should be assessed in every patient. This is best performed by attempting to displace the distal ulna from the sigmoid notch of the radius in forearm pronation, neutral, and supination. If the ulna head can be displaced completely, the possibility of instability should be considered.

When associated with an ulna styloid fracture, especially those occurring at the base of the styloid, stability will be restored following internal fixation of the styloid. This is best accomplished through a separate incision along the diaphysis of the distal ulna; the surgeon should keep in mind the more anterior location of the styloid process. Also, the surgeon should identify and protect the dorsal sensory branch of the ulnar nerve, which divides into three branches at or about the level of the ulnar styloid. Internal fixation can be accomplished in several ways, including via K wires along with a tension band, a small screw, or combination of screw and tension band. (Fig. 13.21).

When the distal radioulnar joint is unstable without an associated ulna-styloid fracture, alternative treatment options include postoperative immobilization of the wrist and forearm in an above-elbow splint for 4 weeks, cross pinning the ulna to radius for a similar period and application of an above elbow splint; or open repair of the triangular fibrocartilage complex also followed by forearm immobilization for 4 to 6 weeks.

A less common situation may be found with an unstable ulna-neck fracture, which may also require internal fixation. Alternatives will include an intramedullary smooth pin placed percutaneously or an ORIF with a small plate (33).

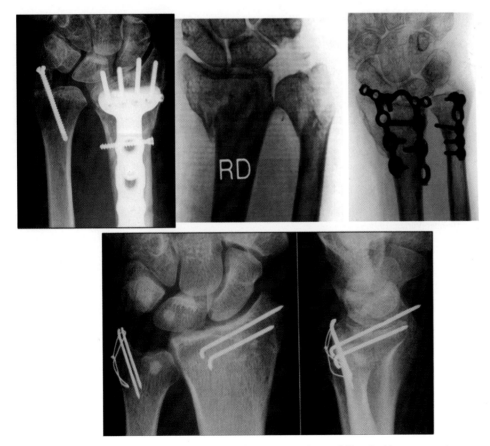

Figure 13.21. The ulna styloid and/or neck fracture can be stabilized with a screw, tension band wire, or plate.

POSTOPERATIVE MANAGEMENT

We prefer to support the wrist in a bulky postoperative dressing combined with a volar plaster splint for the initial 7 to 10 days postsurgery. During this period, the patient is encouraged to mobilize their upper limb, regain digital mobility, and incorporate their hand and limb in activities of daily living. In those patients in whom distal radioulnar-joint instability was present, the forearm is also immobilized for 14 to 21 days. During this initial recovery period, anti-edema measures should be encouraged including elevation, digital mobilization, and elastic wrapping if indicated.

Following discontinued postoperative immobilization and evaluation and instruction by an occupational or physical therapist, active wrist and forearm range of motion is initiated. Resistive activities are withheld until healing is assured (ordinarily after 6 to 8 weeks). Patients often need exercises for strength and motion for at least 3 months postsurgery with a functional end point often reached only after 12 to 18 months.

COMPLICATIONS

The complications following operative treatment of distal radius fractures are well recognized. They include loss of fixation, infection, nerve compression, complex regional-pain syndrome, digital and/or wrist stiffness among others (34–36). Careful patient selection, pre-operative planning, technical care in fixation and careful postoperative management will help minimize these adverse outcomes.

RECOMMENDED READINGS

1. Axelrod TS, McMurty RV. Open reduction and internal fixation of comminuted, intra-articular fractures of the distal radius. *J Hand Surg Am* 1990;15(1):1–11.
2. Bradway JK, Amadio PC, Cooney WP. Open reduction and internal fixation of displaced, comminuted intra-articular fractures of the distal end of the radius. *J Bone Joint Surg Am* 1989;71(6):839–847.
3. Carter PR, Frederick HA, Laseter GF. Open reduction and internal fixation of unstable distal radius fractures with a low-profile plate: a multicenter study of 73 fractures. *J Hand Surg [Am]* 1998;23(2):300–307.
4. Catalano LW III, Cole RJ, Gelberman RH, et al. Displaced intra-articular fractures of the distal aspect of the radius: long-term results in young adults after open reduction and internal fixation. *J Bone Joint Surg Am* 1997;79(9):1290–1302.
5. Cole RJ, Bindra RR, Evanoff BA, et al. Radiographic evaluation of osseous displacement following intra-articular fractures of the distal radius: reliability of plain radiography versus computer tomography. *J Hand Surg [Am]* 1997;22(5):792–800.
6. Fernandez DL, Geissler WB. Treatment of displaced articular fractures of the radius. *J Hand Surg [Am]* 1991; 16(3):375–384.
7. Fernandez DL, Jupiter JB. *Fractures of the distal radius: A practical approach to management.* New York: Springer-Verlag; 1995.
8. Finsen V, Aasheim T. Initial experience with the Forte plate for dorsally displaced distal radius fractures. *Injury* 2000;31(6):445–448.
9. Fitoussi F, Chow SP. Treatment of displaced intra-articular fractures of the distal end of the radius with plates. *J Bone Joint Surg Am* 1997;79(9):1303–1312.
10. Jupiter J, Ring D. Surgical treatment of redisplaced fractures of the distal radius in patients older than 60 years. *J Hand Surg* 2002;27:714–724.
11. Ring D, Jupiter JB. Percutaneous and limited open fixation of fractures of the distal radius. *Clin Orthop* 2000; 375:105–115.
12. Ring D, Jupiter JB. Plate fixation of distal radius fractures. *Tech Orthop* 2000;15:328–335.
13. Ring D, Jupiter JB. Dorsal and volar plating of distal radius fractures. *J Bone Joint Surg Am* 2004;86:1646–1652.
14. Ring D, Jupiter JB, Brennwald J, et al. Prospective multicenter trial of a plate for dorsal fixation of distal radius fractures. *J Hand Surg Am* 1997;22(5):777–784.
15. Rogachefsky RA, Lipson SR, Applegate B, et al. Treatment of severely comminuted intra-articular fractures of the distal end of the radius by open reduction and combined internal and external fixation. *J Bone Joint Surg Am* 2001;83(4):509–519.
16. Schneeberger AG, Ip WY, Poon TL, et al. Open reduction and plate fixation of displaced AO Type C3 fractures of the distal radius: restoration of articular congruity in eighteen cases. *J Orthop Trauma* 2001;15(5):350–357.
17. Trumble TE, Schmitt SR, Vedder NB. Factors affecting functional outcome of displaced intra-articular distal radius fractures. *J Hand Surg [Am]* 1994;19(2):325–340.
18. Knirk JL, Jupiter JB. Intra-articular fractures of the distal end of the radius in young adults. *J Bone Joint Surg Am* 1986;68(5):647–659.

19. Melone CP Jr. Articular fractures of the distal radius. *Orthop Clin North Am* 1984;15(2):217–236.
20. Trumble TE, Culp RW, Hanel DP, et al. Intra-articular fractures of the distal aspect of the radius. *J Bone Joint Surg Br* 1998;80:582–600.
21. Freedman DM, Dowdle J, Glickel SZ, et al. Tomography versus computed tomography for assessing step off in intraarticular distal radial fractures. *Clin Ortho* 1999;361:199–204.
22. Drobetz H, Kutscha-Lissberg E. Osteosynthesis of distal radial fractures with a volar locking screw plate system. *Int Orthop* 2003;27(1):1–6.
23. Harness N, Ring D, Jupiter JB. Volar Barton's fractures with concomitant dorsal fracture in older patients. *J Hand Surg* 2004;29:439–445.
24. Jupiter JB, Fernandez DL, Toh CL, et al. Operative treatment of volar intra-articular fractures of the distal end of the radius. *J Bone Joint Surg Am* 1996;78(12):1817–1828.
25. Keating JF, Court-Brown CM, McQueen MM. Internal fixation of volar-displaced distal radius fractures. *J Bone Joint Surg Br* 1994;76(3):401–405.
26. Rikli DA, Regazzoni P. Fractures of the distal end of the radius treated by internal fixation and early function: a preliminary report of 20 cases. *J Bone Joint Surg Br* 1996;78(4):588–592.
27. Auge WK II, Velazquez PA. The application of indirect reduction techniques in the distal radius: the role of adjuvant arthroscopy. *Arthroscopy* 2000;6(8):830–835.
28. Mudgal C, Hastings H. Scapho-lunate diastasis in fractures of the distal radius: pathomechanics and treatment options. *J Hand Surg [Br]* 1993;18(6):725–729.
29. Orbay JL. The treatment of unstable distal radius fractures with volar fixation. *Hand Surg* 2000;5(2):103–112.
30. Harness N, Jupiter J, Fernandez D, et al. Loss of fixation of the volar lunate facet after volar plating of distal radius fracture. *J Bone Joint Surg Am* 2004;86:1900–1908.
31. Melone CP Jr. Open treatment for displaced articular fractures of the distal radius. *Clin Orthop* 1986;202:103–111.
32. Chin KR, Jupiter JB. Wire-loop fixation of volar displaced osteochondral fractures of the distal radius. *J Hand Surg [Am]* 1999;24(3):525–533.
33. Ring D, McCarty P, Campbell D, et al. Condylar blade plate fixation of unstable fractures of the distal ulna associated with fracture of the distal radius. *J Hand Surg* 2004;29:103–109.
34. Cooney WP III, Dobyns JH, Linscheid RL. Complications of Colles' fractures. *J Bone Joint Surg Am* 1980;62(4):613–619.
35. Frykman G. Fracture of the distal radius including sequelae—shoulder-hand-finger syndrome, disturbance in the distal radio-ulnar joint and impairment of nerve function: a clinical and experimental study. *Acta Orthop Scand* 1967;108:5–153.
36. Jupiter JB, Fernandez D. Complications of distal radius fractures: instructional course lectures. *J Bone Joint Surg* 2001;83:1244–1265.

Lower Extremity

14

Femoral Neck Fractures: Open Reduction Internal Fixation

Edward Rainier G. Santos and Marc F. Swiontkowski

INDICATIONS/CONTRAINDICATIONS

The primary indication for open reduction and internal fixation (ORIF) of a femoral neck fracture is a displaced fracture that is not satisfactorily reduced using closed means. It can be done in a patient of any age who has adequate bone density. Garden's radiographic index for acceptable reduction is useful in determining the need for ORIF (1). On the antero-posterior (AP) view, the angle between the central axis of the medial trabeculae of the head and the medial cortex of the proximal femoral shaft should be maintained. It should measure between 180 degrees and 160 degrees. Values more than 180 degrees and less than 160 degrees indicate unacceptable valgus and varus alignment, respectively. On the lateral view, the alignment index should be within 20 degrees of the normal 180-degree value. According to this index, fractures that are not satisfactorily reduced by closed means have been shown to be at greater risk for avascular necrosis and osteoarthrosis and are therefore best treated with ORIF.

The benefits of open reduction are twofold. First, the limited anterior capsulotomy results in evacuation of the fracture hematoma, thus decreasing intracapsular pressure. This will improve circulation to the femoral head, thereby decreasing the possibility of osteonecrosis (2). Because no significant blood supply is carried to the femoral head from the anterior capsule, an anterior approach to the femoral neck causes no additional harm to the circulation of the femoral head (3). Second, open reduction allows direct visualization of the fracture site, thereby facilitating optimal fracture reduction prior to fixation. The accuracy of reduction and the density of the femoral head and neck have been shown to be the two most important factors in achieving stability after internal fixation of a femoral neck fracture. Even fractures that appear reasonably well reduced under fluoroscopy can be markedly displaced upon direct visualization, particularly in rotation.

Because the fracture renders the femoral head relatively ischemic, internal fixation should be considered a relative orthopedic emergency (2). Attempts to perform the surgery within 8 hours in the highest risk groups (patients younger than 50 years, including children) have improved outcomes (2,4).

The contraindications for ORIF of a femoral neck fracture include advanced rheumatoid arthritis or moderate osteoarthritis of the adjacent hip joint, poor bone density, limited life expectancy, pathologic fractures related to metastatic disease, and the presence of severe psychiatric disease. These patients are better treated by arthroplasty.

PREOPERATIVE PLANNING

History and Physical Examination

A complete history and physical examination, including pre-injury functional assessment, are vital in preoperative evaluation. It should be determined whether a high-energy or low-energy force caused the injury. Femoral neck fractures are typically the result of a low-energy mechanism in elderly patients, whereas high-energy forces are often the cause in younger individuals. Multiply injured patients must be rapidly evaluated and cleared in terms of abdominal, chest, or head injury.

The presence of multiple medical co-morbidities, poor function, or both directs the surgeon towards arthroplasty. Patients with major medical co-morbidities benefit from treatment of their associated medical condition up to 48 hours before surgery (5). Elderly and sick patients often benefit from arthroplasty. It is also important to determine the preoperative level of function. A previous history of significant hip pain, which may point to a possible preexisting arthrosis in the hip joint, should make the surgeon lean toward arthroplasty.

In patients with multiple orthopedic injuries, the femoral neck fracture should be prioritized over most other closed injuries. Approximately 3% to 5% of patients with diaphyseal fractures of the femoral shaft will have a concomitant femoral-neck fracture (2). High-quality hip and knee radiographs should be taken in all patients with diaphyseal fractures of the femur.

Physical examination is directed toward evaluating the amount of deformity and presence or absence of any neurovascular deficits. Range of motion is typically painful and should not be performed. Associated injuries should be ruled out. It is usually sufficient to immobilize the limb using pillows under the knees, as traction has not been shown to provide any significant benefit. In fact, traction tightens the anterior capsule, resulting in an increase in intracapsular pressures that may further compromise the femoral head circulation (6).

Imaging Studies

Adequate radiographic evaluation is necessary in patients who are deemed candidates for surgery. Specifically, assessment of bone density using Singh's index is useful for purposes of patient selection (7). Standard radiographic examination of femoral neck fractures should consist of an AP and cross-table lateral radiograph. An additional pelvis AP view aids in evaluation of bone density, defines the neck shaft angle, and provides a comparison to the uninjured hip. This is particularly useful in cases where there is extensive comminution of the femoral neck.

Preoperative computed tomography (CT) scanning may be useful in further delineating the amount of comminution of the fracture and the degree of displacement of the fragments. Furthermore, in multiply injured patients, CTs have often been obtained for purposes of evaluation of the abdomen and pelvis and should be reviewed in advance of stabilization of the fracture. Bone scans and magnetic resonance imaging (MRI) have not been reliable in determining viability of the femoral head and in identifying those who will develop post-traumatic osteonecrosis, and are therefore not useful, in the short-term, in selecting patients for either ORIF or arthroplasty (8,9).

SURGERY

General, epidural, or spinal anesthesia may be used. Spinal and epidural anesthesia are the best choices for older patients with medical problems. Patients may be positioned with the extremity draped freely on a radiolucent table (Fig. 14.1A) or on a fracture table in the supine position. If the latter is chosen (which is the best method for obtaining high-quality lateral radiographs), only light traction should be applied. This allows some ability to manipulate the leg during surgery. If the former is chosen, the lateral image is obtained by externally rotating the limb after achieving temporary fixation. Before prepping and draping, the surgeon must ensure that accurate AP and lateral fluoroscopic images are easily obtainable.

Prophylactic first-generation cephalosporins are started preoperatively. The surgical approach is then done through a straight lateral skin incision centered over the greater trochanter. In obese or muscular patients, the proximal end of the incision must be curved anteriorly toward the gluteal pillar of the iliac crest. This allows easier dissection of the distal interval between the tensor fascia lata and gluteus maximus muscles (see Fig. 14.1B).

The deep fascia is divided in line with the skin incision, after which the interval between the tensor fascia and gluteus medius muscles is developed (Watson-Jones approach) (see Fig. 14.1C,D). The hip capsule is then identified by sweeping the pericapsular fat medially and inserting a Hohmann retractor along the anterior acetabular rim (see Fig. 14.1E). The capsule is then opened along the axis of the femoral neck (see Fig. 14.1F). This can be done with minimal soft-tissue stripping, allowing the surgeon to assess the reduction of the femoral fracture directly and under fluoroscopic guidance. A small blade on a long handle can be used under fluoroscopic control to limit the deep dissection.

An intracapsular hematoma under significant pressure is encountered in approximately 15% of patients regardless of the amount of fracture displacement or age of the patient (10). The surgeon must be convinced that the fracture is anatomically reduced before using the limited open technique. When an open reduction is necessary, the capsule is dissected from the intertrochanteric ridge, and its edges tagged with a no. 1 nonabsorbable suture for retraction. A head lamp is very helpful to provide illumination. Another useful technique to aid reduction is placement of a 5-mm Schanz pin in the lateral aspect of the proximal femur distal to the planned insertion of the cannulated screws (see Fig. 14.1G). The fracture is manually distracted by lateral and distal traction on the pin, and the proximal fragment is lifted anteriorly with a blunt curved instrument or a Steinmann pin used as a joystick in the femoral head. The fracture reduction is completed by internal rotation of the distal fragment and by lifting the upward on the Schanz pin and applying a compressive force perpendicular to the plane of the fracture. Provisional fixation is achieved using three K wires or cannulated 3.2-mm guide wires placed with the aid of biplanar image intensification (see Fig. 14.1H). Definitive fixation is achieved with cannulated or noncannulated screws (see Figs. 14.1I and 14.2). Several biomechanical studies (11,12) have shown no benefit from using more than three screws when an anatomic reduction is achieved. Furthermore, there is no advantage in postreduction stability among similar implants. A sliding hip screw has not been shown to increase mechanical stability when anatomic reduction has been achieved. However, this device may be of some benefit when the reduction is not anatomic because it relies on the side-plate fixation to the femoral shaft to resist angular displacement of the fracture rather than the cancellous bone of the femoral head and neck.

In patients with posterior comminution, the reduction can often be obtained by aligning the anterior cortices of the femoral neck. In these cases, it is helpful to insert the anterosuperior screw first because it helps to minimize fracture angulation when more posterior screws are inserted and tightened. A sliding hip screw may also be used when comminution is present to avoid angulation when the fracture is compressed.

Closure is begun with reapproximation of the capsule with a limited number of nonabsorbable sutures. The vastus lateralis is allowed to fall back into place, and the fascia is reapproximated over a drain with interrupted absorbable sutures. The subcutaneous fat is reapproximated with a limited number of absorbable sutures and the skin is reapproximated with a nylon 3-0 suture or staples. Intravenous first-generation cephalosporins are continued for 24 hours postoperatively.

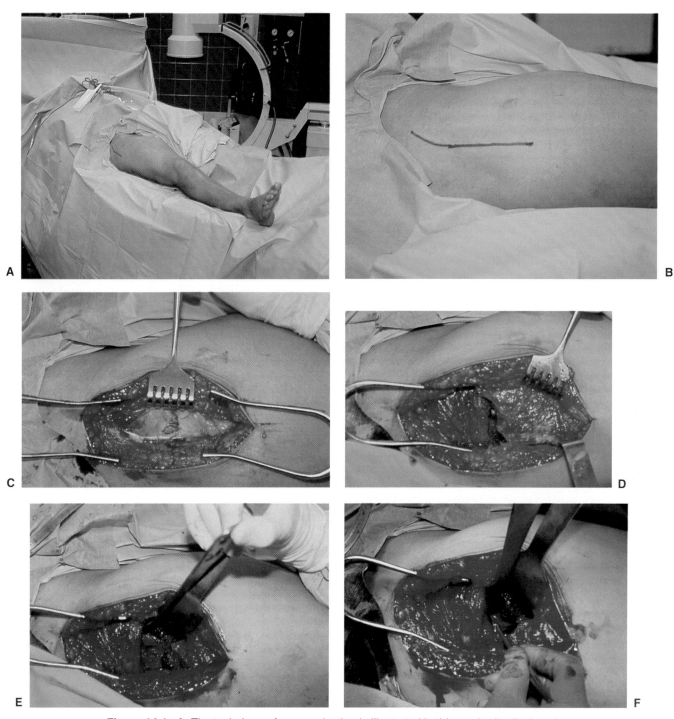

Figure 14.1. A. The technique of open reduction is illustrated in this markedly displaced femoral-neck fracture. Positioning of the patient supine on a radiolucent table; as an alternative, a fracture table can be used. **B.** The skin incision is 8 to 10 cm long and centered over the Precter trochanter. This patient's foot is to the reader's right. **C.** After incising the fascia lata, the surgeon develops the interval between the tensor and gluteus medius muscles. This is visible in the proximal (left side) portion of the wound. **D,E.** The final exposure of the anterior aspect of the hip fracture is accomplished, first by elevating the vastus lateralis off the intertrochanteric ridge **(D)** and then by sweeping the pericapsular fat medially and inserting a Hohmann retractor along the anterior aspect of the acetabulum **(E). F.** The hip capsule is incised in line with the neck of the femur, and any collected intracapsular hematoma is evacuated. (*continues*)

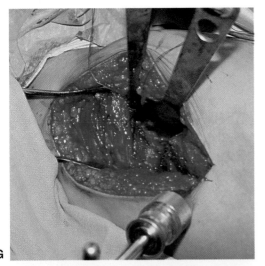

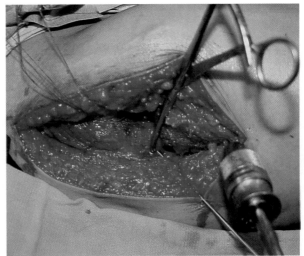

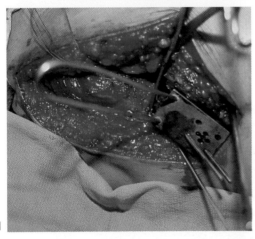

Figure 14.1. (*continued*) **G.** The reduction maneuver is performed with traction via a Schanz pin in the proximal femur with posterior translation of the shaft relative to the neck with a spiked pusher. The final reduction of the displaced neck fracture is accomplished by internal rotation of the leg by using the Schanz pin. **H.** The first guide wire is inserted after an anatomic reduction is documented with biplanar fluoroscopy and confirmed under direct vision. **I.** A second guide wire is placed parallel with the first by using a drill guide.

RESULTS

For displaced femoral-neck fractures, a 90% union rate is expected, and there is a 20% to 30% chance of osteonecrosis. Only 70% of patients older than 65 years reach their prefracture functional level. A 12% risk of death related to the fracture (excess of mortality over age-matched controls) should be expected.

POSTOPERATIVE MANAGEMENT

Patients are rapidly mobilized and are instructed in protected weight-bearing with crutches or a walker, allowing progress in weight-bearing as comfort dictates. Koval et al (13) have shown that elderly patients will increase their weight bearing on the injured hip as comfort allows. Patients who are able to maintain limited weight bearing (up to 50% of body weight) on the injured limb should continue to do so for 12 weeks. In patients older than 60 years, this is generally accomplished with a walker, whereas younger patients generally use crutches. In patients with upper-extremity injuries or those who do not have enough upper-extremity strength and balance to use crutches or a walker, postoperative care must be individualized. Early, excessive, weight bearing has been shown to increase the risk of redisplacement of the fracture, and in these cases the patient may need a wheelchair for a short period. Physical therapy consultation for gait retraining is appropriate. Range-of-motion exercises are generally unnecessary.

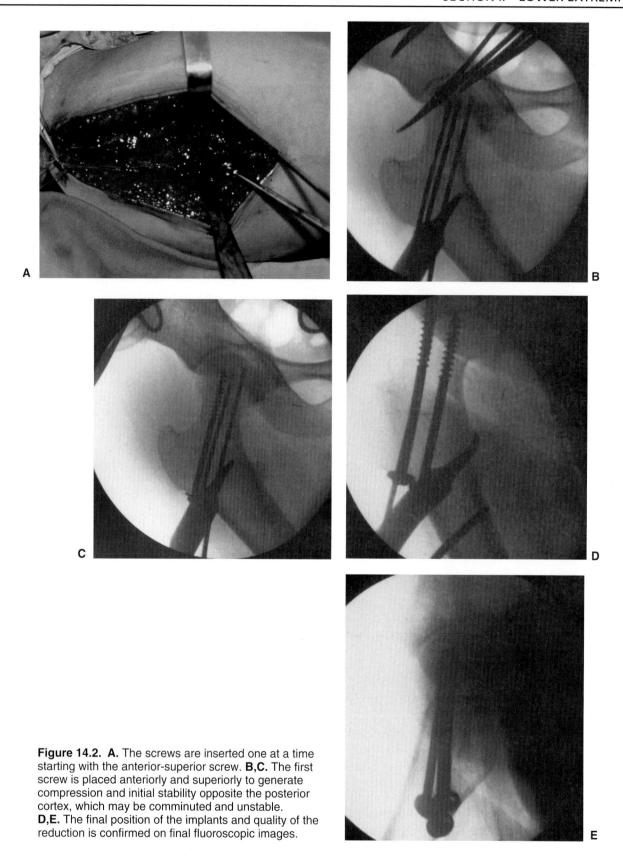

Figure 14.2. A. The screws are inserted one at a time starting with the anterior-superior screw. **B,C.** The first screw is placed anteriorly and superiorly to generate compression and initial stability opposite the posterior cortex, which may be comminuted and unstable. **D,E.** The final position of the implants and quality of the reduction is confirmed on final fluoroscopic images.

The postoperative management should also include deep venous thrombosis (DVT) screening and prophylaxis until the patient is mobile. A Doppler duplex scan is obtained within the first 36 postoperative hours and then weekly thereafter until the patient is fully mobilized. Enoxaparin (Lovenox) and low-dose warfarin (Coumadin) are equally efficacious for prophylaxis. Follow-up radiographs should be obtained monthly until the fracture is healed. Patients are seen annually for at least 3 years to rule out the presence of post-traumatic osteonecrosis.

COMPLICATIONS

The most common complications after internal fixation of femoral neck fractures are avascular necrosis and nonunion (2). In a meta-analysis on the outcome after displaced femoral-neck fractures, the risk of avascular necrosis in older patients was 16 %, and the risk of nonunion was 30% (14). The rate of nonunion in younger patients ranged from 0% to 86%, and avascular necrosis was 20% to 59%. These complications are related to the degree of initial displacement, the accuracy of reduction, and timing of the surgical intervention. In a more recent meta-analysis utilizing only controlled trials, weighted-mean revision rates after internal fixation were 18.5% and 9.5 % for nonunion and avascular necrosis, respectively (15).

Avascular necrosis is not always devastating functionally. In one series, nearly all patients younger than 50 years had symptoms severe enough to require additional surgery, whereas older patients required reoperation in only 30% to 50% of cases (16). Therefore, symptoms are related to functional demand and can be successfully treated with arthroplasty.

Nonunion after femoral neck fractures can be treated with corrective osteotomy or joint arthroplasty. In physiologically younger patients, nonunion can be treated with a closing wedge valgus osteotomy and fixation with a 120-degree blade plate. Marti et al (16) reported on 50 patients who underwent osteotomy, 37 of whom were followed up for a minimum of 7 years and achieved an average Harris hip score of 90. In an interesting result, 22 of these patients had radiographic evidence of avascular necrosis, illustrating that this complication is not always functionally devastating. Less common complications include infection, DVT, pulmonary embolism, loss of reduction, and subtrochanteric fracture through the lateral screw holes in the lateral cortex of the proximal femur. Loss of reduction is almost always related to poor bone quality or poor reduction, and it should be treated with repeat reduction and internal fixation (usually by switching to a sliding hip screw) if the patient's bone density is good, and with a cemented prosthesis if bone density is poor. Deep infection is managed with early aggressive surgical debridement, culture-specific antibiotics, and closure over a drain. Hip motion should be limited until the wound is sealed.

RECOMMENDED READINGS

1. Keller CS, GS Laros. Indications for open reduction of femoral neck fractures. *Clin Orthop* 1980;152: 131–137.
2. Swiontkowski MF. Intracapsular fractures of the hip. *J Bone Joint Surg Am* 1994;76(1):129–138.
3. Trueta J, Harrison MH. The normal vascular anatomy of the femoral head in adult man. *J Bone Joint Surg Br* 1953;35(3):442–461.
4. Szita J, Cserhati P, Bosch U, et al. Intracapsular femoral neck fractures: the importance of early reduction and stable osteosynthesis. *Injury* 2002;33:41–46.
5. Kenzora JE, McCarthy RE, Lowell JD, et al. Hip fracture mortality: relation to age, treatment, preoperative illness, time of surgery, and complications. *Clin Orthop* 1984;186:45–56.
6. Anderson GH, Harper WM, Connolly CD, et al. Preoperative skin traction for fractures of the proximal femur: a randomised prospective trial. *J Bone Joint Surg Br* 1993;75(5):794–796.
7. Singh M, Nagrath AR, Maini PS. Changes in trabecular pattern of the upper end of the femur as an index of osteoporosis. *J Bone Joint Surg Am* 1970;52(3):457–467.
8. Stromqvist B. Femoral head vitality after intracapsular hip fracture: 490 cases studied by intravital tetracycline labeling and Tc-MDP radionuclide imaging. *Acta Orthop Scand* 1983;200: 1–71.
9. Speer KP, Spritzer CE, Harrelson JM, et al. Magnetic resonance imaging of the femoral head after acute intracapsular fracture of the femoral neck. *J Bone Joint Surg Am* 1990;72(1):98–103.
10. Drake JK, Meyers MH. Intracapsular pressure and hemarthrosis following femoral neck fracture. *Clin Orthop* 1984;182:172–176.

11. Springer ER, Lachiewicz PF, Gilbert JA. Internal fixation of femoral neck fractures: a comparative biomechanical study of Knowles pins and 6.5-mm cancellous screws. *Clin Orthop* 1991;267:85–92.
12. Swiontkowski MF, Harrington RM, Keller TS, et al. Torsion and bending analysis of internal fixation techniques for femoral neck fractures: the role of implant design and bone density. *J Orthop Res* 1987;5(3):433–444.
13. Koval KJ, Sala DA, Kummer FJ, et al. Postoperative weight-bearing after a fracture of the femoral neck or an intertrochanteric fracture. *J Bone Joint Surg Am* 1998;80(3):352–356.
14. Lu-Yao GL, Keller RB, Littenberg B, et al. Outcomes after displaced fractures of the femoral neck: a meta-analysis of one hundred and six published reports. *J Bone Joint Surg Am* 1994;76(1):15–25.
15. Bhandari M, Devereaux PJ, Swiontkowski MF, et al. Internal fixation compared with arthroplasty for displaced fractures of the femoral neck: a meta-analysis. *J Bone Joint Surg Am* 2003;85:1673–1681.
16. Marti RK, Schuller HM, Raaymakers EL. Intertrochanteric osteotomy for non-union of the femoral neck. *J Bone Joint Surg Br* 1989;71(5):782–787.

15

Femoral Neck Fractures: Arthroplasty

Jeffrey O. Anglen

Fractures of the hip occur in two distinct anatomic locations in the proximal femur. Intertrochanteric (or pertrochanteric) fractures involve the area of the bone that is mostly or entirely outside the hip joint capsule, where the soft-tissue attachments provide good blood supply for healing and for ligamentotaxis. Fractures of the femoral neck occur through bone inside the capsule, where sparse soft-tissue attachments and the synovial fluid environment make healing slower and less reliable. Intertrochanteric fractures are routinely and successfully treated with reduction and internal fixation, and nondisplaced or impacted femoral-neck fractures are reliably handled with fixation in situ. However, the treatment of displaced femoral-neck fractures involves several controversies.

The first controversy regards whether to reduce and fix the fracture or to excise and replace the femoral head. Reduction and fixation of a displaced femoral-neck fracture is a technically demanding surgical procedure. It allows the patient to retain his/her own femoral head, and thereby avoid problems specific to prosthetic replacement such as dislocation, loosening, wear, or breakage, which may necessitate revision surgery. This has led some authors to propose an age-based protocol: younger patients (<50 years) are treated with reduction and fixation, elderly patients (>70 years) get arthroplasty, and those in between get individualized decisions based on general health, activity level, and bone quality (1). A wide range of implant failure, displacement, and re-operation rates for internal fixation have been reported in the literature (2,3). A meta-analysis of 13 studies in the Cochrane database concluded that internal fixation was associated with less operative trauma than replacement (decreased operative time, blood loss, transfusion, and infection) but a higher need for re-operation. No clear differences in hospital stay, mortality, or functional outcome were found (4). A more recent meta-analysis of 14 studies showed that those treated with arthroplasty had a significantly reduced risk of re-operation, blood loss, long operative times, and infection. However, this study, in contradistinction to the previous review, found that patients who had received arthroplasty had a slightly higher early-mortality rate than those who were treated with fixation (5). A study using cost-analysis methodology suggested that arthroplasty was the most cost-effective treatment when complications, mortality, and re-operation rate are evaluated at 2 years postoperation, but the best functional results are achieved with a healed femoral neck that does not have concomitant osteonecrosis (6).

There are different options with regard to the type of arthroplasty to be performed for femoral neck fracture. Total hip replacement (THR) can be performed for patients with acetabular damage, preexisting degenerative arthritis, or a systemic arthritic disease such as rheumatoid arthritis. Although some authors (7–9) have suggested that THR has better functional results with lower complications than hemi-arthroplasty, others have found that THR after acute fracture has significantly poorer outcomes, in terms of dislocation and revision rates, than primary THR (5,10,11). Those reports are retrospective, uncontrolled, and based on few cases. Two, prospective, randomized studies have compared THR with hemi-arthroplasty, and showed conflicting results. One study (12) revealed no difference between the two procedures, while the other (13) suggested that THR had a lower revision rate and higher hip scores. The study showing differences in acetabular replacement also demonstrated differences in stem fixation between the two groups.

Hemi-arthroplasty can be performed with either a modular unipolar or bipolar endoprosthesis. The bipolar design was developed to reduce metal on cartilage motion and friction, and thereby decrease acetabular wear and erosion, a postulated cause of postoperative pain. At the same time as the bipolar head design, modern modular-stem designs were introduced, complicating analysis. Several studies have shown good results for bipolar endoprostheses, particularly when they were cemented in place (14–16). However, cadaveric and radiographic studies revealed that motion occurs primarily at the outer bearing, particularly when the prosthesis is loaded (as in walking), reducing the likelihood for protection of the acetabular cartilage (17,18). In addition, multiple-prospective comparison studies have failed to show any significant difference in outcome between the bipolar and the unipolar designs (2,19–22). A prospective study reporting outcomes of 270 patients found significantly higher hospitalization costs (30%) for patients receiving a bipolar prosthesis compared to those receiving a unipolar implant (23). The type of implant was chosen by the surgeon, and there were some differences in the two patient populations.

A large number of hip arthroplasty systems are commercially available in the United States, and many offer hemi-arthroplasty components. Femoral stems come in many designs, made of a variety of different metals, and with a variety of surfaces and coating. Many of these stems are substantially more expensive than the basic Austin-Moore (fenestrated) or Thompson (nonfenestrated) design that has been in use for decades, and none has been proven superior.

Another controversy concerns the use of cement fixation for the stem. While operation without cement is faster, avoids the cardiovascular morbidity related to methylmethacrylate, and may make subsequent revision of the stem (if needed) easier, stability is decreased and the patient is slower in returning to activity. A retrospective study of 451 cases comparing the Bateman bipolar prosthesis inserted with or without cement found less thigh pain (13% vs. 46%) and higher Harris hip scores (86% vs. 79%) in the cemented group, with no difference in mortality (16). In a prospective, randomized, trial in which bipolar heads were used, the group whose hips were not cemented had significantly more pain and need for walking aids (24). A recent analysis of 18 published studies found that the use of cement resulted in longer operative times and more blood loss, but better postoperative mobility and less pain; no differences in mortality or general complications were found (25). Sixteen of the 18 studies reviewed concluded that cement should be used routinely, and the authors of the review agreed. A meta-analysis in the Cochrane Library found that there was "limited" evidence that cementing the stem of a hemi-arthroplasty would lead to less pain and improved mobility, but concluded that the data was insufficient to determine whether that advantage was offset by other disadvantages of cementing, such as increased mortality (20). If the stem is inserted without cement, use of an intramedullary corticocancellous bone plug, prepared for the head of the femur, may decrease the rate of subsidence and subsequent thigh pain (26).

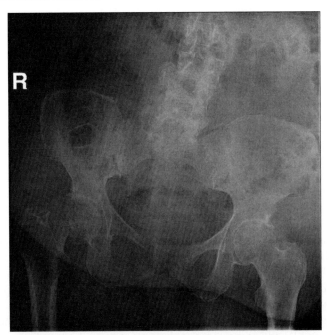

Figure 15.1. An AP pelvis radiograph of a 74-year-old woman with a displaced fracture of the right femoral neck. The position of the proximal femoral shaft explains the shortening and external rotation typically seen on physical examination.

INDICATIONS

Hemi-arthroplasty is indicated for displaced femoral-neck fractures in physiologically older adult patients (some have suggested approximately 70 years of age), or in younger patients with limited life span due to systemic disease, impaired ability to heal fractures, or irreparably damaged femoral heads (Fig. 15.1). Nondisplaced or impacted fractures are better treated with fixation in situ using cannulated screws. Fractures with preexisting arthritic changes or insufficient acetabular structure should be treated with total hip arthroplasty. Fractures in moribund, severely demented, or nonambulatory patients with limited life expectancy may be treated nonoperatively with analgesia.

PREOPERATIVE PLANNING

Patient evaluation includes a thorough history and physical exam, which may be difficult in many elderly, debilitated patients. The circumstances surrounding the fall should be elicited, seeking evidence of a syncopal episode, medication error, or exacerbation of a chronic medical condition that would require further workup. Evidence of an unsafe environment or elder abuse may require social work evaluation. A complete medical history and review of systems may reveal information that impacts the timing of surgery or the choice of anesthetic technique. On physical examination, the injured leg is typically shortened, externally rotated and painful with motion. The examination should include evaluation for other typical insufficiency fractures, such as the distal radius, pelvis, or spine and for fall-associated traumatic conditions such as subdural hematoma. The involvement of a medical consultant, particularly one who knows the patient, is useful. Laboratory studies should include a complete blood count, analysis of serum electrolytes, a blood sample for type and cross match, chest radiograph, and electrocardiogram.

Adequate anteroposterior (AP) radiographs of the hip and proximal femur are necessary to plan for the procedure. Lateral films are difficult to obtain due to patient discomfort and are often of poor quality. Obesity and osteopenia frequently combine to thwart adequate visualization, and repeat films with less penetration may be helpful. Traction and/or rotation films may be helpful to evaluate the fracture line, although traction and internal rotation may restore the position of the femur and make the orientation look normal. Sizing templates for the prosthetic system can be used to estimate the size of the prosthesis necessary. Particular attention should be paid to the level of the neck cut and the size of the femoral head because length discrepancies and size mismatch are associated with poor outcomes (27).

OPERATIVE PROCEDURE

The procedure can be performed under general or spinal anesthesia. Regional technique may offer less risk of some anesthetic complications, but several large retrospective, non-randomized studies of hip fracture surgery have failed to show any difference in mortality, morbidity, or functional outcome (28–31).

Preoperative intravenous antibiotics are given at least 30 minutes, but less than 120 minutes, prior to incision. Usually 2 g of a broad spectrum cephalosporin (e.g., cefazolin) are given, unless the patient is allergic or there is another specific reason to give a different drug.

The operation can be performed through anterior, lateral, or posterior approaches to the hip. One study of relatively poor methodological quality compared anterior to posterior approaches and found (for unexplained reasons) significantly increased mortality in the posterior group (32), and some older studies suggested a higher dislocation rate with posterior approach (33,34). More recent meta-analysis for comparison of lateral and posterior approaches for total hip arthroplasty has yielded no major differences in function or complication rates (35). The surgeon should use the surgical approach with which she/he feels most comfortable.

For the posterior approach to the hip, the patient is placed in the lateral decubitus position after induction of anesthetic. Padding is placed on all bony prominences (Fig. 15.2). A bean bag is used to maintain position, and the down-side arm is placed out in front of the body. An axillary roll may be used. The down-side leg is padded and secured to the bed with straps or tape. The chest may be secured in like fashion, but care should be taken not to make the chest strap too tight. Efforts are made to orient the pelvis directly lateral.

The hip and leg is scrubbed and painted with antiseptic circumferentially from above the iliac crest to the toes, and the draping is applied to allow adequate exposure posteriorly and proximally. The leg is covered with a stockinette to the mid thigh and secured with Coban

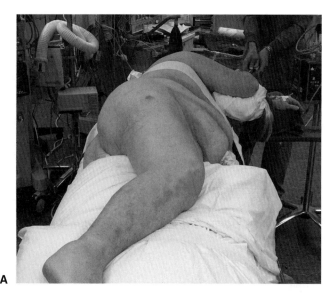

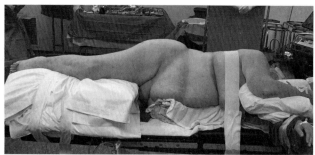

A   B

Figure 15.2. The patient is positioned in the lateral decubitis position on a bean bag with care taken to pad all boney prominences. A pillow is placed between the arms and the legs.

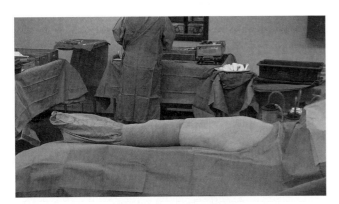

Figure 15.3. The entire leg and hip are draped free, as shown in this image from a patient other than the one in Figure 15.1. A stockinette is used to the mid thigh.

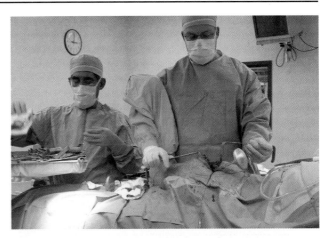

Figure 15.4. The position used by the assistant to support the leg and retract the tissues. It is important to be careful not to contaminate the patient's leg against the assistant's face or mask.

(Fig. 15.3). The incision is marked on the skin and then adherent antiseptic-impregnated plastic drapes may be applied to cover the exposed skin completely, including the medial thigh and groin.

The surgeon stands behind the patient while the assistant stands on the opposite side. This allows the assistant to keep his/her hands free while supporting the leg with the hip extended, knee flexed, and the femur externally rotated (Fig. 15.4). The incision is centered on the greater trochanter and extends distally along the lateral aspect of the femur for approximately 10 cm. Proximally the incision extends approximately 45 degrees toward the posterior, superior, iliac spine for approximately 10 cm (Fig. 15.5). With an obese patient, larger incisions will be necessary. The subcutaneous tissue is divided in line with the incision, and hemostasis is accomplished with electrocautery. The fascial level is identified and opened sharply with knife or Bovie, and the incision is extended distally in the fascia posterior to the iliotibial band and proximally, splitting the gluteus fascia and muscle bluntly. The trochanter is exposed (Fig. 15.6).

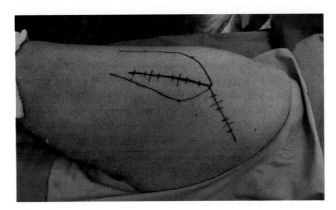

Figure 15.5. The incision is centered on the trochanter and marked on the skin.

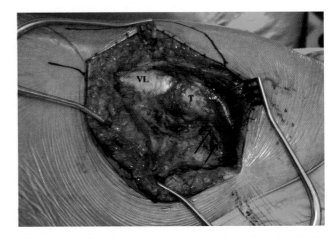

Figure 15.6. The incision has been made and the fascia divided. As the surgeon would view the field: Distal is to the left, and proximal is to the right; anterior is up and posterior is down. The *arrows* indicate the posterior edge of the medius tendon inserting onto the trochanter. VL, vastus lateralis; T, trochanter.

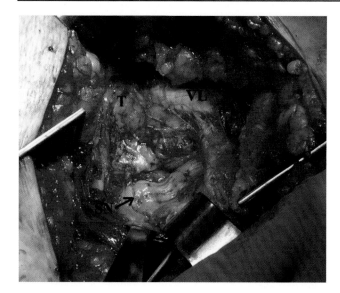

Figure 15.7. The sciatic nerve is seen passing proximal to distal (left to right) posterior to the quadratus femoris muscle in this image from another patient. T, trochanter; VL, vastus lateralis; SN, sciatic nerve.

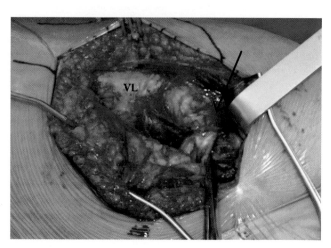

Figure 15.8. In this picture, distal is to the left, and proximal to the right. The piriformis tendon is indicated by the clamp behind it. The *arrow* identifies the tip of the trochanter. VL, vastus lateralis.

The sciatic nerve is palpated posterior to the quadratus femoris and its position clearly noted (Fig. 15.7). Awareness of the nerve position is maintained throughout the operation, and it is protected from tension by extension of the hip and flexion of the knee. The piriformis tendon is identified by palpation posterior to and underneath the edge of the gluteus medius, which is attached to the trochanter (Figs. 15.8 and 15.9). The tendon is separated from the underlying capsule by gentle spreading the right angled clamp and by passing a soft tissue elevator between the short rotators and the capsule surface (Fig. 15.10). A tag suture is passed through the tendon approximately 1.0 cm from its insertion and looped around the tendon to grasp it. The tendon is divided with the Bovie near the insertion. As an alternative, and to increase postoperative hip stability, the tendon can be retracted and attempts made to preserve it throughout the procedure (36). The conjoined tendon of the obturator internus

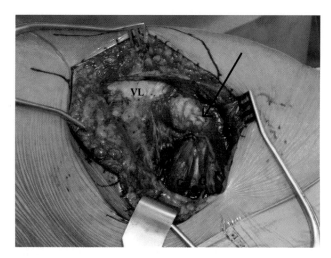

Figure 15.9. The short external rotators of the hip. In this picture distal is toward the left and proximal is toward the right. The arrow indicates the tip of the trochanter with gluteus medius attaching. VL, vastus lateralis; G, gemelli (superior and inferior); O, obturator internus; P, piriformis.

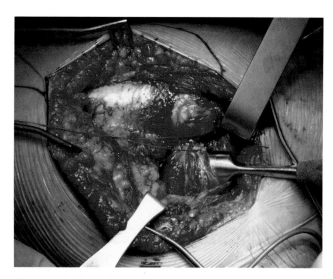

Figure 15.10. Defining the capsular plane with an elevator. Note the tag suture placed in the conjoined tendon of the external rotators.

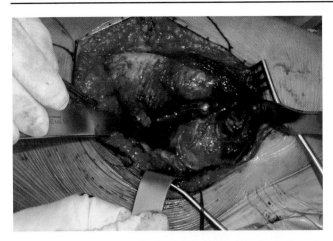

Figure 15.11. The capsule is exposed by retractors placed above and below it after the external rotator muscles are retracted.

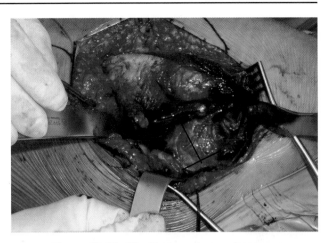

Figure 15.12. The H-shaped capsulotomy.

and the gemelli muscles (see Fig. 15.9) is identified in like fashion, tagged, and divided. Note that this tendon is frequently on the undersurface of the musculature and must be located by palpation rather than by direct vision. When these two tendons are reflected, the sciatic nerve usually passes behind the conjoined tendon and attached muscles, and is in front of the piriformis tendon/muscle. However, there is substantial variation among patients and one must be on the lookout for a split sciatic nerve on either side of either tendon.

Once the tendons are reflected, the hip joint capsule is cleaned of attachments by gentle scraping with the soft-tissue elevator. Homan retractors are used to define the capsular plane superior and inferior (Fig. 15.11). Internal rotation of the femur facilitates full exposure of the posterior capsule. The capsule is opened by incising parallel to the neck of the femur, and perpendicular at either end, to form a sort of H capsulotomy (Fig. 15.12). The labrum is protected and retained. Retraction of the capsular flaps reveals the femoral head and neck, and the fracture is obvious. Homan retractors can then be placed inside the capsule (Fig. 15.13). The labrum is not incised.

The fracture is opened by rotation, in opposite directions, of the femur and the head, exposing the broken surface of the head. A corkscrew tool (Fig. 15.14) is screwed into the cancellous bone of the head and used to gently lever it out of the acetabulum. The

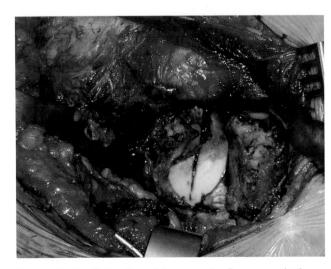

Figure 15.13. Retraction of the capsular flaps reveals the femoral head. The head is marked by the Bovie used to cut the capsule.

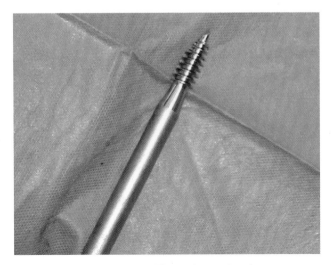

Figure 15.14. The corkscrew tool.

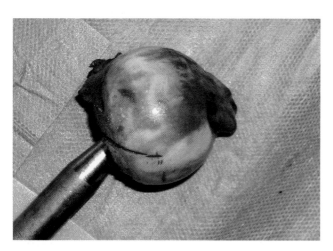

Figure 15.15. The impaled femoral head is removed by levering the corkscrew tool and cutting the ligamentum teres with heavy scissors.

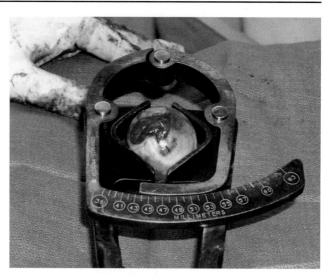

Figure 15.16. Measuring the diameter of the removed femoral head to help select the appropriate prosthetic head size.

ligamentum teres is cut with curved mayo scissors, and the head is removed (Fig. 15.15). In difficult cases, the head can be removed in pieces with a rongeur or by gently cutting it with careful use of osteotomes. If the head can be removed intact, the diameter can be measured for guidance in selecting a prosthetic head (Fig. 15.16).

Once the head is removed, the broken femoral neck is addressed. The hip is internally rotated to bring the neck up and out of the socket (Fig. 15.17), and the neck cutting guide is used to mark the angle of the cut approximately 1 to 2 cm (traditionally taught as one fingerbreadth) above the lesser trochanter (Fig. 15.18). By using preoperative planning templates, surgeons will have previously indicated the correct level for the incision; if uncertain, he/she should use fluoroscopy and a radio-opaque marker or should just cut a little less. Cutting the neck too short is associated with residual pain and loosening of the stem (27). Fluoroscopy can be used to verify the level of the neck cut (Fig. 15.19). Care is taken to cut the neck in neutral or slight anteversion, depending upon the design of the stem used. Frequently, posterior comminution of the neck fracture will be found (Fig. 15.20). With the head and neck removed, the acetabular sizers can be used to verify the correct diameter head for the prosthesis. The head should sit securely within the acetabulum, with contact

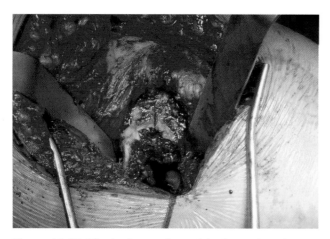

Figure 15.17. The broken surface of the femoral neck.

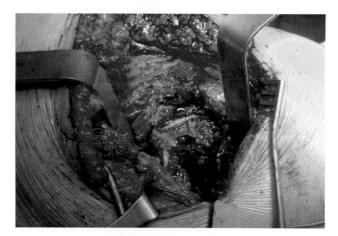

Figure 15.18. The level and angle of the femoral neck cut is marked with the Bovie based on the use of an angle guide and palpation of the lesser trochanter.

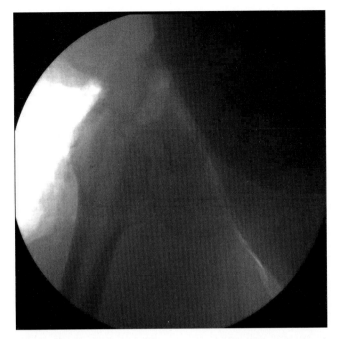

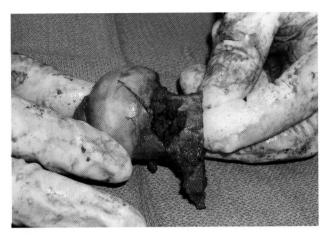

Figure 15.19. Fluoroscopic image taken to confirm the level of the neck cut.

Figure 15.20. After the neck cut has been made, the two pieces are held together at the fracture site, showing comminution and bone loss in the neck posteriorly.

all around the surface and not just on the rim, and should rotate smoothly without toggle. Prosthetic head size greater than 2 mm smaller than the contralateral side is associated with pain and loosening (7,27). An oversized head has also been associated with poor postoperative results with regard to pain (7).

Attention is turned to preparation of the proximal femur. A box osteotome or "cookie cutter" is used to open the metaphysis, with the surgeon taking care to start the cut well lateral to avoid varus alignment of the stem, and with awareness of the rotation to ensure the correct 10 to 15 degrees of anteversion (Fig. 15.21). This can be confusing because of the

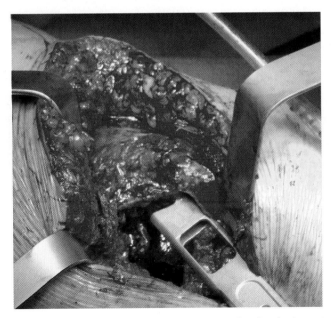

Figure 15.21. Use of the box osteotome, or "cookie cutter," to begin the entry into the femoral metaphysic. Internal rotation of the instrument with relation to the femur will place the prosthetic stem in retroversion; external rotation leads to anteversion.

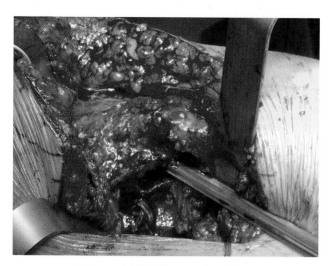

Figure 15.22. The canal seeker.

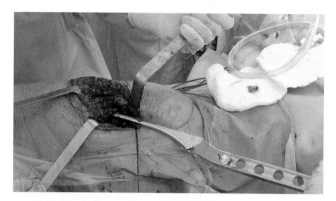

Figure 15.23. The broach prepares the shape of the intramedullary canal to accept the stem. Take care to avoid varus alignment by holding the handle laterally during insertion.

posterior position of the surgeon, and it is worth taking time to ensure correct starting position. Internal rotation of the instrument will lead to retroversion of the prosthesis, which may increase the risk of postoperative dislocation. A canal seeker with blunt tip and side cutting flutes may be used to begin a path down into the intramedullary canal (Fig. 15.22). Depending upon the instrumentation for the brand of stem being utilized, reamers and/or broaches are used to create a space for the stem (Figs. 15.23 and 15.24). The broach should be used gently to avoid exploding the metaphysis and breaking the proximal femur. It is inserted with gentle taps of the mallet, and after going in a bit, it should be extracted and then reinserted deeper. The surgeon should pause when the fit is tight to allow hoop stresses to relax through viscoelasticity. Patience is a virtue here. The in and out motion will help to avoid incarceration. The broach is not a file and should not be used as one. It is a device for shaping the intramedullary canal. The surgeon should avoid varus alignment. Attention must be paid to the soft tissues to avoid damage from the broach. A trial stem is inserted, and a trial head component is attached. The hip is gently reduced by having the assistant apply traction and slow external rotation, while the surgeon applies pressure to the head and holds the capsular flaps out of the way (Fig. 15.25). A portable radiograph is taken (Fig. 15.26). The hip is moved through a range of motion with the trial components in place to assess stability. If acceptable, the hip is dislocated and the trial components are removed.

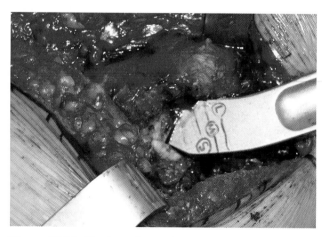

Figure 15.24. The broach may have marks that indicate the correct depth of insertion, and there may be different options for neck length.

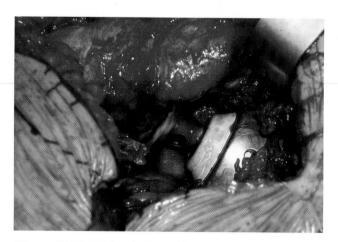

Figure 15.25. Trial reduction with trial components to assess stability and range of motion as well as obtain intraoperative radiographs.

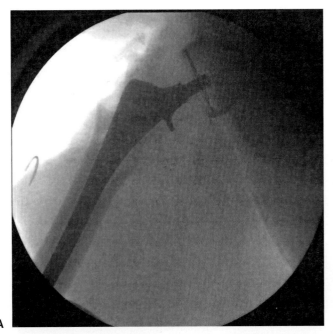
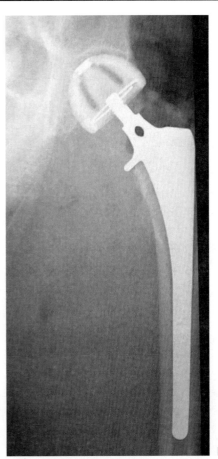

A   **B**

Figure 15.26. Radiographic evaluation of the trial component fit. **A.** A fluoroscopic image with the trial components in place. The stem fills the canal well, there is no varus alignment, and the collar rests on the calcar cut. The trial head sits well in the acetabulum. **B.** A portable radiograph taken in the operating room to demonstrate fit of the trial components.

If cement is to be used, the canal is plugged with plastic restrictor or a bone plug from the metaphysis at the correct depth to allow for a few millimeters of cement distal to the tip of the stem. The acetabulum is protected with sponges. The canal may be irrigated with jet lavage, brushed to clean marrow contents, and dried with sponges. Cement is injected from the distal to proximal with a pressurized cement gun, and the stem is inserted in the correct version. It is held still while the cement hardens. Excess cement is removed with curettes. If cement is not used, a corticocancellous plug, approximately 2 mm wider than the femoral canal, may be made from the head of the femur. This plug is inserted into the canal cortical side distal and advanced with the broach just proximal to the anticipated tip position for the prosthesis. The stem is inserted and advanced with the mallet driving the plug distally (Fig. 15.27) (26). Care should be taken to seat the collar of the prosthesis all the way down onto the bone of the femoral neck osteotomy (calcar) because failure to do so is associated with postoperative pain and loosening (27).

The modular unipolar or bipolar head is inserted and seated fully with gentle taps of the mallet. Reduction is performed gently. Repeat radiographs can be done with the final components in place (Fig. 15.28). Stability is checked by placing the hip through a range of motion and gently stressing the reduction. The hip should flex beyond 90 degrees, adduct beyond neutral, and externally rotate 15 to 20 degrees without dislocating.

The capsular flaps are closed around the prosthesis with heavy suture (Fig. 15.29). The short external rotators are reattached to their insertions with nonabsorbable suture placed through bone. Usually, the heavy needle can be driven through the bone of the trochanter

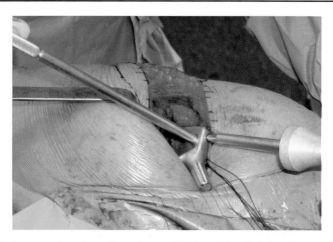

Figure 15.27. A cementless insertion of press-fit stem. Care is taken to maintain the correct version during stem insertion.

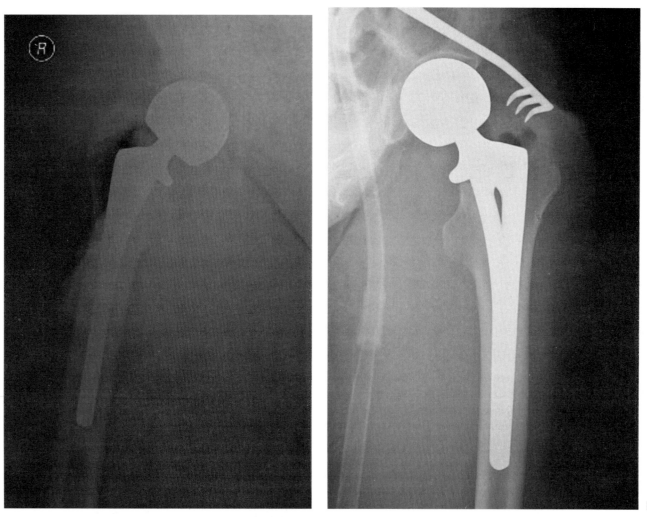

A   B

Figure 15.28. Intraoperative portable radiographs of the final prosthesis for a **(A)** cemented and **(B)** cementless prosthesis.

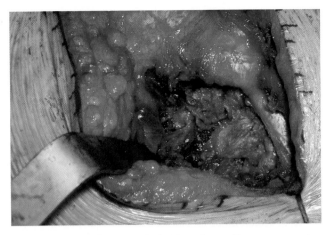

Figure 15.29. The capsule is closed over the components.

by hand or with light taps of the mallet. The fascia lata is closed with interrupted absorbable sutures and then the incision is closed in layers. Sterile dressings are applied and a hip abduction pillow is placed.

POSTOPERATIVE REGIMEN AND REHABILITATION

Prophylaxis against deep venous thrombosis (DVT) is believed to be appropriate by many physicians, although there is controversy regarding the method. Mechanical devices such as foot or calf pumps may be used. Antibiotics are usually continued for 24 hours after surgery and then stopped. The patient is mobilized from the bed on postoperative day one and taught appropriate transfer techniques. Patients may begin weight bearing as tolerated. The abduction pillow and hip positioning precautions are enforced strictly for 6 weeks. Transfer techniques and ambulation are taught. Physical therapists and social workers can help assess the patient's abilities and needs for placement decisions. Limited evidence suggests that protein and energy supplementation may reduce unfavorable outcomes (not including mortality) in the recovery of hip fracture in elderly patient (37).

RESULTS

Pain

Pain in the thigh or groin is reported by 10% to 32% of patients after cemented hemi-arthroplasty, and by 25% to 70% of patients after uncemented hemi-arthoplasty (16,24,38). Analgesic use is reported by 26% to 35% of patients (38,39). There does not seem to be any difference in postoperative among those with unipolar and bipolar prostheses (22). If the size of the prosthetic head is larger or smaller than 2 mm of the natural head, increased postoperative pain may result (7,27).

Hip Scores

In one study of 451 fractures treated with bipolar endoprosthetic replacement, 83% of those with cemented hemi-arthroplasties had Harris scores of Good and Excellent, while 50% of uncemented stems received a good and excellent score (16). A retrospective study of 53 independently mobile patients treated with cemented bipolar prostheses showed a strong correlation of modified Harris hip score with prefracture levels of mobility and independence. Seventy-three percent of fully independent patients who could walk a mile before their fracture had Good and Excellent hip scores at follow-up, while of those who needed help shopping or could walk less than 100 yards, 0% to 9% had a good or excellent outcome (14).

Ambulation

Overall, approximately 50% to 60% of hip fracture patients regain their prefracture ambulatory status within a year (29). The percentage of patients who achieve unassisted community ambulation (able to get around outside the home) has been reported as 11% to 30% (7,39–41). One study found that 30% of postsurgery patients with cemented prostheses needed a higher level of walking aid than before injury; 60% of patients with uncemented prostheses needed similar assistance (24). Use of a cane or walking stick was required in 17% to 62% of patients with uncemented prosthesis and 40% to 50% of patients with cemented prosthesis; walker or crutch use was required for 15% to 35% and 27% to 40% of patients with cemented and uncemented prostheses, respectively (7,38,39). The percentages of persons who had ability to ambulate outside the home dropped from 92% before the injury to 70% to 75% after the operation (21,22). At an average follow-up of 10 years, only 31% of the patients in one study retained the ability to ambulate in the community (40). Seventy-five percent of patients with pre-injury senile dementia lost the ability to ambulate at all (42). However, 11 out of 28 (39%) patients who had been independent in all activities of daily living (ADLs) and could walk more than 1 mile before their injury had a strong chance of regaining the ability to walk a mile after cemented bipolar endoprosthesis (14).

Independence

Thirty-two percent to 64% of postoperative patients are discharged to their own homes (38,39,41,42), while 15% to 40% of those who were independent before fracture end up in some sort of institution after the surgery (29). A living situation with a lower level of independence is the result for 11% to 40% of patients with a cemented prosthesis, and is the case for 18% to 56% with an uncemented prosthesis (24,25). One study found that the percentage of patients who were independent in basic activities of daily living (dressing, bathing, feeding) dropped from 80% to 90% pre-injury to 60% postoperatively, and that those independent in instrumental activities of daily living (shopping, housework, laundry) dropped from 40% to 60% to approximately 20% (22).

Radiographic and Histologic Examinations

Significant loosening or subsidence of the stem is common, occurring in up to 50% of cemented stems and found over 90% in some series of uncemented stems (16). Acetabular erosion is also seen, particularly in active patients. The rate of protrusio acetabuli is 5% to 26% after 5 years (9). The proposed difference between bipolar and unipolar prostheses has not been convincingly demonstrated.

At 5 years, a nearly complete loss of acetabular cartilage has been seen on histological examination of biopsy specimens from patients undergoing revision due to groin pain. The loss of cartilage correlated with duration of articulation with the prosthesis (43).

Revision

In the first 2 years after hemi-arthroplasty, recurrent or irreducible dislocation is the most common reason for revision. After 2 years, pain associated with loosening, subsidence, or erosion is more common. The rate of revision after long-term follow-up varies from 3% to 24% (5,7,9,40,44) with an average of approximately 11% for all types considered. Gebhard et al (7) found that cemented endoprostheses were revised nearly 8% of the time, while uncemented prostheses had a 13% revision rate; approximately 2% of those with total hip arthroplasty also needed revision. With modular components, the revision from either bipolar or unipolar endoprosthesis to total hip arthroplasty can be accomplished without removal of the stem.

COMPLICATIONS

The early mortality rate (under 3 months) for patients after hemi-arthroplasty for femoral neck fracture has been reported from 5% to 23% (5,38). As reported in most studies, patient mortality at 1 year is between 17% and 34% in most studies (4,5,19,20,23,44,45) but has been reported as higher (5,38) and lower (22). One prospective study of octogenarians found that 30% of postoperative patients had 1-year mortality (19). At 4 months postoperation, mortality is significantly higher in patients with dementia than in those without it (33% vs. 12%) and at 1 year the difference is 44% versus 20% (42). Due to the elderly nature of the patient population, mortality increases over time. In one study, only 6% of female patients who were over 70 years old at the time of surgery survived 6 years after it (44). As one would expect from the patient population, medical complications are common in the postoperative period, including urinary and respiratory tract infections, DVT and pulmonary embolism, cardiac failure, arrhythmia or infarction, stroke, gastrointestinal bleeding, and renal failure. A prospective outcome study of 270 patients revealed a 16% rate of major medical complication and a 35% rate of minor medical complication (23).

Surgical complications are less common, occurring in approximately 5% to 10% of patients; the numbers vary according to the research question asked. Intra-operative fracture of the femur may occur from vigorous broaching or forceful reduction and may necessitate a change to a longer stem and concomitant internal fixation. Dislocation rates have been reported from 1% to 9% (4,7,20,36,44,46). However, no differences have been found in dislocation rate between bipolar and unipolar prostheses. One study has suggested that dislocation of a bipolar more frequently requires open reduction, but the numbers from the study are too small for significance to be calculated (20). Bipolar dislocations do not necessarily are not always address through open reduction. THR for fracture may have a higher dislocation rate than hemi-arthroplasty (4,5,11), but this is not a universal finding (7,9). Dislocation after hemi-arthroplasty is a significant event, and according to a retrospective study of 1,000 patients (47), is associated with a mortality of 65% within 6 months. Dislocation is more common after posterior than anterior or anterolateral surgical approaches (7,36), but preservation of the capsule and labrum improves stability and lowers the dislocation rate (36). Incorrect sizing of the prosthetic head has been implicated as a predisposing factor to dislocation (7). In most series, wound hematoma occurs in 3 to 4% and infection is seen in approximately 2% of patients. Deep infection, which has been reported to occur in 0 to 18% of patients (5), requires further surgery and often results in Girdlestone hip resection.

RECOMMENDED READINGS

1. Swiontkowski MF. Current concepts review: intracapsular fractures of the hip. *J Bone Joint Surg* 1994;76: 129–138.
2. Davison JN, Calder SJ, Anderson GH, et al. Treatment for displaced intracapsular fractures of the proximal femur: a prospective randomized trial in patients aged 65 to 79 years. *J Bone Joint Surg* 2001;83(21): 206–212.
3. Toh EM, Sahni V, Acharya A, et al. Management of intracapsular femoral neck fractures in the elderly; is it time to rethink our strategy? *Injury* 2004;35:125–129.
4. Masson M, Parker MJ, Fleischer S. Internal fixation versus arthroplasty for intracapsular proximal femoral fractures in adults (Cochrane Review). In: *The Cochrane Library*. Issue 3. Chichester, UK: John Wiley & Sons, Ltd; 2005.

5. Bhandari M, Devereaux PJ, Swiontkowski MF, et al. Internal fixation compared with arthroplasty for displaced fractures of the femoral neck: a meta-analysis. *J Bone Joint Surg Am* 2003;85(9):1673–1681.
6. Iorio R, Healy WL, Lemos DW, et al. Displaced femoral neck fractures in the elderly: outcomes and cost effectiveness. *Clin Orthop* 2001;383:229–242.
7. Gebhard JS, Amstutz HC, Zinar DM, et al. A comparison of total hip arthroplasty and hemi-arthroplasty for treatment of acute fracture of the femoral neck. *Clin Orthop* 1992;282:123–131.
8. Healy WL, Iorio R. Total hip arthroplasty: optimal treatment for displaced femoral neck fractures in elderly patients. *Clin Orthop* 2004;429:43–48.
9. Rodriguez-Merchan E. Displaced intracapsular hip fractures: hemiarthroplasty or total arthroplasty? *Clin Orthop* 2002;399:72–77.
10. Greenough CG, Jones JR. Primary total hip replacement for displaced subcapital fracture of the femur. *J Bone Joint Surg Br* 1988;70:639–643.
11. Gregory RJ, Gibson MJ, Moran CG. Dislocation after primary arthroplasty for subcapital fracture of the hip: wide range of movement is a risk factor. *J Bone Joint Surg Br* 1991;73:11–12.
12. Dorr LD, Glousman R, Hoy AL, et al. Treatment of femoral neck fractures with total hip replacement versus cemented and noncemented hemiarthroplasty. *J Arthroplasty* 1986;1:21–28.
13. Skinner P, Riley D, Ellery J, et al. Displaced subcapital fractures of the femur: a prospective randomized comparison of internal fixation, hemiarthroplasty and total hip replacement. *Injury* 1989;20(5):291–293.
14. Dixon S, Bannister G. Cemented bipolar hemiarthroplasty for displaced intracapsular fracture in the mobile active elderly patient. *Injury* 2004;35:152–156.
15. Lestrange NR. Bipolar arthroplasty for 496 hip fractures. *Clin Orthop* 1990;251:7–19.
16. Lo WH, Chen WM, Huang CK, et al. Bateman bipolar hemiarthroplasty for displaced intracapsular femoral neck fractures: cemented versus uncemented. *Clin Orthop* 1994;302:75–82.
17. Chen SC, Badrinath K, Pell LH, et al. The movements of the components of the Hastings bipolar prosthesis. *J Bone Joint Surg Br* 1989;71:186–188.
18. Tsukamoto Y, Mabuchi K, Futami T, et al. Motion of the bipolar hip prosthesis components: friction studied in cadavers. *Acta Orthop Scand* 1992;63(6):648–652.
19. Calder SJ, Anderson GH, Jagger C, et al. Unipolar or bipolar prosthesis for displaced intracapsular hip fracture in octogenarians: a randomized prospective study. *J Bone Joint Surg Br* 1996;78(3):391–394.
20. Parker MJ, Gurusamy K. Arthroplasties (with and without bone cement) for proximal femoral fractures in adults (Cochrane Review). In: *The Cochrane Library*. Issue 2. Chichester, UK: John Wiley & Sons, Ltd; 2004.
21. Raia FJ, Chapman CB, Herrera MF, et al. Unipolar or bipolar hemiarthroplasty for femoral neck fractures in the elderly? *Clin Orthop* 2003;414:259–265.
22. Wathne RA, Koval KJ, Aharonoff GB, et al. Modular unipolar vs. bipolar prosthesis: a prospective evaluation of functional outcomes after femoral neck fracture. *J Ortho Trauma* 1995;9(4):298–302.
23. Kenzora JE, Magaziner J, Hudson J, et al. Outcome after hemiarthroplasty for femoral neck fractures in the elderly. *Clin Orthop* 1998;348:51–58.
24. Emery RJH, Broughton NS, Desai K, et al. Bipolar hemiarthroplasty for subcapital fracture of the femoral neck: a prospective randomized trial of cemented Thompson and uncemented Moore stems. *J Bone Joint Surg Br* 1991;73(2):322–324.
25. Khan RJK, MacDowell A, Crossman P, et al. Cemented or uncemented hemiarthroplasty for displaced intracapsular fractures of the hip: a systematic review. *Injury* 2002;33:13–17.
26. Kligman M, Zecevic M, Roffman M. The effect of intramedullary corticocancellous bone plug for hip hemiarthroplasty. *J Trauma* 2001;51:84–87.
27. Sharif KM, Parker MJ. Austin Moore hemiarthroplasty: technical aspects and their effects on outcome, in patients with fractures of the neck of femur. *Injury* June 2002;33(5):419–422.
28. Gilbert TB, Hawkes WG, Hebel JR, et al. Spinal anesthesia versus general anesthesia for hip fracture repair: a longitudinal observation of 741 elderly patients during 2-year follow-up. *Am J Orthop* 2000;29:25–35.
29. Koval KJ, Aharonoff GB, Rosenberg AD, et al. Functional outcome after hip fracture: effect of general versus regional anesthesia. *Clin Orthop* 1998;348:37–41.
30. Koval KJ, Aharonoff GB, Rosenberg AD, et al. Hip fracture in the elderly: the effect of anesthetic technique. *Orthopedics* 1999;22:31–34.
31. O'Hara DA, Duff A, Berlin JA, et al. The effect of anesthetic technique on postoperative outcomes in hip fracture repair. *Anesthesiology* 2000;92:947–957.
32. Parker MJ, Pervez H. Surgical approaches for inserting hemiarthroplasty of the hip (Cochrane Review). In: *The Cochrane Library*. Issue 3. Chichester, UK: John Wiley & Sons, Ltd; 2004.
33. Bochner RM, Pellicci PM, Lyden JP. Bipolar hemiarthroplasty for fracture of the femoral neck: Clinical review with special emphasis on prosthetic motion. *J Bone Joint Surg Am* 1988;70:1001–1010.
34. Chan RNW, Hoskinson J. Thompson prosthesis for fractured neck of femur: a comparison of surgical approaches. *J Bone Joint Surg Br* 1975;57:437–443.
35. Jolles BM, Bogoch ER. Posterior versus lateral surgical approach for total hip arthroplasty in adults with osteoarthritis (Cochrane Review). In: *The Cochrane Library*. Issue 3. Chichester, UK: John Wiley & Sons, Ltd; 2004.
36. Martinez AA, Herrera A, Cueneca J, et al. Comparison of two different posterior approaches for hemiarthroplasty of the hip. *Arch Orthop Trauma Surg* 2002;122:51–52.
37. Avenell A, Handoll HH. A systematic review of protein and energy supplementation for hip fracture aftercare in older people. *Eur J Clin Nutr* 2003;57:895–903.
38. Lennox IAC, McLauchlan J. Comparing the mortality and morbidity of cemented and uncemented hemiarthroplasties. *Injury* 1993;24(3):185–186.
39. Partanen J, Jalovaara P. Functional comparison between uncemented Austin-Moore hemiarthroplasty and osteosynthesis with three screws in displaced femoral neck fractures: a matched pair study of 168 patients. *Int Orthop* 2004;28:28–31.
40. Clayer M, Brucker J. The outcome of Austin-Moore hemiarthroplasty for fracture of the femoral neck. *Am J Orthop* 1997;26(10):681–684.

41. Heikkinan T, Wingstrand H, Partanen J, et al. Hemiarthroplasty or osteosynthesis in cervical hip fractures: matched pair analysis in 892 patients. *Arch Orthop Trauma Surg* 2003;122(3):143–147.

42. van Dortmont LMC, Douw CM, van Breukelen AMA, et al. Outcome after hemi-arthroplasty for displaced intracapsular femoral neck fracture related to mental state. *Injury* 2000;31:327–331.

43. Dalldorf PG, Banas MP, Hicks DG, et al. Rate of degeneration of human acetabular cartilage after hemiarthroplasty. *J Bone Joint Surg Am* 1995;77:877–882.

44. Wachtl SW, Jakob RP, Gautier E. Ten-year patient and prosthesis survival after unipolar hip hemiarthroplasty in female patients over 70 years old. *J Arthroplasty* 2003;18(5):587–591.

45. Lu-Yao GL, Keller RB, Littenberg B, et al. Outcomes after displaced fractures of the femoral neck: a meta-analysis of one hundred and six published reports. *J Bone Joint Surg Am* 1994;76(1):15–25.

46. Goldhill VB, Lyden JP, Cornell CN, et al. Bipolar hemiarthroplasty for fracture of the femoral neck. *J Orthop Trauma* 1991;5(3):318–324.

47. Blewitt N, Mortimore S. Outcome of dislocation after hemiarthroplasty for fractured neck of the femur. *Injury* 1992;23(5):320–322.

16

Intertrochanteric Fractures: Use of a Sliding Hip Screw

Kenneth J. Koval

INDICATIONS/CONTRAINDICATIONS

The primary goal of fracture treatment is to return the patient to his/her prefracture level of function. There is general agreement that in the patient who sustains an intertrochanteric hip fracture, this can best be accomplished through surgery. Nonoperative management is appropriate only in nonambulators, often with multiple medical co-morbidities, who experience minimal discomfort from the injury. Occasionally, younger healthy patients who have a completely nondisplaced intertrochanteric fracture can be managed nonoperatively; however, these patients must be closely followed to detect evidence of fracture displacement. All patients treated nonoperatively should be rapidly mobilized to avoid the complications of prolonged recumbency, such as decubitus, deep venous thrombosis (DVT), aspiration, and the like.

Numerous authors have proposed classification schemes for intertrochanteric fractures; however, the most important aspect of any classification is the determination of fracture stability. Stability is provided by the presence of an intact posteromedial cortical buttress. Unstable fracture patterns include those with loss of the posteromedial buttress, fractures with subtrochanteric extension, and reverse obliquity fractures.

I currently use a sliding hip screw with a two-hole side plate for stable intertrochanteric hip fractures and an intramedullary nail for unstable fracture patterns, particularly in younger individuals. Following fixation of intertrochanteric fractures with a stable fracture pattern, there should be minimal fracture settling, limb shortening, or medialization of the distal fragment. I prefer a variable angle hip screw (VHS) (EBI, Parsippany, NJ) because it allows some adjustment of the fracture alignment once the screw and plate assembly has been implanted (Fig. 16.1). The use of this implant also helps with inventory control as a single plate can allow a range of plate angles, from 89 to 159 degrees. For unstable fracture patterns, I prefer use of an intramedullary hip screw (IMHS) device because it prevents excessive fracture collapse and deformity. The lag screw portion of the intramedullary devices can telescope within the nail only until the femoral head and neck segment abuts the intramedullary nail.

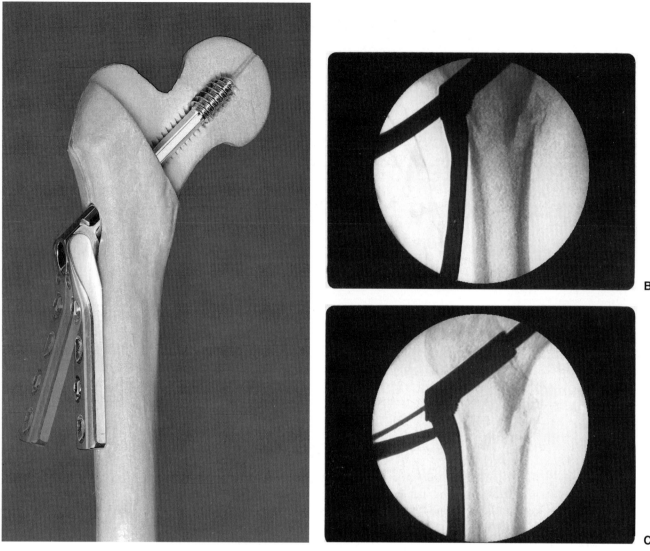

Figure 16.1. A. Photograph of the VHS system demonstrating the adjustability of the plate angle. **B.** Radiographs after initial plate placement and **(C)** after use of the mechanism to bring the plate to the lateral femoral cortex.

PREOPERATIVE PLANNING

The range of clinical deformity of the involved lower extremity varies depending on fracture displacement and comminution. Nondisplaced fractures may present with virtually no clinical deformity, while displaced fractures present with the classic shortened and externally rotated extremity. Range of motion of the hip can be painful and should be avoided. Neurovascular injuries are rare, but a careful evaluation should be performed. Hip fractures following high-energy trauma require a careful work-up to rule out the possibility of associated injuries.

Standard radiographic examination for patients with suspected hip fractures include an anteroposterior (AP) view of the pelvis, and an AP and cross-table lateral of the injured proximal femur (Fig. 16.2). A cross-table lateral radiograph is necessary to evaluate the posteromedial cortex for signs of comminution. In situations where the fracture geometry is not clear due to deformity, an AP view of the hip internally rotated 15 to 20 degrees may be helpful (Fig. 16.3). An AP view of the contralateral side is helpful, particularly as a means of assessing the size and angle of the implant for intramedullary fixation.

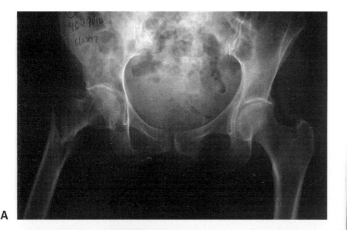

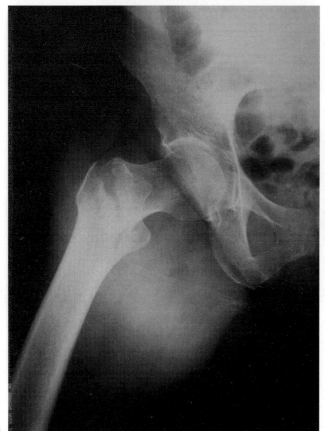

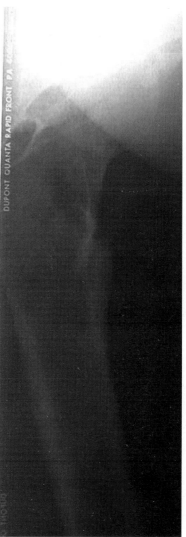

Figure 16.2. A. AP view of the pelvis.
B. An AP and **(C)** cross-table lateral
view of the hip revealing a right intertrochanteric fracture.

SURGERY

Following satisfactory general or spinal anesthesia, the patient is positioned supine on a
fracture table, with care taken to pad and protect the labia or scrotum against the peroneal
post. Once the patient is properly positioned, a mobile c-arm intensifier is positioned to
allow visualization of the hip in AP and lateral planes. Most intertrochanteric hip fractures
can be reduced using gentle longitudinal traction with the leg externally rotated followed
by varying degrees of internal rotation. The uninvolved leg must be positioned so that it
does not block positioning of the image intensifier for a lateral view (Fig. 16.4).

The surgeon must confirm satisfactory fracture reduction before prepping the patient and
be certain that nonobstructive, biplanar, radiographic visualization of the entire proximal
femur, including the hip joint, is obtainable (Fig. 16.5). Inadequate visualization of the
entire proximal femur can result in technical errors, such as inappropriate lag screw

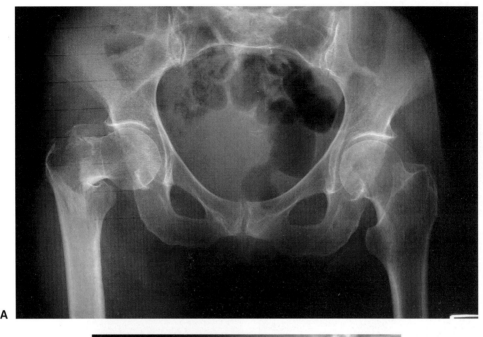

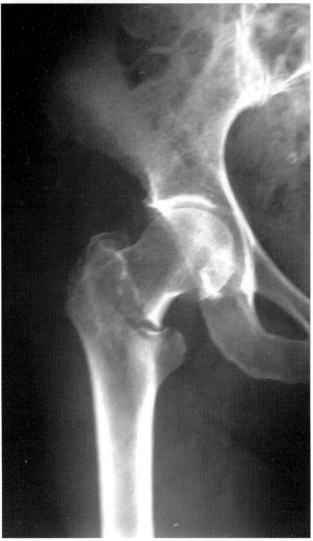

Figure 16.3. Use of internal rotation with gentle traction to evaluate a right, proximal, femur fracture.

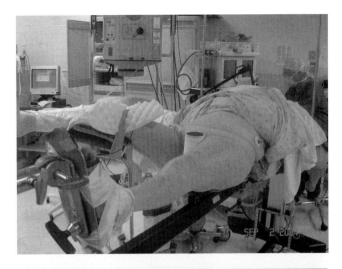

Figure 16.4. Patient positioning for stabilization of a left intertrochanteric fracture with the uninvolved leg flexed, abducted, and externally rotated.

Figure 16.5. Positioning of the image intensifier for **(A)** AP and **(B)** lateral radiographic views. **C.** AP and and **(D)** lateral radiographs of a reduced intertrochanteric fracture prior to patient draping.

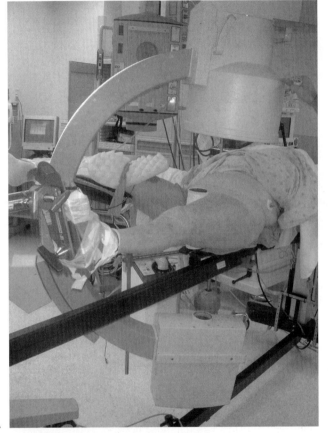

A

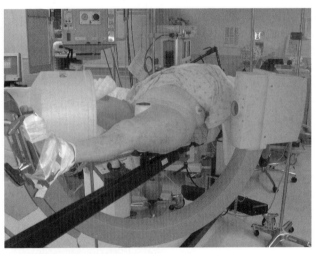

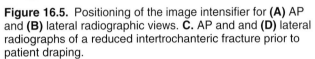

B

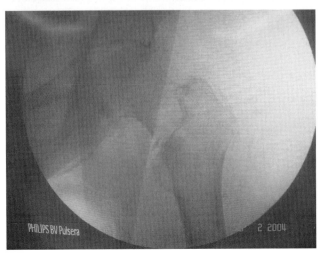

C

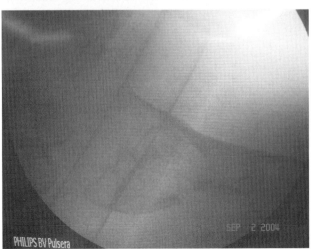

D

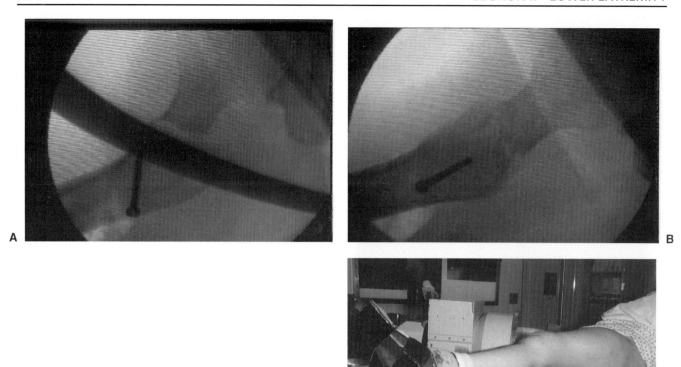

Figure 16.6. A. Posterior sag after intertrochanteric fracture reduction can be corrected with use of a **(B,C)** crutch placed under the proximal thigh.

positioning or length. Varus angulation often results in guide pin positioning in the inferior femoral neck and superior femoral head. The surgeon must be prepared to deal with residual varus angulation, posterior sag, or malrotation. Varus angulation can usually be corrected by placing additional traction on the lower extremity to disengage the fracture fragments. Occasionally, one may need to abduct the lower extremity to correct a varus malreduction. If residual varus remains, one should check the position of the fracture fragments on the lateral radiographic view, as posterior sag may prevent adequate fracture reduction. In this situation, traction should be released and the fracture manipulated to disengage the fragments. Attempting fracture fixation with varus angulation or posterior sag can lead to difficulty centering the lag screw in the femoral head.

Posterior sag requires manual correction using a crutch, bone hook, or periosteal elevator (Fig. 16.6). If unrecognized, posterior sag can result in guide pin positioning in the anterior femoral neck and posterior femoral head. After a satisfactory reduction has been achieved, I rotate the lower extremity under fluoroscopy to determine whether the fracture fragments move as a single unit. In those patients where the femoral shaft moves independently of the proximal fragment, excessive internal rotation of the leg should be suspected. In these cases, the lower extremity should be placed in neutral or slightly external rotation. Once the fracture is fully reduced, the patient is prepped and draped.

APPROACH AND IMPLANT INSERTION

A straight lateral incision is made starting just distal to the greater trochanter and extending distally in line with the femoral shaft (Fig. 16.7). The length of the incision depends upon the patient's size. The iliotibial band is exposed and incised in line with its fibers (Fig. 16.8). The vastus lateralis is elevated from the intermuscular septum and the lateral aspect

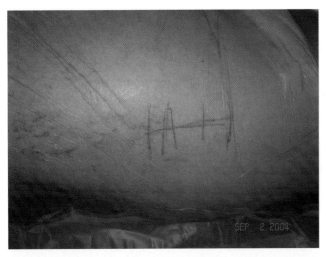

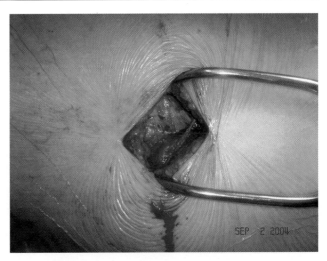

Figure 16.7. A straight 3- to 4-cm lateral incision is initiated just distal to the greater trochanter and is extended distally in line with the femoral shaft.

Figure 16.8. Exposure of the iliotibial band.

of the proximal femur dissected of soft tissue (Fig. 16.9). Using image intensification, a guide pin is inserted into the femoral neck and head using an angle guide. Most commercially available sliding-hip screws are available in plate angles of from 125 to 155 degrees, of which the 135- and 150-degree devices are the most popular. I usually select a 135-degree device because its use facilitates lag screw placement into the desired central portion of the femoral head, and because of its entry point in metaphyseal cancellous bone, it decreases the stress riser effect of a higher-angle device.

The Variable Angle Hip Screw system allows guide pin insertion into the femoral neck and head using either an angle guide or freehand technique with later adjustment of the plate to accommodate the selected angle. I prefer to use the angle guide because it helps ensure placement of the guide pin at the desired 135 degree angle and to a check to proper fracture reduction; inability to place the guide pin into the center of the femoral head and neck using this angle should alert the surgeon to the possibility of a fracture malreduction.

The position of the guide pin is adjusted until it lies in the center of the femoral head and neck on both the AP and lateral planes within 5 to 10 mm of the subchondral bone (Fig. 16.10). Central and deep placement allows lag screw purchase in the best bone available as well as allows maximal collapse of the screw before its threads engage the plate barrel.

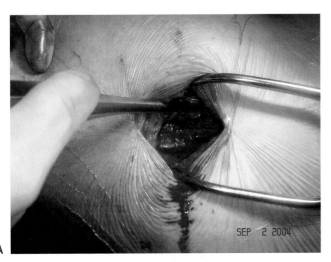

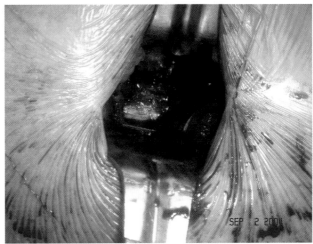

A   B

Figure 16.9. A. After incising the iliotibial band, the surgeon exposes the vastus lateralis and then elevates it from the lateral aspect of the proximal femur. **B.** Homan retractors are placed under the vastus lateralis, exposing the lateral femoral shaft.

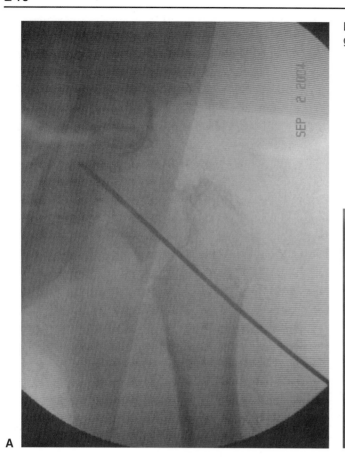

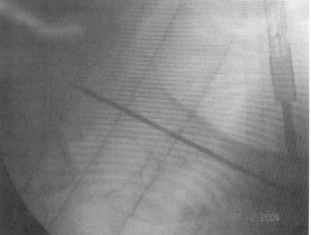

A   B

Figure 16.10. **A.** AP and **(B)** lateral image-intensifier radiographs of the inserted guide pin.

Baumgaertner et al popularized the concept of tip-apex distance (TAD) to determine the ideal position of the lag screw within the femoral head. This measurement, expressed in millimeters, is the sum of the distances from the tip of the lag screw to the apex of the femoral head on both the AP and lateral radiographic views (after controlling for radiographic magnification) (Fig. 16.11). Peripheral malposition of the lag screw is not differentiated from shallow lag screw positioning; only the actual distance from the tip of the lag screw to the apex of the femoral head is considered.

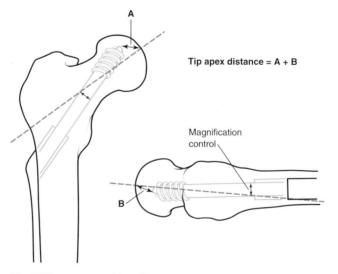

Figure 16.11. The TAD, expressed in millimeters, is the sum of the distances from the tip of the lag screw to the apex of the femoral head on both the AP and lateral radiographic views.

The benefit of utilizing the TAD was demonstrated by Baumgaertner et al in a series of 198 intertrochanteric fractures treated with a compression hip screw. In their series, 16 (8%) fractures had loss of fixation secondary to lag screw cutout of the femoral head. However, no lag screw cutout occurred when the TAD was 27 mm or less, regardless of patient age, fracture stability, quality of fracture reduction, or type or angle of implant used. Conversely, lag screw cutout rate increased to 60% when the TAD was greater than 45 mm. Using multivariate, logistic, regression analyses, Baumgaertner et al demonstrated that screw position as measured by the TAD was the strongest (though not the only) independent predictor of lag screw cutout. (Unstable fractures and increasing patient age were also predictive of lag screw cutout.) They therefore recommended that if guide pin location yields a TAD of more than 25 mm, the surgeon should reassess the fracture reduction and/or reposition the guide pin.

When the guide pin is confirmed to be in the desired position, it is advanced to the level of the subchondral bone and the length of the lag screw is measured (Fig. 16.12). Reaming of the femoral neck and head over the guide pin is performed under image intensification to the desired final position of the lag screw (Fig. 16.13). I recommend that the reamed tract be tapped, even in the elderly, to prevent femoral head rotation during lag screw insertion (Fig. 16.14). The lag screw is then inserted to within 1 cm of the subchondral bone (Fig. 16.15).

The side on which the fracture occurs (left or right) may contribute to malreduction with a sliding hip screw. In most intertrochanteric fractures, the proximal fragment tends to be displaced anteriorly. All lag screws are placed in a clockwise fashion. As the lag screw is advanced on left-sided intertrochanteric fractures, the clockwise rotation may further displace the fracture, while on the right side, the screw may help reduce the fracture. This phenomenon was demonstrated in a retrospective study in which 11 of 30 unstable left-sided intertrochanteric fractures were found to be malreduced with an anterior spike, while none of 26 right-sided fractures showed an anterior spike.

When the proper position of the lag screw within the femoral head is confirmed, a two- to four-hole side plate is placed over the screw (Fig. 16.16). I prefer use of a two-hole keyed, side plate. In a keyed system, the lag screw is captured within the barrel such that the screw can slide along the barrel but cannot rotate. This mechanism theoretically improves rotational stability of the femoral head and neck better than a nonkeyed system in which the lag screw can rotate within the plate barrel. The advantage of a nonkeyed system is that the free rotation of the plate over the lag screw facilitates plate insertion.

The surgeon must also ascertain that there is adequate room for sliding within the lag screw/barrel. Loss of sliding capability may be related to excessive postoperative impaction or jamming of the lag screw within the plate barrel. Kyle et al, in a biomechanical

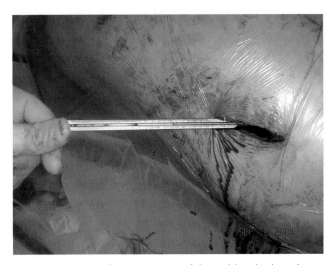

Figure 16.12. Measurement of the guide wire length.

Figure 16.13. A. Reaming of the femoral neck and head over the guide pin is performed under image intensification **(B)** to the desired final position of the lag screw.

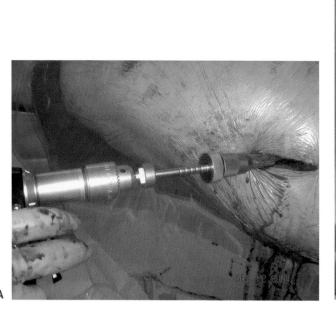

A

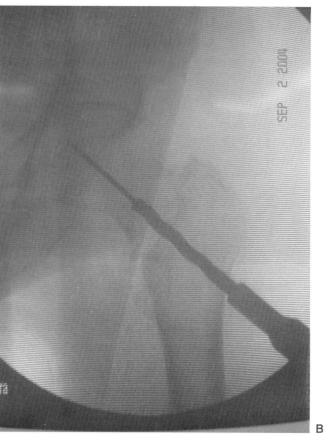

B

Figure 16.14. A. Tapping of the proximal femur under image intensification to the **(B)** final, seated, lag-screw position to prevent femoral head rotation during lag screw insertion.

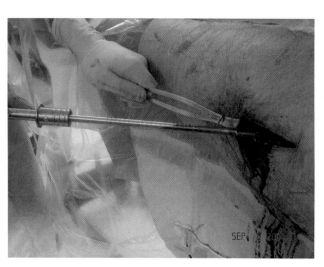

A

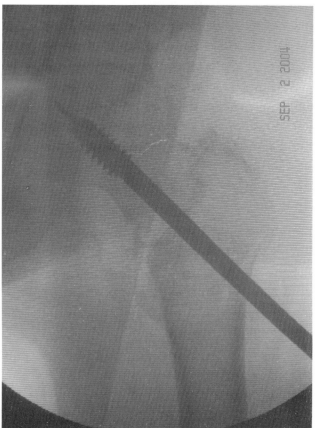

B

Figure 16.15. Insertion of the lag screw to within 1 cm of the subchondral bone.

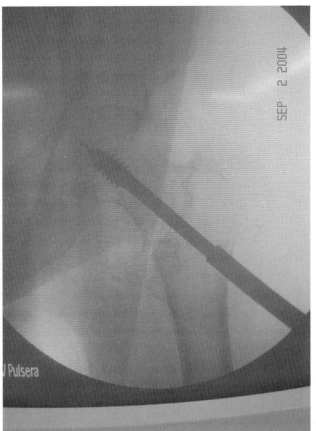

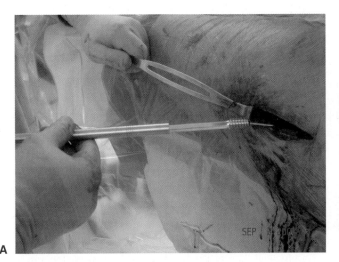

A

B

study, demonstrated that jamming of the lag screw within the plate barrel can occur when the force of contact between the lag screw and barrel lip is greater than the sliding forces in line with the lag screw. The amount of bending of the lag screw is inversely related to the amount of lag screw-plate barrel engagement and results in impingement of the screw at the barrel junction. Because bending of the lag screw is more likely to occur with use of a short-barrel side plate, a regular- length barrel side plate is preferred for most intertrochanteric fractures.

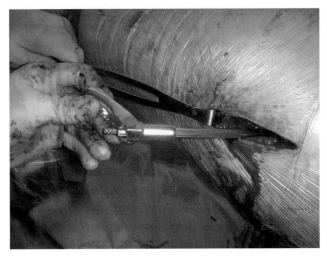

Figure 16.16. Placement of a two-hole side plate over the lag screw.

Gundle et al reported on a prospective series of 100 consecutive patients who sustained an unstable intertrochanteric fracture that a stabilized with a sliding hip screw. In fractures stabilized with <10 mm of available slide, the risk of fixation failure was more than three times greater than those fractures with ≥10 mm of available slide. Based on the specifications for the particular lag screw and side plate used in the Gundle et al study (Synthes DHS with a 32-mm barrel and 32 lags screw length), Gundle et al advocated use of a short-barrel side plate when using lag screws of ≤85 mm. This concern is less with use of the VHS because the VHS has a single side-plate barrel length of 24 mm and a lag-screw thread length of 22 mm. Even with an 80 mm total lag-screw length, 34 mm (80 − 46 = 34 mm) would be available to slide.

The side plate is impacted against the lateral cortex of the proximal femur. With the VHS system, if the side plate does not parallel the lateral cortex, one can adjust the plate angle using a screw driver to move the mechanism that controls the side plate–barrel angle (Fig. 16.17). Once the plate has been inserted and placed against the bone, it is loosely clamped to the femoral shaft and the fracture is impacted by releasing the traction on the extremity and gently displacing the femoral shaft toward the proximal fragment. This impaction maneuver is thought to enhance fracture stability. The plate-holding screws are then inserted (Fig. 16.18). The need for a compression screw is determined by direct visualization of the lag screw within the plate barrel; a compression screw is inserted if there is risk of postoperative screw-barrel disengagement. A compression screw is not used routinely because it often loosens (even during uneventful fracture healing) and can become a source of lateral thigh pain.

POSTOPERATIVE MANAGEMENT

Patients should be assisted by a physical therapist out of bed on the first postoperative day and allowed to ambulate with weight bearing as tolerated. It is difficult if not impossible for elderly patients to make significant progress in a rehabilitation program if weight bearing is restricted. In addition, there is little biomechanical justification for restricted weight bearing after hip fracture because activities such as moving around in bed and use of a bedpan generate forces across the hip approaching those resulting from ambulation. All patients should have thromboembolic and 24 to 48 hours of broad spectrum antibiotic prophylaxis.

After hospital discharge, patients are seen at 2, 6, and 12 weeks, and then at 6 months, 12 months and yearly. At follow-up, an AP view of the pelvis, and an AP and cross-table lateral of the fractured hip are taken. Patients initially receive at-home physical therapy for gait training and range of motion exercises of the hip and knee; they are then referred to outpatient physical therapy. Once there is radiographic evidence of fracture healing, muscle strengthening exercises are initiated.

More than 95% of intertrochanteric hip fractures can be expected to unite uneventfully. Evaluation of functional recovery following hip fracture has become increasingly important because success is measured by return to prefracture levels of function. Forty percent to 60% of hip fracture patients are able to return directly home after hospitalization. Factors predictive of a hospital to home discharge are younger age, prefracture and early postfracture independent ambulation, ability to perform activities of daily living (ADLs), and the presence of another person at home. Forty percent to 60% of patients will regain their prefracture ambulatory status within one year after fracture. The factors associated with regaining prefracture ambulatory status following hip fracture include: younger age, male sex, and the absence of preexisting dementia. The vast majority of patients will require assistance in performing ADLs. Of those who were independent in ADLs before fracture, only 20% to 35% will regain their prefracture ADLs independence. The factors reported to be predictive of recovery of ADLs are younger age, absence of dementia or delirium in nondemented patients, and greater contact with one's social network.

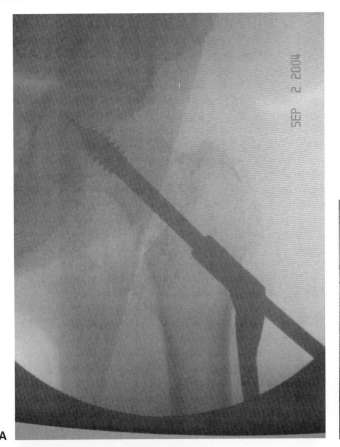

A

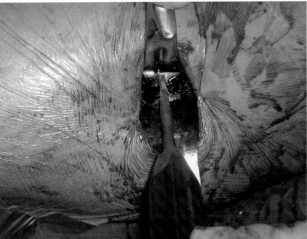

B

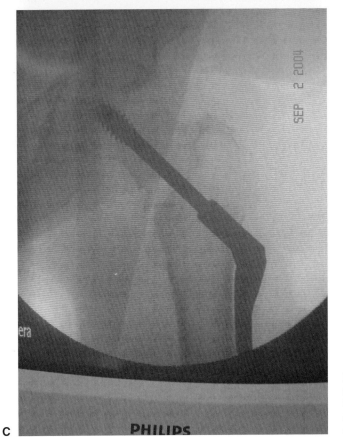

C

Figure 16.17. The side plate is impacted against the lateral cortex of the proximal femur. With the VHS system, **(A)** if the side plate does not parallel the lateral cortex, **(B)** one can adjust the plate angle using a screw driver to move the **(C)** worm gear that controls the side plate–barrel angle.

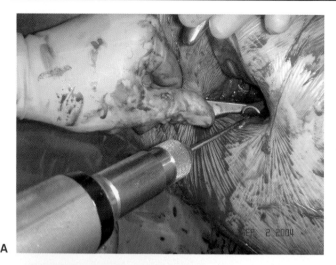

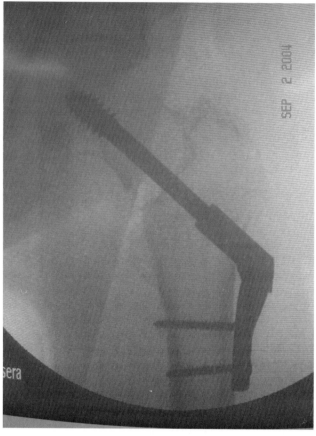

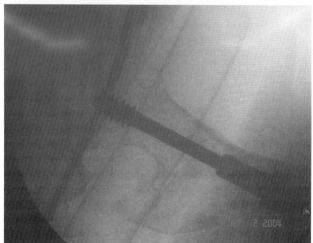

Figure 16.18. A. Insertion of the plate-holding screws and **(B)** final AP and **(C)** lateral radiographs.

COMPLICATIONS

One year mortality following intertrochanteric fracture is similar to that reported after femoral neck fracture and ranges from 14 to 36%. Most authors agree that the highest risk of mortality occurs within the first 4 to 6 months following fracture. After the first year, the mortality rate approaches that of age- and sex-matched controls who have not sustained a hip fracture. The incidence of wound infection has decreased significantly with the use of prophylactic antibiotics; most recent studies have reported an incidence of less than 3%. Risk factors include urinary tract infection, decubitus ulcers, prolonged operating time, disorientation that interferes with proper wound care, and proximity of the incision to the perineum.

The surgical complications most frequently encountered are varus displacement of the proximal fragment with loss of fixation, malrotation deformity and nonunion. Varus displacement following internal fixation usually occurs in unstable fractures, with the lag screw "cutting out" through the anterosuperior portion of the femoral head (Fig. 16.19). This complication can result from (a) placement of the lag screw into the anterosuperior aspect of the femoral head, (b) inability to obtain a stable reduction, (c) excessive collapse of the fracture such that the sliding capacity of the device is exceeded, (d) inadequate screw-barrel engagement that prevents sliding, or (e) severe osteoporosis that precludes secure fixation. When this complication occurs, management choices include acceptance of the deformity; a second attempt at open reduction and internal fixation (ORIF), which may require methylmethacrylate; or conversion to a unipolar or bipolar endoprosthesis or total hip arthroplasty. Acceptance of the deformity should be considered in nonambulatory patients

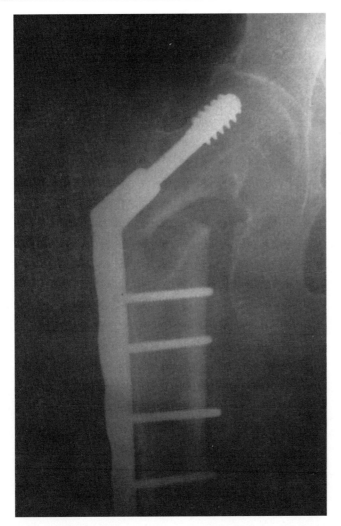

Figure 16.19. Loss of reduction after surgery with resultant varus displacement of the proximal fragment and screw cutout.

who are poor surgical risks. When reoperation is indicated, conversion to a hemiarthroplasty or total hip replacement (THR) is usually performed.

Malrotation deformity usually results from internal rotation of the distal fragment at the time of internal fixation. In unstable fractures, the proximal and distal fragments may move independently. In these cases, the distal fragment should be internally fixed in neutral to slight external rotation. Nonunion occurs in less than 2% of cases. In some cases, with good bone stock, repeat internal fixation combined with a valgus osteotomy and bone grafting can be considered. However, in most elderly patients, conversion to a calcar replacement arthroplasty will be preferred.

RECOMMENDED READING

Baumgaertner MR, Chrostowski JH, Levy RN. Intertrochanteric hip fractures. In: Browner BD, Levine AM, Jupiter JB, Trafton PG, eds. *Skeletal trauma*. Vol. 2. Philadelphia: W.B. Saunders; 1992:1833–1881.

Baumgaertner MR, Curtin SL, Lindskog DM, et al. The value of the tip-apex distance in predicting failure of fixation of peritrochanteric fractures of the hip. *J Bone Joint Surg* 1995;77:1058–1064.

Bolhofner BR, Russo PR, Carmen B. Results of intertrochanteric femur fractures treated with a 135-degree sliding screw with a two-hole side plate. *J Orthop Trauma* 1999;13(1):5–8.

Chaim SH, Mukherjee DP, Ogden AL, et al. A biomechanical study of femoral neck fracture fixation with the VHS Vari-Angle Hip Fixation System. *Am J Orthop* 2002;(Suppl 1):22–24.

Evans E. The treatment of trochanteric fractures of the femur. *J Bone Joint Surg* 1949;31:190–203.

Gundle R, Gargan MF, Simpson AH. How to minimize failures of fixation of unstable intertrochanteric fractures. *Injury* 1995;26:611–614.

Kim WY, Han CH, Park JI, et al. Failure of intertrochanteric fracture fixation with a dynamic hip screw in relation to preoperative fracture stability and osteoporosis. *Int Orthop* 2001;25(6):360–362.

Koval KJ, Friend K, Aharonoff G, et al. Weight bearing after hip fracture: a prospective series of 596 geriatric hip fracture patients. *J Orthop Trauma* 1996;10(8):526–530.

Kyle RF, Gustilo RB, Premer RF. Analysis of six hundred and twenty-two intertrochanteric hip fractures. *J Bone Joint Surg Am* 1979;61(2):216–221.

Kyle RF, Wright TM, Burstein AH. Biomechanical analysis of the sliding characteristics of compression hip screws. *J Bone Joint Surg* 1980;62(8):1308–1314.

McLoughlin SW, Wheeler DL, Rider J, et al. Biomechanical evaluation of the dynamic hip screw with two- and four-hole side plates. *J Orthop Trauma* 2000;14(5):318–323.

Mohan R, Karthikeyan R, Sonanis SV. Dynamic hip screw: does side make a difference? Effects of clockwise torque on right and left DHS. *Injury* 2000;31:697–699.

Rha JD, Kim YH, Yoon SI, et al. Factors affecting sliding of the lag screw in intertrochanteric fractures. *Int Orthop* 1993;17(5):320–324.

17

Intertrochanteric Hip Fractures: Intramedullary Hip Screws

Michael R. Baumgaertner and Sudeep Taksali

INDICATIONS/CONTRAINDICATIONS

The number of hip fractures in the United States is estimated at 250,000 per year and will double by the year 2040. Fifty percent of hip fractures are intertrochanteric, of which 50% to 60% are classified as unstable. These fractures typically occur in elderly females, with 90% of fractures occurring in patients older than 65 years. The etiology of intertrochanteric hip fractures is typically attributed to low-energy falls in the setting of osteoporosis.

The stability of the intertrochanteric fracture drives both the treatment strategy and the surgical outcome. Unstable fractures have significant disruption of the posteromedial cortex, including subtrochanteric extension, or are reverse obliquity fractures. Stable two-part fractures, once reduced, will resist medial and compressive loads, whereas unstable fractures will have a tendency to collapse into varus.

Intramedullary hip screws (IMHS) are indicated for all unstable intertrochanteric hip fractures and are ideal for subtrochanteric and reverse obliquity fractures. An additional indication is an impending or pathologic fracture of the proximal femur. Multiple studies have indicated that the IMHS offers no advantage over a sliding hip screw and side plate in a stable fracture pattern. However, its utilization with stable fractures will provide a means to improve and streamline one's technique when dealing with the more challenging unstable fracture patterns.

Contraindications to using an IMHS include all femoral neck fractures, deformities of the femoral shaft, and hip ankylosis. An additional contraindication is the young patient because an excessive amount of trabecular bone is removed from the trochanteric block to accommodate these relatively large implants.

The IMHS combines a sliding hip screw with an intramedullary nail. Implant insertion can be performed in a closed, percutaneous manner, allowing minimal surgical insult to the fracture zone and reduced perioperative blood loss. The device functions as an intramedullary buttress, effectively reestablishing the mechanical support of the postero-medial cortex and thus preventing excessive shaft medialization. By avoiding violation of the fracture zone, the surgeon facilitates fracture union.

PREOPERATIVE PLANNING

Elderly patients will typically present after a fall with the affected limb shortened and externally rotated. It is important to obtain a thorough medical and social history as well as determine if the patient has an oncologic history. It is equally important that a complete physical examination is performed with care to examine the condition of the skin overlying the hip and to rule out any associated injuries.

The diagnosis of an intertrochanteric hip fracture is generally confirmed with standard anteroposterior (AP) and lateral radiographs. These radiographs should include at least the proximal half of the femur because deformities of the shaft may preclude the use of an intramedullary device. Internal rotation and traction radiographs can further aid in understanding the pathoanatomy.

Close perioperative medical management of patients with intertrochanteric hip fractures is critical to obtaining a successful postoperative outcome because the patient population is medically complex. Some issues of particular importance are the patient's nutritional status, management of urinary tract infections, hemodynamic stability, coagulopathy, deep vein thrombosis (DVT) prophylaxis, and perioperative antibiotics. Typically, optimization should not be prolonged, as mortality is increased when surgery is delayed beyond 48 to 72 hours from admission.

Careful examination of the preoperative radiographs as well as the unaffected hip will help guide appropriate implant selection with respect to the neck angle, diameter, and screw length. We typically use a 135-degree neck angle with a 95-mm lag screw. It is important to note that the IMHS is not designed to fill the canal. A long stem device should be considered in the setting of a pathologic fracture or fractures with significant subtrochanteric extension.

SURGICAL TECHNIQUE

We generally use a fracture table and position the patient supine (Fig. 17.1A). A well-padded post is placed in the perineum. The affected side is secured to the traction assembly. We prefer to use the heel stirrup and metatarsal bar as opposed to putting the foot in the Velcro-strapped boot. The heel and the forefoot are cushioned with an ABD pad, and heavy cloth tape is used to secure the foot to the stirrup (Fig. 17.1B). By locking the transverse tarsal joint and dorsiflexing the ankle, we gain greater control over the extremity for firm traction and internal/external rotation. The affected extremity is adducted with the torso shifted away from the surgical side. The unaffected extremity can be placed in the well leg holder with the knee flexed and the hip flexed and internally rotated. This allows for unhindered access for the image intensifier so that lateral radiographs of the fracture zone can be obtained (Fig. 17.1C). Unfortunately, this visualization may occasionally come at a price: There is no countertraction on the well leg. As a result, when strong traction is applied to the fracture, the pelvis has a tendency to rotate around the perineal post. This produces abduction of the operative side and can significantly hamper achieving the correct starting point, leading to a varus reduction (Fig. 17.2).

An alternate method of positioning the patient allows countertraction on the pelvis by placing both extremities parallel in foot traction. The extremities are "scissored," with the operative side slightly flexed at the hip and the well side extended to allow for lateral plane fluoroscopic imaging (Fig. 17.3).

Once the patient has been appropriately positioned on the table, the extremity is manipulated. The primary goal is to gain access to the starting point; secondarily, we attempt fracture reduction. Most stable fracture patterns will reduce with axial traction and internal

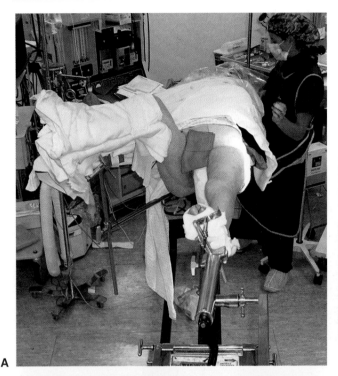

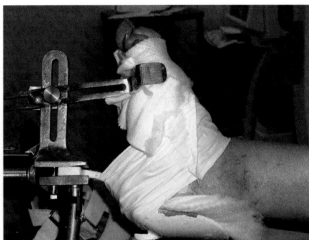

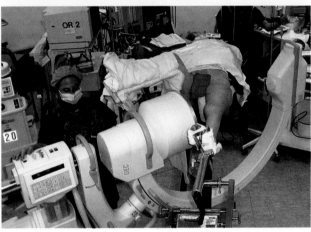

Figure 17.1. **A.** In the typical position, the patient is supine on the fracture table with the torso windswept and the affected extremity secured to the traction assembly. The well leg is flexed and internally rotated at the hip to allow for unimpeded bi-planar imaging. **B.** The foot is secured to the stirrup with the metatarsal bar and held in dorsiflexion. **C.** Patient is positioned so that a lateral radiograph can be readily obtained.

rotation of the femur. However, unstable intertrochanteric hip fractures may require different maneuvers, such as slight external rotation. Prior to draping the field, we confirm that we can see the following areas via fluoroscopy: the anterior cortex of the proximal femur, the fracture zone, the anterior neck, the entire circumference of the femoral head, the posterior neck, and the trochanter.

In considering an ideal reduction, we determine an acceptable neck-shaft angle to be 130 to 145 degrees. More valgus is allowed because it reduces the bending forces on the implant and may offset the limb shortening that occurs with fragment impaction. Angulation greater than 15 degrees, as seen on the lateral view, is unacceptable.

Once a provisional reduction has been attempted, skin surfaces should be prepped in standard sterile fashion. Care should be taken to prep to the level of the knee in the event that a long nail is used such that a distal interlocking screw can be placed. We use a sterile shower- curtain type drape but add an extra sterile layer proximally to protect against puncture hole contamination from the instrumentation.

Before incision, the tip of the trochanter and the femoral shaft axis are marked in both planes with the skin marker (Fig. 17.4). This provides a visual aid for the correct insertion

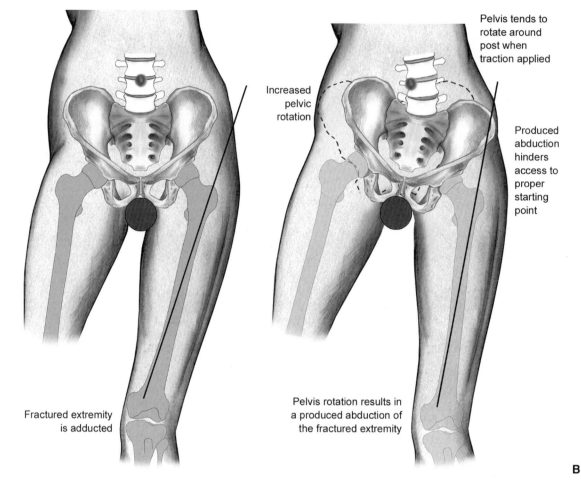

Increased
pelvic
rotation

Pelvis tends to
rotate around
post when
traction applied

Produced
abduction
hinders
access to
proper
starting
point

Fractured extremity
is adducted

Pelvis rotation results in
a produced abduction of
the fractured extremity

A   B

Figure 17.2. With the application of unopposed traction, the pelvis rotates around the perineal post. The hip abducts, hampering access to the starting point.

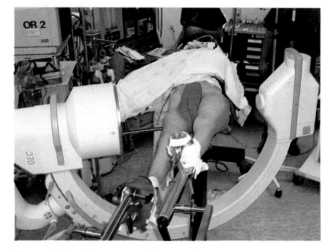

Figure 17.3. Alternate method of positioning with the legs scissored. This position provides countertraction on the pelvis and still allows for lateral plane imaging.

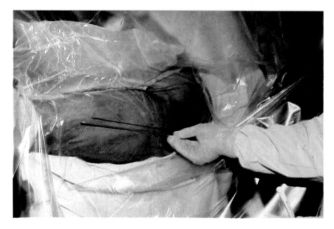

Figure 17.4. Marking of the femoral shaft axis and the tip of the trochanter.

of the guide pin and the IMHS. In addition, this helps reduce fluoroscreening time. Typically, prior to skin incision, the implant and insertion jig are preassembled per the preoperative plan. It is very helpful to insert and partially advance the set-screw that locks the nail to the sleeve prior to implantation because later it is often difficult to place through the percutaneous wound (Fig. 17.5).

Prior to creating the entrance channel, the reduction should be verified with bi-planar imaging. Using a freehand technique, we insert a 3.2-mm guide pin percutaneously (Fig. 17.6), about 3 to 4 cm proximal to the trochanter, engaging the bone at or just medial to the tip of the greater trochanter. This location will counteract the tendency toward varus and increased neck-shaft offset as well as minimize any damage to the gluteus medius insertion (Fig. 17.7). Based on the lateral view, the guide pin should be centered in the canal (Fig. 17.8A), and based on the AP, it should be aimed slightly medial (Fig. 17.8B).

Prior to making the incision, we inject a few milliliters of local anesthetic with epinephrine proximal to the greater trochanter. We then make a 2 cm incision and cut down with a no. 10 blade along the guide pin, through fascia, and directly onto the greater trochanter (Fig. 17.9).

With the guide pin in place, we ream over the pin with the proximal reamer (Fig. 17.10A). We then ream to a depth such that the widest part of the reamer has reached the lesser trochanter (Fig. 17.10B); it is unnecessary to ream to the isthmus. The surgeon must be certain that the reamer is cutting a channel for the implant rather than simply displacing the fragments as it passes into the canal (particularly if the guide pin is in the fracture line). Placing firm medial-directed pressure on the trochanteric mass, as well as medial/lateral translational forces applied to the rigid reamer as it is repeatedly advanced and retracted,

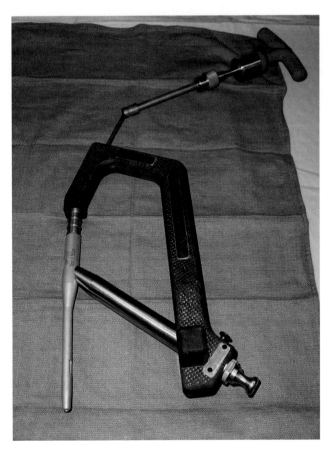

Figure 17.5. The implant and insertion guide are pre-assembled. The torque-limiting screwdriver is engaged in the nail.

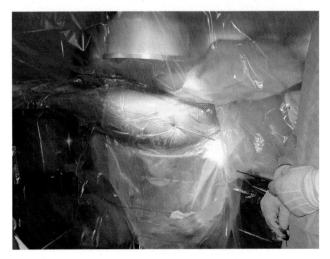

Figure 17.6. Percutaneous, freehand insertion of the guide pin at the tip of the greater trochanter.

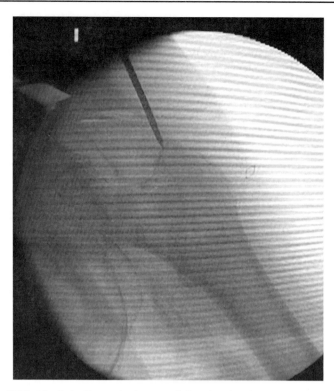

Figure 17.7. Ideal starting point just medial to the tip of the greater trochanter.

can insure appropriate canal preparation (Fig. 17.11). Inadequate entrance-site preparation is much more problematic than generous reaming in this patient population, particularly if one wants to modify the neck-shaft axis after nail insertion.

We then insert the assembled nail into the intramedullary canal. Only hand force should be required; hammering risks iatrogenic fracture (Fig. 17.12). Usually the nail need not be inserted over a guide pin. Bi-planar fluoroscopy should be checked at this point to ensure

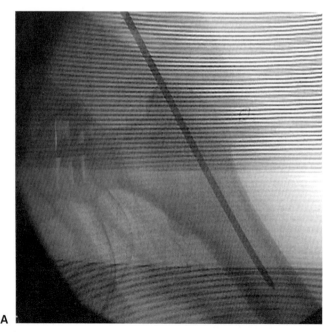

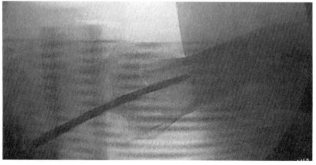

Figure 17.8. **A.** Ideal guide pin location on the AP view: centered in the intramedullary canal. **B.** Ideal guide pin location: centered on the lateral view.

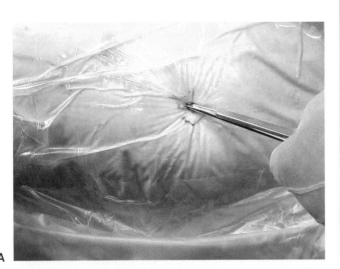

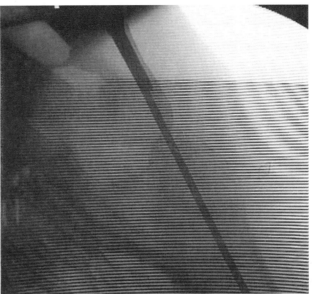

A   B

Figure 17.9. A. Incision is made directly over the guide pin through the skin and fascia.
B. The scalpel is advanced to the level of the tip of the greater trochanter.

that the nail is not exiting the canal through the fracture and that the nail is seated to an adequate depth. If the nail does not fully advance but does not appear "tight" on the AP image, the surgeon should check the lateral image to see if the tip of the nail is impinging on the anterior cortex because most nail systems do not have a sagittal bow to the nail. Also, soft tissue should be checked to ensure that it is not restricting the entrance site. A combination of eccentric entrance site reaming (primarily anterior), soft-tissue release, isthmic (flexible) reaming, or implant downsizing will invariably solve the problem.

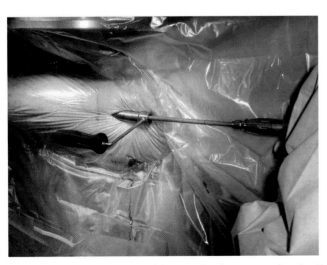

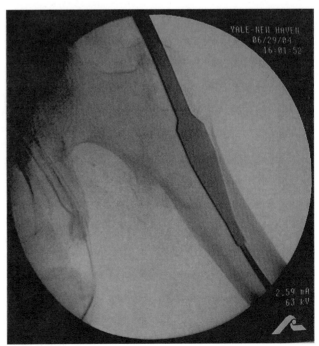

A   B

Figure 17.10. A. Insertion of the proximal reamer using the tissue protector sleeve. (We usually do not use the sleeve and minimize soft-tissue trauma by simply running the reamer in reverse until it has entered the bone [see Fig. 17.11].) **B.** Insertion of the proximal reamer so that the widest part is at the level of the lesser trochanter.

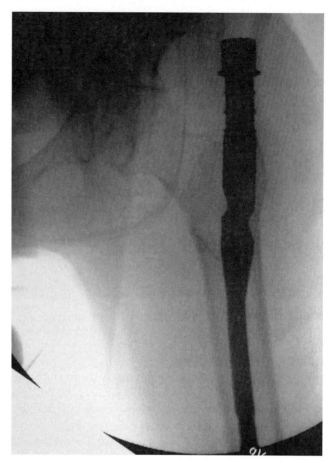

Figure 17.12. The nail is fully seated in the canal.

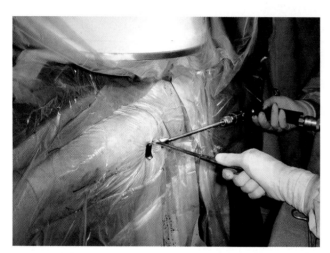

Figure 17.11. Firm medial pressure is placed to prevent lateral fracture displacement and to assure that a channel for the implant is created.

To help the surgeon predict the proper location for skin incision and subsequent lag-screw insertion, some systems have a tower attachment that can be used to preview the position of the guide pin for the sliding hip screw (Fig. 17.13A). Through this positioning guide, a 3.2-mm guide pin can be placed anterior to the patient's soft tissue. Otherwise, one can estimate the location and again inject with local anesthetic and make a 2-cm skin incision. The surgeon should be certain to split through the fascia lata so that the sleeve can be placed flush against the lateral cortex of the femur (Fig. 17.13B). Taking into account the anteversion of the neck, the surgeon should advance the appropriate guide pin through the jig and nail up into the femoral head.

This is the stage of the operation where we confirm and often improve the reduction. On the lateral view, any "sag" or translation needs to be addressed. Anterior translation of the insertion jig, and hence the shaft which it controls, is often helpful. This effect can be enhanced in the setting of a difficult reduction with percutaneous manipulation of the head-neck fragment (Fig. 17.14). In particularly difficult fractures, the proximal fragment can be manipulated and then pinned to the inferior acetabulum. For interpretation of the AP view, the guide pin acts as an excellent reference because it is 135 degrees to the shaft. If it is parallel but simply too superior in the head, the neck-shaft axis is acceptable, and pin removal with nail advancement and pin reinsertion will solve the malposition. However, if the neck and guide pin are not parallel, the fracture is most likely malreduced in varus. The reduction can be improved with increased traction, or perhaps more effectively, by abduction of the extremity. With the nail inserted, hip adduction is no longer mandatory, or necessarily desirable. As long as the entrance site was adequately reamed, this simple maneuver will increase the neck-shaft angle without significantly displacing the medial fracture line or increasing offset.

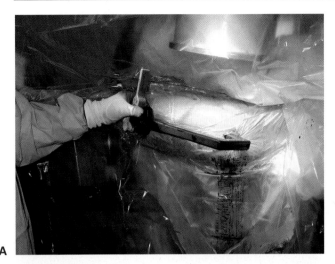
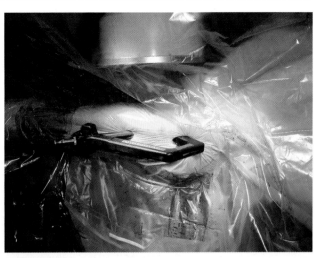

A   B

Figure 17.13. A. Tower attachment with guide pin allows preview of lag screw placement prior to skin incision. **B.** Jig assembly for guide pin placement into the head.

With the nail seated to the appropriate depth, a 3.2-mm guide pin is inserted centrally and very deep using both the AP and lateral x-rays for guidance (Fig. 17.15A,B). The guide pin placement should then be confirmed to have the optimal tip-apex distance (TAD) of 5 to 10 mm from the articular surface of the femoral head (see Fig. 17.15C).

Once satisfied with the reduction and a deep, centrally placed guide pin, we add an auxiliary stabilizing pin for all unstable fractures (Fig. 17.16). This auxiliary pin is directed through the jig such that it avoids the path of the lag screw and locks the jig to the head-neck fragment. The auxiliary pin serves as an antirotation device during screw insertion as well as an independent stabilizer should the guide pin be inadvertently removed while the surgeon is reaming for the lag screw.

With the guide pin seated deep and central in the femoral head, we ream 5 mm short of the subchondral bone. We take the instability of the fracture into account in setting the reamer depth because markedly unstable fractures are often found to be distracted following reduction maneuvers and will shorten with the compression provided by the reamer itself. Reamer progress is monitored with spot fluoroscopic images to identify inadvertent binding and advancement of the guide pin as well as to prevent overpenetration. An obturator should be used during reamer removal to prevent loss of the guide pin. We seldom use a tap because of the bone quality typically seen in this patient population.

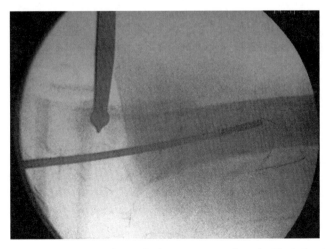

Figure 17.14. A ball-spike pusher is applied percutaneously to facilitate fracture reduction.

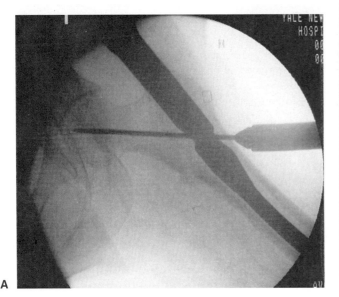

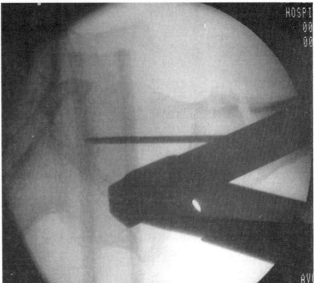

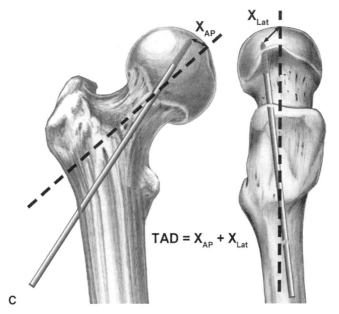

Figure 17.15. A. Appropriate guide pin placement on the AP x-ray. **B.** Appropriate guide pin placement on the lateral x-ray. **C.** The technique to measure TAD.

$$TAD = X_{AP} + X_{Lat}$$

The lag screw length is chosen such that the distal aspect of the fully seated screw lies 5 to 8 mm recessed into the centering sleeve, exactly as one would do when using a barrel and side plate. For a 135-degree nail, a 95-mm screw is almost always appropriate. The lag screw is then inserted over the guide pin (with the centering sleeve mounted onto the jig for systems that employ this sliding adjunct). Once the lag screw has reached the appropriate depth (Fig. 17.17A) and the reduction is verified, the centering sleeve should be advanced though the lateral cortex and into the nail using the sleeve pusher (Fig. 17.17B).

The head-neck fragment is typically torqued somewhat as the screw is seated into the dense subchondral bone. On right hips, screw insertion tends to extend the fragment, which often helps correct mild extension deformities at the fracture. However, for left-side fractures, the clockwise seating of the screw flexes the hip and worsens any extension deformity at the fracture. We scrutinize the fracture on the lateral fluoroscopic image while slightly rotating the screw insertion wrench back and forth (which controls the head-neck fragment) to identify the optimum reduction (Fig. 17.18). The reduced position is then maintained while the AP image is obtained to confirm the reduction. The sleeve is then

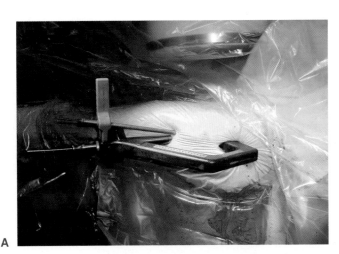

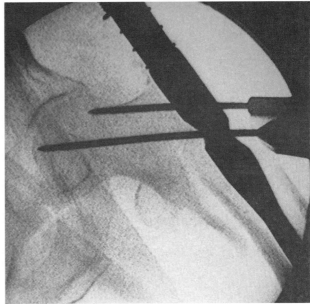

A   B

Figure 17.16. **A.** Certain implant systems provide a targeting attachment to place the auxiliary stabilizing pin. **B.** An auxiliary stabilizing pin is added to help control rotation. It is placed out of the path of the lag screw.

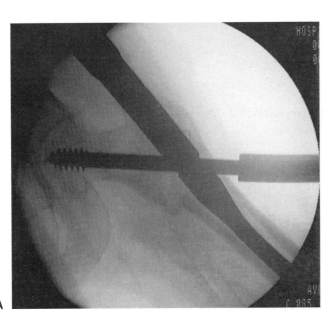

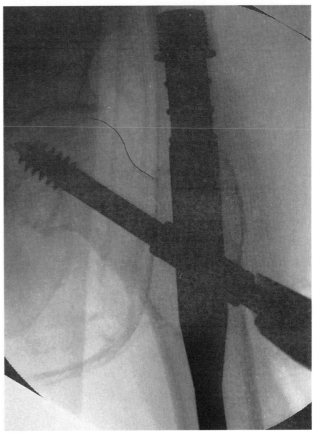

A   B

Figure 17.17. **A.** The lag screw is seated to the appropriate depth. Image was taken prior to centering of sleeve insertion. **B.** The centering sleeve is advanced through the lateral cortex and into the nail using the sleeve pusher.

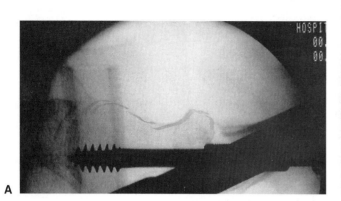
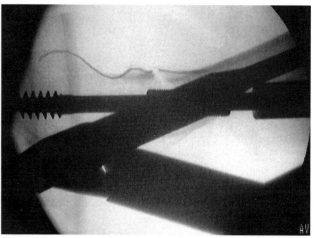

Figure 17.18. A. Lag screw insertion in a left hip showing worsening of extension deformity. **B.** Rotation of the screw results in fracture reduction.

locked to the nail when we tighten the previously inserted set screw with the torque-limited driver (Fig. 17.19). This locks in the rotational reduction but allows unimpeded sliding of the screw in the sleeve.

For most cases, we insert a compressing screw to initiate sliding and increase the immediate stability of the fracture (Fig. 17.20). This also prevents the rare but catastrophic complication of proximal disengagement of the screw from the nail.

For length-stable fractures, traction should be released from the extremity prior to considering a distal interlocking screw. We then assess rotational stability by securing the distal extremity and follow by gently rotating the insertion jig. If the femur moves as a unit, we do not distally lock (Fig. 17.21). If there is any question of motion, a single screw is placed in the dynamic slot using the alignment jig. For length-unstable fractures, two interlocks are placed through the insertion jig, or for the longer nails, by freehand techniques.

Closure is routine, though we feel it is important to place a deep, strong suture to close the tensor fascia proximal to the trochanter at the nail insertion site. This proximal wound is at risk of contamination from a disoriented elderly patient's wandering fingers (Fig. 17.22). A dry sterile dressing is applied with care in consideration of the elderly patient's fragile skin.

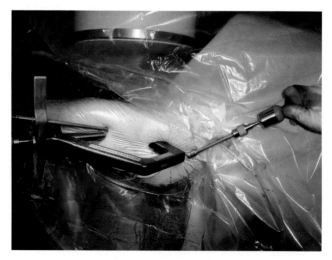

Figure 17.19. The sleeve is locked to the nail by tightening the previously inserted set screw with the torque-limited driver.

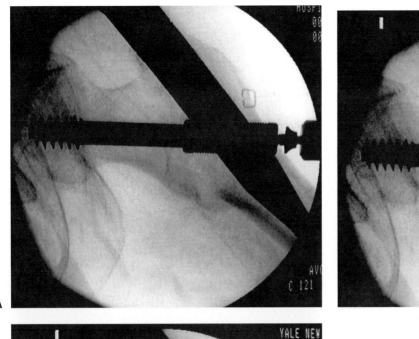

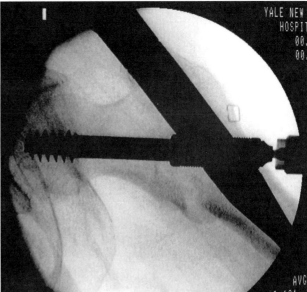

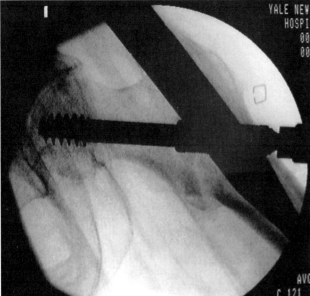

Figure 17.20. A–C. A demonstration of compression screw insertion. Note how the fracture reduces with the applied compression.

RESULTS

In a prospective study performed by the primary author, no difference was demonstrated in comparing an IMHS versus compression hip screw (CHS) with respect to complications. However, we were able to demonstrate decreased fluoro time, decreased operative time, and decreased blood loss. In a prospective study, Hardy et al demonstrated that patients receiving an IMHS had improved early mobility and decreased limb shortening. As surgeons have become more familiar with instrumentation techniques and newer generation nails are released, the rate of surgical complications reported in the literature has decreased.

POSTOPERATIVE MANAGEMENT

Patients are managed postoperatively with 24 hours of antibiotic prophylaxis, generally with a first-generation cephalosporin. Prophylaxis against DVT is carefully considered

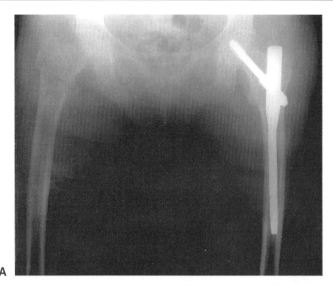

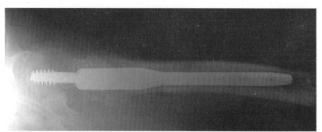

A   B

Figure 17.21. A,B. AP and lateral postoperative radiographs.

with a combination of sequential compression devices and pharmacologic prophylaxes. All patients are allowed to weight bear to tolerance, although we may limit the amount of ambulation in the cognitively impaired patients with severely unstable patterns. Patients will ambulate with a physical therapist beginning on postoperative day 1 or 2. Patients are typically discharged to a short-term rehabilitation facility on postoperative day 3 or 4. We see patients at 10 to 14 days to rule out wound healing problems and at 6 and 12 weeks to confirm clinical and radiographic union. Patients who sustain low-energy intertrochanteric hip fractures should be evaluated and treated for osteoporosis.

COMPLICATIONS

Most complications can be avoided by following proper surgical technique and appropriate implant selection. The most common complication is implant cutout. A varus neck-shaft angle universally leads to an increased TAD and an increased offset when an intramedullary device is used. In a study performed by the primary author, cutouts were shown to be related to implant position as measured by the TAD. At TAD <25

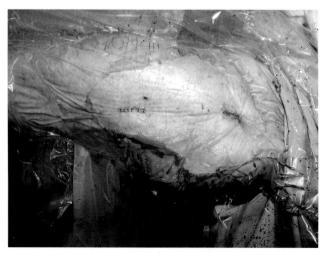

Figure 17.22. The two small skin incisions with staple closure.

mm, failure rates approach zero, but at TAD >25 mm, the chances of failure increase rapidly.

Additional complications include femoral shaft fracture, periprosthetic fracture, painful hardware, and nonunion. A number of techniques, such as conversion to a hip replacement, re-osteosynthesis with a long stem IMHS, or open reduction and internal fixation (ORIF), can be used to address these problems. Fortunately, these complications are uncommon with proper surgical technique and new generation devices.

RECOMMENDED READING

Baumgaertner MR, Curtin SL, Lindskog DM. Intramedullary versus extramedullary fixation for the treatment of intertrochanteric hip fractures. *Clin Orthop* 1998;348:87–94.

Baumgaertner MR, Curtin SL, Lindskog DM, et al. The value of the tip-apex distance in predicting failure of fixation of peritrochanteric fractures of the hip. *J Bone Joint Surg Am* 1995;77:1058–1064.

Hardy DC, Descamps PY, Krallis P, et al. Use of an intramedullary hip-screw compared with a compression hip-screw with a plate for intertrochanteric femoral fractures: a prospective, randomized study of one hundred patients. *J Bone Joint Surg Am* 1998;80: 618–630.

Lindskog DM, Baumgaertner MR. Unstable intertrochanteric hip fractures in the elderly. *J Am Acad Orthop Surg* 2004;12:179–190.

18

Hip Arthroplasty for Intertrochanteric Hip Fractures

George J. Haidukewych

The vast majority of intertrochanteric hip fractures treated with internal fixation heal. However, certain unfavorable fractures patterns, fractures in patients with severely osteopenic bone, or patients with poor hardware placement, can lead to internal fixation failure (nonunion). Randomized prospective studies of displaced femoral-neck fractures in elderly osteoporotic patients have shown a high complication rate associated with internal fixation of these injuries. For this reason, most surgeons favor arthroplasty, which has a documented excellent success rate and offers the advantage of early weight bearing. This has led some surgeons to consider the use of a prosthesis in the management of selected, osteoporotic, intertrochanteric, hip fractures. In theory, this may allow earlier mobilization and minimize the chance of internal fixation failure and need for re-operation. The use of arthroplasty in this setting, however, poses its own unique challenges including the need for so-called "calcar replacing" prostheses and it raises questions regarding the need for acetabular resurfacing and the management of the often-fractured greater trochanteric fragment. The purpose of this chapter is to review the indications, surgical techniques, and specific technical details needed to achieve a successful outcome. Also addressed are the potential complications of hip arthroplasty for fractures of the intertrochanteric region of the femur.

INDICATIONS

The vast majority of intertrochanteric hip fractures, whether stable or unstable, will heal uneventfully with accurately placed internal-fixation devices. When the procedure is done correctly, the fixation failure rate should be minimal. European studies have found that hip arthroplasty can lead to successful outcomes; however, there is a higher perioperative mortality rate among these patients compared to those who undergo internal fixation. Therefore, the indications for hip arthroplasty for peritrochanteric fractures include patients with neglected intertrochanteric fractures when attempts at open reduction and internal fixation (ORIF) are unlikely to succeed; pathologic fractures due to neoplasm; internal fixation failures or established nonunions where the patient's age and remaining proximal-bone stock precludes a revision internal-fixation attempt; (very rarely) in patients with severe preexisting, symptomatic osteoarthritis of the hip; and an unstable fracture pattern. Recent studies have documented that hip arthroplasty for salvage of failed internal fixation provides predictable pain relief and functional improvement.

PATIENT EVALUATION AND PREOPERATIVE PLANNING

Because these patients are typically elderly and frail with multiple medical co-morbidities, a thorough medical evaluation is recommended. Preoperative correction of dehydration, electrolyte imbalances, and anemia is important. In general, surgery is performed within 48 hours of injury to avoid prolonged recumbency.

Plain anteroposterior (AP) and lateral radiographs of the hip, femur, and pelvis are important for preoperative planning. If the surgeon has any concern of a pathologic fracture, computed tomography (CT) or magnetic resonance imaging (MRI) scanning can occasionally be helpful. If a pathologic fracture due to metastasis is diagnosed, full-length femur radiographs are even more critical in evaluating any distal lesions that would need to be addressed. Appropriate imaging of the proximal fragment is important to allow templating of the femoral component for length or offset and to determine whether any proximal calcar augmentation will be necessary to restore the normal neck-shaft relationship. Careful scrutiny of the hip joint is necessary to detect evidence of acetabular degenerative change that would make total hip arthroplasty more attractive than hemi-arthroplasty. A final decision is often made intraoperatively after visual inspection of the quality of the remaining acetabular cartilage. If previous hardware from internal fixation is present, specific screwdrivers and a broken screw removal set, with or without the use of fluoroscopy, may assist the surgeon in hardware removal. It is wise to have implant-specific extraction tools available. Obtaining the original operative note can assist the surgeon in determining the implant manufacturer if it is not recognized from the radiographs.

Often it is difficult to ascertain preoperatively whether hemi-arthroplasty or total hip arthroplasty is appropriate, and whether cemented or uncemented femoral component fixation is indicated. I prefer to have both acetabular resurfacing and femoral-component fixation options available intraoperatively. Although having such a large inventory of implants available for a single case is laborious, it is wise to be prepared for the unexpected situations that can be found during these challenging reconstructions.

To evaluate infection as a potential etiology for failed internal fixation, I recommend that a complete blood count with differential, a sedimentation rate, and a C-reactive protein be obtained preoperatively. I have not found aspiration to be predictable in the setting of fixation failure and rely on preoperative serologies and intraoperative frozen-section histology for decision making.

SURGICAL TECHNIQUE

The exact surgical technique will vary, of course, based on whether the reason for performing the arthroplasty is an acute fracture, a neglected fracture, a pathologic fracture, or a nonunion with failed hardware. However, many surgical principles are commonplace regardless of the preoperative diagnosis.

The patient is positioned in lateral decubitus position on the operating room table, and an intravenous antibiotic, typically a first-generation cephalosporin, is given. Careful padding of the down axilla, peroneal nerve area, and ankle can minimize the chance of a neurological or skin pressure problem due to positioning. A stable horizontal position can guide the surgeon to appropriate pelvic positioning, which will facilitate proper acetabular-component implantation. Several commercially available hip positioners are available to simplify accurate and stable pelvic positioning. Consideration should be given to the use of intraoperative blood salvage (cell saver), as these surgeries can be long and bloody.

The leg is prepped and draped in the usual fashion, and if possible, the previous incisions are used. If no previous incision is present, then a simple curvilinear incision centered on the greater trochanter will suffice. The fascia is incised in line with the skin incision and the status of the greater trochanter is evaluated. If the greater trochanter is not fractured, either an anterolateral or posterolateral approach can be used effectively based on surgeon preference. In the acute fracture situation it is always preferable, if possible, to leave the abductor–greater trochanter–vastus lateralis complex intact and immobilized in a long sleeve as much as possible during the reconstruction.

In nonunions or neglected fractures, the trochanter may be malunited and preclude access to the intramedullary canal. In this situation the so-called "trochanteric slide" technique may be useful (Fig. 18.1). This technique of preserving the vastus-trochanter-abductor sleeve may minimize the chance of so-called "trochanteric escape" and should be used whenever possible.

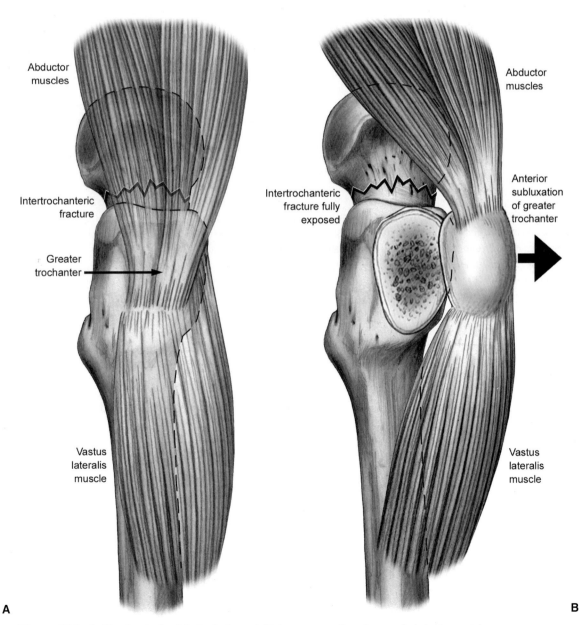

Figure 18.1. A. Trochanteric slide technique, initial exposure: the sleeve of abductors and vastus lateralis are in continuity. **B.** Trochanteric slide technique, deep exposure. Note continuity of the musculotendinous sleeve with mobilization of the greater trochanter.

If hardware is present in the proximal femur, it is wise to dislocate the hip prior to hardware removal. The torsional stresses on the femur during surgical dislocation can be large, especially in these typically stiff hips, and iatrogenic femur fracture can occur with attempted hip dislocation. If previous surgery has been performed, I prefer to obtain intraoperative cultures and frozen section pathology. If there is evidence of acute inflammation or other gross clinical evidence of infection, then I recommend removal of all hardware, careful debridement of all tissues, and resection of the proximal femoral-head fragment with placement of an antibiotic impregnated polymethacrylate spacer. The reconstruction is then performed in a delayed fashion after a period of organism-specific intravenous antibiotics based on the sensitivities obtained from deep intraoperative cultures.

The hip can be dislocated either anteriorly or posteriorly, depending upon surgeon preference and the status of the abductor mechanism. The proximal fragment is excised, and the acetabulum is circumferentially exposed. The quality of the remaining acetabular cartilage is evaluated. If the cartilage is in reasonable condition, then a hemi-arthroplasty can be used with good results. Appropriate attention to head size with hemi-arthroplasty is important as an undersized component can lead to medial loading, instability, and pain, while an oversized component can lead to peripheral loading, instability, and pain as well. If preexisting degenerative change or the acetabular cartilage damaged is noted from prior hardware cutout, a total hip replacement is preferable. Of course, even in the setting of normal-appearing acetabular cartilage, an acetabular component may provide more predictable pain relief, and this decision should be at the surgeon's discretion. The acetabulum is reamed carefully because these hips do not have the thick, sclerotic subchondral bone commonly found in patients with degenerative joint disease. The acetabulum is reamed circumferentially until a bleeding bed is obtained. Either cemented or uncemented acetabular component fixation can be used with good results. I prefer uncemented acetabular fixation due to the versatility it allows with multiple liner, bearing surface, and head size options; I also typically augment initial cup fixation with screws.

Attention is then turned to the femur. It should be emphasized that the femoral side of the reconstruction is typically more challenging in this setting. The general principles of femoral reconstruction are summarized diagrammatically in Figure 18.2. It is important to carefully evaluate the level of bony deficiency medially. Typically, bone loss from the fracture or a nonunion results in a bony deficiency well below the standard resection level for a primary total-hip arthroplasty. Therefore, a calcar prosthesis is usually necessary to restore leg length and hip stability. Femoral components with modular calcar augmentations are available and allow intraoperative flexibility in restoring the hip center. A large posteromedial fragment may be reduced and stabilized with cerclage wires or cables, which will help the surgeon judge appropriate femoral component seating height. In the acute fracture situation, reduction by wire or cable can potentially result in bony healing, thereby restoring medial bone stock.

Sclerotic hardware tracks, fracture translation, callus, and so forth can alter the morphology of the proximal femur. These alterations can deflect reamers and broaches leading to intraoperative fracture or femoral perforation. I have found it useful to use a large diameter burr to provisionally shape the funnel of the proximal femur. Once these sclerotic areas have been opened, standard reamers and broaches can be used to prepare the canal more safely.

If previous hardware has been present, then it is recommended that a stem length is chosen that bypasses the most distal stress riser (i.e., screw hole) in the shaft by at least two cortical (diaphyseal) diameters. Because most adult femoral shafts are approximately 30 mm in diameter, templating for 6 cm of bypass is a good general guideline for stem length. Either cemented or uncemented femoral-component fixation can be effective in this type of reconstruction and is, of course, based on surgeon preference and assessment of the intraoperative bone quality. If an uncemented femoral component is chosen, it is wise to select an extensively coated design that can achieve distal diaphyseal fixation. This strategy will allow the surgeon to bypass stress risers effectively and not rely on proximal boney support for implant stability. Cemented fixation may be advantageous for elderly patients with capacious, osteopenic femoral canals. Regardless of whether cemented or uncemented

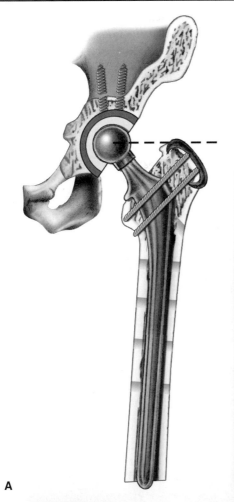

A

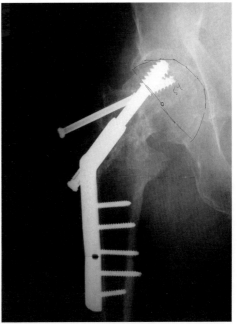

B

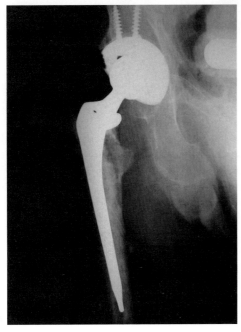

C

Figure 18.2. A. Illustration summariz-
ing the general principles of femoral
reconstruction for intertrochanteric fracture or salvage of failed internal fixation.
Note the restoration of appropriate
femoral-component height using a
calcar-replacing stem. Referencing the
tip of the greater trochanter as a guide
to restoring the center of rotation. Secure fixation of the greater trochanter
has been obtained as is typical: with a
cable through and a cable below the
lesser trochanter. Note the stem length
chosen to bypass all cortical stress risers by a minimum of two diaphyseal
diameters. **B.** Preoperative nonunion
and hardware cutout after ORIF of an
intertrochanteric fracture. Note the
acetabular erosion superiorly from the
lag screw. **C.** Postoperative reconstruction with a total hip arthroplasty with
particulate bone grafting of the superior
acetabular cavitary defect.

fixation is used intraoperatively, radiographs are recommended to assure appropriate alignment and bypass of previous stress risers and to rule out iatrogenic fracture or extravasation of cement. Extravasated cement can be a cause of late periprosthetic fracture, and it is recommended that careful removal of extravasated cement be performed. Small, medial, screw-hole extravasations can typically be ignored as long as they are bypassed sufficiently by the femoral component.

A helpful guide to the appropriate height of calcar reconstruction is the relationship between the center of the femoral head and the tip of the greater trochanter: It should be essentially coplanar. Although this may be difficult to assess in the presence of a trochanteric fracture, usually, the greater trochanteric fragments are still somewhat attached and can be used as a gross guide for evaluating the appropriate level of calcar buildup. Trial reduction is performed, and leg lengths and hip stability are assessed. Again, intraoperative radiographs should be obtained. The author typically obtains an intraoperative radiograph after the real acetabular component and the trial femoral component are in place, and then once again after all of the real components are implanted and greater trochanteric fragment fixation, if necessary, is complete.

Regardless of the method of stem fixation chosen, it is wise to use autogenous bone graft obtained from the resected femoral-head fragment to fill any lateral cortical defects from prior hardware as well as the interface with the greater trochanter and the femoral shaft, if necessary. Countless methods of greater trochanteric fixation have been described elsewhere in the literature, with mixed results. In general, the use of multiple wires or a cable claw technique is preferred. Regardless of the method chosen, the greater trochanteric fixation should be stable through a full range of motion of the hip. The fascia, subcutaneum, and the skin are closed per surgeon preference. Representative cases emphasizing these principles are shown in Figures 18.2, 18.3, 18.4, and 18.5.

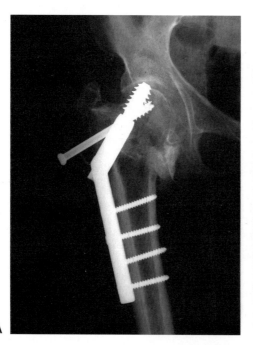
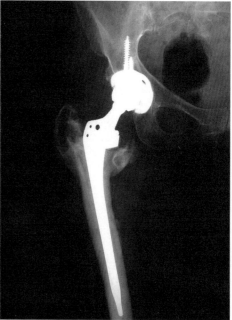

A   B

Figure 18.3. A. Preoperative failed ORIF with proximal fragment translation and screw cutout. **B.** Postoperative reconstruction with a total hip arthroplasty with calcar augmentation to restore appropriate femoral-component height, thereby restoring leg length and hip stability.

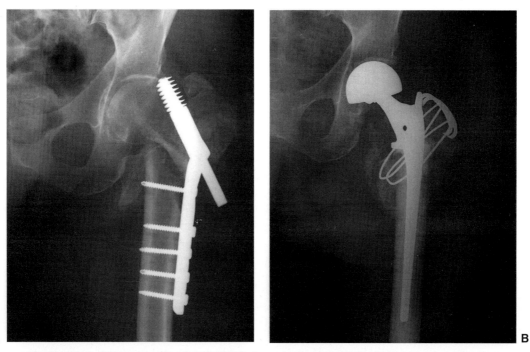

Figure 18.4. A. Preoperative failed ORIF of a reverse obliquity fracture. Note the difficulty in managing the greater trochanter in this situation. **B.** Postoperative reconstruction with calcar-replacing bipolar hemi-arthroplasty through a trochanteric slide technique.

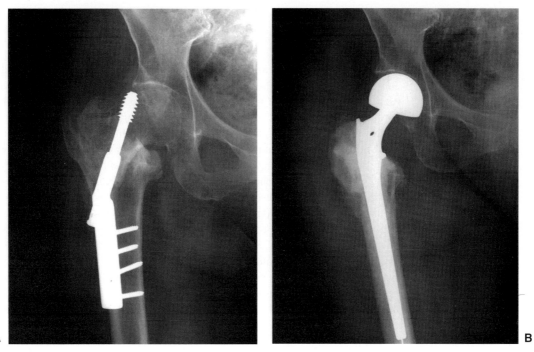

Figure 18.5. A. Preoperative failed ORIF with screw cutout. The acetabular joint space is well preserved. **B.** Postoperative radiograph demonstrating a cemented calcar-replacing bipolar hemi-arthroplasty.

REHABILITATION

In general, weight bearing can progress as tolerated after surgery; however, the surgeon should individualize the rehabilitation regimen based on patient compliance quality of intraoperative component-fixation achieved, and most importantly, the status of the greater trochanter. If trochanteric fixation was required, the selective use of an abduction orthosis, partial weight bearing for 6 weeks, and avoidance of abductor strengthening until trochanteric union has occurred are recommended. Sutures are typically removed at 2 weeks and periodic radiographs are obtained to evaluate component fixation and trochanteric healing status. Clinical and radiographic follow-up is typically performed at the discretion of the treating surgeon; for younger patients, follow-up visits are preferred at 6 weeks, 12 weeks, and 1, 2, and 5 years postoperatively, then every 2 years thereafter. For asymptomatic elderly patients with transportation difficulties, of course, the follow up periods are typically modified to 6 weeks, 3 months, one year, then every 5 years thereafter.

RESULTS

There are several reports of arthroplasty for intertrochanteric fracture in the literature. They generally document the efficacy of arthroplasty as an alternative treatment for the acute fracture; however, complications still remain concerning. Most reports regard salvage of failed internal fixation. Haidukewych and Berry reported on 60 patients undergoing hip arthroplasty for salvage of failed ORIF. Overall, functional status improved in all patients, and the 7 year survivorship free of revision was 100%. Pain relief was predictable. Dislocation was not problematic; however, persistent trochanteric complaints and problems obtaining bony trochanteric union were common. Both bipolar and total hip arthroplasties performed well. Calcar-replacing designs and long stem prostheses were necessary in the majority of cases.

COMPLICATIONS

Medical complications are common due to the debilitated, older patients undergoing these surgeries. Thromboembolic prophylaxis, perioperative antibiotics, and early mobilization are recommended. If a long-stem cemented implant is used, intraoperative embolization and cardiopulmonary complications can occur. It is important to lavage and dry the canal thoroughly prior to cementing in these frail patients, and little, if any, pressurization should be used. Infection and dislocation are surprisingly rare after such reconstructions in which modern techniques and implants are used. Dislocations are managed with closed reduction and bracing as long as the trochanteric fragment fixation remains secure.

Trochanteric complaints, including bursitis, hardware pain, and nonunion are the most common complications after these reconstructions. Patients should be counseled preoperatively that such chronic complaints are very common. Bony union will occur in most but not all trochanteric fragments. Stable trochanteric fibrous unions in good position will often be asymptomatic and not require treatment. Displaced trochanteric escape, if symptomatic, is typically treated with a repeat internal fixation attempt with some form of bone grafting. The best treatment is prevention, with extremely secure initial trochanteric fixation, the use of the trochanteric slide technique if mobilization of the trochanter is required, liberal use of autograft bone at the trochanter-femur interface, and careful postoperative rehabilitation.

SUMMARY

Hip arthroplasty is a valuable addition to the armamentarium of the surgeon treating intertrochanteric hip fractures. In general, it is reserved for neglected fractures, pathologic fractures due to neoplasm, salvage of internal fixation failure and nonunion, and (rarely) for fracture in patients with severe, symptomatic, preexisting degenerative change. Attention to specific technical details is important to avoid complications and provide a durable reconstruction. Trochanteric complications are common, but functional improvement and pain relief are predictable.

RECOMMENDED READING

Chan KC, Gill GS. Cemented hemiarthroplasty for elderly patients with intertrochanteric fractures. *Clin Orthop* 2000;371:206–215.

Eschenroeder HC Jr, Krackow KA. Late onset femoral stress fracture associated with extruded cement following hip arthroplasty. *Clin Orthop* 1988;236:210–213.

Green S, Moore T, Proano F. Bipolar prosthetic replacement for the management of unstable intertrochanteric hip fractures in the elderly. *Clin Orthop* 1987;224:169–170.

Haentjens P, Casteleyn PP, DeBoerk H, et al. Treatment of unstable intertrochanteric and subtrochanteric fractures in elderly patients: primary bipolar arthroplasty compared with ORIF. *J Bone Joint Surg* 1989;71(8):1214–1225.

Haentjens P, Casteleyn PP, Opdecam P. Primary bipolar arthroplasty or total hip arthroplasty for the treatment of unstable intertrochanteric or subtrochanteric fractures in elderly patients. *Acta Orthop Belg* 1994:60:124–128.

Haentjens P, Casteleyn PP, Opdecan P. Hip arthroplasty for failed internal fixation of intertrochanteric and subtrochanteric fractures in the elderly patient. *Arch Orthop Trauma Surg* 1994;113:222–227.

Haidukewych GJ, Berry DJ. Hip arthroplasty for salvage of failed treatment of intertrochanteric hip fractures. *J Bone Joint Surg* 2003;85:899–905.

Haidukewych GJ, Berry DJ. Revision internal fixation and bone grafting for intertrochanteric nonunion. *Clin Orthop* 2003;412:184–188.

Haidukewych GJ, Israel TA, Berry DJ. Reverse obliquity of fractures of the intertrochanteric region of the femur. *J Bone Joint Surg* 2001;83:643–650.

Harwin SF, Stern RE, Kulich RG. Primary Bateman-Leinbach bipolar prosthetic replacement of the hip in the treatment of unstable intertrochanteric fractures in the elderly. *Orthopedics* October 1990;13:1131–1136.

Kim Y-H, Oh J-H, Koh Y-G. Salvage of neglected unstable intertrochanteric fractures with cementless porous-coated hemiarthroplasty. *Clin Orthop* 1992;277:182–187.

Knight WM, DeLee JC. Nonunion of intertrochanteric fractures of the hip: a case study and review. *Orthop Trans* 1982;16:438.

Kyle RF, Cabanela ME, Russell TA, et al. Fractures of the proximal part of the femur. *Instr Course Lect* 1995;44:227–253.

Lifeso R, Younge D. The neglected hip fracture. *J Orthop Trauma* 1990;4:287–292.

Mariani EM, Rand JA. Nonunion of intertrochanteric fractures of the femur following open reduction and internal fixation: results of second attempts to gain union. *Clin Orthop* 1987;218:81–89.

Mehlhoff T, Landon GC, Tullos HS. Total hip arthroplasty following failed internal fixation of hip fractures. *Clin Orthop* 1991;269:32–37.

Parvizi J, Ereth MH, Lewallen DG. Thirty day mortality following hip arthroplasty for acute fracture. *J Bone Joint Surg* 2004;86:1983–1986.

Patterson BM, Salvati EA, Huo MH. Total hip arthroplasty for complications of intertrochanteric fracture: a technical note. *J Bone Joint Surg* 1990;72:776–777.

Rodop O, Kiral A, Kaplan H, Akmaz I. Primary bipolar hemiarthroplasty for unstable intertrochanteric fractures. *Int Orthop* 2002;26:233–237.

Sarathy MP, Madhavan P, Ravichandran KM. Nonunion of intertrochanteric fractures of the femur. *J Bone Joint Surg* 1994;77:90–92.

Stoffelen D, Haentjens P, Reynders P, et al. Hip arthroplasty for failed internal fixation of intertrochanteric and subtrochanteric fractures in the elderly patient. *Acta Orthop Belg* 1994;60:135–139.

Tabsh I, Waddell JP, Morton J. Total hip arthroplasty for complications of proximal femoral fractures. *J Orthop Trauma.* 1997;11:166–169.

Wu CC, Shih CH, Chen WJ, et al. Treatment of cutout of a lag screw of a dynamic hip screw in an intertrochanteric fracture. *Arch Orthop Trauma Surg* 1998;117:193–196.

19

Subtrochanteric Femur Fractures: Plate Fixation

Michael J. Gardner, Eric E. Johnson, and Dean G. Lorich

INDICATIONS/CONTRAINDICATIONS

Open reduction and internal fixation (ORIF) with a fixed-angle plate, while used less commonly today, is an excellent method of treatment for selected subtrochanteric femur fractures (1–13). The blade plate has traditionally been used most commonly, but with the recent development and refinement of locking screw-plate technology, fixed-angle screw-plate constructs are being used more frequently. Plate fixation has a long history of successful application for proximal femur fractures, but instills a certain degree of anxiety among many surgeons. Outside of trauma centers, fixed angle plates are infrequently used implants. However, these implants offer several advantages when compared with other forms of fixation for proximal femoral fractures (4). They can be used in severely comminuted fractures, ipsilateral hip and shaft fractures, and subtrochanteric fractures with extension into the base of the neck or peritrochanteric region.

Blade plates and locking plates possess many unique qualities found with few other implants. They offer excellent stability and rotational control in complex fractures, can be used after corrective osteotomy about the hip, provide immediate fracture compression through surgeon- controlled application, and can offer valuable salvage options for failed fixation of other devices used in the proximal femur. Like any technically demanding procedure, immediate and long-term outcomes are optimized with experience and mastery of the surgical technique. Fixed-angle plating is an excellent implant when using indirect reduction and biological plating of both proximal and distal femoral fractures (4,14,15). Indirect reduction and fixation with these devices provide mechanically sound stabilization, allowing rapid mobilization and early, protected, weight bearing.

Fixed-angle plating, with either a standard blade plate or a fixed-angle locking-screw plate system, is indicated for many of proximal femoral fractures, including subtrochanteric and subtrochanteric-intertrochanteric fractures, fractures with extension into the basilar femoral neck, and some combined femoral-shaft and femoral-neck fractures. Alternative implants for these fractures include dynamic condylar screw devices and reconstruction cephalomedullary nails (5,9,12,16,17). Relative contraindications to traditional fixed-angle plate osteosynthesis for subtrochanteric fractures include elderly patients with osteoporotic bone whose poor bone quality may compromise extramedullary fixation stability; unreliable patients who cannot comply with protected, postoperative, weight bearing; and surgeons unfamiliar with the technique.

In general, two operative techniques are available for reduction of the proximal femur with fixed-angle plates: direct or indirect reduction. Direct reduction is recommended when the injury involves two main, large fragments (proximal and distal shaft fragments) and only one or two butterfly fragments with minimal comminution. Anatomic reduction and individual lag-screw fixation of the large butterfly fragments can usually be achieved without difficulty (16). Indirect or biological reduction is the preferred technique when moderate to severe comminution is present. In the latter case, anatomic reduction of individual fragments is technically impossible, and the required soft-tissue stripping of the fragments leads to devascularization. The goal of indirect reduction is to restore anatomic length, axis alignment, and rotation of the extremity, using both the implant and a femoral distractor in concert (4). The most appropriate method of fixation is a bridging technique in which a long plate, with relatively few, well-spaced, possibly locking, screws are used. Indirect reduction also relies upon the ability of the surgeon to tension the soft-tissue envelope with distraction of the fracture back to length with minimal disturbance of the surrounding fracture hematoma and periosteum.

PREOPERATIVE PLANNING

Accurate preoperative planning is critical when a fixed-angle plate is to be used for proximal femoral fractures. The surgeon should be familiar with implants and techniques of the AO/ASIF group before attempting this procedure. To avoid intraoperative complications, the surgeon must address several key points in preoperative planning of plate osteosynthesis. If a blade plate is being planned, the correct insertion site of the blade, the appropriate length of both the blade and the plate portion of the device, and the number of lag and plate compression screws are important to consider. If a locking plate will be used, the surgeon should consider the proximal or distal position of the plate that is necessary to allow correct placement of the screws into the femoral neck and understand that the length of the plate is crucial. The first step in planning osteosynthesis is to reconstruct the proximal femoral fracture by drawing all the individual fracture fragments into a reduced position. Frequently, multiple radiographs of the involved side are required because of fracture fragment displacement and rotation (Figs. 19.1 and 19.2).

In blade plating, the key to a good reduction is correct placement of the blade, and thus the next step is to determine the correct entry site of the seating chisel in the lateral greater trochanter. Most commonly, this is just proximal and lateral to the most prominent portion of the greater trochanteric ridge (Fig. 19.3). Using this landmark will, in the majority of cases, place the blade in the inferior portion of the femoral head and proximal to the inferior aspect of the femoral neck.

To assist in planning the subtrochanteric fracture reduction, AO blade-plate templates can be used to estimate the blade length and side-plate size. Blade lengths are available in 10-mm increments, starting at 50 mm, and side plate lengths are determined by the number of holes, which range from 5 to 26 holes with special order implants. The blade portion of the plate should reach to within 1.0 to 1.5 cm from the inferior central portion of the femoral-head articular surface. Estimation of the side plate length and number of screw holes below the most distal extent of the fracture is possible from the preoperative plan. At least four screws engaging eight cortices are necessary distal to a comminuted subtrochanteric fracture. Alternatively, the plate length may be increased, and screws may be spaced out along the length of the shaft fragment. This approach distributes the deforming forces over a greater distance and leads to a more stable construct. After planning the reduction of the fracture fragments into an acceptable position and tracing the most appropriate plate template over the reconstructed femur, the surgeon confirms the preoperative plan in a step-wise fashion, verifying the implant size, number of screws above and below the fracture, and the correct trochanteric entrance site.

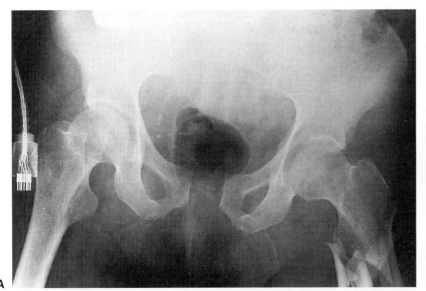
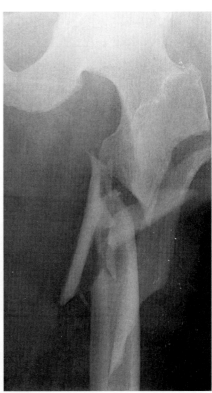

Figure 19.1. A. AP radiograph of the pelvis and **(B)** AP radiograph of the proximal left femur, which shows a comminuted, left, subtrochanteric, femur fracture and diastasis of the pubic symphysis in a 79-year-old man.

When planning preoperatively for a locking screw-plate device much of the templating is similar to process use for a blade plate, with several additional issues requiring attention. Once the fracture is reconstructed on paper the right or left AO template should be selected, and the appropriate plate length can be determined. Plate lengths vary from 2 screws to 16 screws along the shaft of the plate. These newly designed plates have special combination-plate screw holes that allow either 4.5-mm compression screws or 4.0-mm or 5.0-mm locking screws to be inserted. Three fixed-angle screws are used for proximal fixation into the femoral head and neck, at angles of 95 degrees (7.3-mm screw), 120 degrees (7.3-mm screw), and 135 degrees (5.0-mm screw). There is little room for adjustment after inserting these screws once the plate placement is decided, so the correct plate position on the lateral femoral cortex is necessary. As with a blade plate, recent improved understanding in biological plating techniques has indicated that a longer plate with well-spaced screws, leaving several holes unfilled, is preferable.

SURGERY

Surgery is performed by placing the patient in either a lateral decubitus position with cross-table fluoroscopy, or via supine positioning on a radiolucent fracture table. If lateral positioning is used, the extremity is prepped and draped free, allowing manipulation of the fracture fragments and facilitating "frog lateral" views that provide orthogonal x-ray visualization of the fracture and correct position of the plate and screws in the proximal femur.

A direct, lateral, surgical approach to the femur is performed, extending from several centimeters proximal to the greater trochanter to a level distal enough to allow reduction of the side plate to the femoral shaft (Fig. 19.4). After dissection through skin and subcutaneous tissue, the tensor fascia lata is incised and the vastus lateralis is released from the

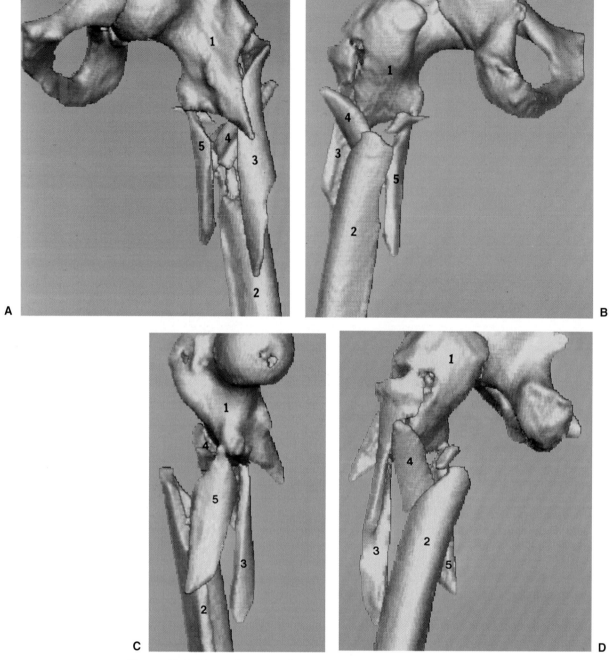

Figure 19.2. Three-dimensional computed axial tomography (CAT) images of the **(A)** anterior, **(B)** posterior, **(C)** medial, and **(D)** lateral views of the subtrochanteric fracture seen in Figure 19.1. These views demonstrate comminution of the lateral, proximal, femoral cortex below the lateral trochanteric ridge. Major fragments are numbered 1 to 5 on all views.

posterior aspect of the femur and intermuscular septum and reflected anteriorly. It is important to adequately expose the greater trochanter. During this dissection, the surgeon should take care to minimize stripping of individual comminuted bone fragments (Fig. 19.5).

After exposure of the trochanter, the femoral cortex immediately distal to the lateral trochanteric ridge is examined. If the cortex at this level is compromised, an important anatomic landmark is lost (see Figs. 19.1 and 19.2). Reconstruction of the proximal, lateral, femoral cortex (see Fig. 19.2, fragment 3, and Fig. 19.3, step 1) to the femoral neck–trochanteric fragment (Fig. 19.2, fragment 1) is crucial if a blade plate is being used

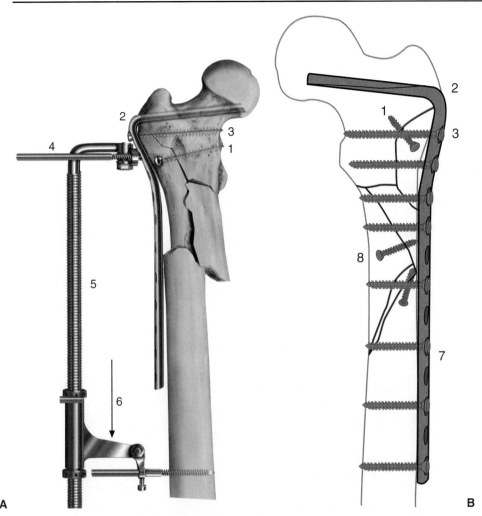

Figure 19.3. A. Steps used to obtain reduction of the subtrochanteric fracture by using the AO/ASIF fracture distractor. Step 1, reconstruction of the proximal, lateral, femoral cortex with a lag screw. Step 2, cutting and seating of the blade plate into the proximal femur. Step 3, insertion of the first screw of the blade plate to stabilize it in the proximal femur. Step 4, placement of the distractor pin holes, the proximal one in the second hole of the plate and the distal one below the end of the plate. Step 5, application of the AO/ASIF fracture distractor to the pins. Step 6, overdistraction of the fracture. **B.** Preoperative plan showing the reconstructed, left, subtrochanteric, femur fracture with individual lag screws and blade-plate template traced over the femoral shaft. The size of the blade, number of holes for the side plate, and entrance site slightly proximal to the lateral trochanteric ridge (steps 1 to 3). Stabilizing the plate to the distal shaft and completion of lag-screw and distal-screw fixation (steps 7 to 8). Direct reduction of this fracture is planned with multiple lag-screw fixation of large butterfly fragments and long oblique fracture under the plate.

because it recreates the entry point reference for the seating chisel (see Fig. 19.3, step 2 and Fig. 19.6). When using a locked plate this step is less critical because the greater trochanter and guide wire position in the neck can be used as a guide for the correct proximal-distal plate position.

Following exposure, the first step when using either implant is to establish fixation into the proximal femoral-head and femoral-neck fragment; this approach will allow for anatomic fracture alignment when the distal fragment is reduced to the plate. For blade plate application, two guide wires are placed initially to direct the insertion of the chisel. The first wire is placed along the anterior cortex of the femoral neck to indicate the degree of anteversion and to dictate the direction of chisel insertion in the anteroposterior (AP) plane. Alterations to the chisel orientation at this stage will affect internal or external rotation of the final fracture reduction. The second wire is placed into the superior portion

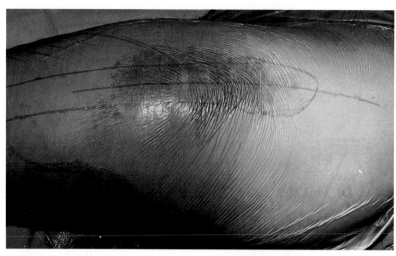

Figure 19.4. The patient is placed in the lateral decubitus position, and a direct lateral approach is made, extending above the level of the greater trochanter to the proximal third of the femoral shaft.

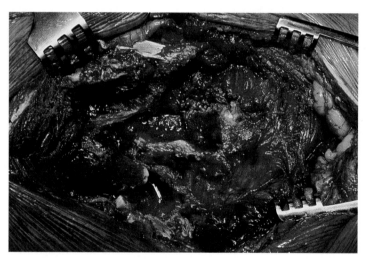

Figure 19.5. Prereduction exposure of the subtrochanteric fracture. Minimal stripping of individual bone fragments is mandatory to ensure viability of fragments after reduction.

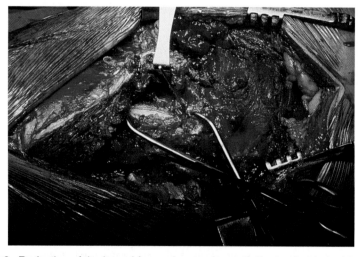

Figure 19.6. Reduction of the lateral femoral cortex beneath the trochanteric ridge is performed by using large reduction forceps and stabilized with K wires or lag screws. Lag screws are preferable for definitive fixation. Reduction of fragments three and four to the main proximal neck–trochanteric fragment reconstructs the lateral, proximal, femoral cortex.

of the greater trochanter at a 95-degree angle to the femoral shaft, and it is advanced into the femoral neck and head. The second wire controls the coronal plane alignment of the chisel position and subsequently the plate position. Miscalculation of this angle will lead to varus or valgus mal-alignment of the fracture site. An angled guide instrument (preset to 95 degrees) can aid in the proper insertion angle of this wire (Fig. 19.7), which should be

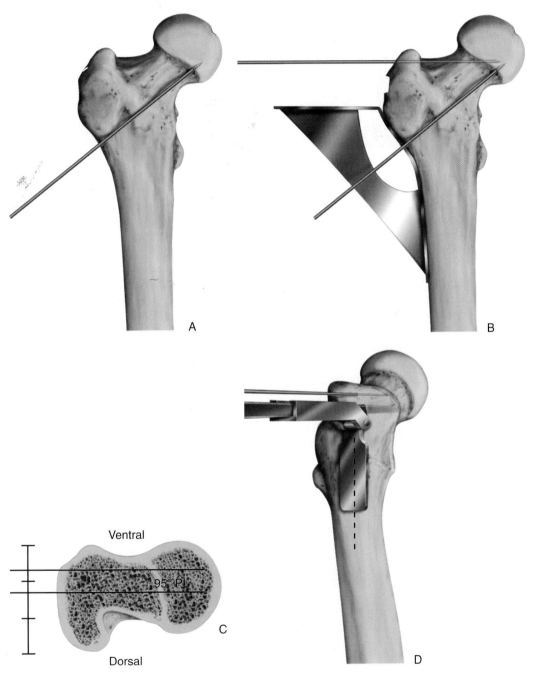

Figure 19.7. Placement of guiding K wires to facilitate cutting of the blade slot into the femoral neck. **A.** Anterior femoral-neck guide wire indicating femoral-neck anteversion. **B.** The 95-degree angled guide and placing the corresponding guide wire into the proximal portion of the femoral neck. **C.** Relation of the femoral neck to the proximal greater trochanter for insertion of the 95-degree fixed-angle blade plate. Note the central femoral neck corresponds to the anterior half of the greater trochanter at this level. **D.** Anterior lateral view of the seating chisel placement, cutting the blade slot into the base of the femoral head (note that the flange of the seating guide is in the midportion of the femoral shaft). Reconstruction of the lateral, proximal, femoral cortex enhances the correct position of the seating-chisel guide.

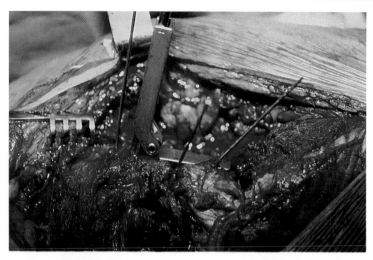

Figure 19.8. Anterior view of the seating chisel and guide parallel to the 95-degree greater trochanteric guide wire.

placed in neutral or slight valgus alignment to ensure avoidance of varus coronal alignment. Other anatomic landmarks include the lateral trochanteric ridge; the lateral, proximal, femoral shaft; and the AP width of the greater trochanter.

The chisel is then inserted through the insertion guide (preset at 95 degrees) under fluoroscopic control. The femoral neck rises from the anterior half of the greater trochanter; therefore, the seating chisel should enter the anterior half of the trochanter just proximal to the lateral trochanteric ridge and not in the anatomic middle of the trochanter (Fig. 19.7). One of the more common errors with the use of a blade plate is penetration of the anterior femoral cortex with the seating chisel, which will result in plate malposition and an external rotation deformity of the distal fragment and extremity when the plate is reduced to the shaft. The weight of the insertion handle has a tendency to fall posteriorly and direct the chisel anteriorly. This chisel movement can be avoided by using frequent AP and lateral fluoroscopic imaging as the chisel is progressively seated into its final position in the femoral neck and head (Figs. 19.8 and 19.9). Constant attention to the angle of insertion, rotation of the chisel, and internal or external torsion of the femur will reduced the risk of technical errors. The seating chisel has an adjustable flange that is placed against the lateral femoral cortex inferior to the trochanteric ridge. This serves as an alignment guide for detection of any internal or external rotation and any flexion or extension of the chisel as it is

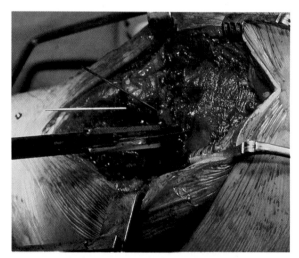

Figure 19.9. Axial view of the seating chisel and its relation to the anterior femoral-neck guide wire.

seated. The chisel must be advanced slowly and backed out frequently to prevent the chisel from becoming stuck in the dense bone of the proximal femur.

Once the chisel is fully seated and removed, the inferior edge of the entry slot is removed with a narrow osteotome to allow the neck at the junction of the plate and blade to be fully inserted. The selected implant is then attached to the insertion handle, and the blade is introduced into the slot in a technique like that to seat the chisel. The surgeon should not assume that the blade will automatically follow the slot to the correct position. Retention of the Kirschner (K) wires as guides will help reproduce the proper insertion of the blade. Misplacement of the blade often occurs secondary to overconfidence and lack of attention at the time of insertion. If an error occurs with placement of the blade portion of the plate, it is possible to remove it and redirect into its proper position. However, only slight corrections may be made and this requires considerable technical skill and experience. One key advantage of the blade plate implant is that the seating chisel does not remove any bone from the femoral head and neck, allowing slight corrections to be made. After the implant is seated in the proximal fragment, it is crucial to insert a screw into the proximal portion of the plate to enhance fixation stability and to prevent the blade from cutting out of the femoral head during reduction of the fracture (see Fig. 19.3, step 3).

Proximal fixation with a locking plate is generally more forgiving than with a blade plate; however, meticulous care must still be taken to prevent fracture malalignment following final reduction. The ultimate plate position, and thus fracture reduction, depends on the placement of guide wires into the femoral head and neck. The fixed-angle wire guides are threaded to the proximal three holes of the plate, and the plate is approximated to the proximal femur. Next, a guide wire is advanced through the most proximal (95-degree) hole. The correct path of this wire is approximately 1 cm inferior to the piriformis fossa into the inferior femoral head on the AP view, and central in the femoral head on the lateral view (Fig. 19.10). A guide wire is inserted into the next distal (120-degree) hole, and because this is in a different plane than the first hole, the surgeon must visualize its position on the lateral x-ray. The third guide wire, in the 135-degree hole, is then placed, which is in the same plane as the first hole and may alternatively be inserted near the end of the procedure without compromising the stability of the construct.

With all three guide wires inserted, the surgeon should recognize that the plate may not be flush with the greater trochanter. Although the plate is precontoured, individual variations may leave the plate slightly proud of the bone. However, due to the angular stability of the screws in the plate, exact plate apposition to the bone is unnecessary for stable fixation. The most important factor is that the guide wires are in the correct position and that the shaft of the plate is in neutral or slight valgus alignment with the femur shaft. Any amount of varus should be avoided. Next, the screw lengths are measured using an indirect device over the guide wires with the wire guides still attached (Fig. 19.11), and the appropriate, fully threaded, cannulated screws (7.3 mm for the two proximal holes and 5.0 mm for the third proximal hole) are selected. These cannulated screws are inserted over the guide wires with the guides removed. To allow for complete engagement of the locking mechanism, the surgeon must seat fully the threads on the undersurface of the screw heads.

After the implant is fixed to the proximal fragment, the ensuing fracture reduction and stabilization is similar for both blade and locking plates. The femoral distractor is applied to span the implant and the fracture, facilitating restoration of length and alignment of the fracture. A distractor or Schanz pin may be placed through a plate hole into the proximal cortex. A similar pin is placed in the distal femoral shaft, perpendicular to the shaft cortex, and below the level of the distal extent of the plate. Either the short or long AO distractor, mounted on these two pins, is appropriate. Slow distraction is applied across the fracture site through the implant until the fracture fragments are slightly overdistracted (Fig. 19.12). As the tension in the soft tissue increases, there is a tendency for the fracture site to deform into varus, resulting in the plate pulling away from the distal shaft fragment. This can be minimized by placing several plate-holding clamps to keep the plate reduced to the shaft cortex as the fracture is distracted (see Fig. 19.12).

In general, with direct reduction techniques, large butterfly-fracture fragments should be reduced to either the proximal or distal main fragment prior to insertion of the implant.

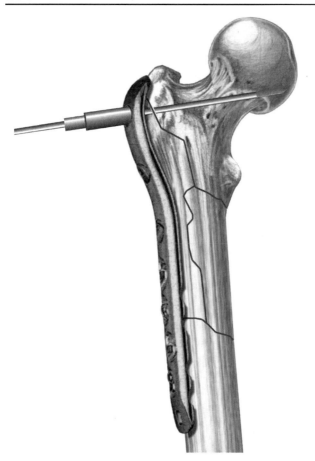

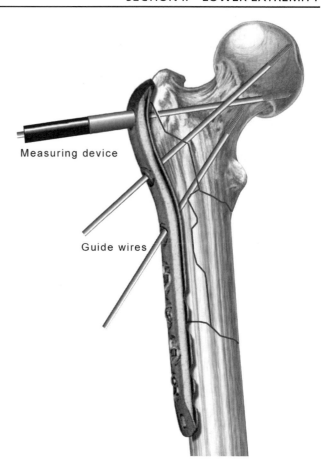

Measuring device

Guide wires

Figure 19.10. Through a threaded wire guide attached to the most proximal hole (95 degrees), a guide wire is inserted so it lies 1 cm inferior to the piriformis fossa and inferior in the femoral head. It should be central on a lateral view.

Figure 19.11. The appropriate screw lengths are measured using an indirect measuring device over the guide wires with the guides still attached to the plate.

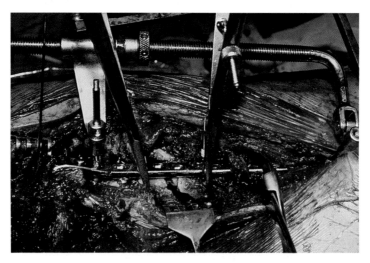

Figure 19.12. Application of the femoral distractor across the subtrochanteric fracture with bone clamps holding the plate to the distal shaft fragment. Slight overdistraction of 5 mm is performed to allow alignment of major fracture lines.

Occasionally, posteromedial fracture fragments involving the lesser trochanter cannot be reduced until the main fragments have been reduced. These large fracture fragments are stabilized by lag screws positioned to avoid interference with the final position of the implant. The distractor allows manipulation of rotation and correction of angular mal-alignment during distraction of the fracture. Once alignment of the fracture is achieved, the distractor is reversed to allow the fracture fragments to return to an anatomic position (Fig. 19.13). Lag screws can be inserted between the two main fragments as the distractor and bone clamps maintain the reduction. The completion of osteosynthesis is achieved by final screw placement in the plate and removal of the clamps and distractor. The locking plate allows compression screws to be used in the distal combination holes to stabilize simple fracture patterns rigidly. Finally, the hip is examined under fluoroscopy to assess the reduction and fixation in both the AP and lateral planes.

When indirect reduction techniques are used in comminuted fractures, realignment is achieved by returning the soft-tissue tension to normal through the use of the distractor and fluoroscopic evaluation of the overall reduction. Indirect reduction demands preservation of fracture hematoma by avoiding direct dissection at the fracture site, and no attempt at interfragmentary compression with lag screws is performed when there are small comminuted fragments (Fig. 19.14). Considerable operative skill is required to estimate accurately the correct fracture length and alignment and the appropriate level of soft-tissue tension. Locking plates are ideal for use in these fractures, and the combination holes should be used in locking mode with 4.5-mm screws placed to bridge the fracture site (Fig. 19.15). Radiographs are obtained to verify correct length and overall reduction. Wounds are closed over suction drains. Closure of the vastus lateralis and tensor fascia lata completes the deep closure, and a compressive dressing is applied to the wound.

POSTOPERATIVE MANAGEMENT

Drains are removed at 24 to 48 hours or when the drainage is less than 30 cc over a 24-hour period. Postoperative prophylactic antibiotics are discontinued when the drains are removed. Range-of-motion exercises are initiated immediately in the postoperative period by using a continuous passive-motion machine. Early mobilization with crutches or a walker is prescribed with only touchdown weight bearing maintained for the first 6 postoperative weeks. Thromboprophylaxis, including pulsatile stockings and anticoagulant therapy, is continued until the patient is able to ambulate independently, usually within 4 to 5 days after surgery. Subcutaneous low-molecular-weight heparin or warfarin therapy is prescribed at the physician's discretion. Radiographs are obtained at monthly intervals and

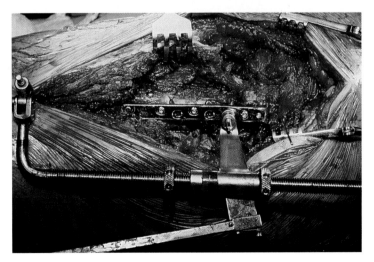

Figure 19.13. Reverse of the overdistraction and settling of the major fracture lines. Once this reduction is achieved, definitive lag-screw fixation is performed between major bone fragments to enhance fixation.

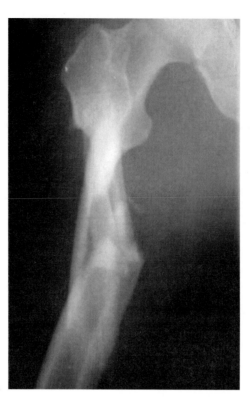
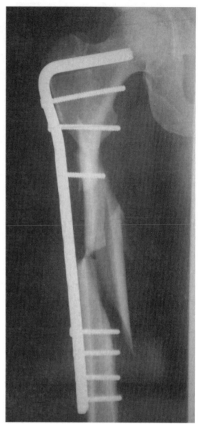

A   B

Figure 19.14. A. A comminuted subtrochanteric fracture is best treated with **(B)** indirect reduction techniques and plate fixation that spans the comminution.

progressive weight bearing is initiated when the radiographs demonstrate callus formation and fracture line healing (Fig. 19.16). Full weight bearing is usually not possible until 12 weeks after a subtrochanteric fracture. Patients may return to further activities once radiographs demonstrate complete fracture healing. Participation in high-risk contact sports is limited for 6 months after surgery. If the mechanical axis, extremity rotation, and length are anatomic, the patient can anticipate an excellent result.

Outcome after blade plate osteosynthesis for subtrochanteric femur fractures varies according to experience of the surgeon and complexity of the fracture (1,4,10,11,18). Direct reduction, with extensive medial dissection and bone grafting has been associated with poor results (16). Kinast et al (4) studied two groups of patients with subtrochanteric femur fractures who underwent either direct or indirect reduction techniques. They found significantly improved healing time and complication rates for indirect reduction over those found for direct reduction. High rates of union and good functional results can be achieved once the technical difficulties and nuances of the technique are mastered. Because the surgeon has only one chance to determine the final fracture alignment apprehension with using blade plates is common. Long-term results following locked plating are still unknown, but locked screws for proximal fixation and distal combination holes may offer a theoretical biomechanical advantage over traditional blade-plate implants.

COMPLICATIONS

Plate fixation of subtrochanteric femur fractures shares problems common to any plate device used for treating hip fractures. Loss of fixation and collapse into varus position can occur with poor implant placement. When locked screws are used, it is crucial to visualize all three proximal screws to ensure penetration into the hip joint has not occurred. The use of these implants in osteoporotic bone has some risk of failure due to poor purchase. Patients who weight bear prematurely may produce hardware failure because of

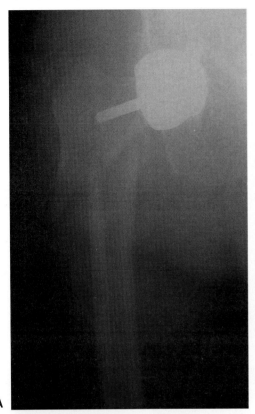

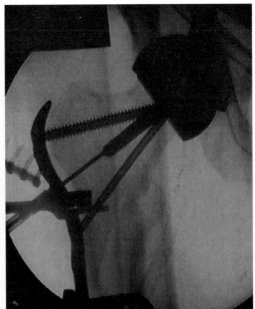

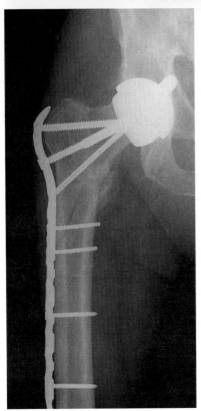

Figure 19.15. **A.** Example of a locking plate for the treatment of a comminuted subtrochanteric fracture around a femoral head prosthesis. **B.** The three proximal guide wires and screws are placed proximally, and the bone is reduced to the plate. An indirect reduction technique was employed in this case, followed by well-spaced locking screws along the shaft of the plate distally. **C.** X-rays at 3 months show maintained anatomic alignment of the fracture and evidence of healing.

the high stress concentrations produced in the subtrochanteric area. The most common complications related to the technique are residual varus malalignment of the fracture, penetration of the femoral neck with the blade or screws, external rotation, and shortening of the extremity. Nonunion rates of up to 16% have been reported (1,4,10,19). Other complications are a direct result of poor insertion technique (including inferior or

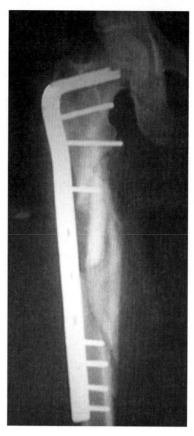

Figure 19.16. Anatomic alignment and healing of a comminuted subtrochanteric fracture.

posterior penetration of the femoral neck, varus or valgus, internal or external torsion), and sagittal plane mal-alignment may occur if attention to the insertion technique is not vigorously observed.

RECOMMENDED READINGS

1. Asher MA, Tippett JW, Rockwood CA, et al. Compression fixation of subtrochanteric fractures. *Clin Orthop* 1976:202–208.
2. Bedi A, Toan Le T. Subtrochanteric femur fractures. *Orthop Clin North Am* 2004;35:473–483.
3. Herscovici D Jr, Pistel WL, Sanders RW. Evaluation and treatment of high subtrochanteric femur fractures. *Am J Orthop* 2000;29:27–33.
4. Kinast C, Bolhofner BR, Mast JW, et al. Subtrochanteric fractures of the femur: results of treatment with the 95 degrees condylar blade-plate. *Clin Orthop* 1989:122–130.
5. Kulkarni SS, Moran CG. Results of dynamic condylar screw for subtrochanteric fractures. *Injury* 2003;34:117–122.
6. Lundy DW, Acevedo JI, Ganey TM, et al. Mechanical comparison of plates used in the treatment of unstable subtrochanteric femur fractures. *J Orthop Trauma* 1999;13:534–538.
7. Lunsjo K, Ceder L, Tidermark J, et al. Extramedullary fixation of 107 subtrochanteric fractures: a randomized multicenter trial of the Medoff sliding plate versus 3 other screw-plate systems. *Acta Orthop Scand* 1999;70:459–466.
8. Neher C, Ostrum RF. Treatment of subtrochanteric femur fractures using a submuscular fixed low-angle plate. *Am J Orthop* 2003;32:29–33.
9. Pakuts AJ. Unstable subtrochanteric fractures: gamma nail versus dynamic condylar screw. *Int Orthop* 2004;28:21–24.
10. Siebenrock KA, Muller U, Ganz R. Indirect reduction with a condylar blade plate for osteosynthesis of subtrochanteric femoral fractures. *Injury* 1998;29:7–15.
11. Whatley JR, Garland DE, Whitecloud T III, et al. Subtrochanteric fractures of the femur: treatment with ASIF blade plate fixation. *South Med J* 1978;71:1372–1375.
12. Vaidya SV, Dholakia DB, Chatterjee A. The use of a dynamic condylar screw and biological reduction techniques for subtrochanteric femur fracture. *Injury* 2003;34:123–128.
13. Sims SH. Subtrochanteric femur fractures. *Orthop Clin North Am* 2002;33:viii,113–126.

14. Fankhauser F, Gruber G, Schippinger G, et al. Minimal-invasive treatment of distal femoral fractures with the LISS (Less Invasive Stabilization System): a prospective study of 30 fractures with a follow up of 20 months. *Acta Orthop Scand* 2004;75:56–60.

15. Syed AA, Agarwal M, Giannoudis PV, et al. Distal femoral fractures: long-term outcome following stabilisation with the LISS. *Injury* 2004;35:599–607.

16. Sanders R, Regazzoni P. Treatment of subtrochanteric femur fractures using the dynamic condylar screw. *J Orthop Trauma* 1989;3:206–213.

17. Borens O, Wettstein M, Kombot C, et al. Long gamma nail in the treatment of subtrochanteric fractures. *Arch Orthop Trauma Surg* 2004;124:443–447.

18. Muller ME, Allgower M, Schneider R, et al. Angled plates. In: Allgower M, ed. *Manual of Internal Fixation: Techniques Recommended by the AO-ASIF Group.* Berlin: Springer-Verlag; 1991.

19. Brien WW, Wiss DA, Becker V Jr, et al. Subtrochanteric femur fractures: a comparison of the Zickel nail, 95 degrees blade plate, and interlocking nail. *J Orthop Trauma* 1991;5:458–564.

20

Subtrochanteric Femur Fractures: Reconstruction Nailing

Thomas A. Russell

INDICATIONS/CONTRAINDICATIONS

Reconstruction or cephalomedullary nails are specialized, antegrade, femoral, intramedullary nails designed to provide fixation into the femoral head and neck for selected, complex, proximal-femoral fractures. Reconstruction nails are a subset of cephalomedullary nails that are distinguished by two proximal interlocking screws that permit sliding lag-screw fixation into the femoral head, which enhance rotational stability in the proximal femur, and distal interlocking screws, which ensure rotational and axial stability. In addition, the geometry of the nail is altered throughout its length with variations in cross section to maximize nail strength and to minimize its stiffness. This modulation in cross section is especially important in the subtrochanteric region where fatigue stresses are relatively high. All reconstruction nails have an anterior bow to facilitate nail insertion.

The original reconstruction nail was the Russell-Taylor Reconstruction Nail (Smith & Nephew, Memphis, TN) introduced in 1986. It was a closed-section implant designed for a piriformis entry. The nail was calibrated to approximate 95% of the intact bending stiffness and 50% of the rotational stiffness in the intact femoral diaphysis. The proximal cross section was modified to enable a higher fatigue life in the subtrochanteric region and was 15 mm in diameter in this area with the diaphyseal diameter available in 12, 13, and 14 mm (Fig. 20.1). This original design was frequently referred to as a "second-generation interlocking nail." Subsequently, newer generations of reconstruction nails have been introduced by various manufacturers. They vary in their proximal geometries, diameter, cross-sectional design, and proximal screw geometries (see Fig. 20.1A–C).

Mechanically, a statically locked reconstruction nail can be used to stabilize injuries from the femoral neck to approximately 4 cm above the knee. Reconstruction nails were originally designed for subtrochanteric femoral fractures, pathologic femoral fractures, and

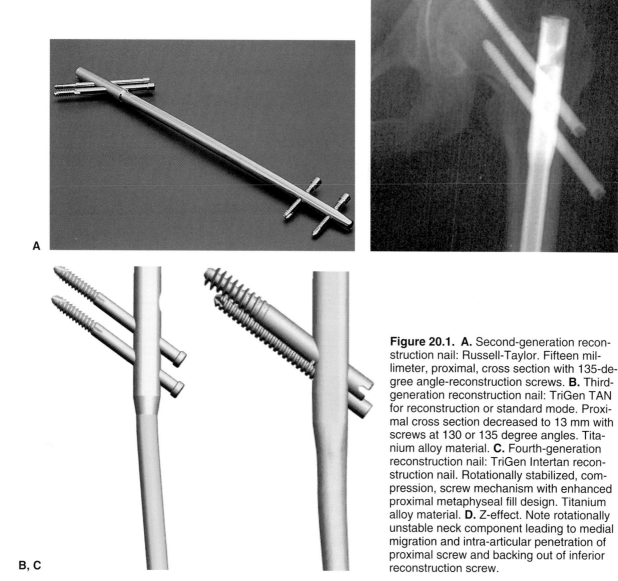

Figure 20.1. A. Second-generation reconstruction nail: Russell-Taylor. Fifteen millimeter, proximal, cross section with 135-degree angle-reconstruction screws. **B.** Third-generation reconstruction nail: TriGen TAN for reconstruction or standard mode. Proximal cross section decreased to 13 mm with screws at 130 or 135 degree angles. Titanium alloy material. **C.** Fourth-generation reconstruction nail: TriGen Intertan reconstruction nail. Rotationally stabilized, compression, screw mechanism with enhanced proximal metaphyseal fill design. Titanium alloy material. **D.** Z-effect. Note rotationally unstable neck component leading to medial migration and intra-articular penetration of proximal screw and backing out of inferior reconstruction screw.

selected, ipsilateral, femoral neck and shaft fractures. Segmental fractures of the femur, in which the proximal fracture extends into the upper femoral metaphysis, are also good indications for reconstruction nails. Reconstruction nail techniques are also used for deformity correction and stabilization of malunions, nonunions, and failed plate fixation of subtrochanteric femur fractures.

A reconstruction nail should not be considered the nail of first choice for diaphyseal fractures of the femur because of the complexity of targeting and placing screws in the femoral head. However, in pathologic fractures and osteoporotic femoral fractures, reconstructions nails are often recommended to prevent subsequent femoral-neck fractures. Reconstruction nailing is contraindicated in children with open, proximal, physeal plates.

Second-generation reconstruction nails with piriformis entry portals should be avoided in displaced femoral-neck fractures and four-part intertrochanteric fractures due to their propensity for fixation loss with rotation and varus loading. This so-called "Z-effect" results in loss of proximal screw fixation with intrusion of the cephalic screw into the joint space and subsequent backing out of the inferior head and neck screw (see Fig 20.1D).

In an effort to minimize fracture deformity and loss of reduction or fixation, third-generation reconstruction nails, such as the TriGen Trochanteric Reconstruction Nail (Smith & Nephew, Memphis, TN) for use with trochanteric entry portal, have been designed.

Russell and Taylor described a classification for subtrochanteric femur fractures based on the presence or absence of fracture involvement of the lesser trochanter/medial calcar and greater trochanter (piriformis fossa) (Fig. 20.2). Fractures involving the lesser trochanter but without extension into the greater trochanter (Russell-Taylor IB), are perhaps the best indication for a piriformis-portal reconstruction nail (Fig. 20.3). Historically, group 1 Russell-Taylor fractures were considered optimal for intramedullary nail techniques with piriformis portal approaches, and group 2 Russell-Taylor fractures were most often treated with plate and screw techniques. Now, almost 20 years since the first reconstruction nail was introduced, the techniques of nailing have undergone such significant improvements that many Russell-Taylor group II fractures can be addressed with an intramedullary hip screw (IMHS) or third-generation trochanteric reconstruction nails.

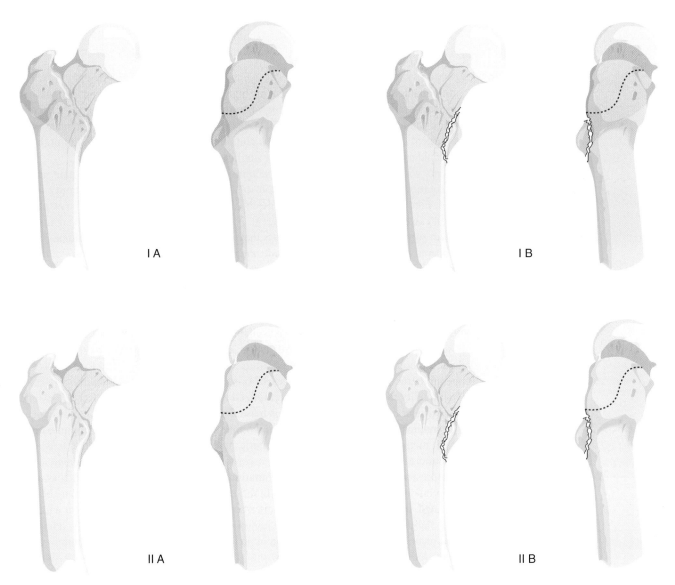

I A   I B

II A   II B

Figure 20.2. Diagram of components of Russell-Taylor IB subtrochanteric pattern with greater trochanter intact and lesser trochanteric fracture.

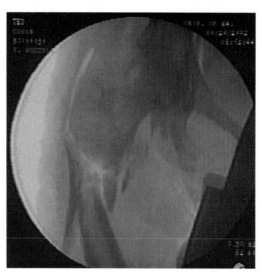

Figure 20.3. Subtrochanteric fracture with intact greater trochanter and fracture of the lesser trochanter.

PREOPERATIVE PLANNING

Subtrochanteric fractures often occur in high-energy trauma in younger patients and lower-energy falls in the elderly. With high-energy subtrochanteric fractures, associated injuries are found in up to 50% of patients. Open subtrochanteric fractures are rare, as are compartment syndromes, but both of these complications increase the morbidity of the injury if rapid assessment and treatment are not instituted.

Patients with subtrochanteric femur fractures invariably have hip or thigh pain, an external rotation deformity, and angulation in the proximal thigh if the extremity is not splinted. Frequently (depending on the mechanism and time elapsed since injury), ecchymosis and swelling of the thigh are apparent. Neurological or vascular injuries are uncommon with subtrochanteric fractures unless they are the result of penetrating trauma.

Preoperative radiographs should include anteroposterior (AP) and lateral views of the entire femur including the hip and knee. The radiographs should be carefully inspected to rule out intra-articular propagation of fractures or concomitant degenerative disease. In patients with complex fracture patterns or extensive comminution, radiographs of the uninjured femur may be used to estimate nail diameter and length. Radiographic templates for planning an operation in which reconstruction nails are available from most of the implant manufacturers.

If surgery is delayed, restoration of length at the fracture site must be obtained with skeletal traction before closed nailing. Failure to restore length may lead to excessive intraoperative traction and resultant pudendal or sciatic nerve injuries.

High-quality radiographs must be scrutinized to determine whether the fracture extends into the greater trochanter and piriformis fossa. With the widespread use of rapid CT scanners in trauma units, inclusion of proximal femur scans of patients with hip injuries is an excellent method for determining trochanteric involvement. In patients with extension of the fracture above the lesser trochanter, a coronal split in the proximal fragment is frequently present. This may result in comminution of the proximal fragment with loss of the entry portal during reaming and nailing. In these cases, reconstruction nailing may be contraindicated. If the fracture is nailed, an open reduction of the proximal fragment with provisional stabilization of the trochanteric region via reduction forceps is strongly advised.

Most reconstruction nails are now available in sizes ranging from 10 to 16 mm in diameter with lengths between 240 and 500 mm. The nails are right-sided and left-sided, to compensate for the anteversion of the femoral neck in relation to the shaft axis in the coronal plane. To facilitate screw entry into the femoral head, the proximal locking-screw holes are oriented anteriorly 8 to 15 degrees in relation to the distal screw holes. When using reconstruction nails, surgeons typically also use two sliding lag screws proximally to maximize purchase in the femoral head and to minimize rotation of the proximal fragment. These lag screws vary between 5 and 8 mm in diameter.

Precise knowledge of the neck-shaft angle of the screws in relation to the nail, spacing between the proximal screws, and their enclosed diameter are important in implant selection. Nail neck-shaft angles vary from 125 to 135 degrees. Higher-angle designs maximize sliding capabilities but are difficult to insert in hips with a relative varus position. Lower-angle designs have higher stresses and less sliding capability but are easier to insert. Most designs are moving toward a compromise of 130 degrees. In most designs, reconstruction nails have an effective spread between the two proximal screws of 11 to 21 mm. Measurement of the preoperative radiographs is necessary to understand the patient's neck-shaft angle and to plan screw spacing and final nail position. Reconstruction nails are typically enlarged proximally to compensate for the higher stresses in the subtrochanteric region. This must be recognized in preoperative planning because additional reaming of the proximal fragment is necessary in relation to the diaphyseal reaming. Distal interlocking screws are usually 4.5 to 6.4 mm in diameter and vary from full-threaded to partially threaded designs.

Appropriate nail length and diameter depend on the size of the patient and the extent of femoral comminution. To minimize the risk of nail failure, the largest implant suitable for the patient should be used such that excessive amounts of cortical bone are not removed. Even when interlocking is used, the nail should fill the medullary canal at the isthmus to minimize translational deformities. For maximal stability, static locking is recommended in acute fractures. The nail tip should extend into the distal femoral metaphysis to avoid stress risers in the diaphyseal area and facilitate distal interlocking.

SURGICAL TECHNIQUE

I currently use the minimally invasive nail-insertion technique (MINIT) in conjunction with the TriGen nail system with both piriformis and trochanteric nail designs. MINITs are designed to protect soft tissues and preserve bone; they are not just percutaneous techniques. They emphasize precise portal placement and preservation, as well as trajectory control, to avoid malreductions and damage to the proximal femur.

Patient Positioning

The supine position for patients is recommended for reconstruction nailing because it is familiar to most surgeons and allows adequate visualization of the hip in both AP and lateral views, which is critical to successful implantation of the device. The lateral decubitus position, which allows better visualization of the entry portal than does the supine position, is helpful with revision nailing, especially in patients who have experienced previously failed nailings due to incorrect entry portals. It is also helpful with reverse obliquity fractures because the lateral position reduces the medial translation of the shaft component.

With the patient in the supine position, the unaffected limb and trunk are abducted while the affected extremity is adducted. To reduce the distal shaft fragment to the proximal fragment, the affected hip is flexed 15 to 35 degrees with maintenance of the heel-to-toe relation (Fig. 20.4). Traction is applied after flexion positioning through the foot holder attached to the fracture table or through a skeletal pin in the distal femur or proximal tibia. Rotational alignment of the proximal fragment is determined with the image intensifier. The distal fragment is rotated to align with the proximal fragment (a true lateral of the knee is confirmed with overlapping of both femoral condyles). The surgeon must remember that femoral-neck anteversion in adults averages 15 degrees in Caucasian populations, but it may be up to 30 degrees in Asian populations. In the supine position, the leg will usually lie in 0 to 15 degrees of external rotation when the distal fragment is correctly rotated. In the lateral decubitus position, the foot and leg should be internally rotated approximately 15 degrees to match the tendency of the femoral head to orient toward the floor in a pendulum-like fashion.

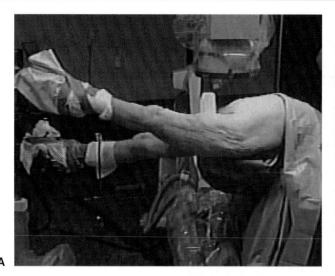

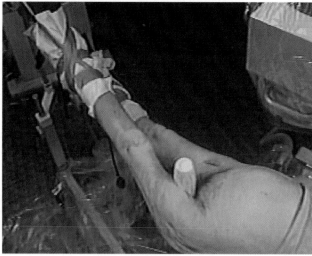

A   B

Figure 20.4. A,B. Supine position with affected extremity in foot traction, adducted for facilitation of entry portal, flexed approximately 15 degrees at the hip, and with knee extended.

Patient Preparation

The patient should be prepped and draped from the iliac crest, including the buttocks and lateral thigh, distally to below the knee. The image-intensifier arm should be covered with a sterile isolation drape. A first-generation cephalosporin (or substitute in the patient with penicillin allergies) is administered. Vancomycin or an aminoglycoside is added if the fracture is open. Usually cephazolin (1 g by IV) is continued for 24 to 48 hours after surgery in patients with closed fractures. Reconstruction nailing of open fractures should be performed only after appropriate debridement and irrigation of the open fracture wound. Delayed nailing is recommended for grade IIIB fractures. Reprepping and redraping of the extremity are required to minimize cross contamination at the nail insertion site.

Surgical Approach (Russell-Taylor Reconstruction Nail 1986)

A 10-cm, oblique, skin incision is made just proximal to the greater trochanter (Fig. 20.5). The fascia of the gluteus maximus is incised, and the muscle is opened in line with its fibers. The subfascial plane of the gluteus maximus is identified, and the trochanteric or piriformis fossa is palpated.

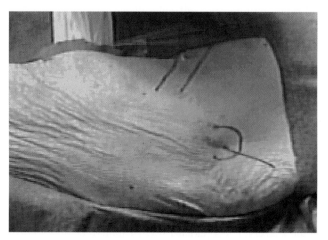

Figure 20.5. Skin incision.

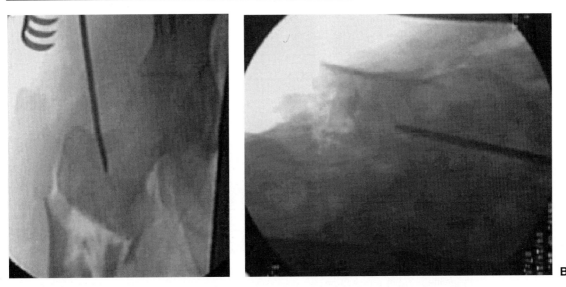

Figure 20.6. A,B. Tip-threaded guide pin inserted into piriformis fossa, centered on lateral view.

Femoral Preparation Establishing the correct portal for nail entry is crucial. Incorrect starting points can lead to angular deformities. For conventional, reamed, piriformis, intramedullary nailing, the correct starting point is in the piriformis fossa. However, for reconstruction nailing, the portal of entry is slightly anterior to the fossa. Because the femoral neck arises from the anterior portion of the proximal femur, moving the starting point 3 to 4 mm anteriorly facilitates proximal screw insertion. A 3.2-mm threaded guide pin is inserted at the entry site and confirmed by fluoroscopy to be in the midline of the femur in both AP and lateral views (Fig. 20.6). The entry portal is enlarged with the cannulated reamer over the guide pin (Fig. 20.7). If the proximal femoral fragment is flexed, externally rotated, and adducted to such a degree that the entry portal cannot be visualized, then the surgeon should manipulate the proximal fragment with a pointed reduction forceps or percutaneously inserted Schanz pin into a position such that the AP projections show a normalized fragment.

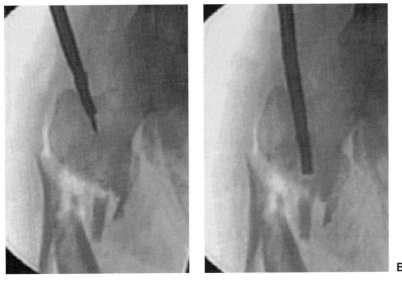

Figure 20.7. A,B. For correct entry portal, the guide wire should be overreamed with an 8-mm cannulated rigid reamer.

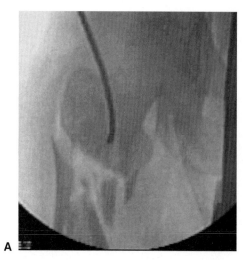
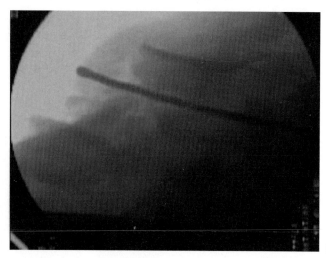

Figure 20.8. A,B. A 3.2-mm guide wire is inserted into fracture site. The tip of wire is bent to facilitate fracture reduction.

To assist in reduction of the shaft fracture, a ball-tipped guide wire is bent at its tip. The wire is advanced to the level of the fracture with the curve opposing the medial cortex. Its position is confirmed within the femur by AP and lateral views taken with the image intensifier (Fig. 20.8). The proximal fragment is reduced to the distal fragment manually or with an internal fracture-alignment device (Fig. 20.9). The guide wire is advanced into the center of the distal fragment until its tip reaches the distal femoral-epiphyseal scar. The position of the guide wire is verified within the femur by image intensification (Fig. 20.10).

The femur is reamed in 0.5-mm increments from 9.0 mm to at least 1.0 mm more than the proposed nail diameter. In patients with a large anterior bow of the femur, as seen on lateral radiographs, or fracture extension into the distal one fourth of the femur, the surgeon should overream 1.5 to 2.0 mm larger than the nail diameter. The final reamer diameter should be verified with the reamer template before nail selection and insertion. A nail that has a larger diameter than the last reamer used should never be inserted. The proximal 8 cm of the femur is reamed to 15 mm in diameter with progressive reamers (starting with a 9-mm reamer) to accommodate the enlarged proximal end of most reconstruction nails (Fig. 20.11). Because the proximal fragment must be reamed substantially, the surgeon must avoid the destruction of the proximal entry portal that can be caused by eccentric reaming, which usually occurs during insertion of the reamer and during its extraction. To avoid this complication, a slotted hammer or other instrument to direct a medial force on the reamer shaft should be used during insertion and extraction (Fig. 20.12).

Verification of the proper nail length may be determined by two separate methods: the guide-wire method or the nail-length gauge. With either method, residual distraction at the fracture site must be eliminated. In the guide-wire method, the distal end of the guide wire is placed between the proximal pole of the patella and the distal femoral-epiphyseal scar, while a second guide wire is overlapped to the portion of the reduction guide wire extending proximally from the femoral entry portal. To determine nail length, the length (in mm) of the overlapped guide wires is subtracted from 900 mm. In another alternative, a nail-length ruler is placed on the skin of the anterior thigh (unaffected femur preoperatively; affected femur intraoperatively) with its distal end between the proximal pole of the patella and the distal femoral-epiphyseal scar. The c-arm is moved to the proximal end of the femur, and the correct nail length is read directly from the stamped measurements on the nail-length ruler.

The medullary exchange tube is placed over the guide wire to maintain fracture reduction while the ball-tip guide wire is replaced with a nail-driving wire (without ball tip). The medullary exchange tube is removed. With the Russell-Taylor system, the reaming guide rod and nail driving rods are identical, so placement of the medullary exchange tube is unnecessary.

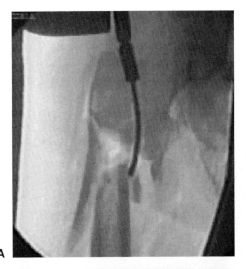

A

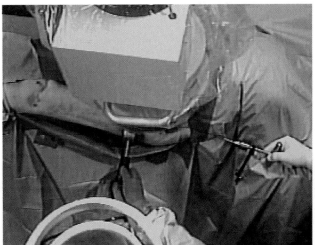

B

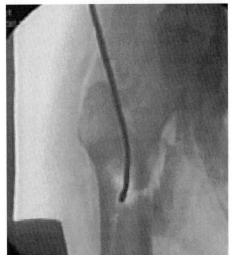

C

Figure 20.9. A–C. Combination of external force, internal guide, and adjustment of fracture table into abduction to accomplish fracture reduction.

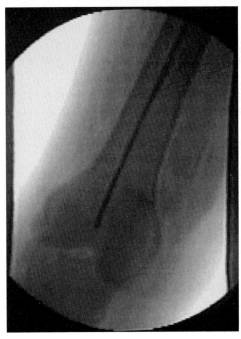

Figure 20.10. Guide wire inserted to knee for reaming and length determination of nail.

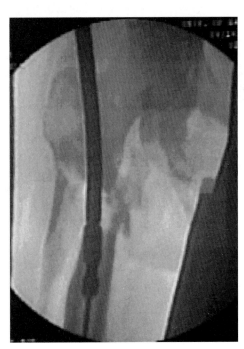

Figure 20.11. Progressive flexible reamers in 0.5-mm increments with proximal 8- to 9- mm overreaming for reconstruction-nail proximal expansion.

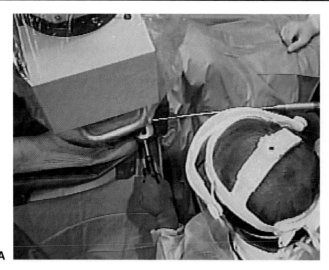
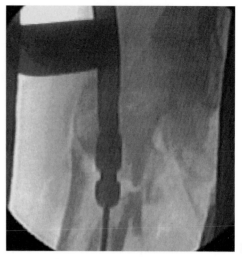

A   B

Figure 20.12. A,B. Slotted hammer is used to insert a medial force on the reamer shaft in which damage to the greater trochanter is avoided during reamer head insertion and extraction.

Nail Insertion The appropriate nail is attached to the proximal driving/proximal drill guide. When assembled properly, the nail will have an anterior bow, and the orientation of the proximal drill guide points laterally.

Either the sliding hammer or supine driver is assembled to the proximal drill guide, and the nail is inserted over the guide wire. The proximal drill guide acts as a handle to control rotation and aid in insertion of the nail (Fig. 20.13). The surgeon must not strike the proximal drill guide directly, because this may deform the targeting device and compromise proximal interlocking. Once the nail has been inserted, the proximal targeting device should be retightened. The nail is driven under radiographic control to within 1 to 2 cm of its anticipated depth.

The anatomy of the proximal femur varies from person to person, so a reconstruction nail is inserted to the point where the upper end of the nail will accommodate two proximal screws into the femoral head. Frequently, minor adjustments in nail position, either proximal or distal, are necessary to line up the holes in the nail within the femoral head and neck. Nail insertion and screw placement can be initially performed with the nail-length ruler and a radiopaque ruler or guide. Its outline is drawn with a skin marker over the femoral head and neck (Figs. 20.14 and 20.15). With the nail nearly fully seated, the inferior drill sleeves are placed into the proximal drill guide to extrapolate the eventual location of the inferior screw.

The c-arm is positioned to obtain a true lateral view of the femoral head and neck. The proximal targeting guide is aligned with the c-arm axis by rotating the proximal drill guide

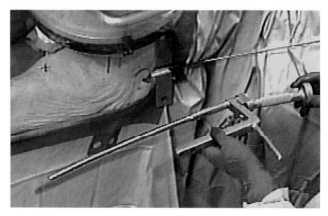

Figure 20.13. Nail assembly with proximal drill guide.

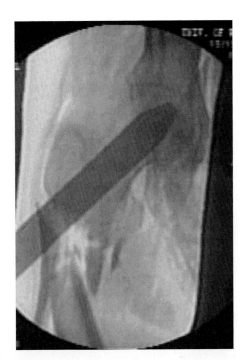

Figure 20.14. Overlay ruler is used to access anticipated final screw-insertion zone.

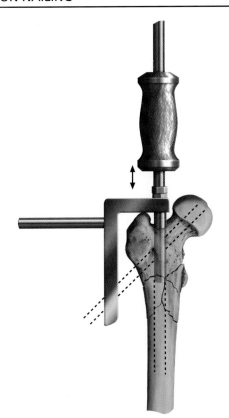

Figure 20.15. Adjust nail-insertion depth for centering of proximal locking screws.

in the transverse plane (Fig. 20.16). If the proximal targeting device is radiopaque, the guide is centralized with respect to the femoral head, bisecting the femoral head in the coronal plane as seen on the true, lateral, c-arm view. The posterior and anterior portion of the femoral head must be seen in relation to the proximal drill guide for the surgeon to confirm that the screws will be contained within the femoral head (Fig. 20.17). Further verification of the proximal guide wires, drill bits, and locking screws may be obtained with oblique c-arm views. With a skin marker, a horizontal line is drawn on the lateral thigh as a reference to correct rotation of the proximal drill guide (Fig. 20.18). The traction is released, and the nail is seated. The intramedullary guide wire is removed from the femur.

Interlocking Screw Technique

Proximal interlocking involves insertion of large cancellous screws. For maximal stability, the proximal interlocking screws should reach the dense subchondral bone of the femoral head. The skin and fascia are incised through the inferior hole of the proximal drill guide. The stacked drill sleeves are inserted through the inferior hole and pushed to bone. The appropriate guide pin is inserted through the drill sleeve and advanced into the femoral head at least 4 mm superior to the calcar and within 5 mm of the subchondral bone of the femoral head. The position of the guide pin within the head is confirmed with AP and oblique lateral views with the c-arm (Fig. 20.19).

If on the true lateral view the guide pin is obstructed by the proximal drill guide but the femoral head is visible anteriorly and posteriorly, then central placement of the pin can be inferred. For further confirmation, the c-arm can be rotated anteriorly and posteriorly from the true lateral position. The second guide pin is placed in the superior hole of the nail, and its location within the femoral head is confirmed with the c-arm. The skin and fascia are incised through the superior hole of the proximal drill guide, and the stacked drill sleeves are inserted

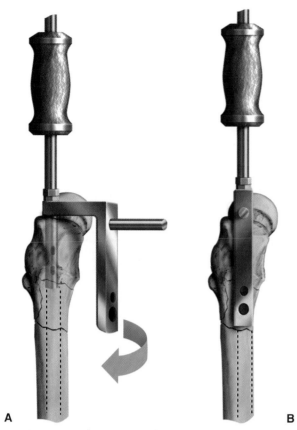

A   B

Figure 20.16. A,B. Rotation of proximal drill guide to center guide for correct anteversion of screws into femoral head; drill guide should bisect the femoral head on the true lateral radiographic view.

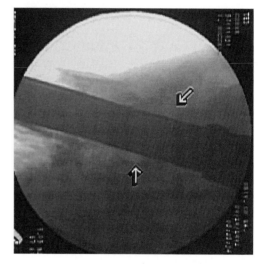

Figure 20.17. Lateral fluoroscopic view with bisection of femoral head through use of drill guide for correct screw position.

through the superior hole. The drill sleeves are pushed to bone. The second proximal guide pin is inserted through the drill sleeve and advanced into the femoral head (Fig. 20.20).

The inferior guide pin and inner drill sleeves are removed if the screw is noncannulated. This leaves a pilot hole to center the large step drill. The appropriate step drill is inserted through the remaining drill sleeve into the femoral head to within 5 mm of subchondral

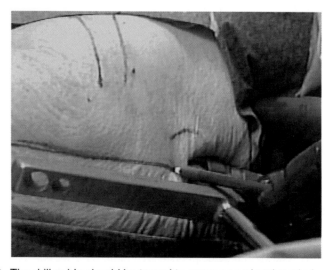

Figure 20.18. The drill guide should be traced to serve as a visual reminder of correct anteversion.

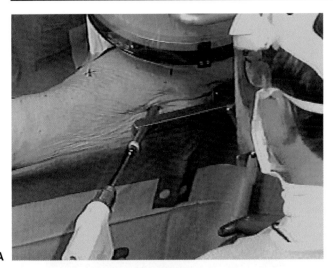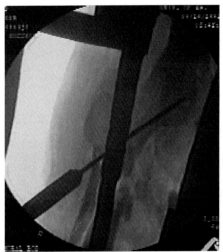

A   B

Figure 20.19. A,B. Inferior guide wire is inserted, and correct placement to within 5-mm of subchondral bone and correct neck-shaft alignment are confirmed.

bone. The surgeon should verify that the drill sleeves are against bone (Fig. 20.21). Screw-length measurement is determined with calibrated drill bits (Fig. 20.22). In another method, length can be assessed with the use of a depth gauge. The appropriate lag screw is inserted through the drill sleeve into the femoral head (Fig. 20.23). To maximize purchase, the threads of the screws must lie totally within the femoral head and not in the femoral neck. The remaining drill sleeves are removed.

The second proximal screw is inserted in a fashion similar to the insertion of the first screw: With the superior hole of the drill guide, a guide pin, if not already in place, is advanced to within 5 mm of subchondral bone. The guide pin and appropriate drill sheaths for noncannulated screws are removed. The step drill is inserted through the drill sleeve into the femoral head to within 5 mm of the subchondral bone. The surgeon should verify that the drill sleeve is against bone. The screw length is determined at this point through use of the calibrated drills or by a depth gauge. The step drill is removed. Tapping is usually recommended, but in dense bone in young patients, it is required (Fig. 20.24). The appropriately sized proximal screw is inserted into the femoral head. The

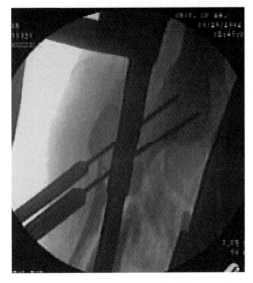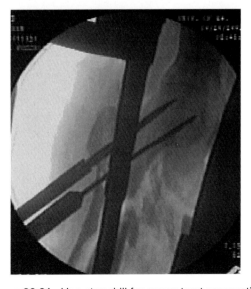

Figure 20.20. Insert second guide wire for centering and stability of proximal guide.

Figure 20.21. Use step drill for screw-tract preparation.

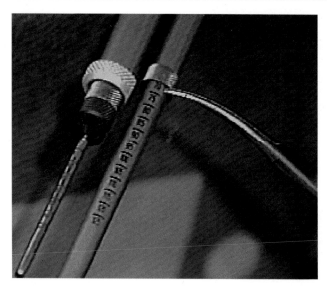

Figure 20.22. Correct screw-length selection is determined from calibrated step drill.

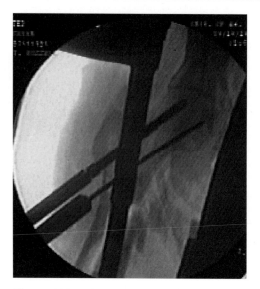

Figure 20.23. Proximal lag screw is inserted.

drill sleeve is removed, and with AP, lateral, and oblique views, the surgeon confirms containment of both screws in the femoral head (Fig. 20.25). For maximal stability, all threads of the proximal locking screws should be within the femoral head. To avoid distraction, screw threads must not be passed across any fracture line. Proximal interlocking is now complete. Insertion of a distal locking screw improves stability and fatigue life of the construct in comminuted fractures, and it decreases the incidence of shortening and malrotation. I prefer a freehand technique or use a radiolucent drill guide for distal interlocking-screw placement (Fig. 20.26).

The proximal drill guide is removed from the nail. The entire femur is scanned with the c-arm to confirm correct screw placement, adequacy of reduction, stability at fracture site, and proper nail length. The wounds are irrigated and closed in layers (fascia, subcutaneous, and skin) in the standard fashion. Sterile dressings are applied. If skeletal traction was used, the traction pin is removed, and the wounds are covered with sterile dressings.

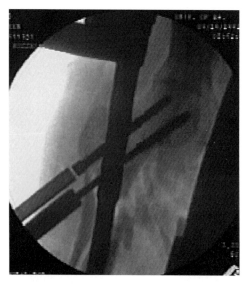

Figure 20.24. Second guide wire is removed and step drill is used for drilling second screw; tapping is frequently required in dense bone.

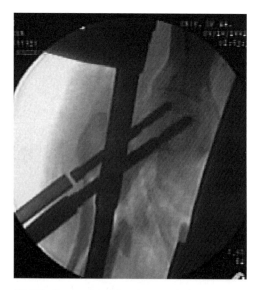

Figure 20.25. Second proximal screw is inserted, and seating is confirmed radiographically.

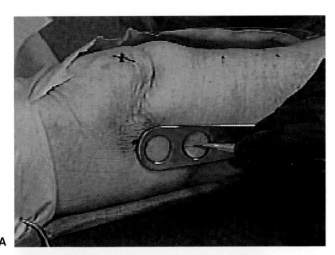

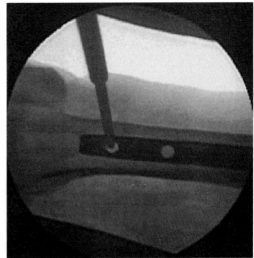

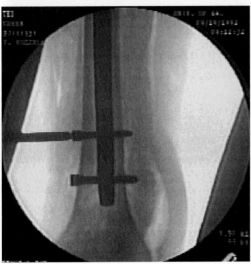

Figure 20.26. A–C. Freehand technique: hole is located with external marker and a stab incision is made over the hole axis; the trocar is inserted to dimple bone; drilling is done for bicortical fixation; screws are inserted.

MINIMALLY INVASIVE NAIL-INSERTION TECHNIQUE WITH THE TRIGEN TROCHANTERIC ANTEGRADE NAIL

Surgical Approach

MINIT allows for less soft-tissue damage and less tissue and bone loss. Pepper et al developed a third-generation nail insertion technique that facilitates either piriformis or trochanteric portal-entry selection. It also allows faster fracture reduction with less chance of damage to the proximal femoral-bone stock when a closed reaming system is used.

The patient is placed supine or lateral with the unaffected limb extended below the affected limb and trunk (Fig. 20.27A,B). The affected limb is adducted 0 to 5 degrees because relatively less adduction is required for a trochanteric portal. The affected hip is flexed 15 to 40 degrees to facilitate the reduction of the distal fragment to the proximal fragment. Traction is applied through a skeletal pin or through the foot with the fracture-table foot holder. The surgeon adjusts the affected limb for length and rotation by comparing it with the unaffected limb. The surgeon further checks rotation by rotating the c-arm to align the femoral neck in anteversion and then making the appropriate correction by the foot, usually 0 to 15 degrees of external rotation.

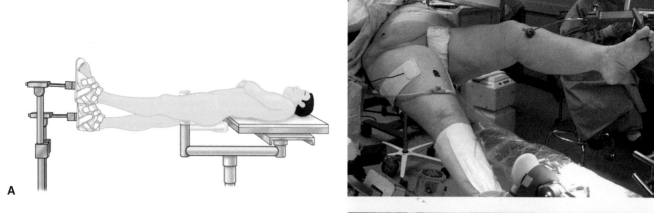

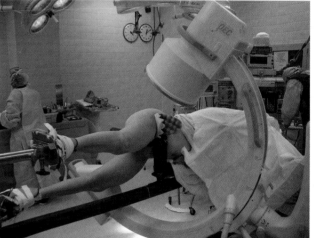

Figure 20.27. Supine position with both feet in traction. **A,B.** Note increased flexion and slight external rotation to better expose subtrochanteric fracture for trochanteric nail portal and **(C)** lateral decubitus positioning.

Lateral decubitus positioning may also be used with the fracture table. It is used when the change of position of the femoral head causes the leg to be internally rotated 10 to 15 degrees (see Fig. 20.27C). The rotation is best checked by visualizing the femoral anteversion proximally and matching it with correct rotation at the knee. The greater trochanter is palpated. Fracture reduction is confirmed possible before skin incision and after c-arm views of good quality are obtained. A 2.5-cm incision is made 3 cm proximal to the greater trochanter in line with the femoral shaft. The incision should be carried through the fascia.

Entry Portal Preparation

To assemble the entry tool and honeycomb insert, the surgeon tightens the entry reamer connector onto the 14.0-mm channel reamer and inserts the 12.5-mm entry reamer until it "clicks" into the assembly. Then, power is applied to the 12.5-mm entry reamer to ream the proximal section of the femur through the entry tool. The entry tool–honeycomb assembly is oriented so that the superior side of the bevel is medial. (This requires setting the entry tool indicator to "R" for a left nail and to "L" for a right nail, which is opposite to the standard femoral antegrade nail [FAN] technique and advanced until it rests against the lateral aspect of the greater trochanter.) Suction is attached to the entry tool to assist in blood evacuation and to minimize blood aerosolization to which the operative team is subjected (Fig. 20.28). The 3.2-mm tip-threaded guide wire is inserted through the honeycomb and advanced 1 cm into the cortex at the tip of the greater trochanter, as seen on the AP view, and in line with the center of the femoral canal as visualized on the lateral view (Fig. 20.29A). With image guidance, a second guide wire may be used to refine the starting portal exactly.

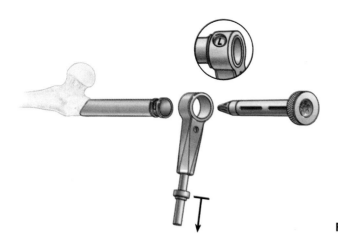

Figure 20.28. Entry portal tool assembly.

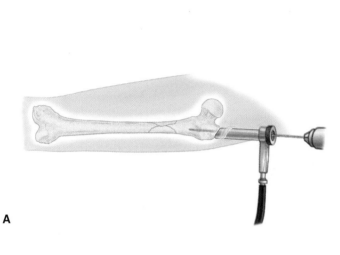

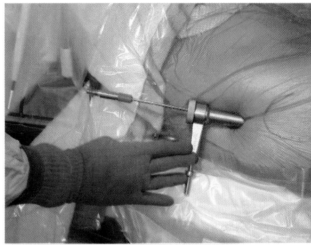

A

B

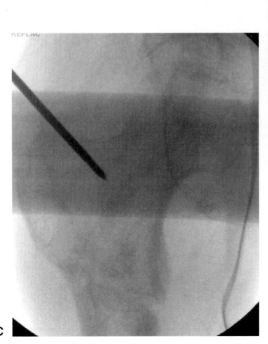

C

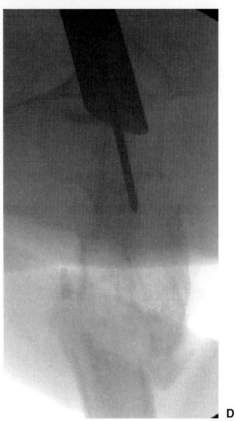

D

Figure 20.29. Guide wire is inserted through entry portal tool. **A.** Guide wire insertion schematic. **B.** Position of guide wire. **C.** Radiographic control ape. **D.** Radiographic control lateral.

Once proper placement of the guide wire has been established, the honeycomb insert should be removed (see Fig. 20.29A–D). The channel reamer assembly is introduced over the tip-threaded guide wire and advanced 1 to 2 cm into bone. The reamer assembly is then manipulated under image guidance until the shaft axis and intended path of the reamer form an angle of approximately 5 degrees in the AP view and is in line in the ML view. The tip of the reamer should be directed to a point just inferior to the normal location of the lesser trochanter as seen on the AP view. Once the correct orientation is obtained, the reamer assembly is advanced to full depth so that it contacts the proximal end of the entry portal tool (Fig. 20.30). This reamer assembly enlarges the proximal femur 1.0 mm over the diameter of the nail head to 14.0 mm. The 12.5-mm entry reamer and guide wire are removed, but the entry tool and 14.0-mm channel reamer is kept in place.

Fracture Reduction Technique

The T handle is snapped onto the reducer, and the reducer is placed through the entry tool and 14.0-mm channel reamer to reduce the fracture. The reducer is advanced down the medullary canal to the fracture site and then the proximal fragment is manipulated with the

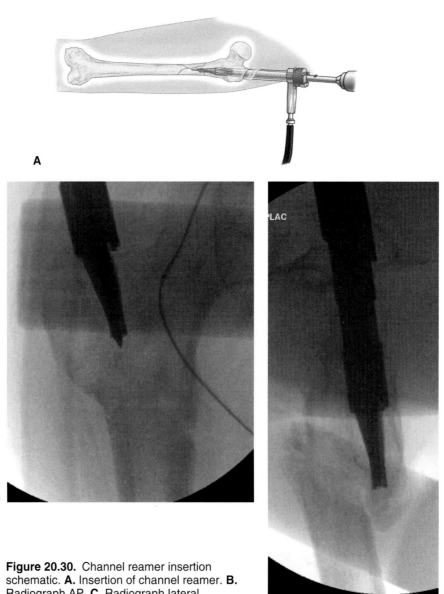

Figure 20.30. Channel reamer insertion schematic. **A.** Insertion of channel reamer. **B.** Radiograph AP. **C.** Radiograph lateral.

entry portal tool and reducer until it is aligned with the distal-fragment medullary canal. The tip of the reducer is rotated into the distal medullary canal to capture the distal fragment (Figs. 20.31 and 20.32). The 3.0-mm ball-tipped guide rod is inserted through the reducer into the distal femur in the region of the old physeal scar. The reducer is rotated to center the guide wire distally in the femur as seen on AP and lateral views.

Medullary Canal Preparation

Canal preparation is surgeon selected depending on the patient requirements and injury. If reaming is planned, progressive reamers should be used through the entry tool. Unreamed nails are selected based on preoperative planning but should be of sufficient size to provide translational fill of the intramedullary canal in the mid diaphysis. Once the guide rod is in place, the reducer is removed, but the surgeon should leave the 14.0-mm channel reamer in place. The channel reamer protects the proximal portal from eccentric reaming, which could lead to a varus reduction (Figs. 20.33 and 20.34). The femoral shaft should be sequentially reamed, through the 14.0-mm channel reamer, to 1.0 mm or more above the chosen nail diameter. For more curved femoral shafts, 1.5 to 2.0 mm of reaming greater than the nail diameter may be required to avoid nail incarceration. In patients who have long femurs, the flex reamer extender may be added to extend the shaft of the flexible reamer for very distal fractures or nails longer than 42 cm.

For 13-mm nails, the 14-mm channel reamer must be removed before the diaphysis is reamed with the 13.5- and 14.0-mm reamer diameters. Usually a 13-mm nail will be reamed at the diaphysis to 14 mm. However, the reamer should be inserted into the femur before reaming is started, and to avoid portal damage, the surgeon should stop reaming before final extraction of the reamer from the medullary canal.

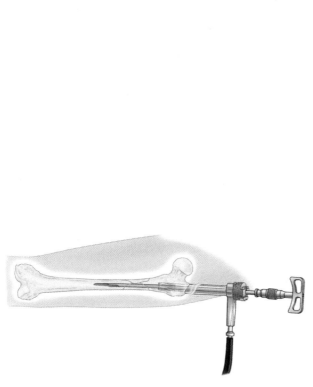

Figure 20.31. Reducer schematic.

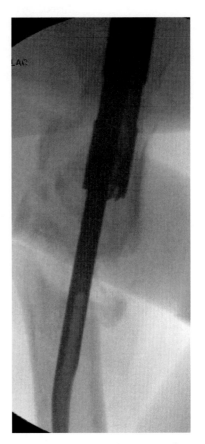

Figure 20.32. Reducer insertion across fracture site.

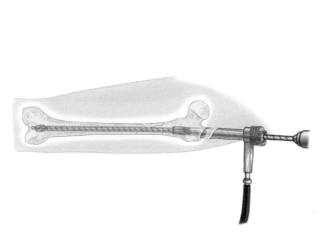

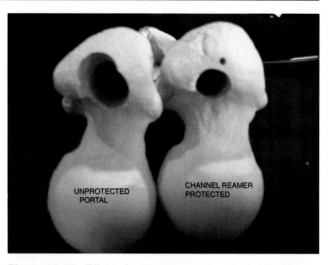

Figure 20.33. Reamer canal preparation through channel reamer to protect the trochanteric region from eccentric reaming.

Figure 20.34. Effect of eccentric reaming on portal with second-generation nail instrumentation with unprotected reaming (*left*) versus minimally invasive channel reamer technique (*right*).

Nail Selection

Nail diameter is determined from image intensifying or templating. A nail that has a larger diameter than the last reamer used should never be inserted. With the distal tip of the guide rod at the desired level of the distal femur, the nail length is measured by positioning the open end of the ruler over the exposed end of the guide rod and pushing the end down to the level of bone through the 14-mm channel reamer. The position of the ruler should be confirmed on the image intensifier. The tip of the ruler should line up with the final position of the proximal end of the nail. This may be predetermined by preoperative templating.

In general, 5 to 15 mm of countersinking below the tip of the greater trochanter allows optimal screw positioning. However, successful positioning also depends on the femoral neck-shaft angle and the screw-nail angle, usually a 130 or 135 degree nail. The nail length is read from the calibrations exposed at the other end of the ruler. The guide rod is left in place for placement of the nail. Exchange of the ball-tipped guide rod is not necessary.

Drill Guide Assembly

The guide bolt is inserted into the drill guide, and use the guide bolt wrench is used to secure the bolt to the nail. The impactor is screwed onto the top of the drill guide to drive the nail into the medullary canal (Fig. 20.35A). The skin protector is inserted into the incision parallel to the entry reamer tool. The entry reamer tool and 14-mm channel reamer are removed. The skin protector will assist in maintaining control of the surrounding tissues and provide continued access to the bone. The nail is advanced over the guide rod with the nail rotated 90 degrees with the proximal guide aimed anteriorly, and the nail is inserted carefully past the fracture; the nail is rotated into correct rotational alignment after it is approximately 50% inserted (see Fig. 20.35B,C). This insertion technique minimizes insertion forces required for nail insertion from the trochanteric portal. The guide rod is removed after the nail is inserted to within 2 cm of the final position of the nail tip and before the locking screws are inserted.

Proximal Interlocking for Reconstruction Mode

For reconstruction proximal locking in a cephalomedullary technique, only one additional instrument is attached to convert the nail into a cephalomedullary construct. This drop is either a 135 or 130 degree guide and may be added after the nail is inserted, or if a

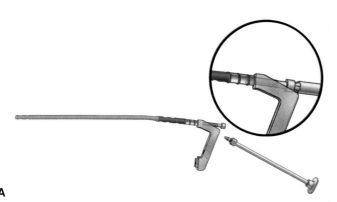

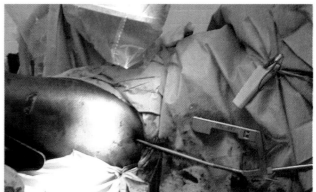

A

B

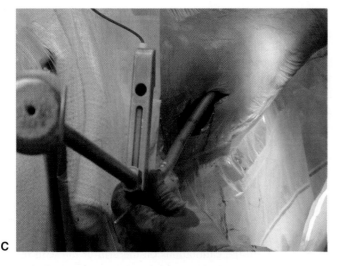

C

Figure 20.35. Nail insertion. **A.** Assembly of nail for insertion. **B,C.** Nail is inserted and internally rotated 90 degrees until 50% of nail is inserted. It is then rotated into final position.

reconstruction nail is planned, before nail insertion. Screws (6.4 mm) (blue) screws are used to lock the 10-mm, 11.5-mm, and 13-mm diameter trochanteric antegrade nails (TAN) implants proximally in the recon mode. The guide bolt is inserted into the drill guide and the guide bolt wrench is used to secure the bolt to the nail. The hip guide is connected to the drill guide. The guide is keyed so that it will only fit one way. The knurled knob is tightened by hand until snug. The end of the guide bolt wrench is used to finish tightening the guide in place (Fig. 20.36).

The alignment of the guide to the screw holes should be checked by the surgeon passing the medium screwdriver through the gold, outer, drill sleeve up into the holes of the nail. The impactor should be screwed onto the top of the drill guide to drive the nail into the medullary canal. The skin protector is inserted in the incision parallel to the entry reamer tool. The entry reamer tool and channel reamer are removed. The skin protector will assist

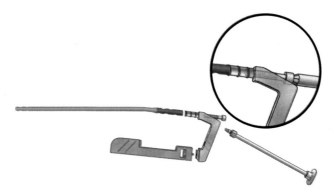

Figure 20.36. Proximal locking recon mode. Recon drop assembly.

in maintaining control of the surrounding tissues and provide continued access to the bone. The nail is advanced over the guide rod and carefully past the fracture. The guide rod is removed after the nail is inserted and before the locking screws are inserted.

Two aspects of screw placement into the femoral head must be noted before drilling into the femoral head: anteversion alignment and depth of nail insertion. To begin, the surgeon rotates the c-arm proximally until a true lateral of the hip is visualized; this gives the correct axis of alignment for anteversion. The handle of the nail guide is rotated until it bisects the femoral head in the lateral view. In this position, the nail and guide are overlaid on the center of the femoral head such that femoral head is visualized anteriorly and posteriorly. This position is marked with a skin marker on the leg parallel to the driving handle. Next, the c-arm is rotated into an AP view through the use of the calibrated notches on the proximal attachment of the nail, which is visualized radiographically.

Preoperative planning with template overlays will aid in determining the depth of nail insertion will center both screws within the femoral head. Usually, the nail will be countersunk 5 to 15 mm below the tip of the greater trochanter. As a rule, the inferior drill is placed first, then the most proximal drill is placed (Fig. 20.37). These screws are angled at 130 or 135 degree in relation to the shaft. If both screws will not seat within the femoral head, too much varus positioning of the proximal fragment has probably occurred, or the proximal nail entry portal is too lateral. With the trochanteric portal, if the varus deformity originates medial to the nail insertion, traction and adduction may correct the varus. An incision is made at the entry holes of the proximal screw sleeves, and the two puncture wounds are connected; a 2.5-cm incision will accommodate the insertion of both screws. The silver, inner, drill sleeve is inserted into the gold, outer, drill sleeve and they are pushed to bone. The 4.0-mm drill bit is inserted into the silver, inner, drill sleeve and power is conducted through the miniconnector.

The surgeon drills into the femoral neck and head to the desired depth and position. The femoral neck is drilled with the 6.4-mm step drill to slightly less than the depth desired. The alignment is checked in the AP view and 15-degree lateral views again before the 6.4-mm drill is removed. The 6.4-mm tap should be used in very dense bone. The depth for the screw length is measured from the calibrations on the drill or tap with respect to the gold, outer, drill sleeve. The appropriate-length 6.4-mm screw is attached to the medium screwdriver. The screwdriver T handle is attached and the captured screw is inserted into the inferior proximal hole. Once the first screw is inserted, the screwdriver should not be disassembled.

The procedure is repeated for the most proximal screw with the long screwdriver (Fig. 20.38). When the proximal screws are tightened for the last time and the screwdriver de-

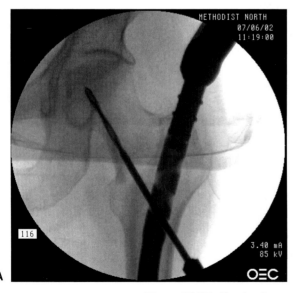
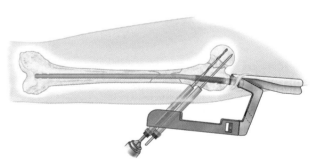

A   B

Figure 20.37. Proximal screw preparation. **A.** Proximal drilling through blue recon drop. **B.** Second drill insertion.

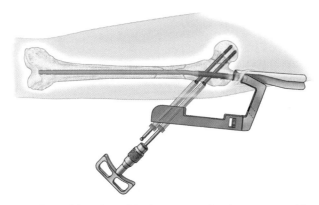

Figure 20.38. Final tightening of both compression lag screws with traction off.

tached from the screws, proximal locking is complete. Distal locking is performed with standard freehand technique. Two distal locking screws are preferred for very comminuted fractures and long spiral-fracture components into the diaphysis. The freehand technique is used with the c-arm placed medial to the patient, allowing for proper image of the femur (Fig. 20.39). Five mm (gold) screws are used to distal lock 10-mm, 11.5-mm, and 13-mm diameter TAN Implants.

Wound Closure

Once implant insertion is complete, the proximal guide is removed with the guide bolt wrench; the wounds are irrigated and closed in a standard fashion. Rotation and final check of length are performed before the patient is transferred off the operative field.

POSTOPERATIVE MANAGEMENT

In the absence of associated injuries, patients are mobilized from the bed to chair and gait trained with a walker or crutches on the first or second postoperative day. Thromboembolic prophylaxis is usually begun 12 hours after surgery with a low-molecular-weight heparin and continued for 7 to 14 days, depending on the patient's mobility. Weight bearing is restricted to 10 to 15 kg on the affected extremity in comminuted fractures. If cortical contact is restored and bone quality is good, weight bearing is permitted as tolerated with crutches or walker. Range-of-motion exercises and straight-leg lifts are started in the first week. Patients are usually discharged to home on the third or fourth postoperative day, when they demonstrate lower-extremity control sufficient for household ambulation with crutches or a walker.

Patients are checked at 3- to 4-week intervals, and radiographs are obtained at each visit. When callus is detected (usually at 4 to 8 weeks), progressive weight bearing is allowed.

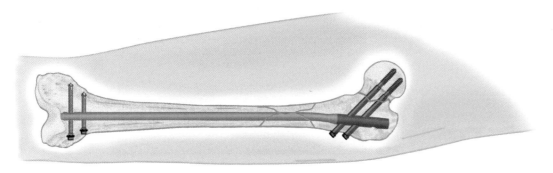

Figure 20.39. Distal interlocking with freehand technique for static construct.

Patients must demonstrate full weight bearing on the affected leg for 60 seconds before crutches are discontinued and have equal abductor strength with standing lateral leg lifts without a Trendelenberg sign. Frequently, the patients have rehabilitated the fractured side but have neglected the opposite side, resulting in a Trendelenberg gait without ambulatory support. A progressive, resistance, exercise program is prescribed, and swimming or stationary bicycling is recommended.

Implant removal is not considered until AP and lateral radiographs shows mature radiographic callus bridging of the fracture site: rarely before 1 year. A general anesthetic is required and usually a 24-hour hospitalization. Patients use crutches after implant removal until their gait returns to the pre-implant–removal status. After implant removal, contact sports are avoided for 3 months.

With isolated fractures, most patients attain community-ambulation status within 6 to 8 weeks with crutches, begin driving motor vehicles at 8 to 16 weeks, and are full weight bearing by 4 to 6 months after injury. Patients can expect functional recovery sufficient to return to their previous occupations in most cases. Union rates after closed reconstruction nailing are 95% to 100% in acute subtrochanteric fractures uncomplicated by other injuries.

There is no current-outcomes research on differing treatments for subtrochanteric femur fractures. As with most hip fractures, avoidance of varus and significant leg-length discrepancies are tantamount to a good result for the patient. Most patients return to their previous occupations and recreational activities if functional restoration is achieved. Most persisting problems are related to associated knee or neurological injuries. Sanders et al proposed a rating system for subtrochanteric fractures, but no comparative series are yet available with this outcome measure.

COMPLICATIONS

Malreduction

Entry-portal creation for the reconstruction nail is significantly more difficult than for standard femoral nailing. When a piriformis portal nail is used, eccentric, lateral, portal placement or portal damage can result in comminution of the medial cortex and varus displacement of the hip with nail insertion (Fig. 20.40). After subtrochanteric fractures, strong

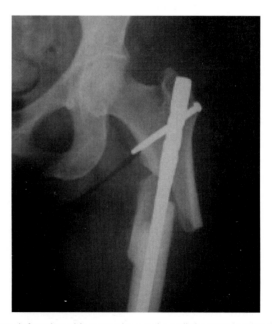

Figure 20.40. Varus deformity with nonunion and medial comminution from eccentric lateral portal with piriformis design nail.

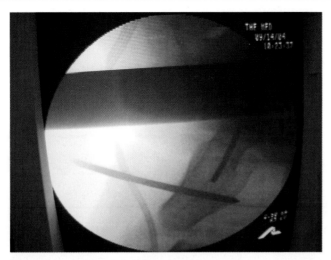

Figure 20.41. Use of Schanz pin inserted percutaneously to facilitate reduction of the proximal fragment.

muscle pull leads to flexion, external rotation, and varus positioning of the proximal fragment. This increases the difficulty in c-arm visualization of the entry portal. The problem may be solved by internally rotating the leg and attempting a closed reduction of the hip or by inserting a pin percutaneously into the trochanteric mass and using this as a joystick to rotate the proximal femur into a more anatomically recognizable position (Fig. 20.41).

If fracture extension or comminution is present medially in obese patients, a straight nail driver will tend to offset the nail laterally and force the hip into varus. This occurs because of driver pressure on the lateral ilium. To restore normal hip alignment, one may use an offset driver and apply pressure medially through the driver the nail is inserted to the correct depth. In an alternative method, nailing in the lateral decubitus position may decrease the tendency toward varus mal-alignment.

Ricci et al reported a 30% malunion rate with proximal fractures with first- and second-generation antegrade-nailing techniques in a level-one trauma center with trauma, orthopedic, staff surgeons. Russell and Taylor studied the problem of malunions and loss of reduction with intramedullary nailing of subtrochanteric fractures. The technical complications relate to nail selection and surgical technique. First, with Russell-Taylor 1B, 2A, and 2B fracture patterns, a cephalomedullary interlocking nail must be used instead of a centromedullary interlocking construct. If fracture lines extend into the medial calcar region or trochanteric area, a single, diagonal, locking screw will not have sufficient stability (Fig. 20.42).

The surgical technique is the second area of difficulty. The problems encountered result from combinations of four errors: incorrect starting point, loss of trajectory control of the reamers in the proximal femur, failure to obtain reduction of the fracture prior to nail insertion, and entry portal damage during fracture reduction and medullary canal preparation.

First, with regard to the correct starting portal, the piriformis portal is very difficult to obtain with patient supine positioning, and the deformity of the subtrochanteric fracture makes the piriformis region very difficult to identify with the image intensifier. Frequently, the surgeon compromises the portal by starting too posterior or too anterior and too far lateral for a conventional piriformis-design nail. In an attempt to reach the medial side of the trochanter, the entry portal is damaged.

Second, the entry site alone does not control the fracture reduction; rather it is the trajectory of the cutting tools that facilitates the reduction of the proximal fragment. If the trajectory is anterior to posterior in the proximal femur, it will induce a varus reduction of the hip upon nail insertion (Fig. 20.43). The MINIT allows precise machining of the proximal fragment to optimize reduction with nail insertion. The channel reamer then protects the portal during fracture reduction and diaphyseal reaming. This precise trajec-

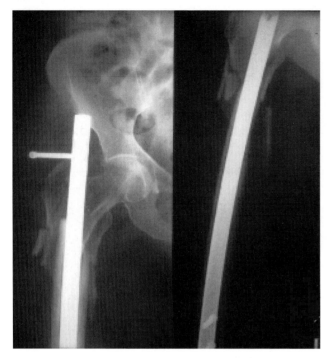

Figure 20.42. Russell-Taylor 1B fracture pattern with failed standard-screw construct in proximal femur. A reconstruction nail construct is recommended for Russell-Taylor IB fractures.

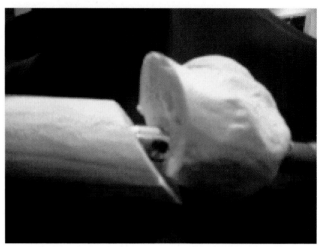

Figure 20.43. Model of varus and flexion deformity of the proximal femur with trajectory of proximal fragment directed posteriorly and lateral placement of the entry portal.

tory control coupled with the protection of the portal with the channel reamer optimizes the fracture reduction made via nail insertion (Fig. 20.44). The development of nails with smaller proximal geometries that make them better suited for a trochanteric portal than the original Russell-Taylor nail, allows nail insertion in between the gluteus minimus and short external rotators such that the MINIT spares the important tendon insertion. In addition, use of these optimized nails means that the trochanteric portal can be

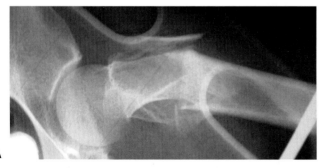
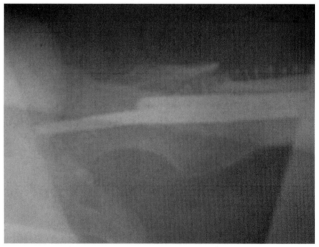

A   B

Figure 20.44. A. Lateral radiograph of subtrochanteric fracture with flexion deformity of proximal femur. **B.** Correction of deformity with channel reamer technique creating an anterior trajectory along anterior cortical wall; note resultant correction of deformity with nail placement.

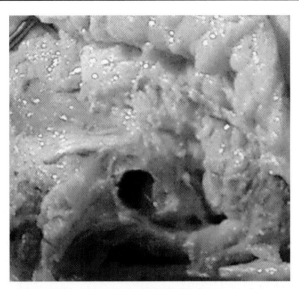

Figure 20.45. New trochanteric portal with MINIT. Placement is just medial to the gluteus medius tendon on the left and anterior to the piriformis tendon insertion inferiorly.

obtained without the excessive varus positioning required with the piriformis technique (Fig. 20.45).

Compared to the data available in the literature, I have observed a significantly decreased malunion rate with the use of MINIT via the channel reamer. In 56 consecutive cases of subtrochanteric fractures, use of the MINIT with the channel reamer resulted in a 95% rate of reduction with less than 5 degrees of deformity in any plane and a 81% rate of normal alignment when MINIT was not used.

Proximal-Screw Placement Errors

Gauging the proper depth of nail insertion to maximize screw centralization of the femoral head can be surprisingly difficult. Preoperative templates can be helpful in determining the diameter of the femoral neck and aid in selection of the proper implant.

Radiographic visualization of the proximal femur, particularly in the lateral projection, may be difficult. Rotation of the c-arm until a true lateral of the femoral head and neck is the key to successful proximal-screw placement. This is facilitated by temporarily rotating the proximal guide anteriorly. Once a true lateral of the femoral neck can be visualized and a reduction confirmed, the handle is rotated posteriorly until the opaque guide bisects the femoral head. This will allow visualization of the femoral head anterior and posterior to the locking guide. When a portion of the femoral head anterior and posterior to the proximal guide handle is visualized, the screws will be contained in the centered position of the femoral head (see Fig. 20.17). I favor screws slightly anterior in the femoral head.

When the patient is in the supine position, the femoral head is anterior to the shaft of the femur, which requires the proximal drill guide to be rotated slightly below horizontal to prevent posterior screw placement in the femoral head. Anteversion built into the nail compensates for the anterior femoral-head offset from the center of the medullary canal. This minimizes the amount of external rotation needed to insert the nail and optimizes distal interlocking so that distal screw insertion is not too posterior at the knee. During insertion, the proximal locking screws tend to be placed in retroversion. Even though 8 to 15 degrees of anteversion (in relation to the distal locking holes) is built into most reconstruction nails, the proximal drill guide should be positioned slightly below the horizontal axis of the limb. Rotational alignment and centralization of the proximal drill guide is confirmed on the lateral c-arm view.

In some patients, placement of two screws within the femoral head may be difficult. The most common causes for this problem are varus reduction of the proximal fragment, a narrow femoral neck, and preexisting coxa vara in reference to the neck-shaft angle of the proximal screws and nail. If the proximal screws transverse an inferior to superior tract in the femoral head or the surgeon perceives that only one screw can be inserted, the fracture is probably in varus.

Another common mistake is inadequate depth insertion of the nail. This can be minimized by preoperative planning and referencing the tip of the greater trochanter to the center of the femoral head. The goal is to try to place the inferior screw just above the medial femoral cortex. If the nail is inserted too deep, it will be difficult to insert the screw or the screw will penetrate the cortex. The guide wire should be placed 4 to 5 mm above the medial femoral neck. In an alternative, a Kirschner (K) wire may be inserted percutaneously anterior to the femoral neck into the desired position and the proximal driving guide inserted by using this reference point.

Frequently during proximal screw insertion, the surgeon will note that the proximal locking screw will not advance past the nail into the femoral neck. This is usually because of the partially threaded proximal screw functioning as a bolt. When all of the threads of the bolt become contained within the proximal nail, no threads are available to pull the nail into the bone. At this point, the surgeon may tap the screw into the femoral head until threads contact bone and start the threading process again.

The proximal screws must provide stable fixation in the operating room. In cases of severe osteoporosis or pathologic lesions in which the screws do not have good fixation, augmentation of proximal screw fixation with nonpressurized methyl methacrylate is advisable.

Infection

Infection is relatively uncommon with closed nailing techniques and probably occurs at a rate of 1% in closed fractures and slightly higher in open fractures. If the implant is stable, incision and drainage of the acute infection and intravenous antibiotics are recommended. Once the fracture has united, the implant should be removed and the canal debrided. A more difficult problem is loss of fixation accompanied with an occult infection. Depending on the type of organism, debridement and exchange nailing and antibiotics may be successful. If a virulent organism is encountered with loss of nail stability, traction or external fixation or both may be required; a higher morbidity expected in this latter situation.

Fixation Disruption

Loss of fixation may occur from failure of screw fixation or nail or screw breakage. Nail breakage usually implies nonunion and fatigue failure. If the problem is aseptic, exchange reamed nailing is recommended. Loss of proximal screw fixation acutely reflects pathologic bone (i.e., osteopenia or neoplasia) or poor initial-screw placement. Late loss of screw fixation implicates nonunion. Revision nailing and bone grafting are required for successful salvage. Distal screw breakage early is usually the result of premature or excessive weight bearing. Length or rotational loss may occur if distal screws are removed prematurely or if the patient engages in excessive weight bearing.

Nonunion

Aseptic nonunions are biologic failures that may or may not be complicated with implant failure. If the existing implant is loose, it should be revised to the most suitable fixation, usually to a larger, reamed, interlocking, reconstruction nail. In hypertrophic nonunions, exchange nailing is frequently all that will be required. When the outcome of these solutions is in doubt or in atrophic nonunions, autologous cancellous iliac-bone graft to the nonunion site with a Phemister–Judet technique is advised.

Functional Loss

Functional loss is usually the result of complications about the hip or knee. Heterotopic ossification is a frequent radiographic finding but rarely symptomatic. Associated patella and peri-articular knee fractures, as well as soft-tissue injuries, can result in the loss of motion after subtrochanteric fractures. Neurological injuries associated with the subtrochanteric fracture are rare but must be evaluated carefully before nailing is done. Sciatic and pudendal nerve injuries observed postoperatively are usually caused by excessive traction required for reduction or compartment syndrome. These injuries do not always resolve with time and therefore may result in significant morbidity.

ILLUSTRATIVE CASES FOR TECHNIQUE

Case I is of a 49-year-old man who experienced parachute malfunction while jumping. On impact, he had a closed, displaced, proximal, femur fracture (Fig. 20.46). The patient underwent reamed, static, reconstruction nailing. His fracture united at 3 months, and he returned to his work without restrictions. This fracture pattern probably represents the ideal indication for a reconstruction nail; that is, it was a subtrochanteric fracture with loss of medial cortical stability and with fracture of the lesser trochanter (Russell–Taylor IB). The fracture did not extend into the piriformis fossa.

Case II is of a 66-year-old female who, after with a fall down stairs, sustained a Russell-Taylor IIB, closed, subtrochanteric fracture (Fig. 20.47). She underwent closed TriGen reconstruction nailing with a trochanteric portal nail. Her fracture united, and she regained independent ambulatory status by 4 months after surgery. This case represents the advantages of a trochanteric portal with the MINIT in comminuted fracture situations.

In case III, a 71-year-old female sustained a nondisplaced femoral-neck fracture that was treated with multiple screws. Two months after the surgery, she fell again, sustaining a subtrochanteric fracture. Her injury was revised with a piriformis entry nail but in a malreduced position. After 1 year, her fracture was successfully revised with a percutaneous osteotomy, autogenous bone grafting with DBM extender, and TriGen Intertan (Smith & Nephew, Memphis, TN) nailing in a reduced position with the channel reamer technique (Fig. 20.48).

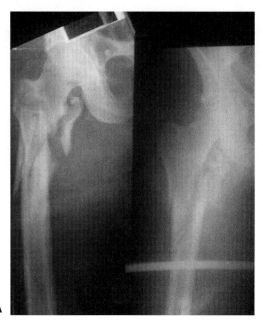
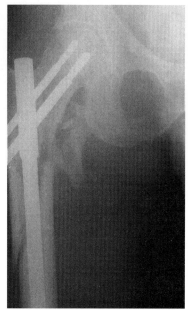

A   B

Figure 20.46. A,B. Subtrochanteric fracture caused from parachuting accident. Stabilization with Russell-Taylor reconstruction nail, static mode.

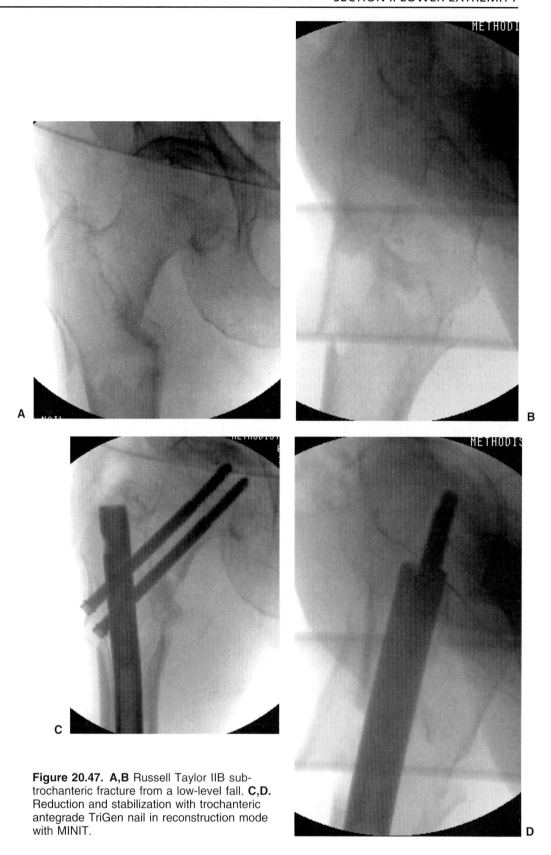

Figure 20.47. **A,B** Russell Taylor IIB sub-trochanteric fracture from a low-level fall. **C,D.** Reduction and stabilization with trochanteric antegrade TriGen nail in reconstruction mode with MINIT.

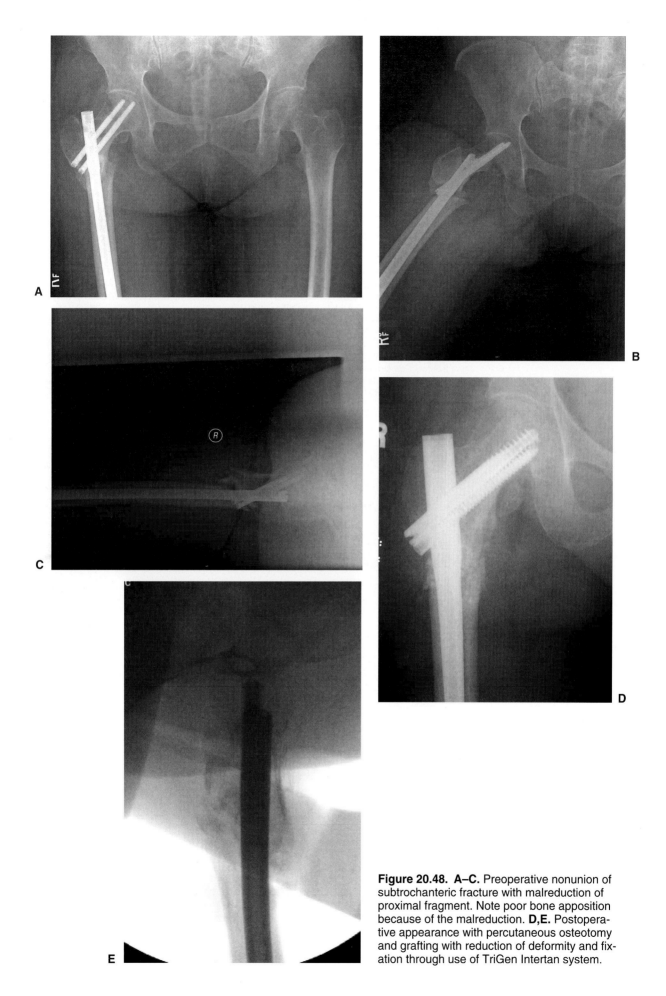

Figure 20.48. A–C. Preoperative nonunion of subtrochanteric fracture with malreduction of proximal fragment. Note poor bone apposition because of the malreduction. **D,E.** Postoperative appearance with percutaneous osteotomy and grafting with reduction of deformity and fixation through use of TriGen Intertan system.

RECOMMENDED READING

Bergman GD, Winquist RA, Mayo KA, et al. Subtrochanteric fracture of the femur: fixation using the Zickel nail. *J Bone Joint Surg Am* 1987;69:1032–1040.

Charnley GJ, Ward AJ. Reconstruction femoral nailing for nonunion of subtrochanteric fracture: a revision technique following dynamic condylar screw failure. *Int Orthop* 1996;20:55–57.

Haidukewych GJ, Israel TA, Berry DJ. Reverse obliquity fractures of the intertrochanteric region of the femur. *J Bone Joint Surg Am* 2001;83A:643–650.

Kitajima I, Tachibana S, Mikami Y, et al. Insufficiency fracture of the femoral neck after intramedullary nailing. *J Orthop Sci* 1999;4(4):304–306.

Pepper J, Russell T, Sanders R, et al. Minimally invasive intramedullary nail insertion instruments and method. US Patent 5,951,561. September 14, 1999.

Ricci WM, Bellabarba C, Lewis R, et al. Angular malalignment after intramedullary nailing of femoral shaft fractures. *J Orthop Trauma* 2001;15:90–95.

Russell TA, Taylor JC. Subtrochanteric fractures. In: Browner B, ed. *Skeletal trauma*. Philadelphia: WB Saunders, 1993.

Sanders R, Regazzoni P, Routt ML Jr. The treatment of subtrochanteric fractures of the femur using the dynamic condylar screw. *J Orthop Trauma* 1989;3:206–213.

Slater JC, Russell TA, Walker BC. Intramedullary nailing of complex subtrochanteric fracture of the femur. Paper presented at: American Academy of Orthopedic Surgeons Orthopaedic Transactions; 1992.

Taylor DC, Erpelding JM, Whitman CS, et al. Treatment of comminuted subtrochanteric femoral fractures in a young population with a reconstruction nail. *Mil Med* 1996;161:735–738.

Waddell JP. Subtrochanteric fractures of the femur: a review of 130 patients. *J Trauma* 1979;19:585–592.

Wheeler, DL, Croy TJ, Well TS, et al. Comparisons of reconstruction nails for high subtrochanteric femur fracture fixation. *Clin Orthop* 1997;338:231–239.

Wiss DA, Brien WW. Subtrochanteric fractures of the femur: results of treatment with interlocking nails. *Clin Orthop* 1992;283:231–236.

21

Femur Fractures: Antegrade Intramedullary Nailing

Bruce D. Browner, Andrew E. Caputo,
Augustus D. Mazzocca, and Donald A. Wiss

INDICATIONS/CONTRAINDICATION

Intramedullary nailing is the treatment of choice for all diaphyseal femoral fractures in adults. Locked intramedullary nailing can be static and dynamic. Static locking involves placement of proximal and distal locking screws, which prevent malrotation and shortening. Dynamic nailing is done with locking screws placed on either the proximal or distal side of the fracture. Because static interlocking does not inhibit fracture healing, all diaphyseal femoral fractures should be statically locked. Occasionally, dynamic locking is indicated for short oblique or transverse mid-diaphyseal fractures without comminution.

Many classification systems have been described for femur fractures. Winquist and Hansen developed a classification based on the amount of comminution (Fig. 21.1). Type I and II fractures are characterized by stable bone contact between the proximal and distal fragments and are considered length stable. Type III and IV comminution results in limited or no contact between the proximal and distal fragments, and static interlocking is required to maintain correct limb length and rotation.

Indications for intramedullary nailing of the femur include simple or comminuted fractures presenting below the lesser trochanter and extending distally to within 7 cm of the knee. Most grade I and II open femoral-shaft fractures can be treated with reamed intramedullary nails. Isolated grade III fractures may be better treated with aggressive wound management, temporary external fixation, and delayed intramedullary fixation. Patients with multiple injuries, including open femur fractures, require early skeletal stabilization to prevent pulmonary compromise. In these circumstances, a nonreamed intramedullary nailing or external fixation may be biologically attractive. However, the mechanical benefits of reaming with insertion of a larger nail, which provides more stability and strength, are sacrificed.

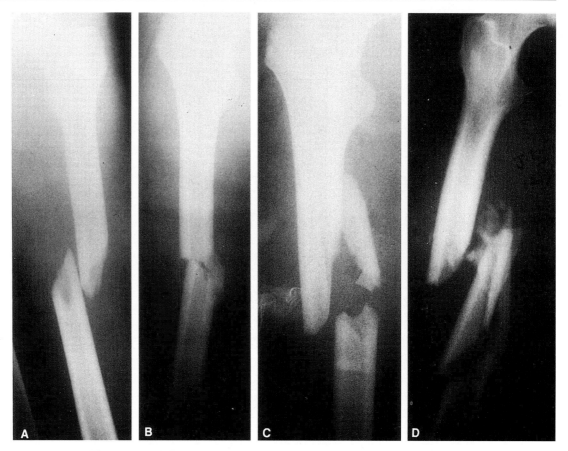

Figure 21.1. Winquist–Hansen fracture classification based on the amount of comminution.

Contraindications to intramedullary nailing include active local or systemic infections. Antegrade nailing in adolescents with open growth plates can damage the blood supply to the femoral head, causing osteonecrosis. These fractures may be better treated through use of flexible intramedullary nails, which are inserted retrograde proximal to the distal femoral-growth plate. Due to a higher incidence of infection when reamed nailing is performed after a prolonged period of initial external fixation, nailing should be used with caution. Other contraindications to nailing include patients with very narrow medullary canals or those with preexisting deformities that would preclude closed nailing.

PREOPERATIVE PLANNING

All patients with femur fractures resulting from blunt trauma should be evaluated for other injuries. Trauma evaluation and resuscitation via a multidisciplinary approach is necessary in patients with multiple injuries. High-quality, full-length anteroposterior (AP) and lateral radiographs of the femur should be obtained to evaluate the fracture (Fig. 21.2). The fracture location and the degree of comminution should be assessed on plain films. Ipsilateral fractures of the hip or femoral condyles must be ruled out before nailing is undertaken. Specific hip or knee films are often necessary for visualizing these fractures. Unrecognized nondisplaced fractures in these areas may displace during nailing. Once recognized, these fractures may be amenable to fixation with percutaneous screws. Osteoarthritis of the hip joint with a flexion contracture may limit hip motion on the traction table and make nailing difficult when the patient is in the supine position. When severe comminution or segmental defects exist, full-length films of the opposite femur may be helpful in determining appropriate length.

Contralateral radiographs also may be used to assess the medullary canal diameter and the degree of curvature of the intact femur. Patients with extremely small intramedullary canals

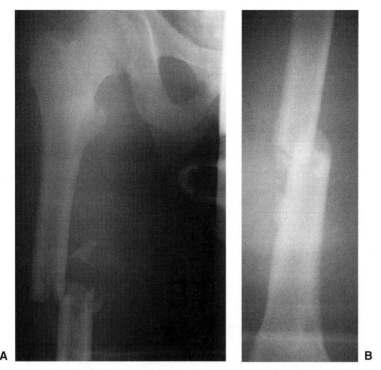

Figure 21.2. AP radiograph of the right femur showing a transverse mid-diaphyseal fracture with minimal comminution.

may require specially sized implants; the size should be determined preoperatively to ensure implant availability. The remodeling process associated with aging and osteoporosis often leads to an increase in the diameter of the medullary canal. In these patients, insertion of very-large-diameter nails is not necessary because stability is better achieved with 12- to 14-mm nails that are statically locked. The increased stiffness of large-diameter nails can cause iatrogenic comminution during insertion into brittle osteoporotic bone. Also, the curve of the implant must match the curve of the femur.

Reestablishing the correct limb length and choosing the nail of appropriate length requires a reference length. We use the distance between the tip of the greater trochanter and the adductor tubercle to determine length. A radiograph of the intact femur with a radiopaque ruler placed along the thigh (Fig. 21.3) should be obtained.

SURGERY

Patient Positioning

Nailing can be performed with the patient in the lateral decubitus (Fig. 21.4) or supine position (Fig. 21.5) with or without a fracture table. The lateral decubitus position allows improved access to the piriformis fossa, especially in large patients or those with ipsilateral hip disease and concomitant decreased range of motion. However, patients with multiple injuries who are placed in the lateral position may experience respiratory compromise. In addition, valgus angulation of the fracture, difficulty determining proper rotation, venous congestion caused by pressure of the perineal post, and greater difficulty inserting distal locking screws are disadvantages to lateral positioning.

Supine positioning of the patient has advantages: ease of setup, less respiratory compromise, better fracture alignment, and easier distal-screw insertion. However, the surgeon will have greater difficulty establishing the correct starting point in the piriformis fossa. With the recent introduction of trochanteric entry nails, this determination has become less of a problem.

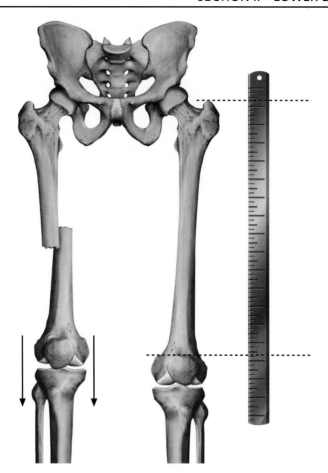

Figure 21.3. Preoperative evaluation of leg length. For simple fractures with limited comminution, the fracture can usually be reduced with minimal problems and the correct limb length restored. In patients with Winquist III and IV fracture comminution, length is reestablished by use of the contralateral intact femur as a reference. The length between the tip of the trochanter and the adductor tubercle is determined. Intraoperatively, the length of the fractured femur is adjusted by using traction to duplicate the correct trochanter–adductor tubercle length. This measurement can be confirmed through use of two overlapping guide wires of the same length.

In the classic procedure, intramedullary nailing is done on a fracture table through which fracture reduction is achieved via sustained longitudinal traction with or without a skeletal pin. A perineal post provides a fulcrum against which traction is applied. The design of most fracture tables allows circumferential access to the extremity for manipulation, surgical exposure, and imaging. The decision to use either a fracture table or a radiolucent table in patients who have experienced multiple traumas and who require simultaneous or sequential surgical procedures should be made on a case-by-case basis.

In an alternative approach, intramedullary nailing can be performed on a radiolucent table. Traction can be applied manually or with the use of a femoral distractor. Nailing can be performed through an antegrade or retrograde approach. The technique works best when nailing is done less than 24 hours after injury. Set up time is minimal, and access to the proximal femur is improved by adducting the limb. Disadvantages with this technique include difficulty visualizing the hip and proximal femur in the lateral projection, difficulty reducing and holding the fracture alignment, risk to the femoral neurovascular structures, and blockage of the operative field by the femoral distractor (Fig. 21.6).

Closed Reduction

Closed reduction is performed via traction through the fracture table and external manipulation. An in-line boot or a proximal-tibial or distal-femoral pin traction is utilized, and

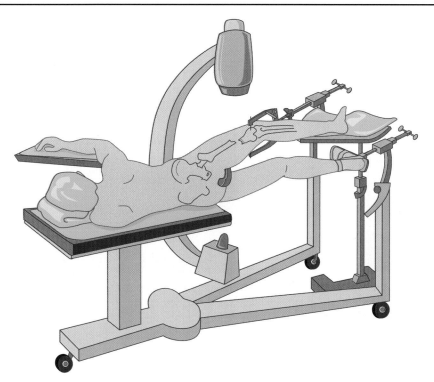

Figure 21.4. Lateral decubitus operative position. Access to the proximal femur is facilitated by increased hip flexion, which minimizes interference of the insertion instrumentation with the patient's torso. A drawback to this technique is that pulmonary function is slightly compromised, the setup is time consuming, and venous congestion can be caused from the peroneal post compressing the medial thigh and femoral vessels.

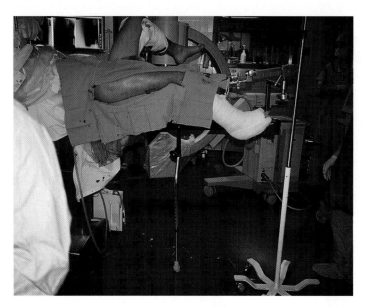

Figure 21.5. Supine operative position. To gain better access to the proximal femur on the operative side, the patient's arm is positioned above the body, and the torso is shifted away from the injured side. The operative limb is adducted at the hip. Rotational alignment is obtained with the knee flexed and the foot hanging free. Traction should be applied by using a Steinmann pin placed at the level of the tibial tubercle. The attachment points for the traction bow should be placed close to the skin to avoid bending the Steinmann pin when traction is applied. Bending of the pin dissipates the traction force and produces difficulties in pin removal. The protruding Steinmann pin should be cut close to the bow and the remaining sharp ends should be covered with tape to avoid injury to health-care personnel.

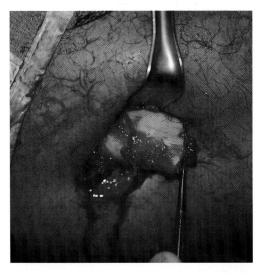

Figure 21.6. Open fracture management. An open fracture wound should be debrided before nailing. The bone ends should be inspected and carefully cleaned with a curette. Surgical extensions of the incision should be closed, and the original wound left open. At the end of the debridement, all of the instruments, gowns, gloves, and drapes should be changed, and the intramedullary nailing should be treated as a separate procedure.

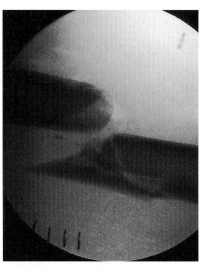

Figure 21.7. Fracture alignment. Once the patient is positioned on the fracture table, the distal fragment is posteriorly displaced.

the fracture alignment is checked with the image intensifier (Fig. 21.7). Occasionally leg manipulation by the surgeon or a crutch may be useful for reduction of an angulated fracture (Figs. 21.8 and 21.9). To minimize the risk of a pudendal nerve palsy, the traction is decreased during the prep, drape, and proximal exposure. Frequently a small-diameter nail may be used in the proximal fragment to reduce a flexed and externally rotated proximal

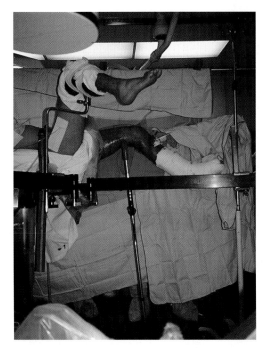

Figure 21.8. Fracture reduction. A crutch is placed between the floor and the posterior aspect of the leg to assist reduction. This places the distal fragment in a neutral position. The push-button expandable crutch allows precise intraoperative adjustment and greater flexibility in reduction.

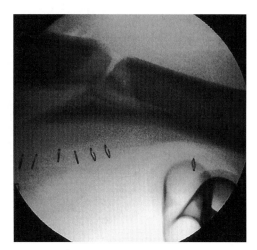

Figure 21.9. Fracture reduction. This lateral view shows the fracture after correction, with use of a crutch, of the posterior displacement of the distal fragment.

fragment. In addition, most implant manufacturers include a small-diameter intramedullary manipulation rod in the nailing sets for this purpose.

Entry Point

To facilitate supine nailing, most implant manufacturers have developed nails designed to enter through the tip of the greater trochanter. While technically easier to use than the classic piriformis entry nails, concerns exist about compromise of the hip abductor mechanism in patients undergoing trochanteric-entry nailing. To date, no long-term outcome studies have been completed on hip function following trochanteric nailing. We are hesitant to recommend its routine use, particularly in young trauma patients, until evidence-based medical studies support its widespread use. For this reason, we still advocate the use of a piriformis entry point for the majority of antegrade nailing procedures.

For a piriformis nailing, the entry point is critical for proper nail placement and fracture reduction. A longitudinal incision 6 to 10 cm is made over the greater trochanter and in-line with the femur (Fig. 21.10). The fascia overlying the abductors is incised, and the muscle is split in-line with its fibers down to the piriformis fossa (Fig. 21.11). A guide pin is placed in the piriformis fossa, and its position is confirmed with fluoroscopy. The tip should be centered directly in-line with the medullary canal as seen in both the AP and lateral views. Medial portal placement should be avoided because it may cause a femoral-neck fracture. Portal placement laterally may lead to comminution and varus alignment in proximal fractures. Once the pin is properly positioned in the piriformis fossa and is confirmed fluoroscopically, the femur is opened with a cannulated drill. In an alternative, an awl may be placed in the piriformis fossa and the proximal femur opened by hand (Figs. 21.12 to 21.20)

Guide-Wire Insertion, Fracture Reduction, and Reaming

A flexible ball-tipped guide wire is placed down the canal under fluoroscopic control. A ball tip is essential to prevent complications while reaming. The distal 2 cm of the tip is typically bent and used to direct the wire into the displaced distal fragment. The guide wire should be placed centrally in the distal fragment because eccentric placement may cause

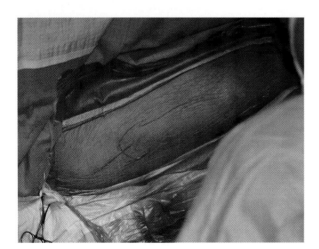

Figure 21.10. Surgical incision planning. A 6- to 10-cm longitudinal incision is made just proximal to the tip of the greater trochanter. To accommodate distal locking, the surgical field must include the distal femur.

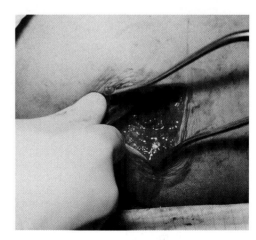

Figure 21.11. Incision and dissection. The incision has been made and the dissection carried through the subcutaneous tissue and the fibers of the gluteus maximus down to the posterior edge of the gluteus medius. The tip of the greater trochanter and the piriformis fossa are localized by digital palpation.

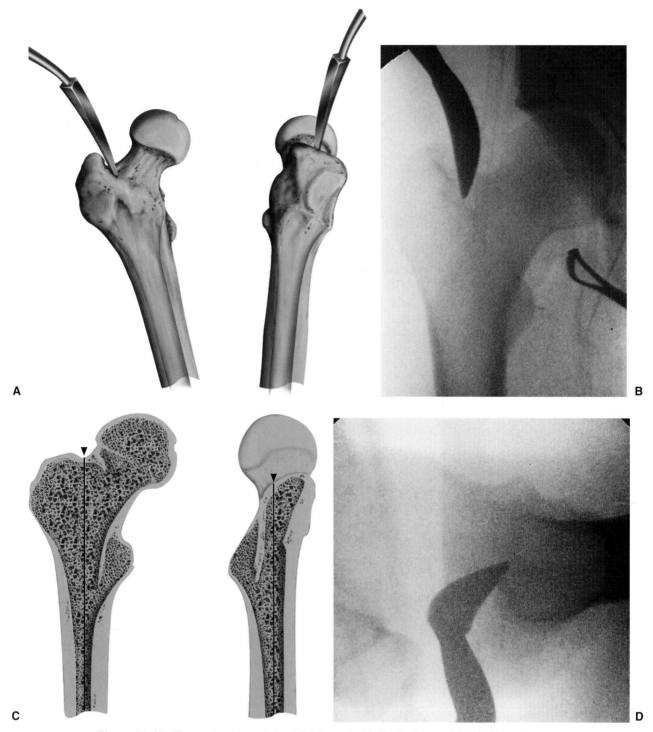

Figure 21.12. Femoral entry-portal establishment with Kuntscher awl. In an alternative technique, a curved awl can be used for establishing an entry portal in the proximal femur **(A)**. Initial position of the awl established by digital palpation should be confirmed radiographically with the c-arm. The AP and lateral views should include images of the greater trochanter, femoral head, and the proximal portion of the medullary canal **(B)**. The surgeon should imagine a line passing down the center of the medullary canal and projecting out the top of the femur **(C)**. The entry portal should be established exactly where this line emerges in the AP view **(D)**.

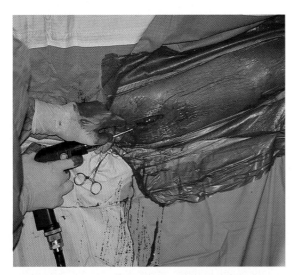

Figure 21.13. Femoral entry portal establishment with cannulated drill. As shown here, a 5/32 inch Steinmann pin is guided radiographically and drilled into the piriformis

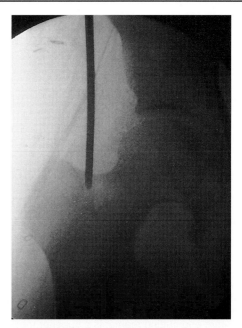

Figure 21.14. Steinmann-pin placement. The correct position of the Steinmann pin as it enters the top of the femur at a point where the line defining the center of the medullary canal would emerge from the top of the bone.

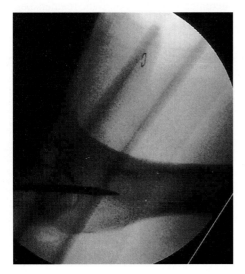

Figure 21.15. Steinmann-pin placement. As in the AP view, the lateral view of the proximal femur shows that the 5/32 inch Steinmann pin penetrates the bone exactly at a point where the line defining the center of the medullary canal emerges from the top of the bone.

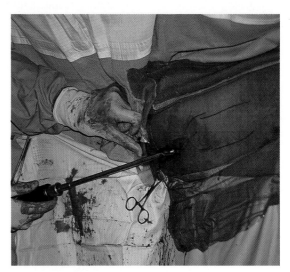

Figure 21.16. Cannulated drill with reamer. The cannulated drill is inserted with the soft-tissue protector in place over the 5/32 inch Steinmann pin.

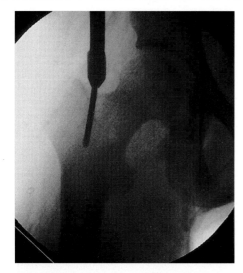

Figure 21.17. Reamer placement. The 13-mm end-cutting reamer is placed over the 5/32 inch Steinmann pin, producing a precisely located entry portal. Power drilling with a sharp 13-mm end-cutting reamer is a superior method for the establishment of an entry portal in the tough proximal-femoral bone in a young patient. The use of this special cannulated reamer over a 5/32 inch Steinmann pin avoids slippage, which can occur with the curved or T-handled awl. The hip must be adequately adducted of the hip.

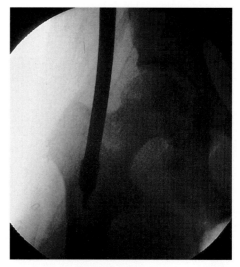

Figure 21.18. Reamer placement. Individual anatomic variations sometimes prohibit directing the 5/32 inch Steinmann pin down into the femur along the axis of the medullary canal. In these cases, the pin should be inserted into the femur only a few centimeters. Once the cannulated drill is passed into the top of the femur, the shaft of the drill can be pushed medially close to the patient to redirect the cutting tip down the medullary canal.

comminution or mal-alignment (Figs. 21.21 to 21.37). The use of a small-diameter, cannulated, intramedullary, manipulation device can be very helpful in aligning the fracture and facilitating guide wire passage.

Initially, a small end-cutting reamer (8.5 or 9.0 mm) is used. Then successive side-cutting reamers, increasing in 1.0-mm increments, are used until the reamers begin cutting

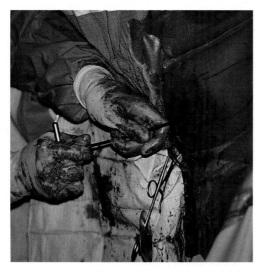

Figure 21.19. Enlargement of the medullary canal with a T-handled awl. Because the shaft of the 13-mm end-cutting entry-portal reamer is rigid, passing the reamer straight down the medullary canal may be impossible. In these cases, a T-handled awl, which has a more flexible shaft, can be introduced to complete the path from the metaphysis into the medullary canal.

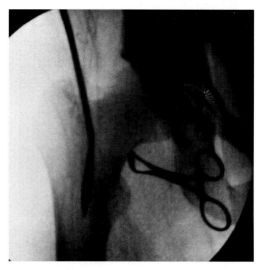

Figure 21.20. T-handled awl. This radiographic view of the proximal femur shows the curved T-handled awl being passed into the medullary canal.

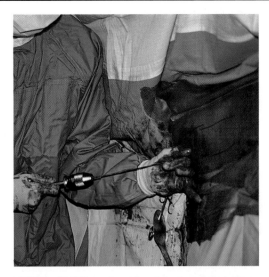

Figure 21.21. Ball-tipped guide-wire placement. The ball-tipped reaming guide wire is held by a T-handled chuck and introduced into the entry portal. The guide wire can be rotated as it is advanced through pressure on the T-handled chuck.

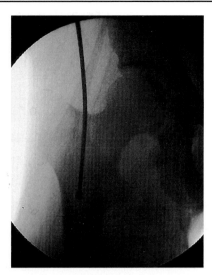

Figure 21.22. Ball-tipped guide-wire placement. Because of the curved bend in the end of the guide wire, the ball tip will sometimes encounter resistance as it is passed through the metaphysis.

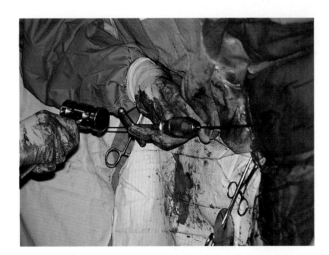

Figure 21.23. Ball-tipped guide-wire placement. The T-handled chuck is clamped onto the guide wire close to the entry wound to optimize control and minimize wire deformation. When a guide wire with a curved tip is used, the T-handled chuck will permit rotational manipulation of the guide wire. Resistance can be overcome by light blows to the T-handled chuck. If great resistance is met, the position of the ball tip should be carefully identified with the image intensifier on AP and lateral views. The tip may need to be withdrawn and repositioned.

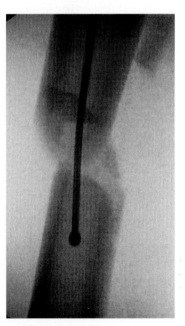

Figure 21.24. Ball-tipped guide-wire placement past the fracture site. If small amounts of residual translation exist at the fracture site, the guide wire may be passed if the surgeon takes advantage of the reestablished bend at the end of the wire. Passage of the guide wire is greatly facilitated by the use of a brief period of live fluoroscopy. Successful passage into the opposite medullary canal can be confirmed by noting that the guide-wire tip is contained within the bone and crosses cortical margins into the soft tissues. To further confirm the location of the guide wire, the surgeon can rotate it. Lateral views are necessary to confirm the correct position of the wire within the medullary canal.

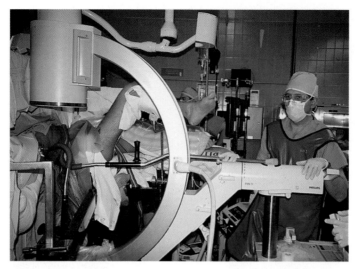

Figure 21.25. Fracture reduction with crutch. When the fracture shows valgus angulation or medial displacement of the distal end of the proximal fragment, an unscrubbed assistant can apply reducing force in the coronal plane via a crutch.

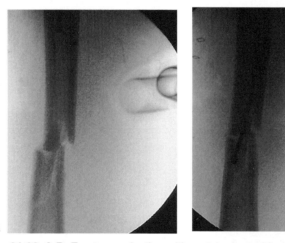

A   B

Figures 21.26 A,B. Fracture reduction with crutch. A combination of maneuvers can be used to reduce the fracture in the sagittal plane. A crutch is often needed to support the distal fragment, which is pulled toward the floor by the two heads of the gastrocnemius muscle. The proximal fragment is pulled anteriorly by the hip flexors. Manual pressure applied on the anterior thigh may assist with reduction. Radiographic conformation of the crutch helps ensure fracture reduction and allows passage of the bead-tipped guide wire.

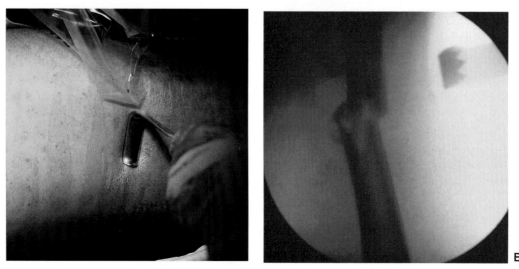

A   B

Figures 21.27 A,B. Fracture reduction with retractors. When the fracture shows varus angulation or medial displacement, reducing force can be applied in the coronal plane through the pressure provided by sterile retractors.

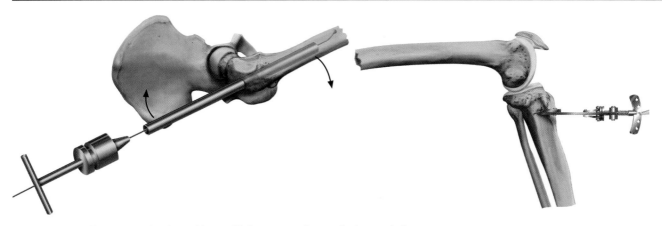

Figure 21.28. Fracture reduction with small-diameter nail or reducing tool. A more powerful reducing force may be applied with the use of a small-diameter nail or reducing tool. When proximal diaphyseal fractures are encountered, this instrument can be used to control the flexed, externally rotated, and abducted proximal fragment during reduction.

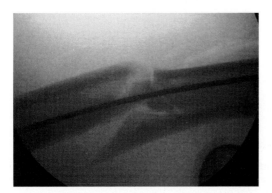

Figure 21.29. Guide-wire passage past the fracture site. Guide-wire passage into the distal fragment is confirmed. Both AP and lateral views should be taken to assure that the wire is in the medullary canal.

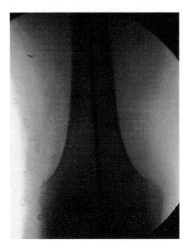

Figure 21.30. Confirmation of proper guide-wire placement. The fracture should be reduced before guide-wire insertion and maintained in this position throughout reaming, nail insertion, and distal screw fixation. Correct reduction is confirmed when the guide wire passes down the center of the medullary canal to the level of the adductor tubercle.

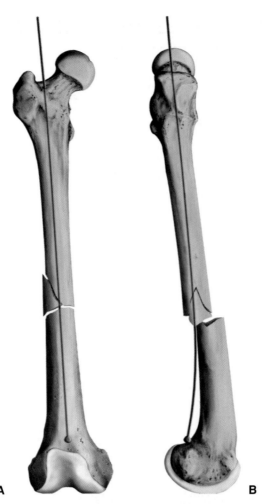

A   B

Figure 21.31. A,B. Proper ball-tip guide-wire placement. A posteriorly placed wire can be seen as central on the AP view. This emphasizes the need to obtain both views to confirm containment of the wire in the medullary canal.

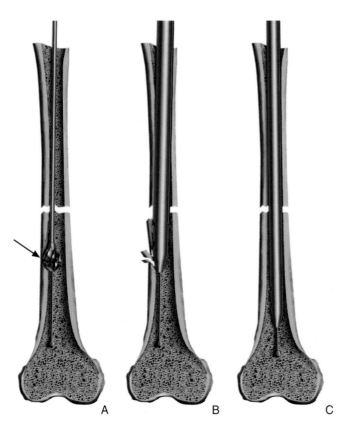

A   B   C

Figure 21.32. Guide-wire placement. Eccentric guide-wire placement can lead to excessive reaming on one cortex and comminution during nail insertion.

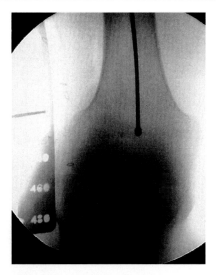

Figure 21.33. Femoral intramedullary nail size. Proposed nail length is based on the measurement from tip of the greater trochanter to the adductor tubercle.

into the endosteal surface, which is perceived as manual resistance and audible chatter. The reamer diameter is then increased in only 0.5-mm increments to minimize heat generation and the likelihood of incarcerating the reamer head in the medullary canal. The reamer should be advanced through the isthmus until resistance is lost, which indicates that the reamer head has entered the widened portion of the medullary canal. Although the ball-tipped guide wire extends the full length of the femur, the cancellous bone in the distal metaphysis should not be reamed. Better fixation will be achieved if the nail can be impacted into cancellous bone. The canal should be reamed 1.0 to 1.5 mm more than the diameter of the desired nail to be inserted. Improvements in metallurgy and manufacturing techniques have enhanced the strength of intramedullary nails, permitting successful fixation with smaller-diameter nails. In most cases, we use 11.0- to 12.0-mm diameter nails in female patients and 11.0- to 13.0-mm-diameter nails for male patients.

The correct length of the fractured femur is reestablished intraoperatively through use of the ball-tipped guide wire and the referenced length previously determined. A second guide wire, equal in length to the ball-tipped guide wire, is inserted into the wound to the level of the entry portal at the top of the femur. A clamp is placed on the guide wire at

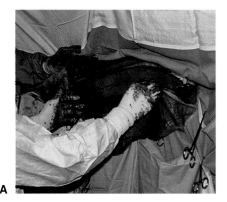
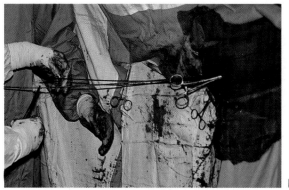

A   B

Figures 21.34. A,B. Ruler measurement. Reestablishing the correct length of the fractured femur and choosing the correct length of the intramedullary nail both require the use of a reference length, which is the distance between the tip of the greater trochanter and the adductor tubercle; this can be measured through use of a radiopaque ruler held lateral to the thigh at the level of the femur.

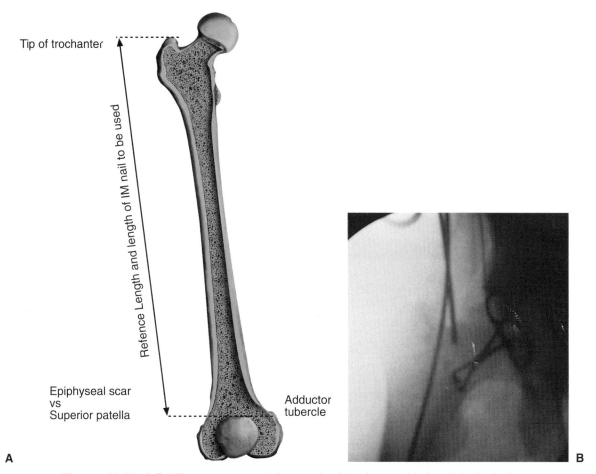

Tip of trochanter

Refence Length and length of IM nail to be used

Epiphyseal scar
vs
Superior patella

Adductor
tubercle

A

B

Figures 21.35. A,B. Wire measurement. A second guide wire equal in length to the ball-tip guide wire is inserted into the wound to the level of the entry portal at the top of the femur. A clamp is placed on the guide wire at the point where it overlaps the tip of the ball-tipped guide wire. The distance between the clamp and the free end of the second guide wire is measured and used as an estimate of the distance from the tip of the greater trochanter to the adductor tubercle. This distance is compared with the reference measurement made preoperatively on the contralateral intact femur. Adjustments must be made with traction to correct any discrepancy with this distance.

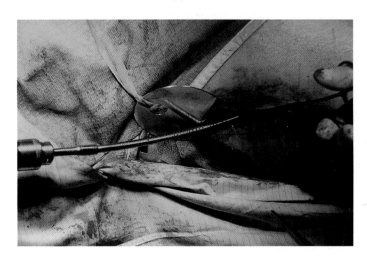

Figure 21.36. Reaming. The soft-tissue protector should always be used to avoid injury to the skin and muscle from the rotating reamer shaft. A lap-pad strap is tied to the protector to prevent it from falling to the floor. When the reamer is pulled back, a Kocher clamp is used to grasp the guide wire; the surgeon must avoid extracting the guide wire across the fracture site. The initial reamer should be a small end-cutting type to create a path for subsequent reamers.

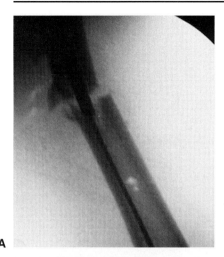
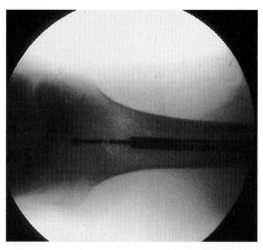

A   B

Figures 21.37. A,B. Reaming. To avoid excessive pressure in the medullary canal, reamers should be sharp, have deep flutes, and have a small shaft relative to the diameter of the reamer head. In addition, the reamer should be advanced slowly, and multiple passes should be made with each reamer size. Side-cutting reamers are used to enlarge the canal to 1.0 mm larger than the intended nail diameter. The diameter of the reamers can be initially increased by 1-mm increments. Once the reamers begin to bite into cortical bone, the reaming diameter should be increased in 0.5-mm increments. If excessive resistance is encountered with a particular reamer, the last diameter that successfully passed should be reintroduced, and several more passes should be made with this reamer to remove additional bone. Overreaming from 1.0 to 2.0 mm is done when the femur has a significant bow, when the isthmus is long and narrow, or if the nail is difficult to drive.

the point where it overlaps the tip of the ball-tipped guide wire. The distance between the clamp and the free end of the second guide wire is measured to estimate the distance from the tip of the greater trochanter to the adductor tubercle. This distance is compared with the reference measurement made preoperatively on the contralateral intact femur. Adjustments must be made with traction to correct any discrepancy with this distance. Many nailing sets come with direct-read, cannulated, depth gauges, which are very accurate.

After reaming, the distal end of the ball-tipped guide wire is positioned corresponding to the distal extent of the desired nail. For the majority of shaft fractures, this corresponds to the adductor tubercle. In distal-third fractures, the ball tip is placed just proximal to the intercondylar notch. In these cases, the surgeon should plan to place two distal-locking screws, which prevent toggle in the distal fragment. Rarely, the nail needs to be customized through trimming of the distal tip, which allows for a more distal locking-screw placement.

For Winquist III and IV fractures, correct limb length is difficult to reestablish by reapproximating the main fragments. For this reason, the traction must be adjusted so that the reference length (greater trochanter to adductor tubercle) determined preoperatively can be reproduced intraoperatively through use of the ball-tipped guide wire and a second guide wire of equal length. Failure to compare the intraoperative length with the reference length may result in the femur being fixed in a shortened or lengthened position.

The ball-tipped guide wire is not designed for nail insertion. The tip of the guide wire is often bent to facilitate cannulation of the distal fragment, and the width of the ball is often wider than the inner diameter of the nail tip. Consequently, the curved ball-tipped guide wire may become trapped if used for nail insertion. In addition, a larger-diameter guide wire that more completely fills the inner diameter of the nail tip is preferable for nail insertion. If the nail is inserted over a thin guide wire, the larger inner diameter at the nail tip can allow the nail to displace into an eccentric position. This can cause inadvertent incarceration on the cortex of the distal fragment. Therefore, a straight, smooth, large, guide wire is necessary. A plastic sheath is used to maintain canal continuity while the ball-tipped guide wire is exchanged for the smooth guide wire (Fig. 21.38).

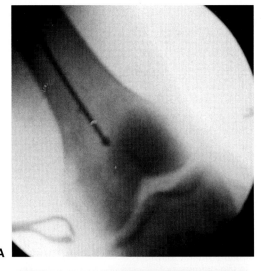

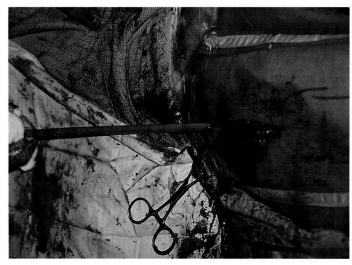

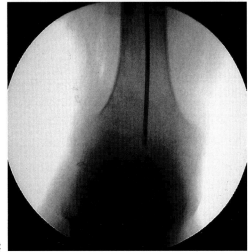

Figures 21.38. A–C. Guide-wire exchange. The purpose of the spherical end on a ball-tipped guide wire is to assist in extracting an incarcerated reamer. However, because of the ball, this wire should not be used for nail insertion. The ball-tipped reaming guide wire is replaced by a slightly larger diameter nonbeaded guide wire (nail-driving guide wire), which fills the nail, minimizing the risk of engaging the cortex of the distal fragment. A plastic exchange tube should be used to avoid displacement of the fracture and to simplify guide-wire exchange. A metallic marker at the tip of the tube allows radiographic confirmation that the tube has passed the fracture site.

Nail Placement

The nail is assembled onto its driver and placed over the smooth-tipped guide wire. To minimize the likelihood of iatrogenic comminution, fluoroscopic control should be used when the nail crosses. The nail is impacted smoothly with a mallet until the proximal nail is flush with or just below the greater trochanter. The distal end of the nail should be inserted to the chosen reference point (adductor tubercle for diaphyseal fractures and adjacent to the intercondylar notch for distal-third fractures) (Figs. 21.39 to 21.42). Most nails are designed with transfixion screws in the coronal plane. To achieve proper rotation, the nail must be controlled with the driver-and- proximal locking device during insertion.

Proximal Locking

Most nail systems incorporate a proximal locking guide connected to the driver. Nail systems are used with either transverse or diagonal, proximal, locking screws (Figs. 21.43 to 21.46). A single cross-locking screw is placed either diagonally from the greater to lesser trochanter or transversely across the femoral diaphysis. Failure to seat the nail fully may lead to superior placement of a diagonal screw, predisposing a loss of fixation or femoral-neck fractures.

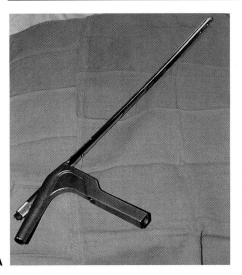
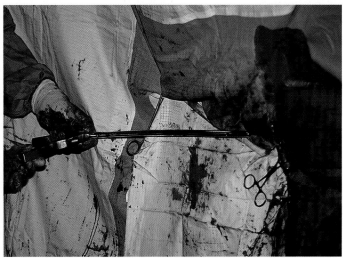

A   B

Figures 21.39. A,B. Intramedullary nail assembly and insertion. The proximal targeting nail and driving device is secured to the top of the nail. The nail driver can loosen after multiple mallet blows during insertion and should be retightened frequently. The nail is inserted over the guide wire into the femur, with the handle of the targeting device projected parallel to the floor so that the proximal and distal screw holes will be located in the coronal plane.

Distal Locking

A number of different methods have been devised to facilitate distal locking (Figs. 21.47 to 21.54). The flexibility of target devices mounted on the image intensifier has caused inaccurate screw insertion. The device, which requires direct attachment to the image intensifier, also lost popularity because surgeons are afraid of voiding the warranty on the image intensifier. A number of manufacturers have designed target devices for distal locking, which attach to the proximal end of the nail. The tendency for open-section intramedullary nails to deform torsionally on insertion has caused concern about the alignment between the target device and the distal screw holes. In addition, the length of these devices makes them subject to displacement and inaccurate screw placement, particularly when used in a patient placed in the supine position. Because of these problems, most

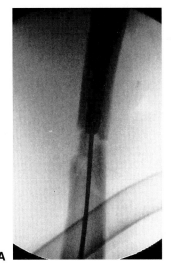
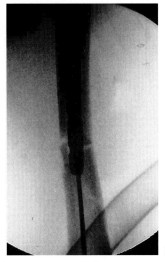

A   B

Figures 21.40. A,B. Intramedullary nail advancement. To avoid incarcerating comminuted fragments that lie in the path of the nail, the proximal end of the nail is pushed medially into the patient such that the distal end of the nail is directed laterally away from the

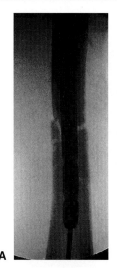
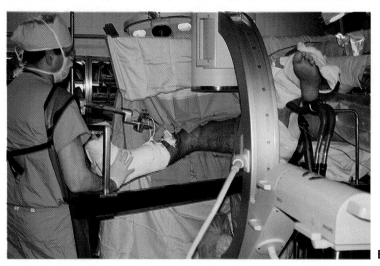

Figures 21.41. A,B. Fracture impaction. Once the nail passes into the distal fragment, traction is released to allow impaction at the fracture site. Impaction is aided by extending the knee and holding the foot firmly. This step is omitted in severely comminuted fractures in which femur length has already been adjusted by traction.

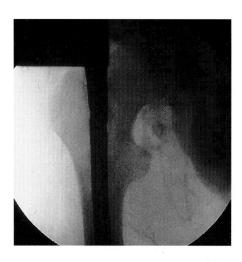

Figure 21.42. Intramedullary nail placement. When the nail is fully inserted, the target device should touch the greater trochanter. Radiographic confirmation of the target device is necessary because soft tissues can impinge and artificially elevate the targeting device, leaving the nail prominent.

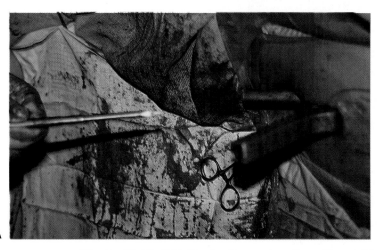
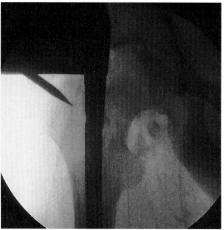

Figures 21.43. A,B. Proximal screw insertion with awl. The path of the proximal screw is diagonal, and the drill bit engages the lateral cortex at an acute angle. This angle can cause distal migration of the drill tip. To avoid this outcome, an awl is used to dimple the cortex before drilling.

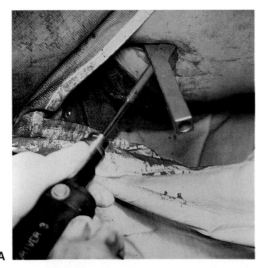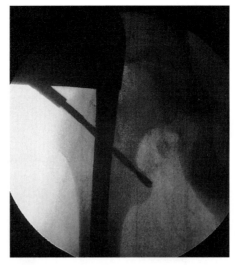

A   B

Figures 21.44. A,B. Drilling the proximal screw hole. On the AP view, the lesser trochanter appears to be in the coronal plane; however, it projects posteromedially. It is not necessary to drill to the apparent tip of the lesser trochanter because the drill bit exits anterior to the lesser trochanter.

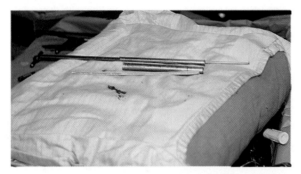

Figure 21.45. Depth gauge and tissue protector. If measuring and hooking the opposite cortex with a depth gauge is problematic, depth can be estimated radiographically. This image shows the difference between the length of the depth gauge and the tissue protector. The tissue protector is 1.0 cm shorter than the sleeve on the depth gauge. To obtain correct the measurement, the surgeon should remove the soft-tissue protector and use the depth gauge with its own sleeve.

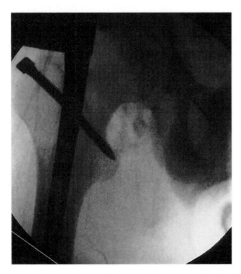

Figure 21.46. Proximal screw placement. Many patients complain of pain at the trochanter because of a prominent head on the proximal screw. To decrease this discomfort, the screw head can be partially buried. It is a self-tapping fully threaded screw, and the nail is threaded so the surgeon can countersink the screw effectively.

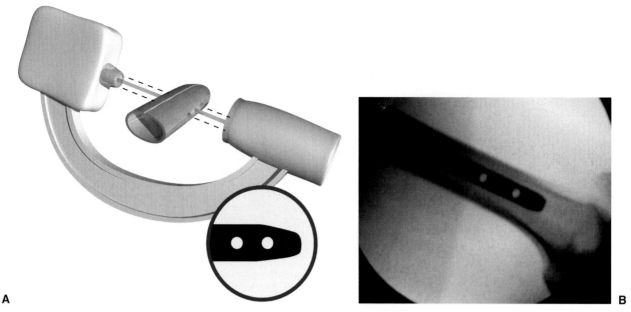

A

B

Figure 21.47. Distal fixation. Correct rotational alignment of the fracture should be confirmed before distal fixation. The c-arm should be positioned to obtain an optimal lateral view of the distal end of the nail. The goal is to pass the beam exactly in-line with the axis of the screw holes **(A)**. This position has been obtained when the holes appear perfectly round **(B)**. An elliptical appearance of the holes suggests mal-alignment of the beam.

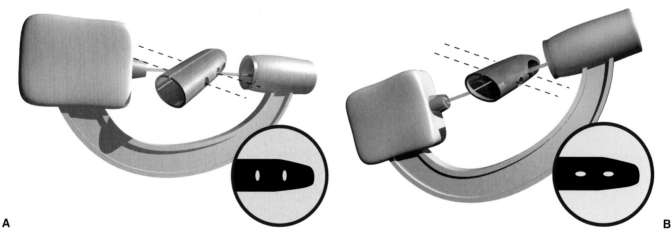

A

B

Figure 21.48. Illustration of oblique, distal, screw holes resulting from rotation.
A. Mal-alignment of the beam in the coronal plane makes the holes appear as vertical ellipses. **B.** Mal-alignment in the sagittal plane makes holes appear as horizontal ellipses.

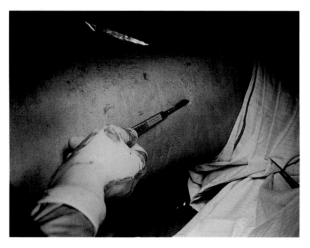

Figure 21.49. Distal entry-hole targeting. The tip of the scalpel is positioned on the skin over the screw hole so that once correct targeting is achieved, an immediate incision can be made.

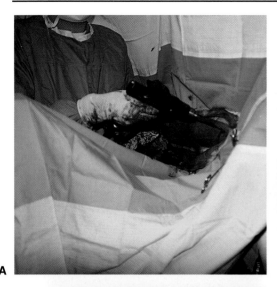

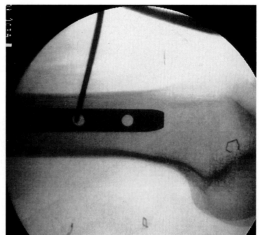

A

B

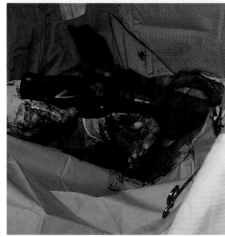

C

Figures 21.50. A-C. Distal entry-hole drilling. The drill is held out of the x-ray beam. The tip of the drill bit is against the lateral cortex and exactly centered on the proximal screw hole. With fluoroscopy off, the drill is lowered in line with the axis of the x-ray beam and screw hole. Continuous pressure must be kept on the tip of the drill as an assistant stabilizes the femur. In addition to these steps, the use of a sharp-tip drill bit helps avoid migration of the drill bit.

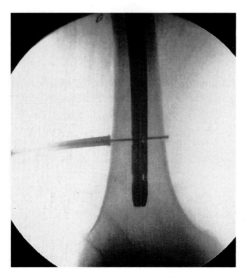

Figure 21.51. Distal fixation-hole depth measurement. Depth measurement for correct screw-length determination. Five millimeters should be added to the screw length to ensure projection beyond the opposite cortex, which will facilitate removal if the screws break.

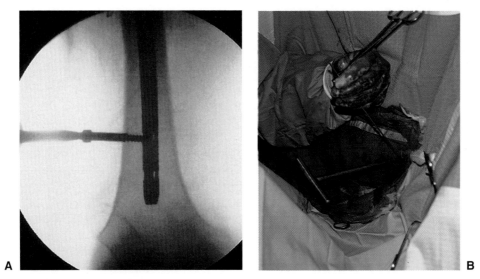

Figures 21.52. A,B. Distal screw insertion. The screw driver is used to define the axis of the first screw, which will be used to assist with the insertion of the second screw.

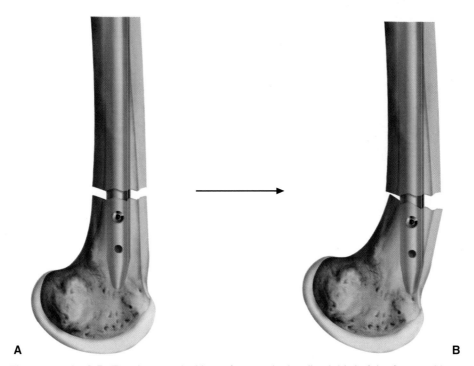

Figure 21.53. A,B. Toggle cross-locking a fracture in the distal third of the femur with a single screw permits the short distal fragment to toggle or rotate on the axis of the screw.

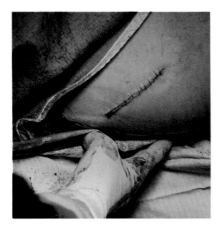

Figure 21.54. Wound closure.

surgeons have resorted to the use of hand-held devices, including drill guides, awls, sharp pins, and drill bits, and the freehand technique. Radiolucent offset drill attachments, which are used in conjunction with standard power drills, have been developed to allow direct drilling under radiographic control.

We routinely use a modified freehand technique for distal interlocking. Imperative to success, the image intensifier must be properly positioned directly perpendicular to the femur and centered over the distal screw holes. With proper positioning, the holes in the distal nail should appear as perfect circles and not as ellipses. A long Kirschner (K) wire is placed on the skin in the center of the hole; its location is confirmed via fluoroscopy. A 2-cm skin incision is made with blunt dissection to the lateral femoral cortex. The wire is then tapped into the bone in the center of the hole, creating a starting point to facilitate drilling. Fluoroscopic confirmation that the drill bit has successfully traversed the nail is essential before the surgeon drills the opposite cortex.

Confirmation of locking screw position is also needed and accomplished via the c-arm. Both screw holes should be filled in distal-third fractures because the diameter of the distal fragment is larger than that of the nail, and fixation with a single screw could lead to rotation of the fragment around the screw and motion at the fracture site. To enhance screw purchase, two distal screws should also be used for any diaphyseal fractures in weak osteoporotic bone. If a reamed nail is used, a single distal screw placed in the more proximal of the two, distal, nail holes is sufficient for fractures in the upper and middle thirds. In these cases, the diameter of the medullary canal at the proximal end of the distal fragment is usually similar in size to the diameter of the nail, preventing distal-fragment rotation.

POSTOPERATIVE MANAGEMENT

Postoperative management depends on the fracture location and amount of comminution, age of patient, preoperative mobility, and extent of coexisting injuries. So that weight will be transmitted through the bone, early weight bearing is encouraged in the patient with a transverse or short oblique fracture in which the contact between the two major fragments is unstable. When comminution prevents transmission of weight through the bone, 6 to 8 weeks of partial weight bearing is recommended to permit callus formation. Patient pain is usually the limiting factor for weight bearing.

The majority of fractures will heal with the nail in the static locked mode. This is advantageous, even in stable transverse fractures, because it helps to control rotation. Dynamization (the removal of proximal or distal screws from a statically locked nail) may be useful to allow impaction in those few fractures that do not show progressive healing 4 to 6 months after nailing.

Physical therapy routinely includes active range of motion, resistive muscle strengthening, gait training, and pool therapy. These therapies speed rehabilitation, enhance fracture healing, and increase the ultimate level of functional recovery.

Patients are seen in the outpatient office 10 to 14 days after surgery for suture removal and wound inspection. AP and lateral radiographs are obtained to inspect the implant position, fracture alignment, and progress of union immediately after surgery and at 6, 12, and 24 weeks. A final set of radiographs is obtained at 6 months to document adequate healing of the fracture. The average uncomplicated femoral-diaphyseal fracture will unite in 3 to 5 months. In the absence of patellar fractures or knee ligament injuries, patients generally achieve excellent recovery of knee motion. Several months of exercise are required to achieve the ultimate range of knee motion. The speed of recovery and degree of motion are enhanced by early physical therapy.

COMPLICATIONS

Malunion

The routine use of static locking has decreased the incidence of the postoperative fracture displacement that leads to malunion. The majority of malunions results when fractures are fixed in a position of mal-alignment. Transverse and short oblique fractures in the isthmus are naturally aligned because of greater endosteal contact with the nail. Fractures above and below the isthmus have a short fragment with a large medullary canal, which predisposes the fragment to angular mal-alignment unless its position is carefully controlled.

During the operation, the surgeon confirms the correct position of the fragment by visualizing the fracture site under low magnification (camera close to the limb) and by ensuring that the guide wire is in the center of the fragment as shown on both AP and lateral views. If the short fragment is held in correct position during guide passage, reaming, and nail and screw insertion, mal-alignment will be prevented. Correct entry-portal placement in the piriformis fossa in-line with the medullary canal is important in preventing varus malunions in proximal-third fractures. In addition to avoiding angular mal-alignment, the correct rotational alignment must be established before nail insertion. In the supine position, diaphyseal fractures are aligned by allowing the knee to flex with the foot hanging to the floor. Proximal placement of the tibial traction pin at the level of the tibial tubercle will facilitate knee flexion, which improves rotational alignment and transmits greater traction force along the femur. More distal placement of the traction pin causes knee extension when traction is applied. This reduces the force transmitted into the femur, reduces the rotational moment arm of the distal fragment, and results in posterior angulation of the femoral fracture.

Malrotation, if recognized early, may be corrected by removal of the distal screws, deformity correction, and reinsertion of the screws. Angulation of 5 to 7 degrees in any plane is usually well tolerated; however, mal-alignment of more than 10 degrees usually requires early revision to avoid late symptoms. Increased comminution associated with nailing is common and is tolerated as long as the comminution is between the static locking screws.

Delayed Union and Nonunion

The use of a closed technique for the insertion of locked nails results in a 1% to 2% incidence of nonunion. Introduction of the nails at a distance from the fracture site avoids direct dissection and periosteal stripping, thereby preserving the fracture biology. Systemic (poor nutrition, diabetes, steroids, smoking, etc.) and local factors (severe periosteal stripping, infection, or vascular injury) can combine to cause delayed union or nonunion. Each of these factors must be taken into consideration and treatment plans developed accordingly.

Pudendal Nerve Palsy

Pudendal nerve palsies usually result from excessive continuous traction on the perineal post. This complication can usually be avoided if the nailing is performed on the day of injury. Only limited traction is needed during this early phase to achieve excellent reductions. When nailing is delayed, sufficient skeletal traction should be applied to overdistract the fracture slightly. This overdistraction should be confirmed through use of a lateral radiograph. The AP view alone should not be used to determine length because the film is usually taken parallel to the surface of the bed rather than the limb, and it can give a false impression of distraction in the presence of overlap. By maintaining preoperative overdistraction, the surgeon can more easily reduce the fracture during nailing without resorting to excessive traction. Pudendal nerve palsies are usually neurapraxia and frequently resolve in 3 to 4 months.

Femoral-Neck Fractures

Most studies on ipsilateral hip and shaft fractures suggest that a femoral-neck fracture more likely represents a missed injury rather than iatrogenic fracture. Radiographs of the hip must be examined carefully to rule out a hip dislocation or femoral-neck fracture. A separate, internal-rotation AP radiograph of the proximal femur can be very helpful in visualizing the femoral neck.

A variety of techniques has been developed to treat these combined fractures. They include insertion of multiple cannulated screws around an existing nail, use of a reconstruction nail, and employment of multiple cannulated screws with a retrograde locked nail.

Infection

Despite the reaming of the medullary canal and the insertion of an implant that extends the length of the femur, infection after closed intramedullary nailing is surprisingly infrequent. The closed technique, which eliminates dissection at the fracture site, contributes to the low incidence of infection and nonunion. When infection does occur, the extent of involvement can vary. The infection may be confined to the superficial layers of the wound or the hematoma at the entry wound or the fracture site. These infections can be treated by intravenous antibiotics and local drainage. Less frequently, the entire medullary cavity is infected. The inner half of the thickness of the cortex, devascularized by the reaming, can become an extensive sequestrum. In this circumstance, treatment requires removal of the nail and repeated reaming to debride the endosteal cortex. A new nail or an external fixator may be necessary if the fracture is not united.

ILLUSTRATIVE CASE FOR TECHNIQUE

A 23-year-old man sustained blunt abdominal trauma and a closed right-femur fracture as a result of a head-on motor vehicle accident. The patient lost consciousness at the site of the accident and experienced mild retrograde amnesia. On initial examination, the physician found an obvious, closed, right, midshaft-femur deformity. The peripheral pulses were intact, and the neurologic examination showed no abnormalities. Cervical spine, chest, and pelvic radiographs were normal. A cranial computed tomography (CT) scan was negative for fracture or intracranial bleed. AP and lateral radiographs of the femur showed a mid-diaphyseal transverse fracture (see Fig. 21.2). The patient had an abdominal injury that required exploratory laparotomy. At surgery, the patient was found to have a complete jejunal transection, which was subsequently repaired. Immediately after the laparotomy, a closed intramedullary nailing was performed with a static locked nail. Because the fracture was mid-diaphyseal, a single distal screw was used for fixation (Fig. 21.55). The patient

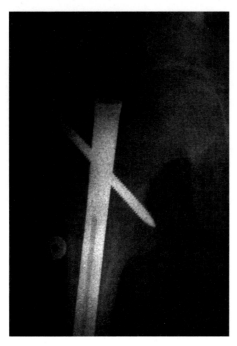

Figure 21.55. Postoperative radiograph.

was mobilized on the second postoperative day. The fracture healed uneventfully in 4 months with excellent restoration of function.

RECOMMENDED READING

Browner BD. *The science and practice of intramedullary nailing*. 2nd ed. Baltimore: Williams & Wilkins; 1996.
Brumback RJ, Reilly JP, Poka A, et al. Intramedullary nailing of femoral shaft fractures, part I: decision making errors with interlocking fixation. *J Bone Joint Surg Am* 1988;70:1441–1452.
Brumback RJ, Stribling EP, Poka A, et al. Intramedullary nailing of open fractures of the femoral shaft. *J Bone Joint Surg Am* 1989;71:1324–1330.

22

Femoral Shaft Fractures: Retrograde Nailing

Robert F. Ostrum and Eric D. Farrell

Retrograde femoral intramedullary nailing has become an accepted method of treatment for femoral shaft fractures, especially those associated with other injuries. Early attempts at retrograde nailing with entry portals through the medial femoral condyle led to comminution and malunion. Moving the starting point to a centromedullary position produced better results with fewer complications. Prior to the introduction of locked plates, internal fixation of comminuted, supracondylar femur fractures was associated with a relatively high incidence of malunion, nonunion, hardware failure, and loss of knee motion. For this reason, a retrograde locking nail was developed. Originally designed as a short nail for distal femur fractures, full-length nails were ultimately developed to manage diaphyseal injuries.

Current indications include diaphyseal femoral-shaft fractures at least 5 cm below the bottom of the lesser trochanter down to the supracondylar femur including fractures with an intercondylar split. Associated musculoskeletal injuries often favor retrograde over antegrade femoral nailing. The ability to do a retrograde nailing in a patient with an ipsilateral acetabulum fracture, which might require a posterior approach, allows for the femoral shaft to be treated and for a pristine area around the posterior trochanter for fixation of the acetabulum fracture.

Ipsilateral fractures of the femur and knee can often be managed through a single, small incision with placement of a retrograde femoral nail and an antegrade tibial nail. In multiply injured patients with other ipsilateral or contralateral lower-extremity fractures, supine retrograde nailing on a radiolucent table allows either simultaneous or sequential fixation of other fractures, saving valuable operating time.

Bilateral femoral-shaft fractures are excellent candidates for retrograde nailing. One of the best indications for a retrograde nail is an ipsilateral hip and shaft fracture. Most authors recommend independent fixation of both injuries with cannulated screws or a sliding hip screw proximally followed by a retrograde nail for the shaft fracture. This approach allows for the best possible treatment of each fracture without compromising fixation of either one.

Relative indications for retrograde nailing include femoral shaft fracture in the obese or very muscular patient or in patients with trochanter lipodystrophy where antegrade nailing may be difficult. Polytraumatized patients often benefit from rapid positioning on a radiolucent table and freeing the area around the pelvis and abdomen for simultaneous treatment by other surgical disciplines. Although antegrade nailing techniques can be done on a radiolucent table rather than a fracture table, it is still more cumbersome than a retrograde approach. The supine position allows for more physiologic treatment of the lungs and brain in a seriously injured patient being resuscitated.

Contraindications to retrograde nailing include patients with open growth plates; previous anterior cruciate ligament reconstruction; or preexisting hardware or prosthesis that would block a retrograde insertion technique. The use of a retrograde nail in complex, grades IIIA and IIIB, open femur fractures is controversial due to the risk of contamination and subsequent infection in the knee joint. Other treatment modalities, such as bridging external fixation, may be more appropriate.

PREOPERATIVE PLANNING

A detailed history and physical examination of the patient should be performed. Many patients with femur fractures have serious associated limb or life-threatening injuries. The condition of the soft tissues and limb compartments, as well as the neurovascular status should be clearly documented.

Full-length radiographs of the entire femur are necessary. Dedicated radiographs of the knee and hip are needed to rule out intercondylar extension or ipsilateral femoral-neck fractures. Displaced intra-articular fractures are often obvious; however, traction views or fluoroscopic radiographs in the operating room may be helpful in identifying subtle injuries to the knee joint. Full-length films also allow determination of the length and diameter of the intramedullary canal. Small women, persons of Asian descent, and those with developmental problems often have very narrow canals. Most manufacturers do not make retrograde nails smaller than 9 or 10 mm in diameter. This must be recognized prior to surgery so that either a nail of appropriate diameter is available or other surgical options are considered. Many studies have shown that the best results following retrograde femoral nailing are achieved with full-length nails inserted to the lesser trochanter. The surgeon should be certain that a full complement of nails is available at the time of surgery.

The decision to use a percutaneous or limited open approach for nail insertion may be dependent on several factors. The presence of an intra-articular split in the femoral condyles should be a priority concern when planning the approach. Visualization and fixation may be compromised by an ill-placed incision. Cannulated screws of similar metallurgy to the retrograde nail should be available, as well as a sliding hip screw for associated hip fractures. When planning for treatment of an ipsilateral femoral-neck fracture, important decisions must be made prior to surgery about the table and patient position during this combined surgical technique. For patients with multiple fractures, as well as a femoral shaft fracture, proper positioning of all involved extremities and adequate prepping and draping can all be done prior to the initiation of surgery if preoperative planning is performed.

SURGERY: PATIENT POSITIONING, TECHNIQUE, AND RESULTS

Nailing is usually performed under general anesthesia, but in isolated injuries in the elderly, a spinal may be utilized. Retrograde intramedullary femoral nailing is performed with the patient supine on a radiolucent table. Some authors prefer a bolster under the torso, but we believe that this can interfere with the determination of appropriate femoral rotation. With few exceptions, we favor a straight supine position and anterior positioning of the patella. The limb is sterilely prepped and draped from the toes to the iliac crest. It is important to have the entire leg exposed to allow for evaluation of length and rotation, as well as placement of proximal anterior-posterior locking screws.

Knee flexion between 40 and 60 degrees is a key part of the case. Too little knee flexion does not allow for correct position of the guide pin or passage of the reamers and nail, which can impinge on the tibial plateau. Too much flexion can cause the patella to obscure the distal-femoral entry site and leads to excessive shortening in comminuted fractures. Appropriate flexion can be maintained with a radiolucent triangle or sheets used as bolsters with the leg maintained in neutral rotation. For the percutaneous approach, a 2- to 3-cm incision is made just medial to the patellar tendon. Alternatively, a patellar tendon splitting approach can be used. Our preference is medial to the tendon because the incidence of anterior knee pain appears to be less with this approach. The fat pad and synovium are bluntly dissected from the intercondylar region by spreading with a scissors. The intercondylar notch is either visualized through a larger incision or palpated through the percutaneous incision. Anterior-posterior fluoroscopy is used, and a trochar-tipped guide pin is positioned in the center of the notch. Rotation of the fluoroscopy unit to a lateral view needs to confirm that the guide pin is centered just at the tip of the inverted V formed by Blumensaat's line. The guide pin is then inserted 4 to 5 cm into the distal femoral metaphysis, with the surgeon making sure that it is centered in both projections (Fig. 22.1). The entry portal is created with the use of a cannulated 12- or 13-mm straight reamer while the patellar tendon is protected with retractors or a sleeve. The guide pin is then removed (Fig. 22.2).

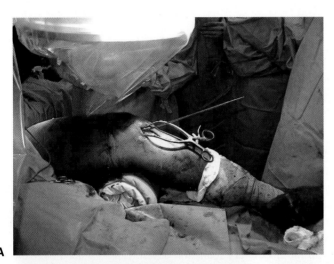

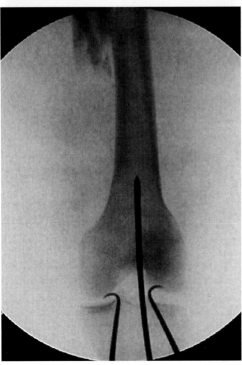

Figure 22.1. **A.** Retrograde nailing through a percutaneous incision and the knee flexed over a bolster at 40 degrees of flexion. Guide pin in place. **B.** Anteroposterior (AP) and **(C)** lateral fluoroscopic views of guide pin placement. Centered on AP view of femoral condyles and at the top of the intercondylar notch; Blumensaat's line is viewed on the lateral view.

A

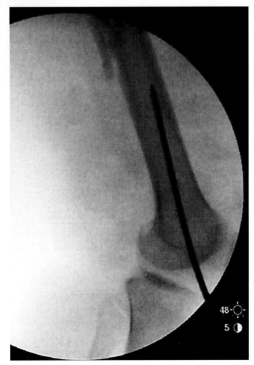

B

C

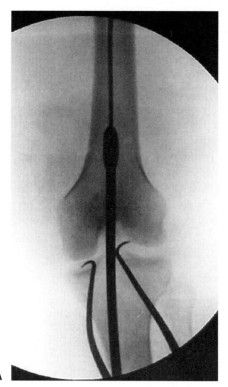

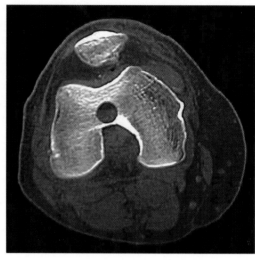

Figure 22.2. A. Rigid reamer inserted over guide pin. **B.** Retrograde nail starting point on computed tomography (CT) scan. Note that it is just above the intercondylar notch.

A 3.2-mm ball-tipped guide wire with a slight bend in the tip is inserted into the distal femur where it was previously reamed. The most difficult part of the surgery may be the reduction of the fracture. Chemical paralysis from anesthesia is helpful to allow for traction on the limb to gain length. Reduction of the fracture can be done by positioning sterile bolsters under the thigh or using external devices to apply forces in the direction appropriate for achieving fracture reduction.

In an alternative approach, an intramedullary reduction device can be placed over the guide rod to manipulate the distal fragment so that it aligns with the proximal fragment, and the guide rod is then inserted up to the intertrochanteric region of the femur. In addition, a terminally threaded guide pin or Schanz pin can be inserted through the cortex and used as a joystick to help with reduction (Figs. 22.3 and 22.4). In some cases, a femoral distractor can be very useful.

Determination of femoral length can then be done with a radiopaque ruler placed on the anterior surface of the leg while slight traction is pulled (Fig. 22.5). The nail should span from 5 mm deep to the articular surface of the knee joint to the level of the lesser trochanter. This span gives the nail a longer working length and better fit in the isthmus to prevent the nail from toggling within the intramedullary canal. Recently, a report on the biomechanics of supracondylar femur fractures suggests that a full-length nail provides better fixation, less of a stress riser at the tip, and minimal windshield-wiper effect in the distal femoral metaphysis.

Adjustments in nail length must be made for comminuted fractures that may be short at the time of nail length determination. Some systems have a reverse depth gauge that can be placed over the guide wire to assess length. For comminuted fractures, the radiopaque ruler can also be placed on the anterior surface of the uninjured limb, and a measurement from the epiphyseal scar distally to the top of the lesser trochanter can give a reasonable estimate and allow for final assessment of nail and femoral length.

Reaming is then performed with flexible reamers and the nail diameter will then be individualized. We usually ream 1 mm greater than cortical chatter and insert a nail 1 mm less than the final reamer size. The plastic intramedullary tube is then used to exchange the ball-tipped guide wire for the stiffer guide wire used for nail insertion. The insertion and

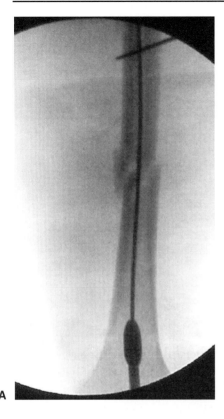

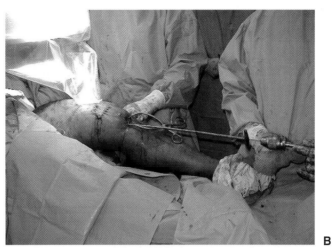

Figure 22.3. A. Radiograph showing insertion of a reduction tool in the distal femur to facilitate fracture reduction with ball-tip guide rod inside of tool. Note Schanz pin proximally placed in segmental piece to aid in reduction. **B.** Reduction tool in distal femur with ball-tip guide rod inside. Lateral traction on the segmental piece through the Schanz pin.

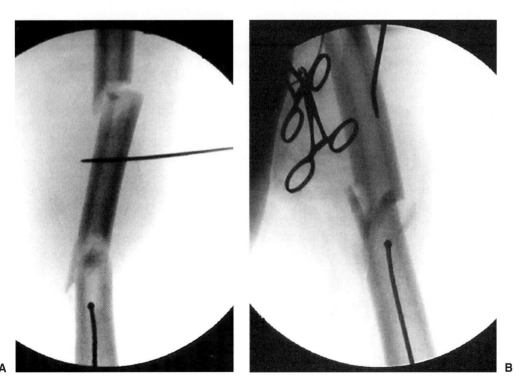

Figure 22.4. A. Ball-tip guide rod in distal metaphysis and **(B)** threaded guide pin in the anterior portion of the segmental fragment to control this segment and help with reduction.

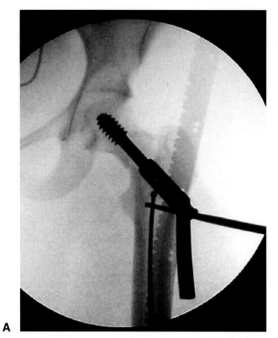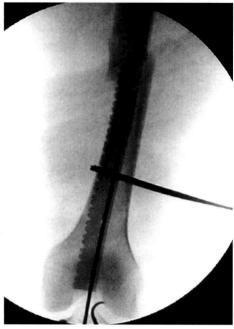

A   B

Figure 22.5. A. Placing guide rod up to lesser trochanter and barrel of sliding hip screw.
B. Measurement of nail length using radiopaque ruler.

targeting guide is inserted onto the nail with the outrigger for distal screw-locking placed
laterally. The nail is then inserted with light blows from a mallet or slap hammer. The
patella is placed in a straight anterior orientation, pointing toward the ceiling.

Recognition of nail insertion depth, femoral length, and rotation are critical steps prior
to final nail seating and locking. There are rings on the insertion jig that may be visible with
the fluoroscope. The most reliable way to assure that the nail is at least 3 to 5 mm deep to
the articular surface is to place the most distal locking screw at or just above the epiphyseal
scar. With most retrograde nails, the most distal screw hole is 15 mm from the tip of the
nail. One distal locking screw inserted percutaneously through the distal locking jig is sufficient for diaphyseal fractures with greater than 50% cortical contact. Two screws should
be used for comminuted and spiral fractures that do not have axial stability (Fig. 22.6). Distal third femur fractures should also have two distal locking screws applied to prevent the
nail from toggling with flexion and extension of the knee. Prior to proximal locking, final
determination of length must be ascertained.

For those fractures that were lengthened during nailing, slight mallet blows on the insertion handle after distal interlocking will close the cortical gap. More commonly, comminuted fractures will shorten during the insertion of the retrograde nail. To help restore
femoral length, a slap hammer device is used after the insertion of the distal interlocking
screws to back slap the nail in the direction of nail removal. Sometimes length can be
sufficiently judged by cortical alignment. When comminution is extensive, preoperative
measurement of the contralateral limb from epiphyseal scar to the top of the lesser
trochanter with placement of the same length nail to those landmarks should give proper
measurement for restoration of femoral length.

Light blows in a reverse direction with the slap hammer will usually not result in over
distraction due to the intact iliotibial band. Once length has been determined to be appropriate, the insertion device can be removed. A fingertip placed in the insertion site should show
that the tip of the nail is 3 to 5 mm deep to the articular surface. The nail should not be prominent by even 1 mm at the notch because this may adversely affect the patellofemoral joint.
With the limb in neutral rotation and the knee bolster removed, fluoroscopy of the proximal
nail holes in an anterior-posterior direction is performed. The perfect circle technique of rotating of the limb or c-arm until round holes are obtained is essential to proximal interlock-

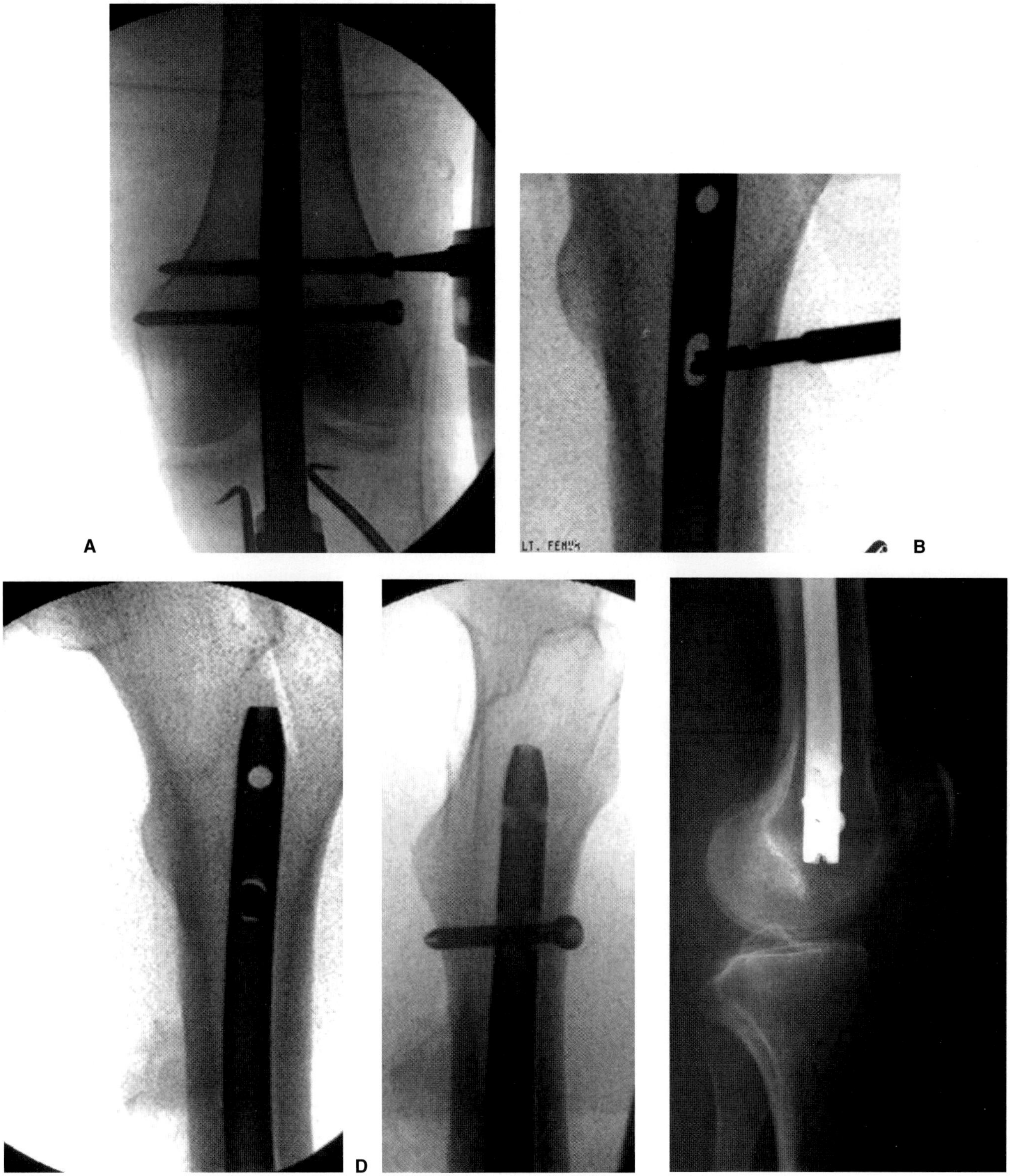

Figure 22.6. A. Placement of distal locking screws using insertion handle outrigger and jig. **B.** Using the free hand perfect circle technique for insertion of the proximal locking screw in the dynamic slot in the nail. **C.** Placement of the proximal locking screw with a locking screwdriver or suture tied around the screw head. **D.** Frog lateral view obtained in operating room to check the length and bicortical location of the proximal screw. **E.** Lateral radiograph demonstrating proper insertion of the retrograde nail deep to the articular cartilage after insertion handle removal.

ing. A 1- to 2-cm anterior incision is made over the screw hole as determined by fluoroscopy. The quadriceps fascia is opened sharply with a knife, and a hemostat is used to spread down to the bone. A trochar, tipped, short, drill bit is inserted at a 45-degree angle onto the anterior femoral cortex such that the tip of the drill is centered in the hole. For those nails with a dynamic slot proximally placed, insertion in this hole can be done proximally or distally, depending on the fracture morphology. For axially stable fractures, the dynamic screw can be placed in the top of the hole to allow for compression with weight bearing. For unstable fractures, the screw can be placed in the bottom of the hole to work as a buttress screw to prevent further shortening. The drill is inserted through the proximal cortex perpendicular to the head of the fluoroscope, and the drill is removed from the drill bit. Fluoroscopy can then be used to evaluate the position of the drill bit in the hole. Minor adjustments to the drill bit can then be made, and once the bit is centered in the hole, a mallet can be used to gently push the bit through the hole in the nail. The drill bit is then attached back onto the drill, and the far, posterior, cortex is drilled. Careful attention should be made to not plunge too deep with this drill bit because the sciatic nerve lies posterior to the femur at this level. A depth gauge is used to determine screw length, and a locking screw driver is used to insert the proximal screw. If a locking screwdriver is not available, then an absorbable suture can be tied to the neck of the screw during insertion to that the screw is not dropped or lost in the soft tissues of the thigh during insertion. Final screw seating should be checked by finger palpation and a cross-table lateral of the limb to assure that the screw is fully seated. Often the screw will tighten when just entering the far cortex and give the illusion of final seating of the screw head. One screw is sufficient for most fractures, with the exception of subtrochanteric fractures where there is limited isthmal fixation of the proximal fragment (see Fig. 22.6).

All wounds are irrigated with sterile saline. The patellar-tendon insertion site is closed in layers with absorbable suture and a routine skin closure. The lateral screw insertion site is closed in layers starting with the iliotibial band and then the subcutaneous tissue and the skin. The proximal locking site is closed only with subcutaneous absorbable suture and skin closure. The wounds are dressed with sterile pads, and a compression bandage is used from toes to groin with tape over the anterior proximal locking site. With the drapes removed, the length, angulation, and rotation of the two limbs are compared. The ipsilateral knee is also examined for ligamentous instability.

POSTOPERATIVE MANAGEMENT

Active range of motion is encouraged in the early postoperative period, and continuous passive motion machines are reserved for multiply injured or head injury patients who are at higher risk for knee stiffness or heterotopic ossification. Full extension and flexion greater than 90 degrees should be obtained between 6 and 8 weeks. Weight bearing can be initiated early in axially stable fractures and is usually delayed 6 to 10 weeks until callus is apparent on postoperative radiographs in unstable fractures. Most fractures heal between 3 and 5 months.

COMPLICATIONS

Nonunion is more frequent when small diameter, noncanal filling nails are employed. Reamed canal-sized implants have been shown to achieve union rates greater than 90%, which equals antegrade nailing. In patients with delays in union, dynamization can be performed on axially stable fractures. This is most commonly performed in fractures that are showing callus but have a gap at the fracture site with a well-fitting nail. Usually, the proximal screw is removed to allow the nail to move in a proximal direction with compression of the fracture site and not toward the knee joint. Pain caused by the distal screw is common and is often caused by screws that are too long, but is found in patients in which screws of the proper length were used. The most distal locking screw is inserted into the trapezoidal distal femur, and screws that appear with their tips just outside the medial femoral cortex are usually too long. Sometimes screw heads are palpable or cause an auditory click on the iliotibial band in thin patients. Distal screws can be removed with an outpatient procedure once union has occurred, or a painful screw may be removed once abundant callus is visible on radiographs. Knee pain is uncommon with proper operative technique. In patients with limited knee motion, we recommend an aggressive physical therapy program for limb rehabilitation. Full extension and flexion to 120 degrees should be expected with a well-placed, retrograde, femoral nail. Residual anterior knee pain is occasionally seen and is most common secondary to trauma and residual weakness in the quadriceps muscle with patellar maltracking rather than impingement from the retrograde nail.

Determination of proper limb length in axially unstable fractures can be a problem with either antegrade or retrograde nailing techniques. For unstable fractures, back slapping of the nail after screw insertion can help overcome shortening (Fig. 22.7). For bilateral fractures, by treating the stable fracture first and then using the same length nail in the same position on the unstable fracture, surgeons will ensure appropriate length of the limb. Fractures at the tip of the implant have been reported in osteoporotic bone with the use of a short nail. Full-length nails are suggested for all fractures, including those in the supracondylar region (Fig. 22.8).

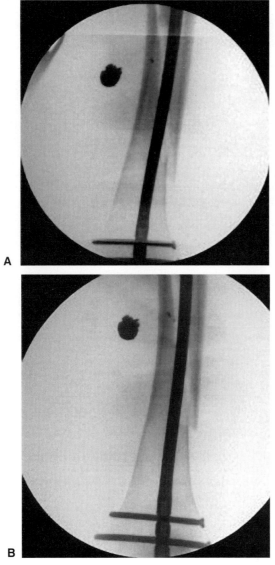

Figure 22.7. **A.** Retrograde nailing of gunshot fracture of femur with axially unstable, long, spiral fracture of the femur. Note shortening of femur after insertion of retrograde nail. **B.** Following distal locking of the insertion jig, back slapping the nail until soft tissues tighten restores femoral length prior to proximal freehand locking.

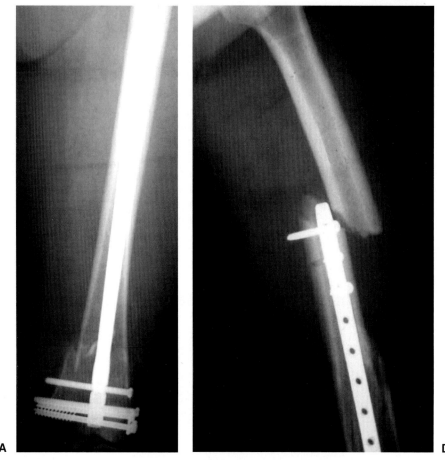

Figure 22.8. A. Intercondylar-supracondylar femur fracture treated with a lag screw and full-length retrograde nail up to lesser trochanter. **B.** Diaphyseal fracture after the patient fell. Note tip of a short retrograde nail.

RECOMMENDED READING

Gregory P, DiCicco J, Karpik K, et al. Ipsilateral fractures of the femur and tibia: treatment with retrograde femoral nailing and unreamed tibial nailing. *J Orthop Trauma* 1996;10(5):309–316.

Herscovici D, Whiteman KW. Retrograde nailing of the femur using an intercondylar notch approach. *Clin Orthop Relat Res* 1996;332:98–104.

Moed BR, Watson JT. Retrograde intramedullary nailing, without reaming, of fractures of the femoral shaft in multiply injured patients. *J Bone Joint Surg Am* 1995;77A:1520–1527.

Ostrum RF. Treatment of floating knee injuries through a single percutaneous approach. *Clin Orthop* 2000;375:43–50.

Ostrum RF, Agarwal A, Lakatos R, et al. Prospective comparison of retrograde and antegrade femoral intramedullary nailing. *J Orthop Trauma* 2000;14:496–501.

Ostrum RF, DiCicco J, Lakatos R, et al. Retrograde intramedullary nailing of femoral diaphyseal fractures. *J Orthop Trauma* 1998;12:464–468.

Ricci WM, Bellabarba C, Evanoff B, et al. Retrograde versus antegrade nailing of femoral shaft fractures. *J Orthop Trauma* 2001;15:161–169.

Sears BR, Ostrum RF, Litsky AS. A mechanical study of gap motion in cadaveric femurs using short and long supracondylar nails. *J Orthop Trauma* 2004;18:354–360.

Tornetta P III, Tiburzi D. Antegrade or retrograde reamed femoral nailing: a prospective, randomised trial. *J Bone Joint Surg Br* 2000;82:652–654.

23

Supracondylar Femur Fractures: Open Reduction Internal Fixation

Sean E. Nork

INDICATIONS/CONTRAINDICATIONS

Distal femoral fractures are common and affect patients of all ages. In older patients, these fractures are frequently the result of a fall from a standing position. However, in younger patients, high-energy mechanisms are common and include motor vehicle crashes, falls from height, and industrial injuries. In these patients, associated ipsilateral extremity injuries frequently occur. The entire lower extremity should be examined to identify any associated open wounds or neurovascular injuries. Although lateral and anterolateral open wounds are more common, medial and posterior open wounds exist and may suggest significant, associated, soft-tissue stripping. Compartmental syndrome, while rare, can occur in association with fractures of the distal femur and should be adequately evaluated.

The vast majority of supracondylar and/or intercondylar, distal, femoral fractures in adults are treated operatively because surgical stabilization allows early knee motion, patient mobilization, and may decrease the incidence of posttraumatic arthritis. Because of the significant muscular attachments surrounding the knee joint, maintenance of the proper anatomical and mechanical axes is difficult with nonoperative treatment. Closed management is usually reserved for elderly patients with significant medical co-morbidities and nonambulatory patients. Significant articular comminution and/or associated bone loss are not considered contraindications to operative treatment.

PREOPERATIVE PLANNING

Unlike many tibial plateau or pilon fractures, the majority of distal femoral fractures can be treated definitively with early operative fixation. If surgical treatment is imminently planned, the limb can be temporarily stabilized with a knee immobilizer, a bulky dressing, or proximal tibial traction. In certain circumstances (open fractures with significant contamination, severe soft-tissue swelling, significant patient co-morbidities, unavailability of the proper implants and/or surgical personnel), surgery may be delayed. Depending on the age of the patient, the amount of shortening and the degree of comminution, a temporary, spanning, external fixation is often recommended.

The initial radiographic evaluation consists of high-quality anteroposterior (AP) and lateral radiographs of the knee joint and the distal femur. Traction films are helpful in comminuted and shortened fracture patterns but may not be tolerated in all patients. Radiographs of the contralateral leg can assist with preoperative planning. Computed tomography (CT) scans can be helpful for understanding the patterns of comminution and for determining the appropriate surgical approach and implants. This is particularly true in high-energy injuries but may be useful in all distal femoral fractures. Coronal plane fractures of the medial and lateral condyles (Hoffa fracture) may be difficult to recognize on the injury and/or traction radiographs. Depending on the location of comminution in the distal femur, the surgical approach may require alteration. Despite numerous classification systems for distal femoral fractures, the AO/OTA system is the most useful, allows effective communication, and may influence surgical treatment (Fig. 23.1).

The distal femoral anatomy must be understood prior to considering a fixation strategy. The distal femur is trapezoidal when viewed from distal to proximal. The lateral metaphyseal surface is angulated approximately 10 degrees while the medial side surface is

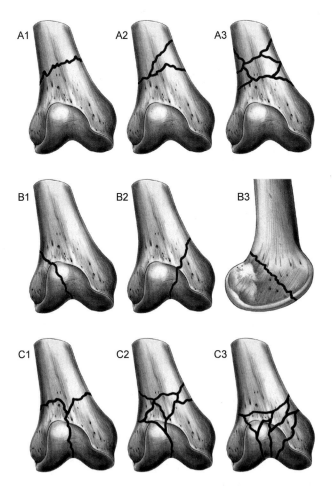

Figure 23.1. The AO/OTA Classification of distal femoral fractures. 33A fractures are extra-articular and can be treated with plates or medullary implants. 33B fractures are articular injuries that are best treated with open reduction and compression across the fracture; locked implants are not indicated for these fractures. 33C fractures require restoration of the articular surface as well as the relationship of the distal articular segment to the shaft of the femur.

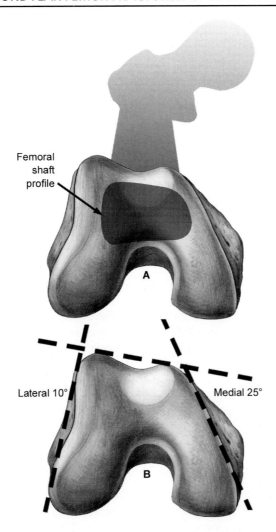

Figure 23.2. The distal femoral anatomy as it relates to plate applications. The lateral metaphysis is angulated 10 degrees from the sagittal plane; the medial metaphysis is angulated 25 degrees from the sagittal plane. To avoid a medial translational deformity of the articular surface, lateral plate applications should follow the sloped, lateral, metaphyseal surface. To ensure that screws are contained within the distal femur, the anterior location of the metaphysis must be appreciated. Anterior implants are shorter than those angulated or placed more posteriorly.

angulated approximately 25 degrees (Fig. 23.2). This combination contributes to the widening of the condyles posteriorly relative to their anterior width. The lateral condyle extends farther anteriorly relative to the medial condyle, producing a posterior slope between the anterior condylar prominences when viewed from lateral to medial. The distal extent of the intercondylar articular surface is best appreciated on the lateral radiograph, which can be useful for determining the safe placement of implants during fixation. The central axis of the femoral shaft normally aligns with the anterior half of the femoral condyles as viewed laterally. This alignment is especially important to assess by surgeons considering the accurate placement of lateral plate constructs.

Comparison radiographs with the contralateral knee are useful for determining the patient's unique condylar width and distal femoral axes. Knowledge of the condylar width can be helpful for planning the length of implants placed in the distal femoral segment. Because of the distal femoral shape, the relative angulation of implants must be considered. Implants placed anteriorly and horizontally will be appreciably shorter than those placed perpendicular to the lateral cortex (and therefore with 10 to 15 degrees of posterior angulation). The mechanical axis of the lower extremity helps determine the proper, anatomic, valgus angulation of the lower extremity. The typical 5 to 9 degrees of anatomical tibiofemoral valgus can be most accurately appreciated from a contralateral extremity radiograph. Similarly, the location of the mechanical axis at the knee joint can be determined intraoperatively. The normal valgus angulation of the distal femur becomes apparent during intraoperative lateral imaging as well. For the femoral condyles to overlap perfectly, the fluoroscopic beam must be appropriately positioned to compensate for the distal femoral valgus.

In general, a formal preoperative plan should be constructed on tracing paper in anticipation of the surgical procedure. This requires the availability of radiographs printed at 100% magnification. With the rapid conversion to digital recording of radiographic images at many hospitals, preoperative templating is quickly becoming a lost art. The outline of the normal distal femur should be drawn first. Then, the injured extremity-fracture fragments should be drawn on a separate piece of templating paper. The fractured segments should then be drawn into the normal outline of the distal femur (with the proper left vs. right reflection) on both the AP and lateral drawings. Based upon the fracture configuration, the bone quality, and the availability of implants, an appropriate fixation construct can be chosen.

Temporary, Spanning, External Fixation

Temporary, spanning, external fixation can be helpful in multiply injured patients and in patients with complex fracture patterns. It usually consists of a knee joint–spanning external fixator with pins placed into the tibia and the femur. Femoral pin placement can be directly anterior, directly lateral, or anterolateral. Regardless of their entry orientation, pins should be placed proximal to the anticipated surgical incision(s) for definitive fixation. Some knee flexion (10 to 20 degrees) is recommended and improves the commonly observed extension deformity of the distal femoral segment.

Fixation Devices

The primary focus of this chapter is on the fixation of combined supracondylar and intercondylar (AO/OTA 33C) distal femoral fractures. However, because of the versatility and number of implants appropriate for fractures of the distal femur, other fracture patterns will be mentioned. Fractures without articular involvement (33A fractures) can be treated with antegrade nails, retrograde nails, and lateral plate constructs. The choice of implant in these injuries is largely dependent upon the surgeon's comfort, the patient's associated injuries, and the predicted management of any potential complications due to the injury or the treatment. Fractures with partial articular involvement (lateral condyle fractures, medial condyle fractures, or tangential fractures of the posterior condyle) can be treated with lag screws, conventional plates, or a combination of both. For fractures with both supracondylar and intercondylar involvement, effective implants include conventional lateral plates (condylar buttress plate, precontoured lateral plates specific for the distal femur), lateral plates with a fixed angle (95-degree angled blade plate, dynamic condylar screw), and lateral locking plates (Fig. 23.3). In general, the surgical tactic and reduction are more important than the implant.

Conventional lateral plates are inexpensive and easy to apply. Angulation of the screws in the distal segment may be advantageous in fractures where multiple lag screws are required to stabilize any articular-surface comminution. The biggest disadvantage is the inability of these implants to prevent postoperative varus deformation due to screw loosening, especially in the distal articular block. This may be most significant in open fractures, patients with osteopenia, and fractures with associated bone loss.

Fixed-angled lateral implants include the 95-degree angled blade plate, the 95-degree condylar screw, and the lateral fixed-angled screw-plate devices. All of these implants have the advantage of minimizing varus deformation by eliminating screw toggling in the distal metaphyseal bone. Blade plates can be placed quite distally and do not remove significant bone from the distal articular segment. However, these implants are technically difficult to place and require a single perfect entry location. This is especially important in distal

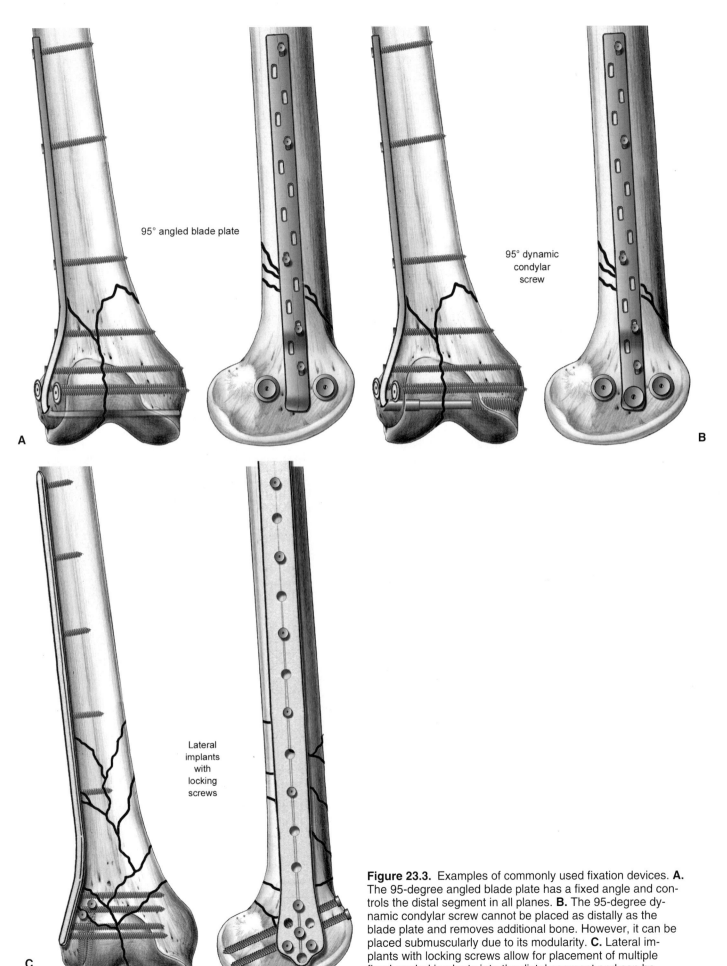

95° angled blade plate

95° dynamic
condylar
screw

Lateral
implants
with
locking
screws

A

B

C

Figure 23.3. Examples of commonly used fixation devices. **A.** The 95-degree angled blade plate has a fixed angle and controls the distal segment in all planes. **B.** The 95-degree dynamic condylar screw cannot be placed as distally as the blade plate and removes additional bone. However, it can be placed submuscularly due to its modularity. **C.** Lateral implants with locking screws allow for placement of multiple fixed-angled implants into the distal segment and can be placed submuscularly.

femoral fractures with associated articular comminution that require a prior surgical stabilization of the multiple articular fragments. These implants may prevent ideal placement of the condylar blade distally. The dynamic condylar screw is easier to implant and allows submuscular implantation. However, this device removes a significant amount of bone and cannot be placed as distally as an angled blade plate. Locking plates, in addition to maintaining the coronal plane reduction, allow for placement of multiple fixed implants (screws) into the distal segment. Thus, they allow for some flexibility in screw location and may be more forgiving. These implants have the further advantage of having specifically designed surgical jigs that enhance submuscular implantation.

SURGERY

Patient Positioning

The patient is positioned supine on a radiolucent table that allows unimpeded fluoroscopic imaging in both planes. A small bump placed beneath the ipsilateral hip should be sized to ensure that the femur is in neutral rotation, assisting with the intraoperative assessment of extremity rotation during and after reduction. The knee is placed in slight flexion over a custom ramp or folded blankets with an additional small rolled bump at the fracture site (Fig. 23.4). This improves the sagittal plane reduction of the fracture by relaxing the primary deforming force of the gastrocnemius. In addition, this position facilitates intraoperative, lateral, fluoroscopic imaging of the proximal thigh without obstruction from the contralateral extremity.

The entire limb is prepped and draped from the ipsilateral pelvis to the toes, allowing intraoperative manipulation of the leg and access to the femur proximally as needed. If traction radiographs in the AP and lateral planes have not been obtained previously, these can be obtained at this time. A sterile tourniquet can be applied proximally if desired.

Incision and Surgical Approaches

The choice of surgical approach is determined by the fracture location and pattern, any associated comminution, the primary reduction techniques, and the implant. In general, an

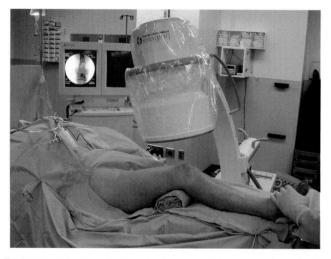

Figure 23.4. Patient positioning. Supine positioning with a bump beneath the ipsilateral hip improves orientation of the limb anatomically relative to the fluoroscopy machine. A bump placed beneath the fracture combined with knee flexion assists sagittal plane reduction of the fracture.

extensile lateral approach can be used for most supracondylar and intercondylar distal femoral fractures (Fig. 23.5). This approach allows access to the lateral femoral condyle, the intercondylar region, and the entire lateral femur. This approach can be useful for both open plating techniques and minimally invasive techniques. The lateral exposure can be limited to that necessary for reduction of the articular surface in cases where submuscular techniques are chosen for stabilization of the articular segment to the femoral diaphysis. A lateral parapatellar approach may be used in fracture patterns with significant intercondylar comminution, coronal plane fractures, or both. Although this approach allows access to intercondylar comminution, trochlear comminution, and most medial and lateral coronal condylar fractures, it is not as easily extended proximally to allow a lateral plate application on the femoral diaphysis. This approach may be most useful is cases where minimally invasive or percutaneous methods are anticipated for plate application proximally (Figs. 23.6 and 23.7). Infrequently, a medial subvastus approach may be required in conjunction with a lateral approach. This approach should be limited to the articular segment, respecting the more proximal, medial, soft-tissue attachments. In all surgical approaches, the posterior and medial soft-tissue attachments to any metaphyseal bone segments should be left intact.

Open Fractures

In open, distal, femoral fractures, as with any open fracture, a thorough debridement of any devitalized tissue is necessary prior to reduction and definitive fixation. The ideal incision for the surgical approach necessary for fracture fixation should first be marked on the skin. The open wound can be incorporated into the incision if appropriate. However, an extensile approach that allows exposure and debridement of the open fracture as well as reduction of the distal femur should be a priority over an objective to minimize the number of scars around the knee. This is particularly true in patients with traumatic open wounds located medially.

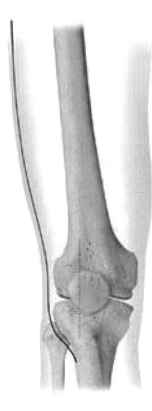
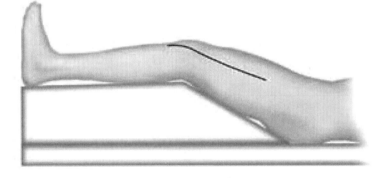

Figure 23.5. An extensile lateral approach is useful for many fractures of the distal femur, especially those that are fixed with a direct application of the plate to the lateral femur.

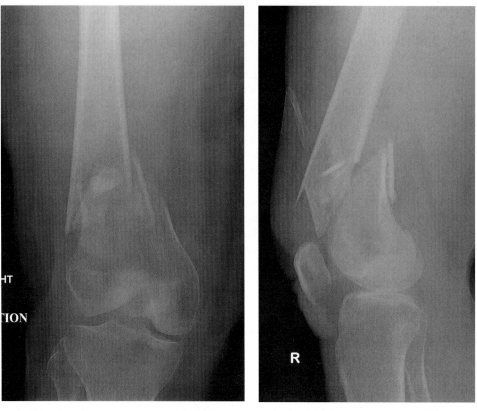

A   B

Figure 23.6. A 33C2 fracture of the distal femur in an elderly patient. **A.** The AP view demonstrates the simple intercondylar component of the fracture. **B.** The lateral view suggests the integrity of the medial and lateral condyles (i.e., no associated coronal-plane fractures).

In general, any bone fragments without soft tissue attachments should be discarded. However, every attempt should be made to retain any articular fracture fragments. If definitive fixation is delayed (either due to the need for a second debridement or due to the combination of fracture complexity and surgical timing), consideration should be given to placing a spanning external fixator as previously described. Antibiotic beads can be placed into any metaphyseal defect that may exist after debridement.

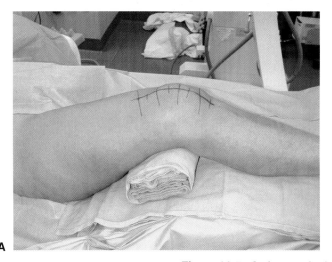
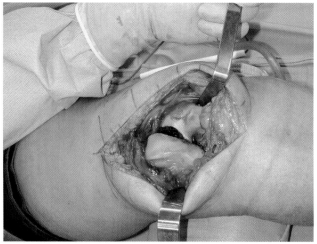

A   B

Figure 23.7. **A.** An anterior incision can be used for a lateral parapatellar arthrotomy. **B.** A limited approach allows excellent exposure of the articular surface in cases where a submuscular approach is anticipated for the lateral-femoral plate application.

Surgical Tactic

By avoiding dissection of the medial soft tissues in the distal-femoral metaphyseal region, healing should proceed predictably in most supracondylar/intercondylar fractures. Therefore, most lateral plate devices will be effective in the majority of fracture patterns. Because of the tendency for these fractures to collapse into varus prior to healing, a fixed-angled implant (angled blade plate or dynamic condylar screw) or a locking implant can be considered for most fracture patterns. The location and severity of articular comminution combined with the implants necessary to reduced them may make the use of certain implants difficult. The use of minimally invasive and percutaneous techniques, which attach the distal, femoral, articular component to the femoral shaft, helps to maintain the blood supply to the metaphyseal fracture fragments (Fig. 23.8). However, an open technique can also be performed in which soft-tissue attachments are respected. As a general rule, the distal, femoral, articular surface is first anatomically reduced and stabilized with multiple lag screws and then the articular block can be reduced and fixed to the femoral diaphysis.

Articular Reduction

Typically, coronal plane fractures are reduced and stabilized prior to reduction of the intercondylar component. For coronal plane fractures of the lateral femoral condyle, the articular surface can be reduced and compressed with a pointed clamp, followed by placement of lag screws (Fig. 23.9). The location and angulation of the fracture plane determine the direction and location of the screws. Usually, 3.5-mm lag screws can be placed from anterior to posterior, perpendicular to the fracture, and angulated approximately 10 degrees from medial to lateral. The screw heads should be countersunk beneath the patellofemoral articular surface when necessary.

For coronal fractures of the medial femoral condyle, angulation of up to 25 degrees from lateral to medial may be required. Two screws are usually adequate for simple coronal plane fractures. The intercondylar fracture can then be reduced and stabilized. All hematoma and loose osseous fragments should be removed from the intercondylar fracture prior to attempting a reduction. Joysticks (2.0-mm to 2.4-mm wires) placed into each femoral condyle can assist with reducing the flexion/extension deformities seen with each condyle. A clamp can then be placed across the fracture, securing the two condyles and compressing the intercondylar fracture. Depending on the location and size of the surgical approach, this clamp may be placed either within the surgical arthrotomy or through small percutaneous stab incisions. The intercondylar fracture can then be secured with multiple 3.5-mm lag screws placed from lateral to medial. These screws should be placed strategically in anticipation of a lateral plate. For fracture patterns with more extensive comminution, 2.0-mm, 2.4-mm, and 2.7-mm screws may be necessary. Intraosseous screws and those placed through the articular surface should be adequately countersunk.

Reduction of the Articular Segment to the Shaft

The entire articular block can then be reduced to the femoral shaft, spanning any areas of metaphyseal comminution. If the metaphyseal fracture component is simple, then a direct, open, lateral reduction can be used. No attempt should be made to reduce the medial metaphyseal components of the fracture. Similarly, if multiple intercalary fracture fragments exist, the temptation to directly reduce and stabilize these components should be avoided. The distal, femoral, articular segment is usually in an extended position relative to the shaft due to the attachment of the gastrocnemius. With increasing longitudinal traction applied to the limb, this deformity frequently increases. A bump placed at the distal femur will allow flexion of the fracture, reducing the extension deformity. If some deformity

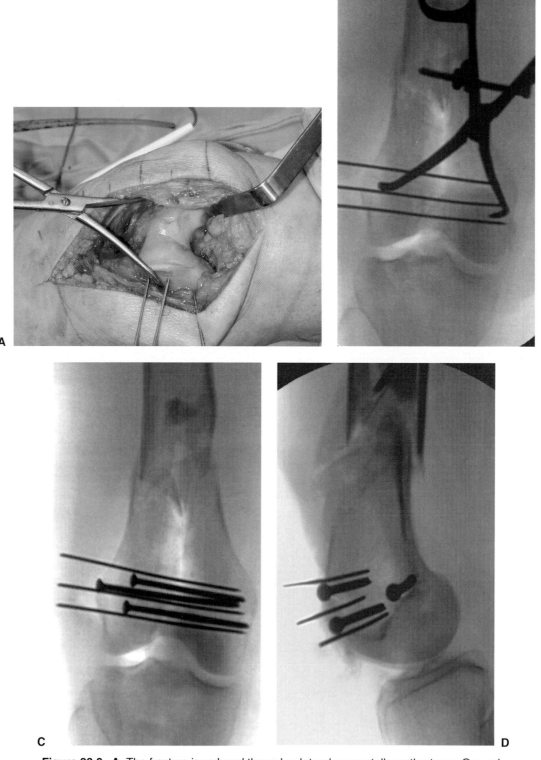

Figure 23.8. A. The fracture is reduced through a lateral parapatellar arthrotomy. One advantage of this approach is that it allows for clamp application within the arthrotomy, as well as visualization of the medial and lateral femoral condyles for reduction of coronal plane fractures (if present). **B.** Multiple K wires can be placed to secure the reduction. **C,D.** Multiple lag screws can then be strategically placed to secure the reduction of the intercondylar fracture. These screws should be placed such that they allow placement of the lateral implant. (*continues*)

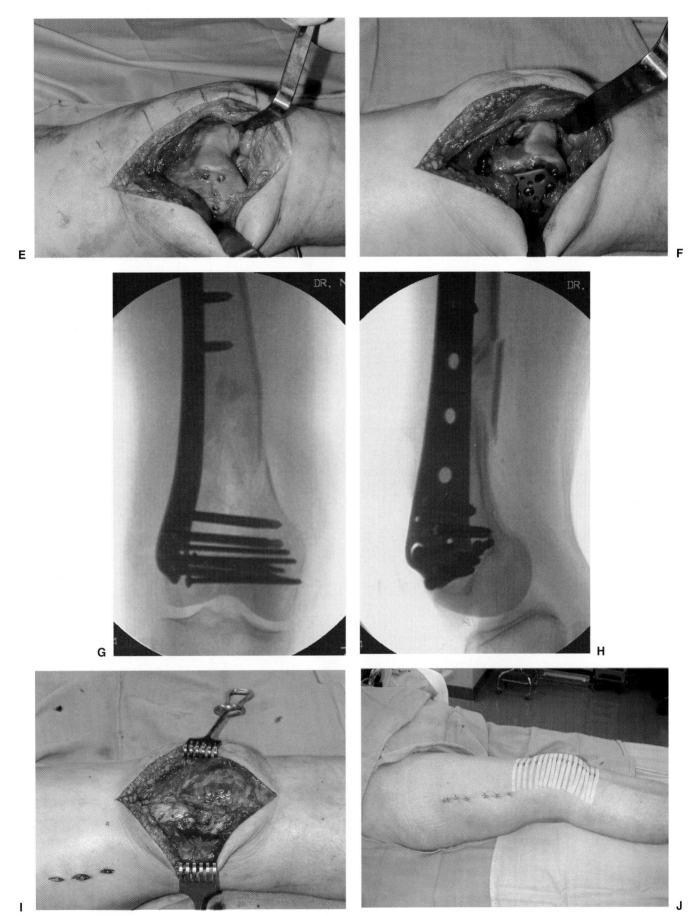

Figure 23.8. (*continued*) **E.** In this case, a lateral locking plate is planned; therefore, these 3.5-mm screws are placed peripherally to allow placement of the plate. **F.** A plate can then be slid in a submuscular fashion and secured to the distal segment. **G,H.** The length and alignment are maintained as the implant is applied to the lateral femur. **I.** The lateral parapatellar arthrotomy is closed and **(J)** the appearance of the limb after wound closure.

persists, joysticks placed from anterior to posterior in the distal segment can be used to restore the proper flexion. The coronal plane alignment can usually be corrected with manual angulation of the extremity.

If a fixed-angled device (such as a 95-degree angled blade plate, a dynamic condylar screw, or a locking condylar plate) is used, the implant is typically fixed to the distal articular block and indirect techniques are used to align this segment with the shaft. The inser-

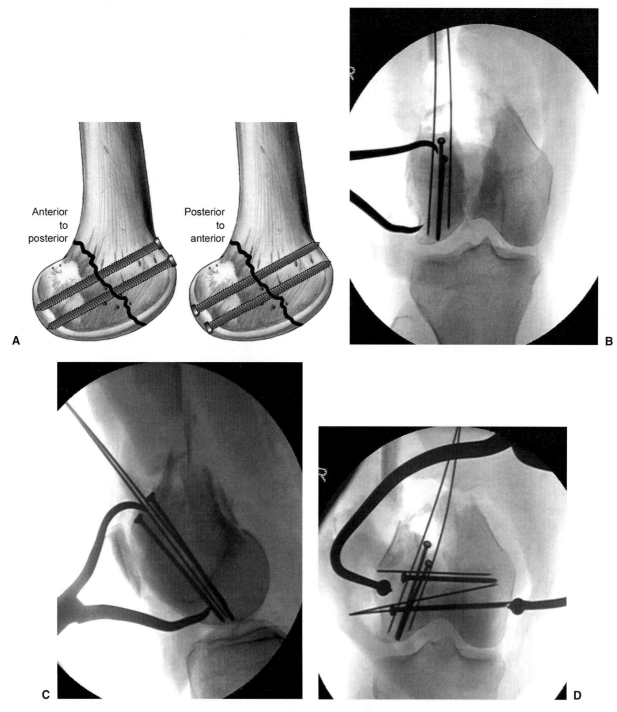

Figure 23.9. Associated comminution in the coronal plane occurs more commonly at the lateral femoral condylar and can be stabilized with lag screws placed perpendicular to the fracture line. **A.** The anterior to posterior direction is usually preferred. In this example, **(B)** the lateral coronal fracture is first reduced and held with a clamp. **C.** Lag screws are then placed perpendicular to the fracture. **D.** The intercondylar component of the fracture can then be reduced, clamped, and temporarily stabilized with K wires. (*continues*)

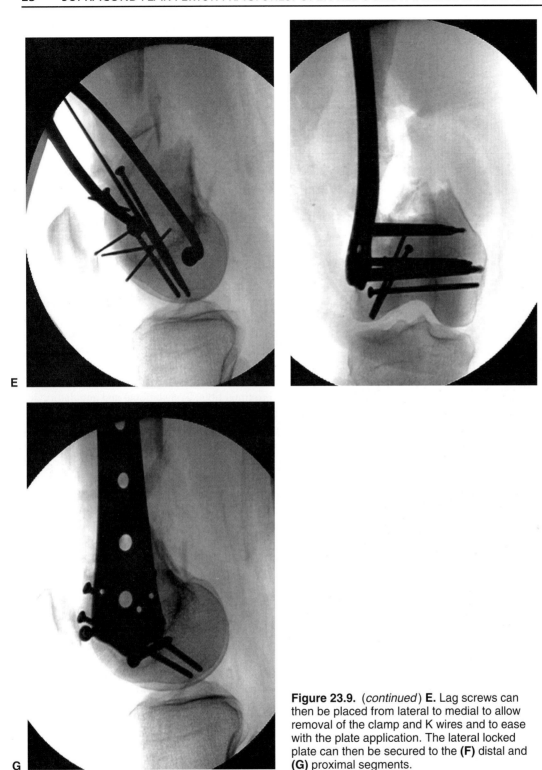

Figure 23.9. (*continued*) **E.** Lag screws can then be placed from lateral to medial to allow removal of the clamp and K wires and to ease with the plate application. The lateral locked plate can then be secured to the **(F)** distal and **(G)** proximal segments.

tion angle, location, and angulation of the implant in the articular segment determine the final reduction of the distal femur. The usual location for insertion is 1.5 cm (angled-blade plate) or 2.0 cm (dynamic condylar screw) proximal to the articular surface and in the middle third of the anterior half of the distal femoral as viewed from the lateral surface. The angle of insertion is parallel to the distal, femoral, articular surface and perpendicular to the lateral femoral metaphysis. Implants placed horizontal relative to the lateral, femoral, distal surface lead to medial displacement and internal rotation deformities.

The shaft can then be reduced to the plate while alignment is maintained. The plate should be of sufficient length such that at least five screw holes are entirely proximal to the fracture. Proximal plate length is more important than the number of screws in the proximal segment. Limb length can be restored using a femoral distractor, the articulated tensioning device, a push screw with a lamina spreader, or with manual traction. When the length is properly obtained, the plate can be secured to the lateral femoral shaft with a reduction clamp. In noncomminuted fractures, the fracture can be compressed using the articulated tensioning device. In most cases, supracondylar comminution exists and the plate is statically fixed to the lateral femur after the proper length is obtained. Three or four bicortical screws maximally spread in the shaft component should be placed. If a long plate is used, the mismatch between the sagittal plane bows that are between the bone and the plate will be accentuated, necessitating a more posterior plate application to ensure that the implant is not off the bone proximally.

Minimally Invasive Reduction Techniques

An accurate articular reduction through an open approach is necessary prior to stabilization of the distal articular block to the shaft (Fig. 23.10). Minimally invasive techniques are useful primarily for reduction of the articular block to the femoral shaft. Virtually all implants can be fixed to the femoral shaft using minimally invasive techniques. Proper length, translation, and alignment should be accurately restored or an open approach is required. Length is best accomplished with either manual traction or a femoral distractor placed anteriorly from the femoral diaphysis to the proximal tibia. Translational and angulatory deformities are best corrected manually with joysticks, mallets, pushers, or bumps. Prior to fixing the implant to the distal articular segment, the plate is slid in a submuscular fashion along the lateral aspect of the femur using a combination of tactile feedback and visual clues from the fluoroscopic imaging. It is important to ensure that the implant is fixed to the midlateral aspect of the femur along its entire length. Frequently, lateral implants are angulated at least 10 degrees posteriorly to ensure proper position in the distal fragment. As a result, fluoroscopic confirmation of proper plate placement on the lateral femur requires limb external rotation.

Unicondylar Fractures

For isolated unicondylar medial or lateral condyle fractures, the surgical approach is dictated by the fracture location. Most lateral condyle fractures (AO/OTA 33B1) can be approached from an extensile lateral approach to the distal femur, similar to that for many supracondylar-intercondylar fractures. However, if extensive involvement of the intercondylar notch is noted on the CT scan, consideration can be given to using a lateral parapatellar approach to better visualize this articular reduction. In medial condyle fractures (AO/OTA 33B2), a medial subvastus approach is extensile proximally and allows excellent visualization of the articular reduction.In either case, the sagittal plane rotation of the condyle must be reduced perfectly at both the proximal cortical exit and the intercondylar articular surface. If significant articular comminution is present, this must be accurately reduced prior to reduction of the major condylar fragment. Temporary Kirschner (K) wire fixations are useful for maintaining these reductions. If visualization is difficult, a knee-spanning femoral distractor can be of assistance. Fixation can usually be accomplished with a combination of lag screws placed perpendicular to the fracture line and an antiglide plate placed proximally (Fig. 23.11).

For lateral condyle Hoffa fractures (AO/OTA 33B3), a lateral approach with a lateral arthrotomy allows visualization of the articular reduction as well as clamp applications for compression and stabilization. For medial condyle Hoffa fractures, a medial subvas-

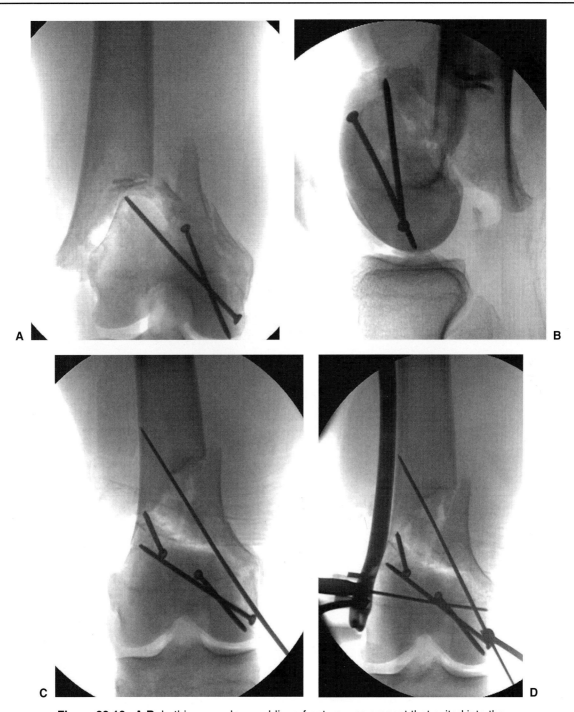

Figure 23.10. A,B. In this example, an oblique fracture was present that exited into the medial femoral condyle. The traumatic, medial, open wound was exploited for the reduction and stabilization of the articular segments. **C.** The relationship between the distal articular segment and the shaft component was established with manual traction and bumps, **(D)** simplifying plate placement across a reduced fracture.

tus approach allows visualization and reduction. These fractures are usually reduced directly at the articular surface and indirectly at the posterior cortical-fracture exit point. The fracture reduction can then be held with K wires placed perpendicular to the fracture line as seen on the lateral fluoroscopic image. The distal, femoral, condylar anatomy suggests that implants for lateral condyle fractures should be angulated approximately

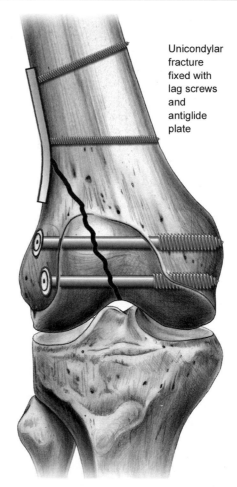

Unicondylar
fracture
fixed with
lag screws
and
antiglide
plate

Figure 23.11. Unicondylar fractures can typically be fixed with lag screws and/or an antiglide plate.

10 degrees laterally in the coronal plane whereas implants for medial condyle fractures should be angulated approximately 25 degrees medially in the coronal plane. Two 3.5-mm lag screws directed from anterior to posterior is usually adequate in uncomplicated fracture patterns.

RESULTS

Open reduction and internal fixation (ORIF) of distal femoral fractures is associated with good results in most patients. By using indirect reduction techniques to span the metaphyseal injury, Bolhofner et al reported high union rates and few complications in a series of 57 patients with distal femoral fractures. No bone grafting was used, delayed unions occurred uncommonly, and no nonunions were seen. The long-term (5 to 25 year) follow-up in a series of 32 patients with intra-articular, distal, femoral fractures was reported by Rademakers et al. They found good results after ORIF and a continued improvement of knee function with time. Furthermore, radiographic evidence of osteoarthritis was not associated with a less favorable result. The use of a lateral locking plate was reviewed in detail by Kregor et al in their series of 103 fractures of the distal femur treated with submuscular plating. They observed fracture union in 98% of closed fractures treated without bone grafting. In addition, no cases of fixation loss in the distal segment were reported.

POSTOPERATIVE MANAGEMENT

The postoperative rehabilitation protocol includes restricted weight bearing for 12 weeks. During that time, patients are allowed unrestricted passive and active knee range of motion combined with extension bracing. Radiographs are obtained in the operating room and at 6, 12, and 24 weeks.

COMPLICATIONS

Intraoperative

The most common intraoperative complication related to ORIF is a malreduction of either the articular surface or the mechanical axis. An accurate reduction requires an appreciation for the anatomy of the distal femoral articular surface as well as the relationship between the distal femoral inclination and the femoral shaft. Restoration of the limb axes as well as the entire articular surface are among the operative goals. Small-fragment and mini-fragment fixations may be required to fix small osteochondral fragments. The relative rotation of the medial and lateral femoral condyles should be accurately restored. Failure to achieve an accurate reduction in a patient with a closed injury is an avoidable complication.

Nonunion/Malunion

Nonunion can occur at any of the original fracture locations and may be extra-articular (supracondylar) or intra-articular (intercondylar or coronal). Supracondylar nonunions occur more commonly than intra-articular nonunions. If indirect reduction techniques are used, the incidence of supracondylar nonunion is low even when bone-grafting materials are not used. Nonunion is associated with certain injury factors, such as open traumatic wounds or bone loss, as well as patient factors, such as smoking or steroid use. Large defects due to open fractures with associated bone loss should be treated with bone grafting at a minimum of 6 to 8 weeks from the time of the initial stabilization. Supracondylar nonunions may be associated with deformity depending on the time from injury and the durability of the implants used to stabilize the distal femur. If no deformity exists, the nonunion can be compressed using a lateral fixed-angled implant. The articulated tensioning device is useful for compressing the nonunion after the implant if fixed to the distal segment. Bone grafting should be used according to the basic principles of nonunion treatment.

Intra-articular nonunions are uncommon and can be minimized with compression at the time of the original fixation. If a nonunion exists and secondary displacement has occurred, an intra-articular osteotomy followed by fixation with compression is required. Bone grafting may be necessary if any bone is lost. However, nonunion is usually due to inadequate fixation at the time of the initial operative procedure. Malunion occurs if the implants are improperly placed (i.e., reduced with deformity) or if the fracture position changes prior to healing. The usual late deformities associated with distal femoral fractures are varus and extension. Locked- or fixed-angled implants may minimize the development of angular deformities in the distal femur. Depending on the amount of angulation and shortening as well as location of the deformity, an osteotomy is usually required for correction.

Knee Stiffness

Loss of flexion may occur following distal femoral fractures. Early and aggressive knee range-of-motion exercises usually prevent this complication. If an extension contracture persists, several options are available. Early contractures may be treated with a combination of a knee manipulation and/or an arthroscopic lysis of adhesions. Care must be taken to gently manipulate the knee to avoid an iatrogenic fracture, especially an avulsion of the tibial tubercle. Most knee contractures require an extensile lateral approach with meticulous dissection of the vastus musculature from the anterior aspect of the femoral shaft. In ideal situations, the periosteum is left attached to the femoral shaft as the quadriceps musculature is dissected. A quadricepsplasty is typically combined with an open arthrotomy with removal of all intra-articular adhesions. Frequent locations of adhesions include the suprapatellar pouch and the medial gutter of the knee. Infrequently, a release of the rectus origin or a v-y quadriceps lengthening may be required to regain knee flexion.

RECOMMENDED READING

Bolhofner BR, Carmen B, Clifford P. The results of open reduction and internal fixation of distal femur fractures using a biologic (indirect) reduction technique. *J Orthop Trauma* 1996;10(6):372–377.

Farouk O, Krettek C, Miclau T, et al. Minimally invasive plate osteosynthesis: does percutaneous plating disrupt femoral blood supply less than the traditional technique? *J Orthop Trauma* 1996;13(6):401–416.

Holmes SM, Bomback D, Baumgaertner MR. Coronal fractures of the femoral condyle: a brief report of five cases. *J Orthop Trauma* 2004;18(5):316–319.

Johnson EE. Combined direct and indirect reduction of comminuted four-part intraarticular T-type fractures of the distal femur. *Clin Orthop* 1988;231:154–162.

Karunakar MA, Kellam JF. Avoiding malunion with 95 degrees fixed-angle distal femoral implants. *J Orthop Trauma* 2004;18(7):443–445.

Kregor PJ, Stannard JA, Zlowodzki M, et al. Treatment of distal femur fractures using the less invasive stabilization system: surgical experience and early clinical results in 103 fractures. *J Orthop Trauma* 2004;18(8):509–520.

Krettek C, Schandelmaier P, Miclau T, et al. Transarticular joint reconstruction and indirect plate osteosynthesis for complex distal supracondylar femoral fractures. *Injury* 1997;28(Suppl 1):A31–A41.

Lewis SL, Pozo JL, Muirhead-Allwood WF. Coronal fractures of the lateral femoral condyle. *J Bone Joint Surg Br* 1989;71(1):118–120.

Ostermann PA, Neumann K, Ekkernkamp A, et al. Long term results of unicondylar fractures of the femur. *J Orthop Trauma* 1994;8(2):142–426.

Ostrum RF, Geel C. Indirect reduction and internal fixation of supracondylar femur fractures without bone graft. *J Orthop Trauma* 1995;9(4):278–284.

Rademakers MV, Kerkhoffs GM, Sierevelt IN, et al. Intra-articular fractures of the distal femur: a long-term follow-up study of surgically treated patients. *J Orthop Trauma* 2003;18(4):213–219.

Sanders R, Regazzoni P, Ruedi TP. Treatment of supracondylar-intracondylar fractures of the femur using the dynamic condylar screw. *J Orthop Trauma* 1989;3(3): 214–222.

Weight M, Collinge C. Early results of the less invasive stabilization system for mechanically unstable fractures of the distal femur (AO/OTA types A2, A3, C2, and C3). *J Orthop Trauma* 2004;18(8):503–508.

Zlowodzki M, Williamson S, Cole PA, et al. Biomechanical evaluation of the less invasive stabilization system, angled blade plate, and retrograde intramedullary nail for the internal fixation of distal femur fractures. *J Orthop Trauma* 2004;18(8):494–502.

24

Patellar Fractures: Open Reduction Internal Fixation

John H. Wilber and Paul B. Gladden

INDICATIONS/CONTRAINDICATIONS

Operative management is the treatment of choice for the majority of displaced patellar fractures. Surgical options include open reduction and internal fixation (ORIF), partial or complete patellectomy, with the choice of treatment dependent on the fracture pattern and the amount of comminution. Although there is no widely accepted classification system for patellar fractures, most are based on an anatomic descriptive classification. Important factors include the location of fracture, direction of fracture lines, and the amount of comminution. In the AO/OTA classification, the patella is delineated as 45 and subdivided into A, B, or C depending on whether the fracture is extra-articular, partial articular without disruption of the extensor mechanism, or complete articular with disruption of the extensor mechanism. For the most part, 45B patella fractures are managed nonoperatively whereas 45A and 45C fractures require surgery.

The patella is an integral component of the extensor mechanism of the knee as well as an articular component of the knee joint. The patella's position in the body and the nature of its role in lower-limb function cause it to be susceptible to injury. Traction forces that pull the patella cephalad are the result of several different vectors caused by contraction of the quadriceps muscle. The quadriceps muscle, extensor retinaculum, along with the iliotibial band, participates in knee extension. The undersurface of the patella, which articulates with the notch of the femur, has the thickest cartilage found in the body. It is this articulation that acts as a fulcrum for extension. Forces measured at the patellofemoral articulation can be over seven times body weight during routine activities such as stair climbing and squatting. Tensile forces can be well over 3,000 N. The importance of the patella for normal knee function cannot be overestimated. Patellectomy results in the loss of the patellar fulcrum, a decrease in the moment arm, and relative lengthening of the quadriceps. This can lead to instability of the knee, extension lag, atrophy of the quadriceps, and loss of extension strength. Therefore, whenever possible, the patella should be repaired rather than excised.

Total patellectomy is generally indicated when the patella is so severely comminuted that an acceptable reduction and stable fixation cannot be achieved with internal fixation.

Partial patellectomy is indicated for cases that have severe comminution of either the inferior or superior pole that is not amenable to ORIF techniques.

ORIF is indicated for displaced patellar fractures that have fragments large enough to be reduced and stably repaired and is the treatment of choice for the majority of displaced patellar fractures in physiologically young patients. Many comminuted fractures can be salvaged. The goal of surgery is to achieve anatomic reduction of the articular surface with restoration of the continuity of the extensor mechanism. Displacement more than 3 mm and articular incongruity of more than 2 mm are considered strong indications for surgical treatment.

Contraindications and relative contraindications to surgical treatment include nondisplaced or minimally displaced stable fracture patterns. Also, contused or injured skin that precludes safe surgical approaches to the fracture, active infection involving the extremity with the patellar fracture, and medical conditions of the patient that would preclude safe surgical intervention are contraindications for surgery.

PREOPERATIVE PLANNING

An accurate history and careful physical examination should be performed. The mechanism of injury may explain the severity of injury as well as the fracture pattern. It is helpful to know whether the injury occurred as a result of a direct blow (e.g., a fall on the knee) or from resisted flexion of the knee resulting in a traction-type injury.

The physical examination must include a thorough evaluation of the extremity, with the surgeon looking for signs of direct trauma and swelling. The presence of fracture blisters, lacerations, abrasions, and contusions should be documented. It is essential to determine whether the fracture is open. Superficial or small wounds should be checked and if necessary carefully explored to determine whether they are in continuity with the fracture or the knee joint. In displaced patellar fractures, a visible or palpable defect is often noted between the fragments, although this may be masked by significant swelling, which develops rapidly. In some cases, a hemarthrosis is not apparent because of a large retinacular tear that allows blood to dissipate into the surrounding soft tissues. The absence of a hemarthrosis does not rule out a patellar fracture.

The continuity of the quadriceps mechanism is evaluated next. A painful, tense hemarthrosis often complicates this part of the examination. Aspiration of the knee with injection of a local anesthetic usually decreases pain. The patient is asked to contract the quadriceps mechanism and attempt to extend the knee fully. The ability to do this does not rule out a patellar fracture because the medial and lateral retinacula may still be intact, providing partial continuity of the extensor mechanism. However, the inability to lift the leg usually indicates that a patella fracture that tears the medial and lateral retinaculum exists. Gentle stress testing of the knee for stability should be carefully performed. Knee flexion should be avoided because this may further displace the fracture in addition to causing significant discomfort to the patient. The peripheral pulses and the compartments of the leg should be evaluated, and a neurologic examination performed.

The initial radiographs to evaluate a painful knee following injury include anteroposterior (AP), lateral, and axial views of the patella. A supine AP radiograph is obtained, centered over the patella (Fig. 24.1). The lateral radiograph can be taken as a cross-table lateral, with the knee slightly flexed. For an axial view, a Merchant's view is most easily and safely obtained in the injured patient (Fig. 24.2). The patient is placed supine on the x-ray table with the knee flexed 45 degrees over the end of the table. The x-ray beam is angled at 30 degrees from the horizontal, and the cassette is placed perpendicular to this x-ray beam 1 foot below the knee. Comparison views of the uninjured knee can be helpful in selected patients (i.e., those with a bipartite patella). Occasionally in patients with complex fracture patterns, a computed tomography (CT) scan is indicated.

Vertical fractures are often missed on both the AP and lateral views and are best visualized on the axial view. Larger displaced-fracture lines can be readily seen, although smaller nondisplaced-fracture lines are often obscured because of the superimposition of the patella on the femur in the AP view. In most cases, the fracture is more comminuted than is

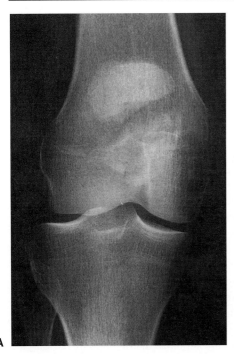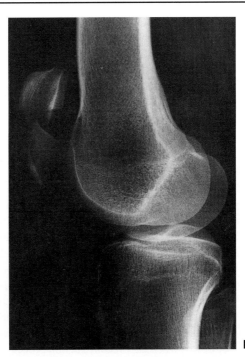

A   B

Figure 24.1. A. AP and lateral radiographs **(B)** showing a transverse fracture of the patella with comminution of the distal fragment. The lateral view shows significant comminution involving the articular surface in addition to displacement of the proximal and distal pole fragments.

apparent on the radiographic evaluation. Displacement more than 3 mm and articular incongruity more than 2 mm are indications for surgery.

Preoperative drawings should be performed for complex fracture patterns. Surgeons should make a tracing on both the AP and lateral views of the uninjured contralateral side and then superimpose the fracture lines from the injured side onto the normal template. The fixation should be drawn and the procedural steps carefully listed. The operating room should be informed of the equipment required based on the preoperative plan. Equipment needed for surgery usually includes various-sized pointed bone-reduction clamps, small curettes, wire cutters, benders, and wire tighteners, and small Kirschner (K) wires. Power drills and wire drivers will also be necessary. Small and mini fragment screws and instruments should be available.

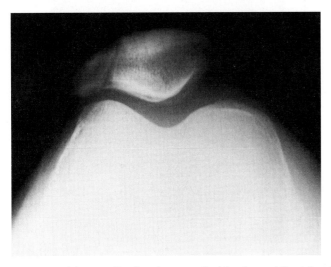

Figure 24.2. Axial view of the patella showing a vertical fracture of the lateral facet of the patella. There is minimal displacement of the fragments.

Surgery can be undertaken as soon as the patient has been prepared and appropriate pre-operative plans completed. If the fracture is open, surgery must be done urgently. Closed fractures should be surgically addressed when the soft-tissue injury and the general condition of the patient permit.

SURGERY

The patient is positioned supine on a standard operating table. Because there is a tendency for the leg to externally rotate, a small bump can be placed under the ipsilateral hip. A tourniquet is placed high on the involved thigh. The procedure can be done under a general or spinal anesthetic. Regional nerve blocks (femoral nerve block) can be very helpful to control post-operative pain. The patient is prepped in a standard fashion, and the leg is draped free by using an extremity drape. The limb is exsanguinated with a sterile Esmarch, and the tourniquet inflated to a pressure appropriate for the size of the leg and the patient's blood pressure. Before inflating the tourniquet, the quadriceps is pulled distally to ensure that it is not trapped under the tourniquet, which can displace the patella proximally, making reduction more difficult. A sterile bump can be placed behind the knee, which allows the knee to flex 15 to 20 degrees. Appropriate antibiotic prophylaxis should be given before inflating the tourniquet.

The skin incision can be either transverse or longitudinal. A longitudinal incision is preferred when more proximal and distal dissection is necessary for the repair of a comminuted fracture and when later reconstruction procedures are anticipated. For cosmetic reasons, the transverse incision is preferred. It also avoids potential damage to the saphenous branch of the femoral nerve.

The incision is carried down through the subcutaneous tissue and the prepatellar bursa. A hematoma is usually encountered as soon as the bursa is opened, and it usually leads directly into the fracture site (Fig. 24.3). Care should be taken to minimize direct dissection of the fracture fragments. The soft tissues surrounding the patella often hold nondisplaced fractures in place, and if these are disrupted, the fragments may displace, creating a more complicated and unstable fracture pattern. The major fracture fragments should be exposed. Clot

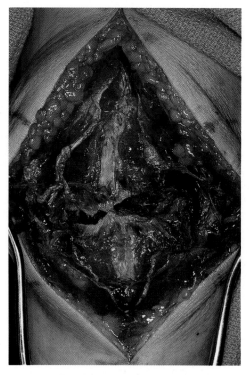

Figure 24.3. Surgical exposure through a vertical midline incision showing the transverse fracture of the patella with medial and lateral retinaculum tears. The soft tissues have been left intact over the surfaces of the patella.

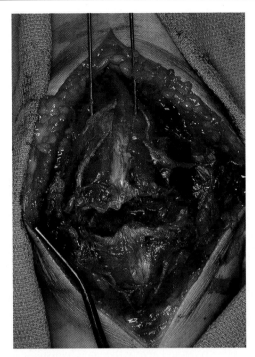

Figure 24.4. The hematoma has been evacuated, and the joint and fracture lines have been debrided. The K wires have been advanced retrograde through the patella, and the patella fragments are now ready to be reduced.

should be removed with a combination of small curettes and the use of a small suction-tip device. Irrigation should be used liberally to help remove the hematoma and small inconsequential comminuted fragments. The extent of the medial and lateral retinacular injuries should be identified and the edges tagged for later repair. The undersurface of the patella, in addition to the patellofemoral groove, should be inspected for evidence of articular damage. The knee joint should be inspected and irrigated to remove any loose fragments.

After the fracture and the knee joint have been thoroughly irrigated, the fracture edges carefully exposed, and the fracture pattern thoroughly delineated, a preliminary reduction is performed. The small bump behind the knee will need to be removed at this time because flexion of the knee will make the reduction more difficult. In the case of a simple, transverse, middle-third fracture, one can proceed directly to the tension band technique. In other more complex fractures, the goal is to try to reduce the fragments to create a two-part transverse-fracture pattern that can then be further stabilized with a tension band technique. For example, if there is a vertical split through either the proximal or distal fragment, the vertical split is first reduced and held temporarily with large, pointed, reduction forceps. This is then temporarily stabilized with a 1.2-mm K wires. Definitive stabilization of this fragment depends on its size and can be done with either K wires or small-fragment or minifragment screws. After this has been performed, the tenaculum clamps and the provisional fixation are removed.

When a transverse fracture pattern has been created, a tension-band wire technique is performed. By using a 2-mm drill, two parallel drill holes are placed in a retrograde fashion through the proximal bony fragment. A 1.6- or 1.8-mm K wire is then advanced through these holes and out through the quadriceps tendon (Fig. 24.4). They are advanced until the sharp tip of the K wire is fully within the proximal bony fragment. The two fracture fragments are then reduced and held with large, pointed, reduction forceps.

Care should be taken to ensure that the articular surface is anatomically reduced by inspecting both the anterior cortical and posterior articular surfaces. The articular surface can be inspected through the preexisting tears in the retinaculum. If there is no significant tear in the retinaculum, a small, medial or lateral arthrotomy should be made to allow inspection or palpation of the articular surface.

The K wires are then sequentially attached to the drill and advanced into the distal fragment (Fig. 24.5). They should be advanced distally at least 1 cm beyond the inferior tip of the patella. Once again, the adequacy of the reduction should be checked. A 30-cm segment of 1-mm wire is passed adjacent to the patella and quadriceps mechanism proximally and distally, passing behind the K wires and closely approximated to both the proximal and distal poles of the patella. If this is not achieved, the wire will not obtain adequate fixation and may loosen, eventually resulting in loss of fixation and reduction. To facilitate passage of the wire, pass a 16-gauge angiocatheter through the quadriceps mechanism just above the superior pole of the patella and behind the K wires (Fig. 24.6). The 1-mm wire is passed through the catheter, which is then removed. The identical technique is performed distally.

To ensure symmetrical tensioning of the wire, a double-loop technique is recommended. A twist is placed in the wire on its continuous side, and on the contralateral side, the two ends of the wires are hand tightened and twisted. Excessive wire is removed. By using either a large needle driver or a large clamp specifically designed for wire tightening, the two ends of the wire are sequentially tightened (Fig. 24.7). The technique of wire tightening is critical. Before twisting, the wire should be tensioned by lifting up on the clamp. The wire is then gently twisted. This will ensure that both wires twist around each other rather than one wire wrapping around the other wire. The wires are sequentially tightened in this manner until adequate compression has been achieved.

Once again, the quality of the reduction is checked, and the knee is gently flexed to check the stability of the fixation (Fig. 24.8). The twisted wire is clipped, and the ends are bent over by using a large needle driver and gently flattened by using a bone tamp and a mallet so that they lie close to the superior surface of the bone. The K wires are bent by stabilizing the wire close to the bone with a needle driver and then using the wire bender, trying to bend the wire to 110 degrees. The excess wire is then cut. The remaining wire is then rotated 180 degrees posteriorly and advanced into the quadriceps mechanism. If it is not advanced into the quadriceps mechanism, it will cause excessive irritation, in addition to having an increased chance of backing out. The distal ends of the wires are then cut so they are not excessively prominent within the patellar tendon. The retinacular defects are repaired with absorbable sutures (Figs. 24.9 and 24.10).

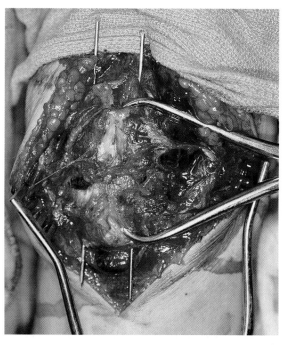

Figure 24.5. The transverse fracture has been anatomically reduced by using a pointed fracture-reduction clamp, and the K wires have been advanced antegrade through the distal fragment. The K wires are parallel to each other.

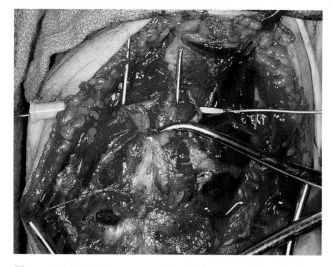

Figure 24.6. A 16-gauge angiocath is passed through the quadriceps tendon behind the K wires and just superior to the patella. The cerclage wire is being passed through the angiocatheter, which will then be removed. An identical procedure is then performed through the distal pole.

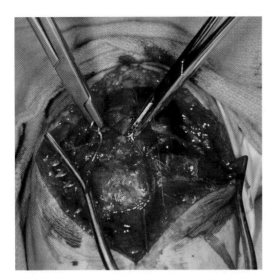

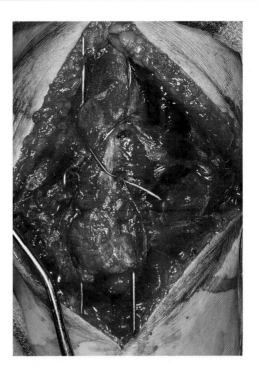

Figure 24.7. A double-tensioning technique is performed by consecutively tightening each side of the tension band wire. The fracture gap can be seen closed down with this technique.

Figure 24.8. The tension band wires have been tightened, clipped short, and bent. The K wires have not yet been shortened, and the retinaculum has not yet been repaired.

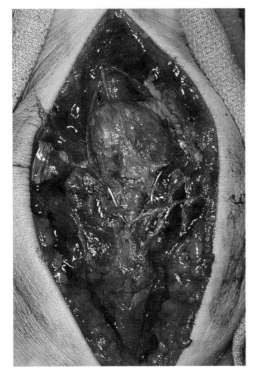

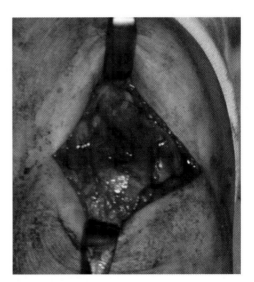

Figure 24.9. The final tension-band construct with the K wires cut and bent and buried within the quadriceps and patellar tendon. The retinaculum has been repaired.

Figure 24.10. Alternative transverse incision with final construct visualized through the wound.

The tourniquet is deflated and hemostasis obtained with electrocoagulation. A suction drain is placed in the knee joint. Closure should be meticulous, including closure of the prepatellar bursa as a separate layer by using 2-0 Vicryl. The subcutaneous tissue is closed by using simple inverted 2-0 Vicryl. Skin closure is dependent on the integrity of the skin. Subcuticular closure gives excellent cosmetic results but should be reserved for those cases without skin injuries and only minimal swelling. If there is concern regarding damage to the skin, nylon sutures should be used. A sterile dressing is applied consisting of fluffs, Webril, and an Ace wrap. The patient is placed into either a knee immobilizer or a hinged knee brace with the knee locked in full extension.

Other variations on the tension-band technique include the use of 4-0 cannulated screws with the tension band wire passed through the cannulated screws and tightened in a standard double-loop technique (Fig. 24.11). In the case of a distal-pole patella fracture, the tension-band wire technique can be used, although the K wires must be placed closer together so that they both capture the distal fragment. An alternative to this is the use of retrograde cannulated or standard 4.0 screws in addition to a tension band technique. With very small fragments, a single screw can be used. In the case of a stellate fracture, circumferential cerclage wire can be helpful to bundle the fracture fragments together (Fig. 24.12). In stellate fractures, it is critical not to violate the soft tissues around the fragments because this will cause significant disruption of the fracture fragments.

POSTOPERATIVE MANAGEMENT

Postoperative care is dependent on the fracture type and the resultant stability after osteosynthesis. The extremity is usually placed in a well-padded compressive dressing and a knee immobilizer or a hinged knee brace locked in extension. In patients with stable fixation, knee motion is begun immediately. On the first postoperative day, the patient is mobilized out of bed to ambulate weight bearing as tolerated with the knee locked in full extension. The hinges can either be loosened or the knee immobilizer removed for range-of-motion exercises. Active flexion and extension are initiated. Quad sets can be started in the immediate postoperative period. The drain is removed at 48 hours, and the patient is usually discharged home shortly thereafter. Patients are seen in follow-up in approximately 7 to 10 days for a dressing change and suture removal. If the wound is well healed, active extension and straight-leg-raising exercises are begun, and the patient is referred to physical therapy. Patients are seen at 4 to 6 week intervals, and radiographs of the patella are obtained out of the brace. If there is radiographic evidence of healing, progressive resistive exercises are started. The patient is progressively weaned from the brace, depending on the motion and strength. Full rehabilitation usually takes 4 to 6 months. If there are any symptoms or signs of loss of fixation during this postoperative period, range-of-motion exercises are stopped, and the patient is immobilized and followed up closely.

In comminuted fractures where the fixation is less secure, early range of motion is not possible. The repair should be protected in either a knee immobilizer or a knee brace with the hinges locked. The braces are removed only for wound checks and extremity cleansing. Quad sets can be initiated, but the repair is protected until there are signs of healing. Range of motion is delayed for 3 to 6 weeks.

COMPLICATIONS

In the immediate postoperative period, the major complications include hemarthrosis and infection. A hemarthrosis can usually be avoided by the use of a postoperative suction drain and a compressive dressing. If the drain was either not used or was removed prematurely, the hemarthrosis can be aspirated. This is necessary only if a tense hemarthrosis causes significant pain or limits rehabilitation.

Infection is a rare but devastating complication. This can usually be avoided by careful timing of surgery and meticulous surgical techniques in addition to the appropriate

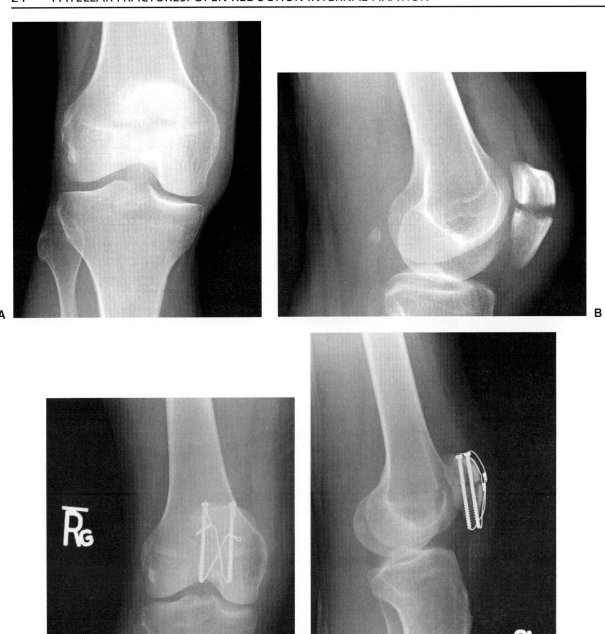

Figure 24.11. A. An AP x-ray of a fractured patella. **B.** A lateral x-ray of a fractured patella. **C.** AP x-ray of ORIF in which cannulated screws and wire have been used. **D.** Lateral x-ray of ORIF in which cannulated screws and wire have been used.

perioperative antibiotics. If infection develops, it should be aggressively treated with antibiotics and debridement with drainage. Physical therapy and early range-of-motion activities should be stopped while treating the infection. If the infection involves the knee joint, it must be drained and irrigated surgically. Culture-specific intravenous antibiotics should be used for 3 to 6 weeks. Internal fixation in general should not be removed until the fracture is healed.

Loss of fixation and reduction are other possible complications after surgical repair of patella fractures. This is more common in complex fracture patterns, in noncompliant

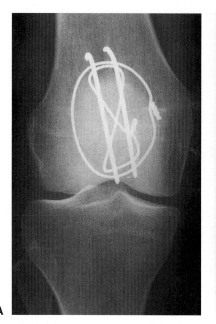
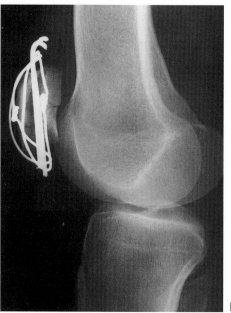

A   B

Figure 24.12. A. Postoperative AP and **(B)** lateral radiographs of a comminuted patellar fracture fixed with a combination tension-band and cerclage-wire technique. The articular surface has been restored anatomically.

patients, and when therapy is overly aggressive. If there are signs of loss of fixation without significant loss of reduction, this can be treated with immobilization. If there are signs of loss of fixation along with loss of reduction, then revision internal fixation is indicated.

Delayed union and nonunion are usually the result of either failure of fixation or inadequate initial reduction. The complications can usually be avoided by good reduction and fixation techniques and close postoperative follow-up. Delayed unions can be treated with repeated cerclage-wire techniques. Significant malunions usually require a patellectomy.

Arthrofibrosis and loss of knee motion are relatively common complications after patella fractures. These complications are more common in severely comminuted fractures and those fractures requiring prolonged immobilization. The majority of patients can be treated with aggressive and persistent physical therapy, although an occasional patient will require manipulation under anesthesia. It is my preference to do an arthroscopic evaluation at the time of manipulation. This allows inspection of the patellar surfaces, a direct lysis of the arthrofibrosis involving the suprapatellar pouch and the lateral gutters, in addition to adhesions from the fat pad into the intercondylar notch. Arthroscopic debridement and manipulation should be followed by aggressive physical therapy to maintain motion and increase strength. Retropatellar arthrofibrosis and patella baja are rare but extremely difficult complications to correct and have a negative effect on patellar function and outcomes.

Posttraumatic osteoarthritis results from either inadequate reduction of the articular surface or injuries to the articular surface that occur at the time of injury. In the early stages, arthroscopy and patellar debridement can decrease some symptoms. Ultimately in the young patient, a patellectomy may be the treatment of choice. In the elderly patient who also has involvement of the medial and lateral compartments, a total knee replacement may be the treatment of choice.

OUTCOMES

Results following patellar fracture treatment are variable and the causes include severity of injury, fracture pattern, articular damage, displacement, preexisting disease, accuracy of reduction, and postoperative regimen. Reliable radiographic (objective) measurements of clinical outcomes do not exist. The best outcomes are seen in patients with anatomic reductions, restoration of normal biomechanics, and preservation of the articular surfaces. Loss of all or even part of the patella may result in loss of extensor strength and function. With the appropriate surgical and postoperative regimen, good functional results can be achieved even in complex displaced fractures.

RECOMMENDED READING

Benjamin J, Dohm M, McMurtry M. Biomechanical evaluation of various forms of fixation of transverse patellar fractures. *J Orthop Trauma* 1987;1:219–222.

Böstman O, Kiviluoto O, Nirhamo J. Comminuted displaced fractures of the patella. *Injury* 1981;13:196–202.

Böstman O, Kiviluoto O, Santavirta S, et al. Fractures of the patella treated by operation. *Arch Orthop Trauma Surg* 1983;102:78–81.

Carpenter JE, Kasman R, Matthews LS. Fractures of the patella: instructional course lectures. *J Bone Joint Surg Am* 1993;75:1550–1561.

Edwards B, Johnell O, Redlund-Johnell I. Patellar fractures: a 30-year follow-up. *Acta Orthop Scand* 1989;60: 712–714.

Goodfellow J, Hungerford DS, Zindel M. Patello-femoral joint mechanics and pathology: 1. Functional anatomy of the patello-femoral joint. *J Bone Joint Surg Br* 1986;58:287–290.

Hung LK, Chan KM, Chow YN, et al. Fractured patella: operative treatment using the tension band principle. *Injury* 1985;16:343–347.

LeCroy CM. Injuries to the patella and extensor mechanism. In: Kellam JF, ed. *OKU Orthopaedic Knowledge Update Trauma*. 2nd ed. Rosemont, IL: American Academy of Orthopaedic Surgeons; 2000:157–166.

Levack B, Flannagan JP, Hobbs S. Results of surgical treatment of patellar fractures. *J Bone Joint Surg Br* 1085;67:416–419.

Lotke, PA, Ecker ML. Transverse fractures of the patella. *Clin Orthop* 1981;158:180–184.

Muller ME, Allgower M, Schneider R, et al. *Manual of Internal Fixation: Techniques Recommended by the AO Group*. Berlin, Germany: Springer-Verlag; 1991.

Smith ST, Cramer KE, Karges DE, et al. Early complications in the operative treatment of patella fractures. *J Orthop Trauma*. 1997;11:183–187.

Torchia ME, Lewallen DG. Open fractures of the patella. *J Orthop Trauma* 1996;10:403–409.

Weber MJ, Janecki CJ, McLeod P, et al. Efficacy of various forms of fixation of transverse fractures of the patella. *J Bone Joint Surg Am* 1980;62:215–220.

25

Knee Dislocations

Anikar Chhabra, Shane T. Seroyer, and
Christopher D. Harner

INDICATIONS/CONTRAINDICATIONS

Traumatic knee dislocations are serious injuries with devastating complications secondary to damage to multiple soft-tissue and stabilizing structures. Associated injuries may include the cruciate ligaments, collateral ligaments, medial and lateral capsular structures, menisci and articular cartilage, as well as neurovascular injuries and compartment syndrome. Traditional nonoperative treatment has resulted in poor outcomes. Surgical treatment remains controversial with respect to timing of surgery, which structures to repair versus reconstruct, and choice of grafts. We believe early surgical repair is indicated in the vast majority of multiligament injuries that result from knee dislocation.

Due to the severity of these injuries, the patient must undergo an extensive preoperative workup to discern the details of his or her injury and to insure he or she is medically stable for surgery. Inherent in this evaluation is detailed attention to factors that may predicate emergent surgical intervention. Evaluation in the trauma bay that reveals an open dislocation, irreducible dislocation, or arterial injury requires an emergency trip to the operating room. In the case of arterial injury, application of a joint-spanning external fixator provides joint stability and protects the vascular graft. Recovery of associated soft-tissue injury determines whether to perform later reconstruction or repair of the ligaments. Following a vascular repair, reconstructive procedures should be postponed until the vascular graft has matured and is not likely to be compromised. After vascular repairs, four-compartment fasciotomies are often required to combat reperfusion injuries.

Elderly, sedentary, or other moribund patients with preexisting functional deficits are not usually candidates for surgical repair and are often better treated with bracing and a functional rehabilitation protocol. Other contraindications to surgery are an active infection, displaced intra-articular or peri-articular fractures of the femur or tibia, and advanced osteoarthritis of the knee.

PREOPERATIVE PLANNING

The preoperative planning for treatment of a knee dislocation begins in the emergency room and requires a very detailed physical exam as well as specific radiological exams, including angiography, to elucidate the extent of the injury. Early vascular surgery consultation is recommended because a normal physical exam does not rule out vascular injury in the acute phase. The physician must also maintain a high index of suspicion for compartment syndrome. The physical exam in these patients can be difficult and inaccurate secondary to pain. Prompt reduction of the dislocation by traction and countertraction under conscious sedation is essential. Appropriate films should be obtained to rule out fractures and to ensure reduction. Stress radiographs may occasionally be used to evaluate varus and valgus instability. Due to the limits of the physical exam, when the patient is medically stable, a magnetic resonance imaging (MRI) scan is necessary to assess the extent of injury and to assist in surgical planning. Soft tissue swelling and generalized edema may hinder the quality of the MRI obtained.

CONTROVERSIES

Numerous controversies remain regarding the surgical management of knee dislocation and include timing of surgery: what structures to repair or reconstruct, the choice of grafts, and the surgical techniques. Recent publications have shown that operative treatment gives better results than nonoperative treatment. Although there are numerous approaches and techniques for these difficult cases, this chapter will present our experience and approach to the knee-dislocation patient.

In studies at our institution, patients who undergo acute ligamentous repair and reconstruction within 3 weeks of injury have done better than patients reconstructed after 3 weeks, as determined by Lysholm and Knee Outcome Survey Activities of Daily Living scores. However, in patients with severe, life-threatening or arterial injuries, or those with open dislocations, ligamentous reconstruction is delayed until soft-tissue swelling has subsided and the patient's condition has improved.

The decision to repair versus reconstruct the soft tissues remains controversial. We believe that the repair and reconstruction of all associated ligamentous and meniscal injuries should be undertaken in patients having surgery. The majority of injuries to the cruciate ligaments are intrasubstance and do not respond favorably to primary repair. An exception to this is when large bony fragments from the tibial insertions of the anterior cruciate ligament (ACL) or posterior cruciate ligament (PCL) are avulsed. In these situations we advocate primary repair by passing large nonabsorbable sutures into the bony fragment and through the bone tunnels in the tibia. In all other situations, we reconstruct ACL and PCL injuries. At our institution we attempt to preserve specific bundles of the PCL that are not injured. In one third of cases, the anterolateral bundle is ruptured, but the meniscofemoral ligament and the posteromedial bundle remain intact. In these cases we do a single bundle reconstruction of the anterolateral bundle.

For medial- and lateral-sided collateral and capsular injuries, we often acutely repair (less than 3 weeks after injury) the injured structures if the tissue quality is adequate. Depending on the stability of the repair, augmentation is often necessary. Chronic injuries (more than 3 weeks after injury) tend to be limited by scar formation and soft-tissue contracture and require reconstruction.

To decrease operative time, limit skin incisions in the traumatized knee, and decrease donor site morbidity, we advocate the use of allografts over autografts in multiple-ligament reconstruction surgery. Inherent in this choice of allografts is the risk of transmissible disease with allografts. This must be discussed with the patient prior to the procedure.

SURGERY

Anesthesia

The choice of anesthetic is made in conjunction with the surgeon, anesthesiologist, and the patient, taking medical co-morbidities, age, and prior history with anesthesia into consiteration. General anesthesia with concomitant IV sedation is most commonly performed. Preoperative femoral and/or sciatic nerve blocks are routinely performed as an adjuvant for postoperative pain relief. A Foley catheter may be placed intraoperatively to monitor fluid shifts during the procedure.

Setup, Patient Positioning, and Exam under Anesthesia

The patient is placed supine on the operating room table. The goal is to allow up to 80 to 90 degrees of static flexion of the knee to be maintained without manual assistance. To do so, a small bump is placed under the patients leg just distal to the greater trochanter with a lateral post placed at the same level. A sterile bump is wedged between the post and the thigh. To maintain flexion, the heel rests on a 4.5 kg sandbag that has been taped to the bed and prevents extension of the leg (Fig. 25.1). Due to the length of time these cases require, we do not use a tourniquet.

After properly positioning the patient on the operating table, a complete ligamentous exam, including anterior and posterior drawer tests, pivot shift, dial test, and posterior drawer with external rotation, is performed. These exam findings are corroborated with MRI findings to establish the proper surgical approach to address the anticipated pathologies.

Anatomic Landmarks and Incisions

Standard, osseous, knee anatomy including patella, Gerdy's tubercle, the fibular head, and medial and lateral joint lines are marked. Special care is taken to palpate and identify the peroneal nerve as it courses around the fibular neck. The dorsalis pedal pulse is palpated and marked for continual monitoring. The standard anterolateral arthroscopic portal is placed just adjacent to the lateral border of the patella tendon, above the joint line. The anteromedial portal is established at the same level, approximately 1 cm medial to the patellar tendon. Additionally, a superolateral outflow portal is established in standard fashion, superior to the patella and posterior to the quadriceps muscle. The posteromedial portal is often required to address the tibial insertion of the PCL, and it is established intraoperatively using an inside-out technique with the aid of a 70-degree arthroscope.

The operative incisions vary according to the structures that require repair. Our standard ACL/PCL tibial tunnel is marked 3 cm longitudinally over the anteromedial proximal tibia, 2 cm distal to the joint line and 2 cm medial to the tibial tubercle. The incision for the PCL femoral tunnel is marked 2 cm medial to the medial articular surface of the trochlea in the subvastus interval. If the injury has an associated medial component, the incision for the tibial tunnels is extended proximally in curvilinear fashion to the medial epicondyle. The incision

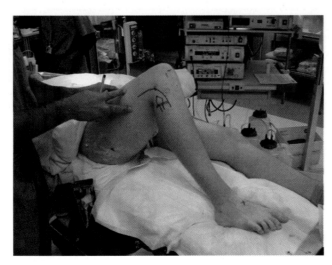

Figure 25.1. Set-up, surface anatomy, and skin incisions with a lateral-sided injury.

for lateral and posterolateral injuries is made, with the knee in flexion, in curvilinear fashion and extends proximally from the lateral epicondyle distally to a location midway between Gerdy's tubercle and the fibular head (see Fig. 25.1) The proximal portion of this incision parallels the plane between the biceps femoris tendon and the iliotibial band. The skin incisions are injected preoperatively with 0.25% Marcaine with epinephrine (1:100,000).

Graft Selection

There are many options for graft selection in the knee injury involving multiple ligaments, most of which are surgeon dependent. The timing of surgery, extent of injury, experience of surgeon, and availability of allograft all factor into the selection process. The inherent advantages to autograft are offset in these complex cases by a choice of allograft, which will provide less donor-site morbidity and decreased operative time. For the ACL graft we currently prefer to use allograft bone-patellar tendon-bone graft. Soft-tissue allograft such as tibialis anterior is also a viable choice. For the PCL, we prefer to use Achilles tendon allograft because of its length, its girth, and the existence of the calcaneal bone plug for femoral fixation (Fig. 25.2). The lateral collateral ligament (LCL) is usually reconstructed with an Achilles tendon allograft with a 7- to 8-mm calcaneal bone plug, which will be fixed in a proximal fibular-bone tunnel at the native LCL insertion site. The posterolateral corner is usually reconstructed with either a tibialis anterior allograft or a semitendinosus autograft.

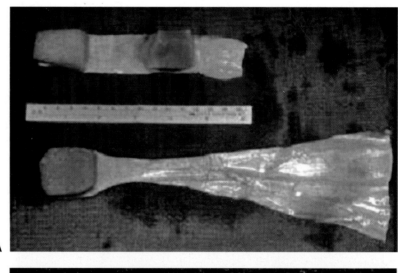

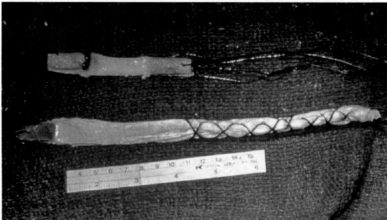

Figure 25.2. Bone–patellar tendon–bone allograft for ACL reconstruction and Achilles tendon allograft for PCL reconstruction: **(A)** before preparation and **(B)** after preparation.

Diagnostic Arthroscopy

To minimize the chance of compartment syndrome, we use gravity inflow irrigation with a superolateral outflow portal rather than a pump. The arthroscopic technique should be abandoned in favor of an open approach should extravasation be noted or a compartment syndrome suspected. A 30-degree arthroscope is introduced through the anterolateral portal and a diagnostic arthroscopy is performed to assess the integrity of the cruciate ligaments, the menisci, and the articular cartilage. A 70-degree scope is now placed through the anterolateral portal to establish the posteromedial portal, which will be used as the working portal for the tibial insertion of the PCL. Extreme caution should be exercised in this area to avoid extension of the debridement beyond the capsule and thus causing injury to the neurovascular structures, which reside approximately 1.5 cm posterior to the tibial insertion of the PCL. The use of the 30- and 70-degree arthroscopes through both the anterolateral and the posteromedial portal will allow for excellent access, visualization, and triangulization of the tibial PCL insertion site. Our attention is now turned to the ACL. We attempt to preserve as much of the ACL footprint as possible for vascular and pro-prioceptive considerations.

Next, we evaluate for any concomitant meniscal or articular cartilage injuries. Peripheral tears will be repaired using our preferred inside-out method, leaving the sutures to be secured with the knee in 30 degrees of flexion after all other grafts have been passed and secured. Central and irreparable tears are debrided back to a stable rim at this time.

Cruciate Tunnel Preparation

We prefer to address the PCL tunnel first because it is the more difficult of the two. With the aid of arthroscopic visualization, a 15-mm offset PCL guide is set between 50 and 55 degrees and passed through the anteromedial portal with the tip of the guide located in the most distal and lateral portion of the native PCL insertion site (Fig. 25.3). A Kirschner (K) wire is passed with a starting point approximately 3 to 4 cm distal to the joint line, and an intraoperative fluoroscopy image is obtained. This K wire is left in place and attention is turned to the ACL tunnel. The ACL guide is set to 45 degrees and inserted through the anteromedial portal. A 3/32- inch guide wire is inserted into the center of the ACL footprint. A fluoroscopic image with the knee in full extension is now obtained to assess the placement of the K wires. The ACL wire should be just posterior to Blumenstaat's line on the lateral, and the PCL wire should be 2 to 3 cm distal to the ACL wire (Fig. 25.4).

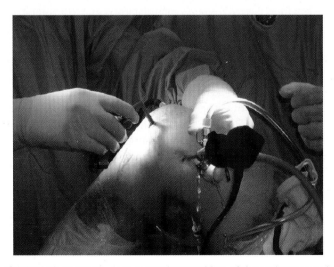

Figure 25.3. Clinical photograph demonstrating position of the arthroscope in the posteromedial portal while drilling the PCL tibial tunnel.

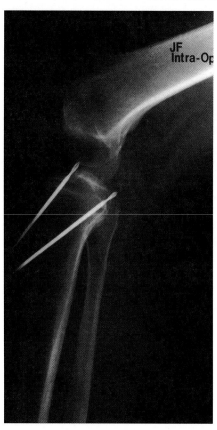

Figure 25.4. Radiographic confirmation of the ACL and PCL tibia-guide wire placement.

After radiographic confirmation of proper K wire positioning, the PCL tibial tunnel is drilled. A curette is placed directly on top of the guide wire, and with direct visualization via a 30-degree arthroscope in the anteromedial portal, a compaction drill bit is passed. The drill is started with pneumatic power, but the drilling is finished by hand after the initial cortex is breeched. Maintaining meticulous attention to the visualization of the K wire tip, we drill 1 mm less than the desired tunnel width. We then dilate, by hand, in 0.5-mm increments. The same technique is used when preparing the ACL tunnel. We desire to have at least a 2-cm bone bridge between the ACL and PCL tibial tunnels.

We now turn our attention to constructing the femoral tunnels. For a single bundle PCL reconstruction, a K wire is passed from the anterolateral portal to a point within the anterior portion of the PCL femoral footprint, which is located approximately 5 to 6 mm from the articular margin. This is overdrilled with a compaction drill to a depth of approximately 25 to 35 mm. If a double-bundle PCL reconstruction is being performed, the anterolateral tunnel is drilled at 1 o'clock, approximately 5 to 6 mm off of the articular cartilage. This allows for anterior placement of the tunnel. The tunnel for the posteromedial graft is much smaller and is drilled in the posterior footprint at approximately the 3 to 4 o'clock position, 1 cm posterior to the anterolateral tunnel. The ACL femoral tunnel is created with the knee hyperflexed. We use a medial portal approach, rather than transtibial, to drill the femoral tunnel. This approach allows positioning and angulation of the femoral tunnel to be independent of the tibial-tunnel angle. In this method, a K wire is placed through the anteromedial portal and into the center of the anatomic insertion of the ACL, approximately 6 to 7 mm anterior to the over-the-top position (at the 1:30 to 2:00 position for left knees or the 10:00 to 10:30 position for right knees). As with the PCL tunnel, the K wire is over drilled with a compaction drill to a depth of 25 to 35 mm, and the hole is expanded to the desired graft size (Fig. 25.5).

The PCL graft is passed first. A malleable 18-gauge wire is passed, in retrograde fashion through the PCL tibial tunnel and retrieved under arthroscopic visualization by a pituitary rongeur inserted through the anterolateral portal. The no. 5 nonabsorbable suture that was

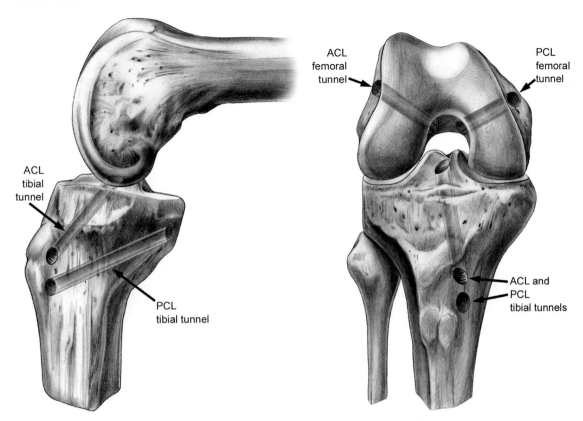

Figure 25.5. Schematic of ACL and PCL tibial and femoral tunnels.

placed through the tibial bone block is now placed through the eyelet on the wire that is external to the anterolateral portal. The other end of the wire is then withdrawn from the tibial PCL tunnel in antegrade fashion bringing the no. 5 suture and tibial portion of the PCL graft with it. For the femoral side of the graft, the no. 5 suture, which had previously been tagged and has remained outside of the anterolateral portal, is place through the eyelet of a Beath pin. The Beath pin is subsequently passed through the anterolateral portal into the PCL femoral tunnel and out the anteromedial thigh. Under arthroscopic visualization, tensioning the sutures and gentle guidance from an arthroscopic probe are used to assist graft passage.

The ACL graft is passed via the medial portal. A Beath pin with a no. 5 suture through the eyelet is passed through the medial portal and out of the femoral tunnel to the anterolateral thigh. With one end of the suture exiting the superolateral portal and one end exiting from the medial portal, a pituitary rongeur is passed retrograde through the tibial tunnel, and the no. 5 suture is withdrawn from medial portal and passed out of the tibial ACL tunnel. This end of the suture is now looped through the tagged femoral end of the ACL graft, and the graft is passed with arthroscopic assistance as described for the PCL graft. The femoral fixation of both grafts is now performed, but tensioning of the tibial grafts is delayed until the end of the case.

There are many options for femoral fixation for ACL and the PCL grafts. Depending on graft type and quality of bone, interference screws or a 4.5-mm AO screw, used as a post, can be used.

Posterolateral Corner Injuries

The lateral incision is used to expose the interval between the posterior edge of the iliotibial band and the biceps femoris, and to allow visualization of the LCL and poplite-ofibular ligament (PFL) insertions (Fig. 25.6). If the injuries to these structures are acute and the soft tissues allow, primary repair can be attempted with a no. 2 braided, nonabsorbable suture (Fig. 25.7). If reconstruction of the LCL is indicated, we prefer to use an

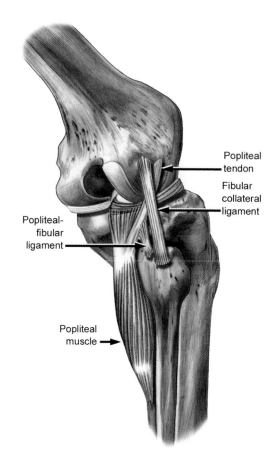

Figure 25.6. Anatomic relationships of the lateral side of the knee. Popliteus tendon (PT). Lateral collateral ligament (LCL). Popliteofibular ligament (PFL).

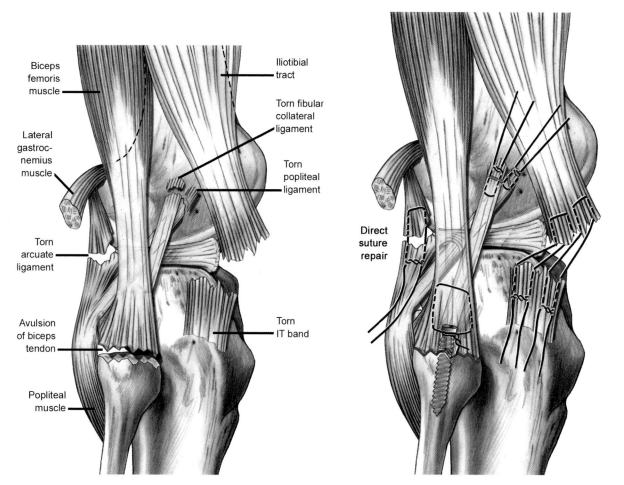

Figure 25.7. Direct repair of the lateral structures.

Achilles allograft, with imbrication of the native LCL by a whipstitch. The tendinous portion of the allograft is secured to the LCL femoral insertion via drill holes or suture anchors. The distal insertion of the LCL on the fibula is dissected free, and a tunnel is drilled along the longitudinal axis of the fibula. The calcaneal bone plug is secured in this bony tunnel with a metal interference screw. It is tensioned with the knee in 30 degrees of flexion (Fig. 25.8).

The main goal of reconstructing the popliteus complex is to restore the static properties of the PFL (Fig. 25.9). We prefer to use a tibialis anterior allograft. The lateral epicondyle is exposed and the popliteus tendon is dissected off. A whipstitch is used to mark the popliteus tendon. A 6-mm tunnel is drilled through the femur at the popliteus insertion site to a depth of 25 to 30 mm. The tunnel is dilated to 7 mm.

The posterior border of the fibula at the PFL insertion is dissected out and exposed with a horizontal incision just below the biceps insertion. The PFL insertion is more proximal and medial on the fibular head than is the LCL. The anterior portion of the fibula is also exposed and a 3/32-inch guide wire loaded on a chuck is passed from anterior to posterior in an attempt to match the oblique angulation of the fibular head. The tunnel for this graft is then drilled over the guide wire by hand with a 6-mm drill and dilated to a diameter of 7

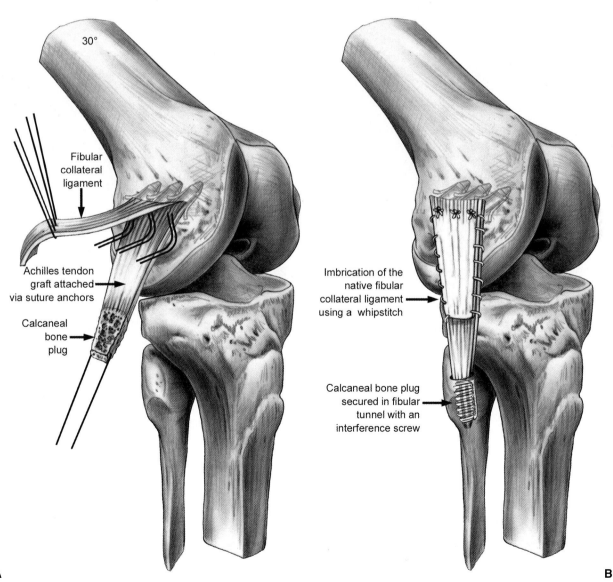

A   **B**

Figure 25.8. LCL reconstruction with Achilles tendon allograft.

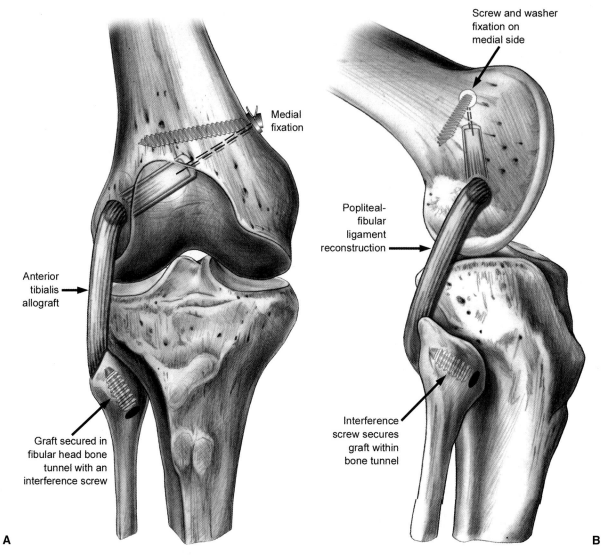

Figure 25.9. PFL reconstruction.

mm. The graft is passed through the tunnel from posterior to anterior with the assistance of a Hewson suture passer. The proximal portion of the graft is then passed underneath and medial to the LCL and inserted via Beath pin into the previously drilled femoral tunnel. Approximately 25 mm of the doubled tibialis allograft is placed into to the tunnel, accompanied by approximately 10 mm of the imbricated popliteus tendon. This graft is secured by tying the sutures over a button place on the medial femoral cortex or tied over a post using a standard 4.5-mm AO screw and washer. This graft is tensioned with the knee in 30 degrees of flexion, using a bioabsorbable interference screw for fixation in the fibular tunnel (Fig. 25.10).

Medial Sided Injuries

The incision for the ACL/PCL tibial tunnels is extended proximal in curvilinear fashion to address medial injury. We feel that concomitant medial collateral ligament (MCL) injuries should only be repaired for a grade III injury in which the medial side opens up in full extension to valgus stress testing. We believe that the posterior oblique ligament

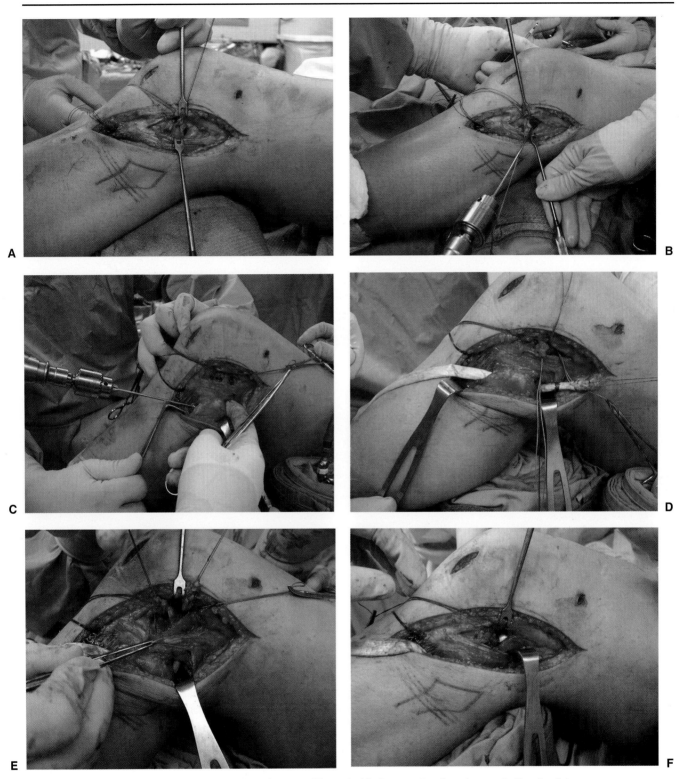

Figure 25.10. Intraoperative pictures of lateral-sided reconstruction demonstrating the following: **(A)** identifying, detaching, and tagging the popliteus tendon; **(B)** drilling of the femoral tunnel; **(C)** drilling of the fibular head tunnel; **(D)** passing the graft through the fibular head; **(E)** passing the graft with the popliteus tendon under the LCL; **(F)** pulling the graft and popliteus tendon through the femoral tunnel. (*continues*)

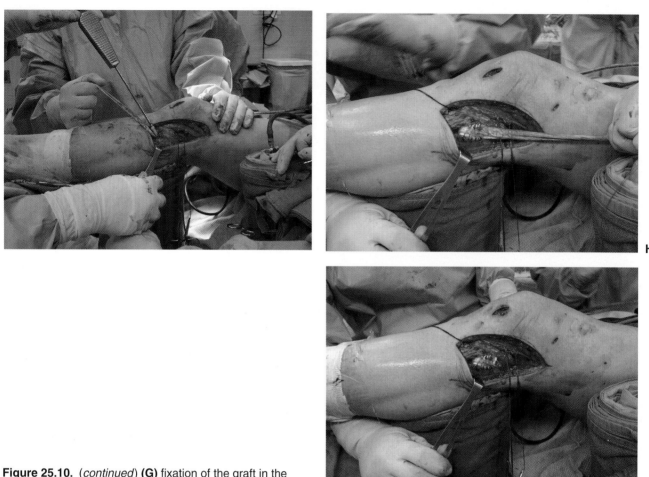

Figure 25.10. (*continued*) **(G)** fixation of the graft in the fibular head after tensioning; **(H)** reinforcing the graft by suturing it onto itself; **(I)** final picture of PLC reconstruction.

(POL), which is confluent with the posterior edge of the superficial MCL, plays an integral role in medial knee stability. If repair is indicated, a plane is established by incising longitudinally between the POL and the superficial MCL. The medial meniscal attachments to the POL are released back to the posteromedial corner of the knee. The peripheral border of the meniscus is rasped to prepare a bed for the repair of the POL. The POL is advanced anteriorly and imbricated to the superficial MCL in pants-over-vest fashion using suture (Fig. 25.11). The meniscus is repaired using full thickness sutures in an outside-in manner. In the acute setting, the MCL can usually be repaired primarily with intrasubstance nonabsorbable suture using a modified Kessler stitch. In the chronic setting, a reconstruction may be required to augment the repair.

Graft Tensioning

Now that all the grafts have been passed, graft tensioning and fixation can be accomplished in the following stepwise manner: Our preference is first to tension and fix the PCL, then the ACL, followed by the lateral structures, and finally the medial structures. The PCL is fixed distally with the knee in 90 degrees of flexion, and a bolster is placed under the tibia to support its weight against gravity. While the assistant is performing anterior drawer, the graft is fixed distally with an interference screw and/or a 4.5-mm AO screw and washer via standard post fixation. The ACL graft is tensioned and fixed distally in full extension with

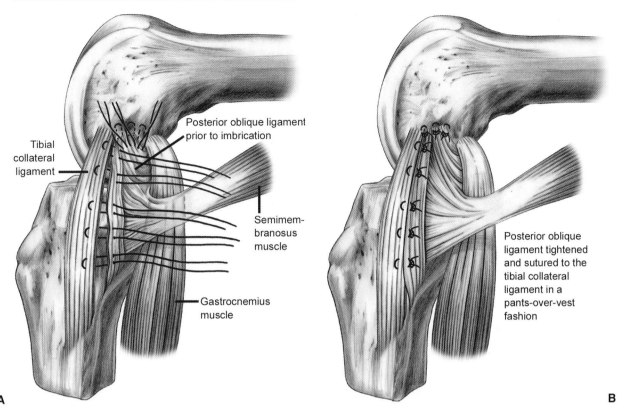

Figure 25.11. POL imbrication procedure.

an interference screw or a screw and washer. The knee is maintained in 30 degrees of flexion for fixation of both the PLC and LCL grafts. The PLC is reduced and fixed with an internal rotation force applied to the tibia relative to the femur. The MCL is fixed in 30 degrees of flexion. (Figs. 25.12 to 25.14).

After tensioning and fixation, the knee is taken through a complete range of motion. An examination for stability is also performed.

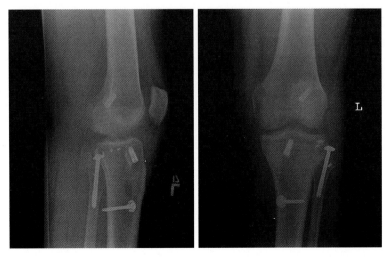

Figure 25.12. Postoperative radiographs of ACL/PCL/LCL reconstruction with PLC primary repair.

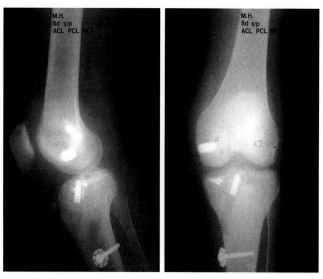

Figure 25.13. Postoperative radiographs of ACL/PCL/MCL reconstruction.

Closure and Postoperative Rehabilitation

The wounds are all well irrigated and a layered closure is performed. A standard sterile dressing is applied and a brace is applied with the knee locked in full extension. Deep venous thrombosis (DVT) prophylaxis is give to high-risk patients.

The brace is maintained, locked in full extension for the first 4 weeks. The goals during the early postoperative period include protecting the healing structures, regaining full passive extension, and maximizing quadriceps firing. Isometric quadriceps sets with the knee in full extension are encouraged in the immediate postoperative period. At the 2 weeks postoperative visit, the physical therapist will begin passive flexion, limited to 90 degrees, while applying an anterior directed force to the proximal tibia to prevent posterior tibial subluxation. Active flexion is prohibited in the first 6 weeks postoperatively to prevent hamstring-induced posterior tibial translation. Crutch weight bearing is progressed from partial weight bearing to as tolerated over the first 4 weeks. If a lateral sided repair or reconstruction was performed, the patient remains doing partial weight bearing until good quadriceps control is regained. At that time, the brace is unlocked and controlled gait training is commenced.

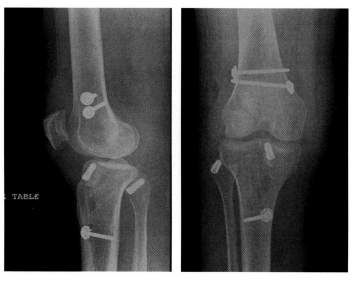

Figure 25.14. Postoperative radiographs of ACL/PCL/PLC reconstruction.

Quadriceps strengthening is progressed from the isometric sets to limited arc, open-chain, extension exercises from 60 to 75 degrees only. Exercises are limited to this motion arc to prevent excessive stress from being placed on the reconstructed grafts. At 6 weeks, passive and active-assisted range of motion and stretching exercises are begun to regain knee flexion. The brace is discontinued after 6 weeks. At 12 weeks, open-chain hamstring exercises may be performed. Patients may return to sedentary work in 2 to 3 weeks or heavy labor in 6 to 9 months. Patients are allowed to return to sports in 9 to 12 months.

COMPLICATIONS

Several potential complications exist, including wound complications, compartment syndrome, neurovascular injury, and residual laxity. Our surgical technique aims at minimizing these devastating complications.

1. Wound complications: Our skin incisions for the procedure are well planned to avoid pitfalls with exposure or wound complications. Consequently, we prefer an arthroscopic approach when possible, and we also prefer using allografts as opposed to autografts. For medial and/or lateral reconstructions, we do not recommend a midline incision because it provides limited access to the collaterals and may be complicated by skin sloughing over the patella. In the rare instance that both medial and lateral incisions are required, then at least 10 cm between incisions is recommended.

2. Compartment syndrome: When performing arthroscopy for multiple ligament surgery, it is important to maintain a low intra-articular fluid pressure to prevent extravasation of fluid. Consequently, we do not use a pump. Extravasation into the leg and thigh may result in a compartment syndrome. Therefore, the leg and thigh are intermittently palpated throughout the case to assure that the compartments are soft. If there is any question about the vascularity or leg compartment pressures, then the arthroscopic irrigation is stopped and the procedure is completed in a dry arthroscopic field or with an open technique. If necessary, compartment pressures are measured and fasciotomies performed.

3. Neurovascular injury: Popliteal neurovascular injury is a devastating complication and possible during creation of the PCL tibial tunnel. Consequently, we use a posteromedial portal to visualize and palpate the posterior cortex. In addition, we use fluoroscopy during placement of the guide wire and drilling of the tunnel, and we protect the guide wire and drill tip from posterior penetration with a curette. During the lateral reconstruction, it is imperative to visualize and protect the peroneal nerve, especially when drilling the fibula. With a medial approach, the saphenous nerve should be identified and protected throughout the case.

4. Residual laxity: Laxity of the grafts will occur if they are not tensioned and secured appropriately. The PCL graft must be secured first to restore the step-off of the tibial plateau. Next, the ACL should be tensioned to ensure reduction of the tibiofemoral joint. The medial or lateral reconstruction is completed last. Strict adherence to the postoperative protocol is critical so the grafts are not stretched.

RECOMMENDED READING

Abou-Sayed H, Berger DL. Blunt lower-extremity trauma and popliteal artery injuries: revisiting the case for selective arteriography. *Arch Surg* 2002;137:585–589.

Almekinders LC, Dedmond BT. Outcomes of operatively treated knee dislocation. *Clin Sports Med* 2000;19:503–518.

Fanelli CG, Edson CJ. Arthroscopically assisted combined anterior and posterior cruciate ligament reconstruction in the multiple ligament injured knee: 2- to 10-year follow-up. *Arthroscopy* 2002;18:703–714.

Fanelli GC, Giannotti BF, Edson CJ. Arthroscopically assisted combined anterior and posterior cruciate ligament reconstruction. *Arthroscopy* 1996;12:5–14.

Harner CD, Hoher J. Evaluation and treatment of posterior cruciate ligament injuries. *Am J Sports Med* 1998;26:471–482.

Harner C, Miller M. Graft tensioning and fixation in posterior cruciate ligament surgery. *Oper Tech Sports Med* 1993;1:115–120.

Harner CD, Waltrip RL, Bennett CH, et al. Surgical management of knee dislocations. *J Bone Joint Surg Am* 2004; 86:262–273.

Hughston JC, Eilers AF. The role of the posterior oblique ligament in repairs of the acute medial (collateral) ligament tears of the knee. *J Bone Joint Surg Am* 1973;55(5):923–940.

Irrgang J, Fitzgerald G. Rehabilitation of the multiple-ligament-injured knee. *Clin Sports Med* 2000;19:545–571.

Mariani PP, Margheritini F, Camillieri G. One-stage arthroscopically-assisted anterior and posterior cruciate ligament reconstruction. *Arthroscopy* 2001;17:700–707.

Meyers MH. Isolated avulsion of the tibial attachment of the posterior cruciate ligament of the knee. *J Bone Joint Surg Am* 1975;57:669–72.

Meyers MH, Harvey JP Jr. Traumatic dislocation of the knee joint: a study of eighteen cases. *J Bone Joint Surg Am* 1971; 53:16–29.

Miranda FE, Dennis JW, Veldenz HC, et al. Confirmation of the safety and accuracy of physical examination in the evaluation of knee dislocation for injury of the popliteal artery: a prospective study. *J Trauma* 2002;52:247–251.

Noyes FR, Barber-Westin SD. Reconstruction of the anterior and posterior cruciate ligaments after knee dislocation: use of early protected postoperative motion to decrease arthrofibrosis. *Am J Sports Med* 1997;25:769–778.

O'Donoghue DH. An analysis of end results of surgical treatment of major injuries to ligaments of the knee. *J Bone Joint Surg Am* 1955;37:1–13.

Richards RS, Moorman CT. Surgical techniques of open surgical reconstruction in the multiple ligament injured knee. *Oper Tech Sports Med* 2003;11(4):275–285.

Shapiro M, Freedman E. Allograft reconstruction of the anterior and posterior cruciate ligaments after traumatic knee dislocation. *Am J Sports Med* 1995;23:580–587.

Shelbourne KD, Porter DA, Clingman JA, et al. Low-velocity knee dislocation. *Orthop Rev* 1991;20:995–1004.

Taylor AR, Arden GP, Rainey HA. Traumatic dislocation of the knee: a report of forty-three cases with special reference to conservative treatment. *J Bone Joint Surg Br* 1972;54:96–102.

Wascher DC, Becker JR, Dexter JG, et al. Reconstruction of the anterior and posterior cruciate ligaments after knee dislocation: results using fresh-frozen nonirradiated allografts. *Am J Sports Med* 1999;27:189–196.

26

Tibial Plateau Fractures: Open Reduction Internal Fixation

J. Tracy Watson and Donald A. Wiss

INDICATIONS/CONTRAINDICATIONS

Fractures of the tibial plateau involve a major weight-bearing joint and may alter knee kinematics. Fractures range from minimally displaced intra-articular injuries with minimal soft-tissue embarrassment to fractures with significant soft-tissue compromise, bicondylar and shaft involvement, and extensive articular disruption. In an effort to preserve normal knee function, the physician must strive to restore joint congruity, preserve the mechanical axis, ensure joint stability, and restore knee motion. These goals may be difficult to accomplish in the face of compromised soft tissues, variable bone quality, and multiple medical comorbidities.

When considering operative management of a tibial plateau fracture, the surgeon should individualize treatment with respect to a variety of factors, such as the patient's age, preexisting levels of activity, medical conditions, and expectations. With regard to injuries, the surgeon should consider the extent of fracture comminution and joint impaction, associated injuries, and most important, the condition of the soft tissue.

The preferred treatment and specific methods of fixation of low-energy tibial-plateau fractures varies widely among surgeons. Numerous authors have reported satisfactory results using both nonoperative and surgical methods for treatment of low-energy tibial-plateau fractures in the elderly and others (1–3). Low-energy tibial-plateau fractures that do not result in joint instability, mal-alignment of the mechanical axis, or axial deformity are best treated nonoperatively.

Contemporary fixation techniques have been developed to improve outcomes in the treatment of high-energy fractures, particularly fractures that occur as a result of high-energy trauma with severe soft tissue compromise in a young patient population. For these complex fracture patterns, little controversy exists regarding the need for operative management. Absolute indications for surgery in these situations include open plateau fractures, fractures with an associated compartment syndrome, and fractures with a vascular injury. Relative indications for surgery include most displaced bicondylar fractures, displaced medial condyle fractures, coronal-plane posterior condylar fracture-dislocations, and lateral plateau fractures that result in axial joint instability (4–8).

The most common contraindication to emergent open reduction internal fixation (ORIF) is a compromised soft-tissue envelope, which can occur in either open or closed fractures. For those fractures, a ligamentotaxis reduction with the application of a temporary external fixator is strongly recommended (7,8). Following the resolution of soft tissue swelling, definitive open techniques that decrease the risk of complications can be undertaken. The spectrum of injuries to the tibial plateau is so great that no single method of treatment has proven uniformly successful. However, by following the principles of sound operative management, a congruous and stable knee joint can be achieved.

PREOPERATIVE PLANNING

History and Physical Exam

A patient with a tibial plateau fracture invariably presents with a painful, swollen knee and is unable to bear full weight on the effected extremity. The magnitude of force delivered to the knee determines the severity of fracture comminution, the amount of articular impaction, and the degree of condylar and shaft displacement. Therefore, the surgeon should determine whether the injury occurred as the result of a high- or low-energy force.

On physical exam, the doctor should focus on the integrity of the soft-tissue envelope particularly following high-energy injuries. Superficial abrasions, deep contusions, hemorrhagic blisters, and massive swelling indicate a severe soft-tissue injury. The presence of some or all of these findings precludes early ORIF techniques. If open wounds are present, their relationship to the fracture site and the knee joint must be ascertained. These areas should be avoided if a surgical approach is to be undertaken (8).

Following high-energy injuries, the peripheral pulses and nerve function as well as the status of the compartments should be evaluated and documented. Compartment pressure monitoring should be done in many patients with high-energy fractures, especially displaced medial plateau, bicondylar, and plateau fractures with shaft dissociation.

In patients with absent or diminished pulses, ankle/brachial indices (ABI) should be obtained. ABIs consist of a systolic blood pressure obtained at the palpated ankle over the palpated posterior tibial artery and a systolic pressure obtained at the elbow over the brachial artery. Under normal circumstances, the ratio of ankle systolic pressure divided by brachial pressure should be greater than 0.9. Values less than 0.9 are indicative of arterial injury, and formal angiography is indicated to determine the level of arterial disruption.

Imaging Studies

Except for very subtle joint injuries, anteroposterior (AP) and lateral radiographs of the knee usually indicate a plateau fracture. Routine radiographs should also include internal and external oblique views. The oblique views often allow physicians to detect subtle degrees of joint impaction or fracture lines not visible on the AP or lateral views.

Traction films are useful in highly comminuted and displaced fractures. Contemporary techniques require the surgeon's precise knowledge of the three dimensional anatomy of the fracture and ligamentotaxis effect; therefore, use of distraction or traction films is helpful in preoperative planning. Computed tomography (CT) scanning with axial, coronal, and sagittal reconstructions is still the image study of choice to delineate the extent and orientation of condylar fracture lines as well as to determine the location and depth of articular comminution and impaction. With low-energy fractures in stable patients, the CT scan can be obtained in a routine preoperative setting. However, for high-energy fractures that require early, spanning, external fixation, the CT scan should be obtained following the distraction treatment. Properly interpreted, CT scans can often influence the choice of surgical approach, including the location of surgical incisions and the insertion points of percutaneous plates and/or screws (8) (Fig. 26.1).

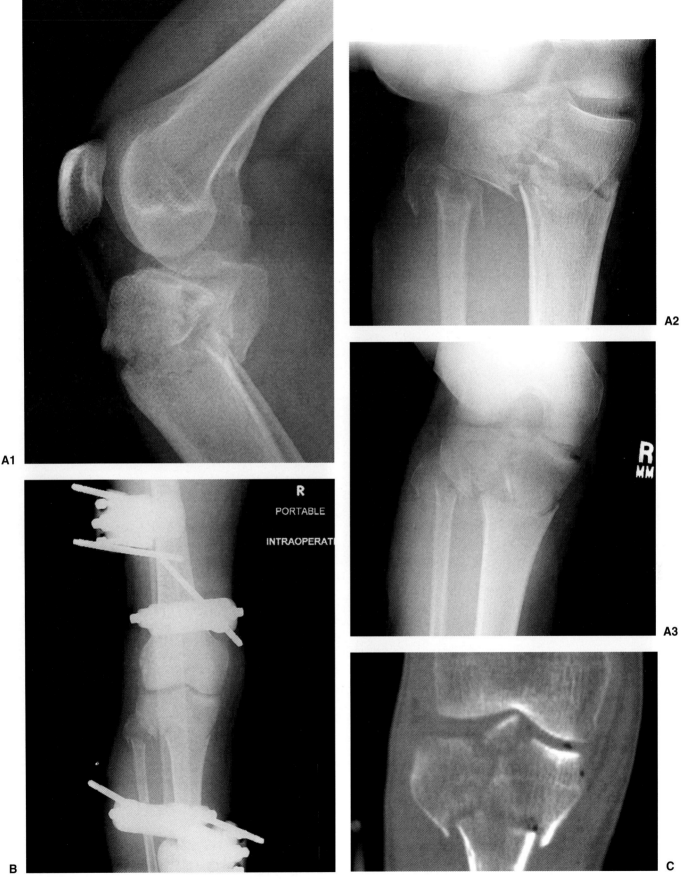

Figure 26.1. A1–3. AP, lateral, and oblique injury x-rays demonstrating a bicondylar fracture pattern. Because of displacement and mal-alignment, the fracture morphology is not clearly seen. **B.** A traction radiograph restores length and allows identification of fracture components. **C.** A traction CT scan demonstrating the fracture morphology. Traction accomplished a near anatomic alignment of medial and lateral condyles, shaft axis alignment, and identified avulsion of the intracondylar eminence.

Because of the high incidence of associated soft-tissue injuries that can occur with tibial plateau fractures, magnetic resonance imaging (MRI) scans can be very helpful. MRI has been shown to be superior to CT scans in assessing soft-tissue injuries. In addition to delineating the fracture and possible meniscal pathology, MRI can detect associated soft-tissue lesions such as tears of the medial collateral ligament or anterior cruciate ligament, which are often seen with lateral plateau fractures. Likewise, tears of the lateral collateral or cruciate ligaments associated with fractures of the medial plateau can be detected through this imaging modality (Fig. 26.2) (9,10).

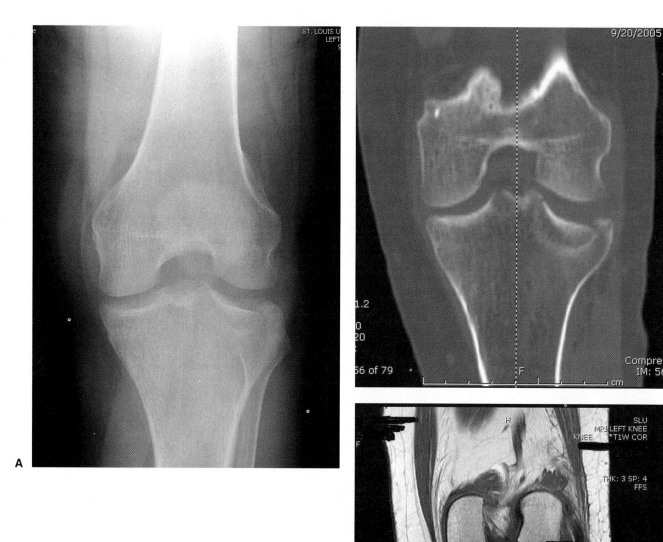

Figure 26.2. A. AP view of Schatzker type III fracture with demonstrated lateral articular impaction. **B.** CT scan demonstrates orientation and depth of articular impaction. **C.** MRI demonstrates not only depth of articular impaction but also denotes peripheral lateral-meniscal tear (*square*).

A preoperative plan and surgical tactic help ensure that the proper implants, reduction tools, bone graft (or bone graft substitutes), and fluoroscopic equipment are available for the surgical procedure.

We stratify tibial plateau fractures according to the Schatzker classification in which these injuries are divided into six distinct subtypes and associated treatment principles (6). In addition, dividing these fractures into low-energy versus high-energy injuries may help in determining the initial degree of soft-tissue compromise (8). Depressed articular fragments will not reduce by manipulation, traction, or ligamentotaxis techniques alone. If articular impaction and subsequent defects are sufficient to produce axial joint instability or mechanical axis deviation with weight bearing, the joint surface should be surgically elevated and supported with graft material and fixation hardware (6). Therefore, the surgical tactic and location of incisions must optimize exposure and reduction techniques.

SURGERY

There is no universal agreement on the amount of articular depression or step off that dictates nonoperative or surgical treatment. Long-term studies with greater than 20-year follow-up have shown an inconsistent relationship between residual osseous depression of the joint surface and the development of osteoarthrosis. However, if joint deformity or depression produces knee instability, the likelihood of a poor outcome is significantly increased (2,3). When forming the goals of surgery, the physician must address the factors that are thought to determine outcomes:

- integrity of the soft tissue envelope,
- the degree of articular depression,
- the extent of condylar separation or widening, and
- the degree of diametaphyseal comminution and shaft dissociation association.

Surgery is performed with the patient under general or spinal anesthesia positioned supine on a radiolucent operating table. Some surgeons prefer a table that has the ability to break so that the knee can be flexed to approximately 90 degrees. We prefer a large bolster or a bean bag patient positioner to elevate the operative extremity when placed under the ipsilateral hip; it allows the knee to be flexed to 90 degrees intraoperatively. A C-arm image intensifier is positioned on the contralateral side. Trial images should be obtained prior to prepping and draping to ensure that accurate AP, lateral, and oblique fluoroscopic images are easily attainable without interference. The entire extremity is then prepped and draped from toes to groin. If an iliac crest bone graft is planned, then the ipsilateral crest is also included in the initial prep and a sterile tourniquet is utilized (Fig. 26.3).

Contemporary implants include 2.7-mm and 3.5-mm low profile sizes, which are precontoured to match the proximal tibial condylar anatomy. The large 4.5-mm and 6.5-mm implants are used less frequently today. Peri-articular plates require less exposure than do their predecessors. Because the majority of plateau fractures involve the lateral condylar surface, a variant of a lateral parapatellar incision is most commonly used for most lateral plateau fractures. This incision can be utilized at its proximal extent to expose only the lateral condyle, but it can also be easily extended proximally and distally when more exposure is needed, such as in an Schatzker V or VI injury.

With medial condylar fractures, the orientation and apex of the medial fracture line determines the location of a possible medial incision. Thus a medial or posteromedial incision may be necessary when treating specific, isolated, medial condylar (Schatzker IV) or bicondylar fracture patterns. With fracture dislocations of the medial condyle in the coronal plane (1), the apex of the fracture line is sometimes oriented directly posterior. In these cases, a direct posterior exposure may be required for fracture stabilization (11).

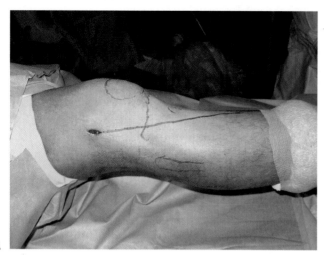

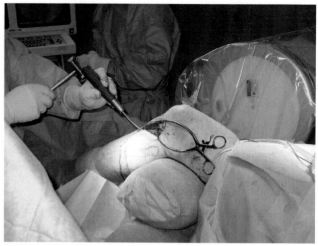

A   B

Figure 26.3. A,B. Position of knee in the operating room. The knee is elevated using a sterile bolster to allow flexion to at least 90 degrees. The ability to achieve 360-degree fluoroscopic visualization is mandatory.

Treatment of Specific Fracture Types

Schatzker Type I. A split or wedge fracture of the lateral tibial plateau is often amenable to a percutaneous fixation (Fig. 26.4). A preoperative MRI should be obtained to assess the integrity of the lateral meniscus. If the meniscus is intact, a closed reduction and percutaneous fixation with cannulated screws or noncannulated cortical screws may be performed (9). Applying longitudinal traction with a varus force may improve the reduction. As an alternative, a laterally based femoral distractor can be used to restore length and alignment through ligamentotaxis. When an acceptable reduction is obtained, the fracture is held with a large pointed forceps placed percutaneously on the medial and lateral condyles to compress the fracture line. Fixation is usually accomplished with two or three 6.5- or 7.0-mm screws placed through small stab incisions, or occasionally through use of multiple 3.5-mm cortical screws (12). The orientation of these screws should be determined preoperatively and based either on the MRI or CT scan (Fig. 26.5).

If the preoperative MRI demonstrates a peripheral meniscal tear or incarceration of the meniscus within the vertical fracture line, or if a closed reduction fails to reduce the fracture adequately, ORIF with meniscal repair or excision is indicated.

In comminuted fracture patterns, when direct cortical apposition (i.e., bone on bone stability following reduction) is not found, a laterally directed buttress or antiglide plate should be used instead of solitary, multiple, lag screws.

Schatzker Type II. Schatzker type II injuries involve a lateral condyle fracture combined with varying degrees of articular surface depression (Fig. 26.6). Preoperative imaging studies are important to determine the degree and location of articular impaction as well as the orientation of the apex of the condylar fracture line. In most cases, the depression is anterior or central and is best approached through an anterolateral incision. The joint surface is visualized through a submeniscal arthrotomy. The lateral menisco-tibial ligament is incised transversely, allowing elevation of the meniscus through the use of several small traction sutures or small angled retractors (Fig. 26.7). A varus stress is applied to open the joint line for visualization of the articular surface of the lateral plateau.

Following joint exposure, the knee is flexed to 90 degrees, which allows additional visualization of the joint surface because the joint is distracted via the weight of the leg. Alternatively a femoral distractor can be used to enhance joint visualization through sustained distraction.

Impacted articular fragments can be reduced by two different techniques. In one method, the condylar fracture line is wedged open like a book. The articular depression is directly visualized and an impactor is inserted from below to disimpact and elevate the

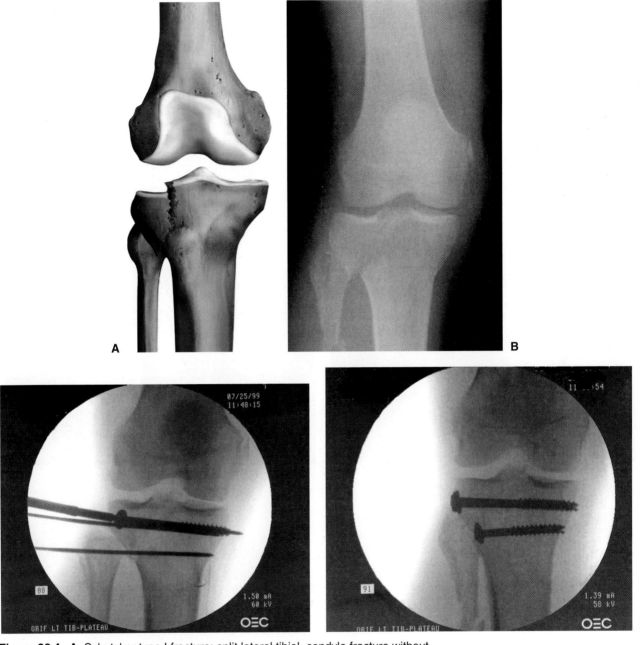

Figure 26.4. A. Schatzker type I fracture: split lateral tibial–condyle fracture without articular impaction. **B.** X-ray demonstrating Schatzker type I injury. **C,D.** Closed reduction accomplished with distraction and varus stress. Guide wires are advanced, followed by cannulated screw fixation. The inferior screw acts as an antiglide washer at apex of fragment.

osteochondral fragments. Once the articular fragments have been repositioned in a congruent fashion, provisional Kirschner (K) wires are used to temporarily stabilize the joint. The elevated osteochondral fragments create a metaphyseal defect that requires support prior to reduction of the condyle. This support is accomplished through placement of graft material beneath the reduced fragment into the subchondral void. Many alloplastic calcium phosphate and sulfate materials are now available for use as substitutes for autograft bone in grafts (13,14). Following graft placement, the split condyle is reduced and held with large reduction forceps (Fig. 26.8). Fixation of the condyle is achieved with a peri-articular plate or lag screws.

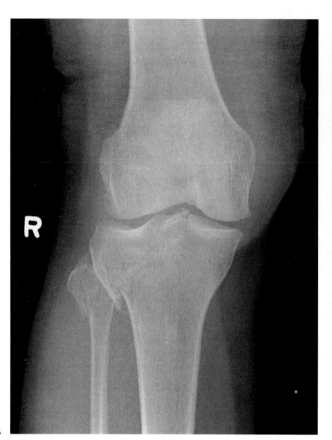

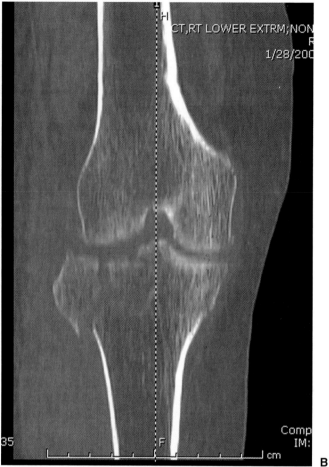

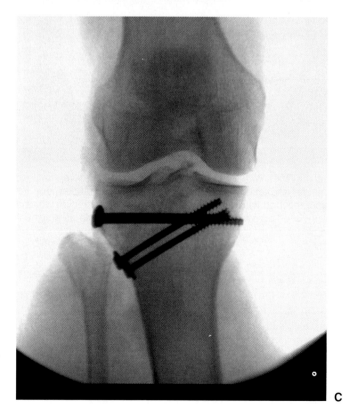

Figure 26.5. A. AP x-ray demonstrating a solitary split in the lateral condyle. **B.** CT scan reveals a sagittal split in the lateral condylar fragment. CT information aids in the orientation of percutaneous screw placement. **C**. Fixation is accomplished percutaneously with small fragment screws and washers functioning as small antiglide plates.

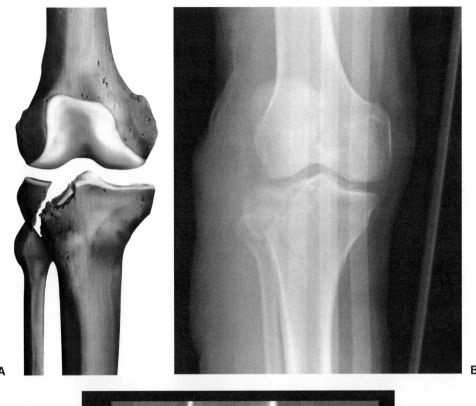

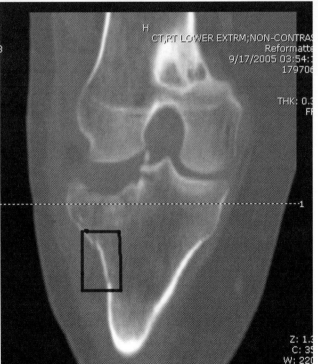

Figure 26.6. A. Schatzker type II injury: Comminution and impaction of the lateral articular surface occurs with a large wedge fracture of the lateral tibial condyle. **B,C.** AP radiograph and CT scan demonstrating the depth and orientation of articular impaction as well as the segmental, lateral-condylar, fracture lines (*square*). This information helps the surgeon determine the length of the incision.

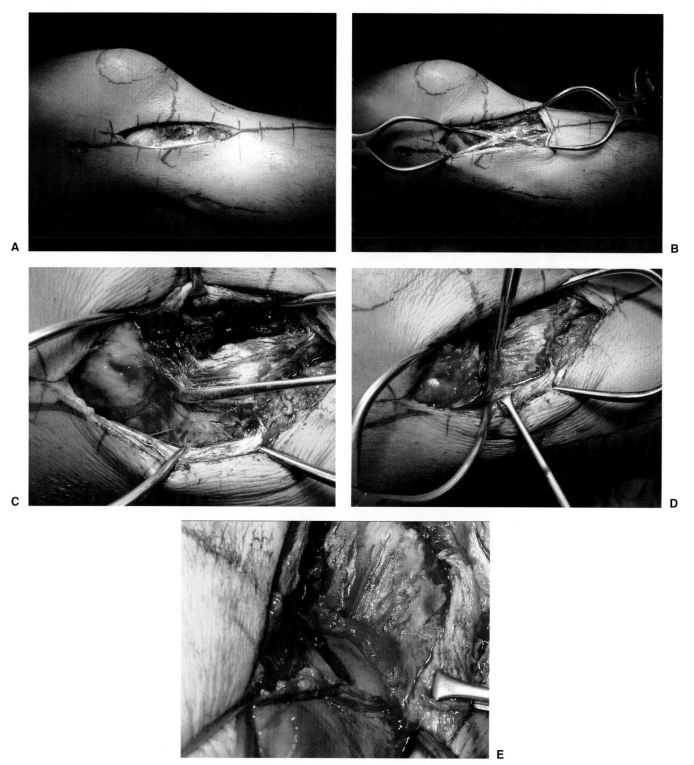

Figure 26.7. A. Standard, lateral, utility incision: The incision begins 1 to 2 cm proximal to the joint line along the midaxillary line in the midportion of the fascia lata. It is carried distally over Gerdy's tubercle and gently angled toward the lateral border of the anterior tibial crest. The incision can be extended proximally or distally as necessary. **B.** The fascia lata is split (retracted for demonstration) in the midline and centered over Gerdy's tubercle. The anterior compartment fascia is incised in continuity just lateral to the anterior tibial crest. **C.** Retracting the anterior (*clamp*) and posterior portions of the fascia lata expose the major fracture line and capsular structures. The meniscal tibial ligament is identified (*elevator*). **D.** The menisco-tibial ligament has been incised below the level of the lateral meniscus. The tibial attachment of the ligament is preserved (*forceps*) to facilitate repair of the peripheral meniscal tear (just proximal to forceps, tear is visible). **E.** Sutures are attached to the meniscus and proximal capsule to facilitate meniscal retraction. The submeniscal arthrotomy allows direct joint visualization. Articular impaction, in continuity with the major fracture line, is visible.

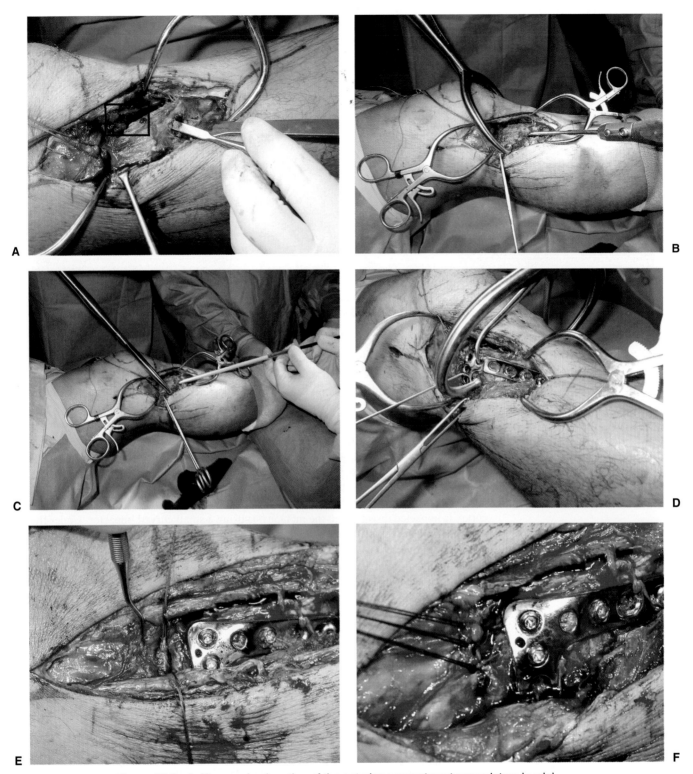

Figure 26.8. A. The proximal portion of the anterior compartment musculature is minimally reflected from the lateral condyle so access is gained to the condylar flare. The major fracture line can be gapped open to gain direct access to the articular impaction through the fracture line (*square*); this technique allows for joint elevation. In an alternative approach, a subcondylar window can be fashioned with multiple drill holes and a small osteotome. **B.** The condyle is reduced and compressed with a large reduction clamp placed percutaneously in the medial and lateral condyle. A curved impactor is used to elevate the depressed articular surface. **C.** The subchondral void is filled with an alloplastic bone-graft substitute, which can be applied in an indirect fashion (injected). The surface is continuously elevated until congruency is achieved. **D.** A precontoured plate is advanced distally in a submuscular fashion. The plate is held in place with large pointed forceps and temporary K wires. **E.** Following application of fixation hardware, the peripheral meniscal tear (*sutures*) is repaired to the capsule. **F.** The submeniscal arthrotomy is closed by suturing the meniscal-tibial ligament. (*continues*)

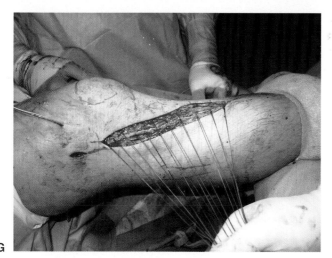
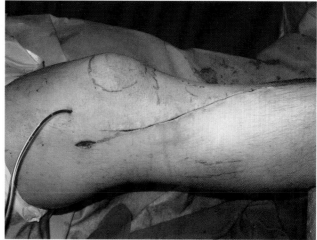

G   H

Figure 26.8. (*continued*) **G.** The fascia lata is closed over suction drains. **H.** Skin closure is accomplished without tension.

Multiple screws can be placed horizontally in the subchondral region as "raft screws." These horizontally directed screws should capture the intact medial cortex. The screws are supported on either side of the impaction by the intact lateral and medial cortices, much like I beams support horizontal rafters on a roof. These raft screws help support the elevated articular surface and prevent late subsidence (Fig. 26.9) (5). The surgeon should carefully repair the menisco-tibial ligament and meniscal tears when present.

In an alternative method, the lateral condyle can be reduced first and held with the large, pointed, reduction forceps. Once the condylar fracture lines have been reduced, the impacted articular surface is addressed indirectly. A 1-cm cortical window in the subcondylar flare is fashioned by connecting multiple, small drill holes with a small osteotome. The cortex is impacted directly into the metaphysis using a small curved impactor. Under fluoroscopic guidance, the impactor is directed to engage from below the depressed osteochondral fragment. The surgeon must disimpact and elevate the fracture fragments en masse by placing graft material continuously beneath the fracture fragment. The pressure from the impactor distributed over a relatively large surface area minimizes fragmentation or splitting of the articular surface. The joint surface is slowly elevated as visualized indirectly by fluoroscopy or directly through the submeniscal exposure. Once articular congruency has been reestablished provisional K wire fixation is utilized. A peri-articular or percutaneous plate with raft screws can be passed directly through the proximal aspect of the incision and distal screws applied through small percutaneous stab wounds (see Fig. 26.8).

Schatzker Type III. Schatzker type III fractures are uncommon and usually occur after a low-energy valgus-stress injury in elderly patients with osteoporotic bone. The articular surface of the lateral plateau is impacted without an associated lateral condylar fracture. A preoperative MRI or CT scan will specifically locate the area of impaction and orientation of the impacted osteochondral fragments. In additional, MRI is helpful in identifying meniscal pathology or incarceration of the meniscus within the depressed articular surface.

The treatment of type III injuries has become relatively less invasive than it has been in the past. This fracture is now treated with small incisions made while the surgeon uses an image intensifier or arthroscopic visualization of the articular surface (Fig. 26.10). A small lateral incision is made over the metaphyseal region of the lateral condyle, and exposure is limited to develop a small, subcondylar, metaphyseal, cortical window. This exposure can also be developed in percutaneous fashion. The window must be of sufficient size to allow grafting and elevation of the fragment from below and the surgeon to assess the reduced surface from above or through arthroscopic visualization. Once reduction of the joint is confirmed, the graft is stabilized by percutaneous raft screws placed in a subchondral location (12,15). As an alternative, cannulated screws can be utilized.

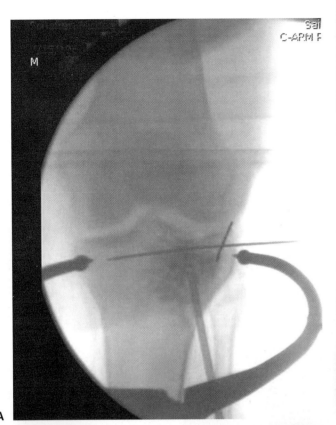

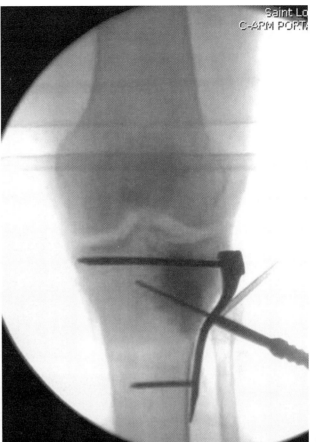

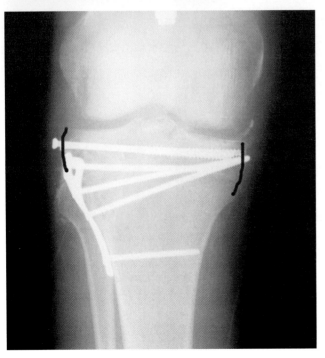

Figure 26.9. **A.** Fluoroscopic visualization shows articular surface elevation and graft placement. **B.** Raft screws are placed through the proximal portion of the plate, capturing the intact medial cortex and thus providing support for the elevated articular surface. **C.** Solitary raft screws placed in a subchondral location support the articular surface. The screws are supported by the reconstructed lateral cortex and the intact medial cortex (*black lines*).

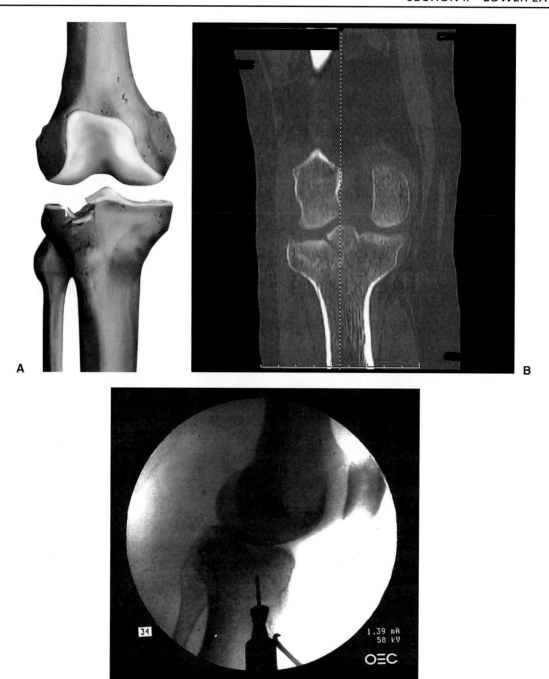

Figure 26.10. A. A Schatzker type III injury involves impaction and comminution of the lateral articular surface. **B.** CT scan of Schatzker type III injury that demonstrates central impaction of the lateral articular surface and preservation of an intact lateral-condylar rim. This particular pattern is amenable to arthroscopic-assisted fixation. **C.** A subchondral window is produced through the use of a cannulated drill with guide wire localized via arthroscopic visualization. (*continues*)

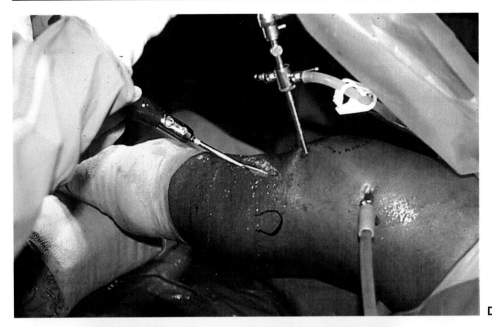

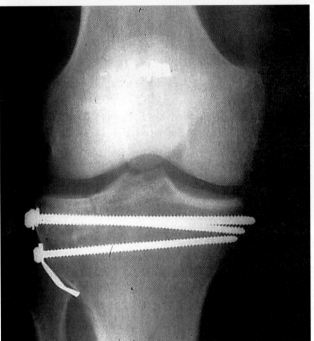

Figure 26.10. (*continued*) **D.** The articular surface is elevated through use of a bone impactor followed by percutaneous raft-screw fixation. **E.** Follow-up x-rays demonstrate healed subchondral surface and maintenance of fracture reduction.

Schatzker Type IV. Fractures of the medial plateau (Schatzker type IV) are usually caused by high-energy trauma and are often associated with neurovascular injuries and significant fracture displacement. They frequently occur with other injuries, such as knee dislocations with ligamentous disruption. A high index of suspicion is necessary to avoid overlooking a limb-threatening injury with this fracture pattern. In fractures with minimal comminution or displacement, closed reduction can be attempted with large reduction forceps. Successful fixation through use of multiple percutaneous screws is usually sufficient. However, most medial plateau fractures are grossly unstable with comminution in the region of the intercondylar eminence and at the distal apex of the condylar fragment (6). For comminuted fracture patterns, a buttress plate rather than lag screws are needed. When the intercondylar eminence is avulsed and includes the anterior cruciate ligament, percutaneous treatment is contraindicated (Fig. 26.11).

Preoperative CT scans are invaluable in determining the apex of the medial-condylar fracture line. The location is highly variable and may be directed posteriorly, posteromedially, medially, or anteromedially. The orientation and location of the medial fracture line dictates

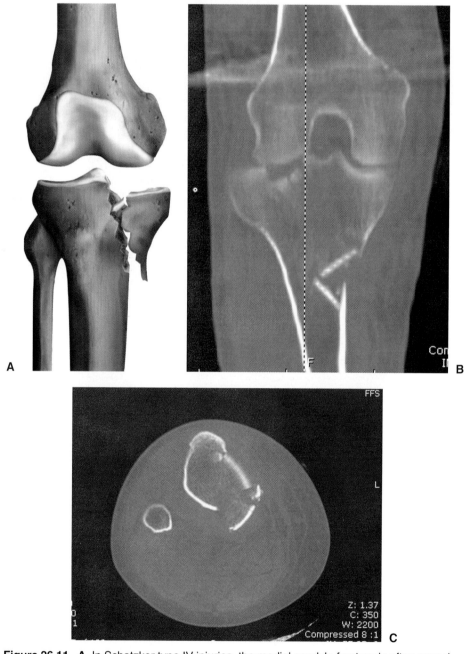

Figure 26.11. A. In Schatzker type IV injuries, the medial condyle fracture is often associated with intracondylar comminution and fragmentation. **B.** Coronal reconstruction demonstrates comminution at the intercondylar eminence and involves the lateral articular surface, which must also be addressed through surgery. **C.** Transverse CT cuts reveal that the apex of the medial condylar fracture is directed posteromedially. Therefore, the incision should be directed in this region and the plate positioned along the posteromedial tibial border.

the location of the surgical incision. To improve the surgical exposure, a preoperative CT evaluation is imperative so the surgeon can place the incision as close to the apex of the major condylar fracture line as possible.

Fixation is accomplished with a small-fragment buttress plate located over the apex of the condylar fracture line. An anteromedial fracture location requires that the anterior pes anserine tendons be posteromedially reflected in continuity with the superficial portion of the medial collateral ligament. The plate lies in contact with the entire metaphyseal surface without entrapping the underlying soft tissue. If the apex is more medially directed, the inferior margin of the pes can be reflected anteriorly and a plate positioned on the posteromedial aspect of the tibia anterior to the medial gastrocnemius muscle (Fig. 26.12).

When the fracture is located in the posterior aspect of the knee, a direct exposure of the posterior medial condyle is accomplished through a posterior approach. The patient is placed prone and a direct medial incision is placed along the posteromedial border of the proximal tibia. The exposure is accomplished by lateral retraction of the medial gastrocnemius and popliteus muscles. This provides direct visualization of the entire posterior aspect of the proximal tibia and facilities direct application of a posterior plate (Fig. 26.13) (11).

Schatzker Types V & VI. The complex plateau injuries designated as Schatzker types V and VI are usually the result of high-energy forces that may compromise the surrounding soft tissues (Fig. 26.14). A staged approach is usually required for successful treatment of these injury patterns (5,7,8). Bridging external fixators should be applied rapidly to restore length and stability. Distraction CT or MRI scans are much more valuable after application of a bridging external fixator. Careful preoperative planning is required and definitive surgery is not undertaken until the soft tissues have recovered. In many cases, surgery may be delayed for 2 or 3 weeks while soft tissues heal (Fig. 26.15).

With the development of precontoured low-profile implants, the necessity for extensile exposure of the upper tibia can be minimized. The routine use of both a medial and lateral plate has also decreased because of the development of locking plates, which allow the stabilization of many medial-condylar fragments from the lateral side alone. In addition, many of these newer implant systems are designed for percutaneous insertion and thus extensile approaches can be avoided.

Schatzker V and VI fractures are frequently comminuted, and the shaft is displaced from the metaphysis. Many locked-plating systems can stabilize the metaphyseal diaphyseal fracture through indirect percutaneous techniques in which one or two femoral distractors maintain the reduction. Large, percutaneously applied, reduction forceps may reduce or improve the position of the intercondylar fracture lines. Based upon preoperative imaging studies, articular impaction is elevated through the surgeon's use of cortical windows placed either medially or laterally in the subcondylar regions.

The universal lateral approach is utilized to expose the proximal aspect of the lateral condyle. Cannulated or 3.5-mm screws can be used to secure the intercondylar reduction after which the condyles must be attached to the tibial shaft. If the soft tissues allow, a locking plate can be slid in a submuscular fashion along the lateral aspect of the shaft. The locking plates are designed to bridge the zone of comminution at the diametaphyseal junction. Many of these implant systems have outriggers that are used to place screws into the distal portions of the plate via small percutaneous incisions (Fig. 26.16) (16). If the condylar fracture fragments are not comminuted and the condyles are well reduced, the medial condyle can be controlled with a laterally based locking plate with locked screws. However, coronal splits of the posterior aspect of the medial condyle cannot be stabilized with a lateral plate alone and require independent fixation. Little data are available to assess accurately the performance and ability of these locking plates to prevent varus deformities of the medial condylar fragment. If anatomic cortical contact can be obtained following reduction, then a laterally based locking plate can be used to maintain both the lateral and medial condylar reduction. However, if the apex of the medial condyle is comminuted or located posteriorly, then this fragment requires support to prevent late varus deformity. This stability is accomplished by placement of an extra periosteal antiglide buttress or small locking plate. A locking plate on the medial side can

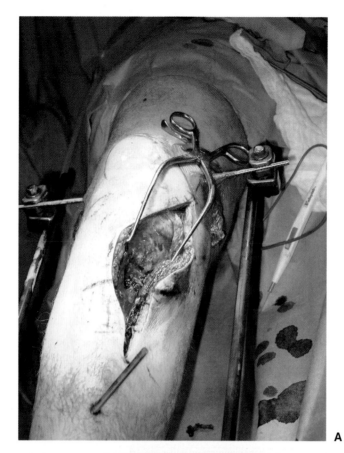

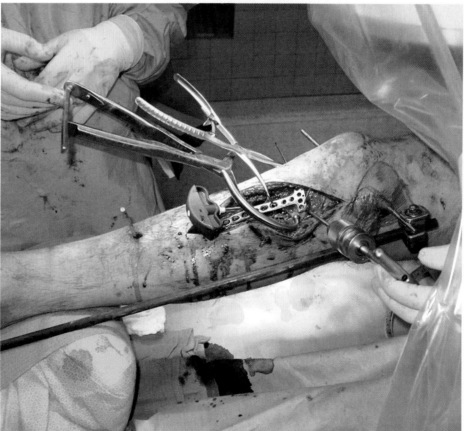

Figure 26.12. A. The medial exposure is directed at the medial aspect of the tibia at the apex of the medial condyle fracture (comminution at the base of the medial fragment determines the location of plate). **B.** Reduction is accomplished with large reduction forceps and a Schantz pin used as a joystick. A trocar is used to insert the bone graft substitute. The plate is positioned directly at the apex of the condylar fracture, bridging the area of comminution. (*continues*)

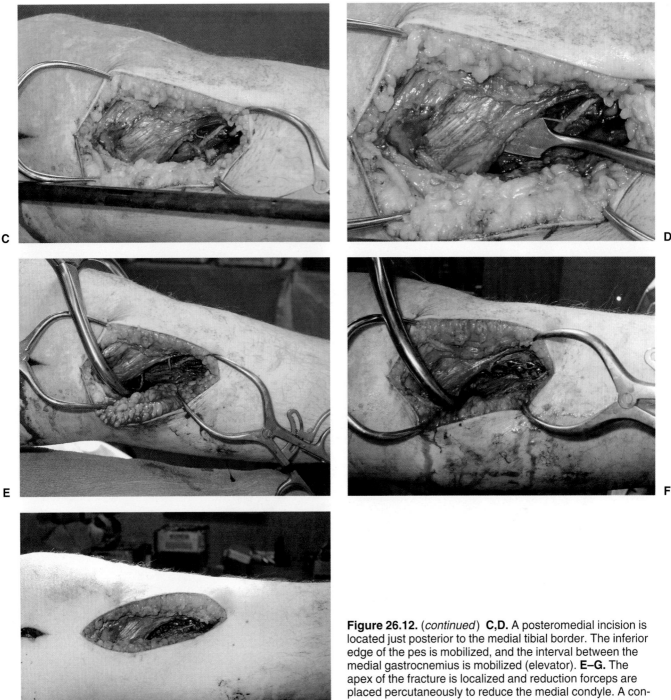

Figure 26.12. (*continued*) **C,D.** A posteromedial incision is located just posterior to the medial tibial border. The inferior edge of the pes is mobilized, and the interval between the medial gastrocnemius is mobilized (elevator). **E–G.** The apex of the fracture is localized and reduction forceps are placed percutaneously to reduce the medial condyle. A contoured plate is then advanced along the medial condylar flare in an extraperiosteal fashion. Following screw application, the surgeon allows the pes to cover the plate, and the wound is easily closed.

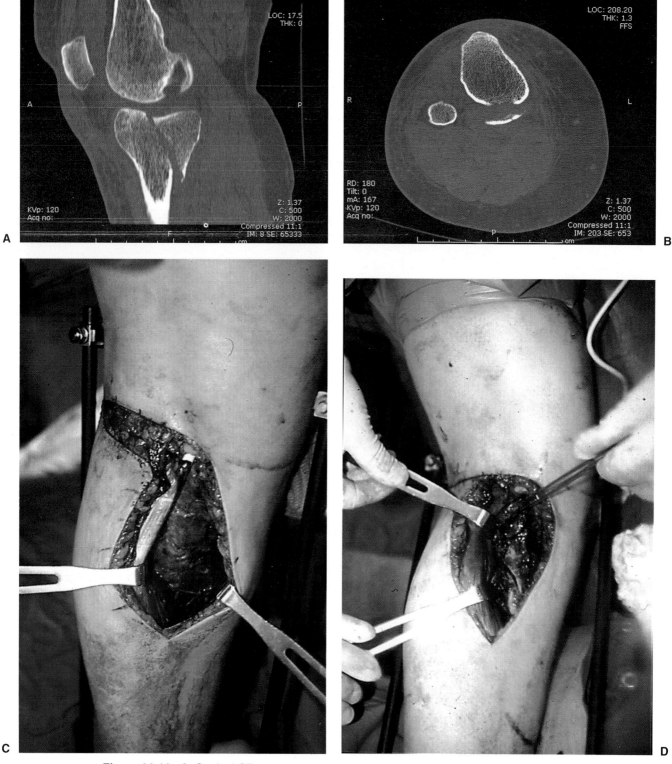

Figure 26.13. A. Sagittal CT cuts reveal a posteriorly directed medial-condyle fracture. **B.** The apex of the fracture line is directly posterior. This placement precludes use of lag screw fixation from front to back. A posterior buttress plate is required to maintain the reduction. **C.** Direct posterior approach allows the surgeon to retract the medial head of the gastrocnemius (under retractor) laterally, exposing the soleus and posteromedial border of the tibia. **D.** The soleus muscle is incised along the medial border of the tibia and then retracted laterally exposing the posterior fracture lines. (*continues*)

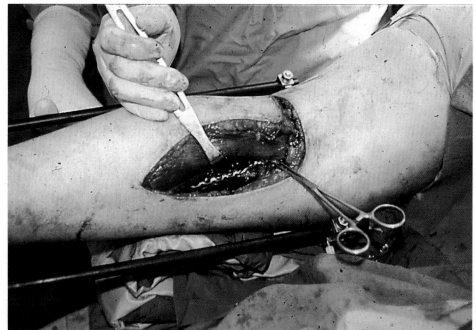

E

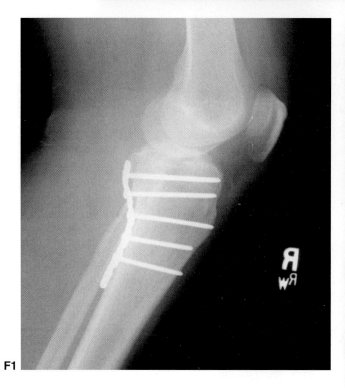

F1

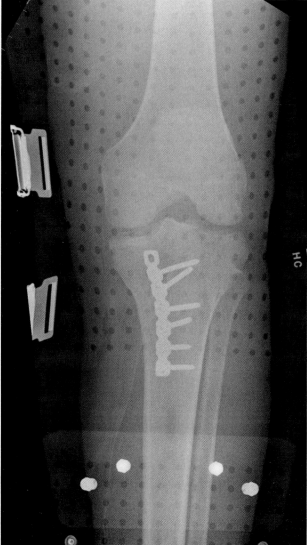

F2

Figure 26.13. (*continued*) **E.** A buttress plate is applied directly to the posterior tibia the posterior capsule, which can also be incised to allow limited visualization of the joint.
F1,2. A reconstruction plate is contoured to buttress the posterior fracture line.

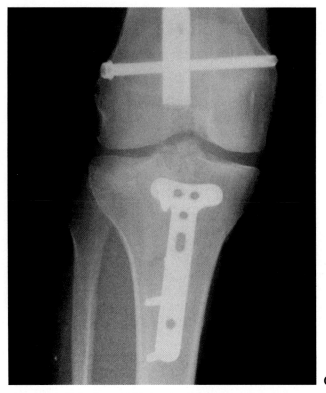

G

Figure 26.13. (*continued*) **G.** A small T plate is directed posteriorly to prevent displacement of this unstable condylar fracture.

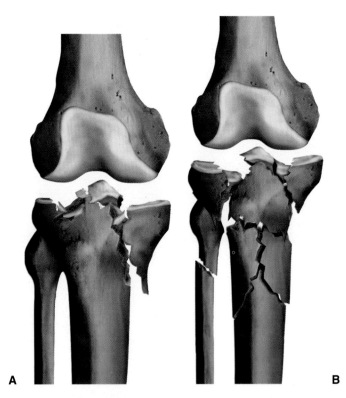

A   B

Figure 26.14. A. A Schatzker type V fracture pattern involves both condyles with lateral joint impaction (high-energy fracture pattern). **B.** This Schatzker type VI fracture involves both condyles as well as complete dissociation of the metaphyseal region from the shaft.

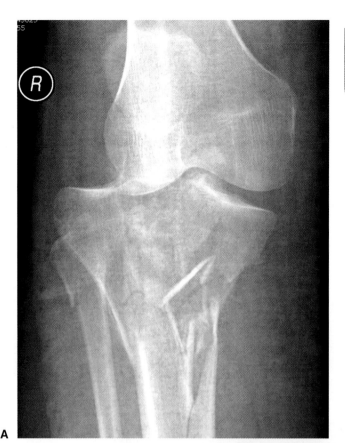

A

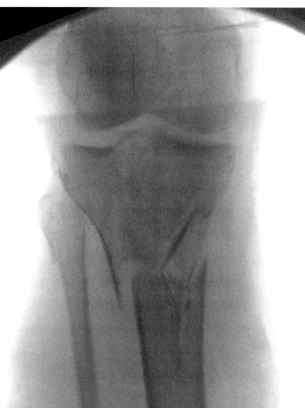

B

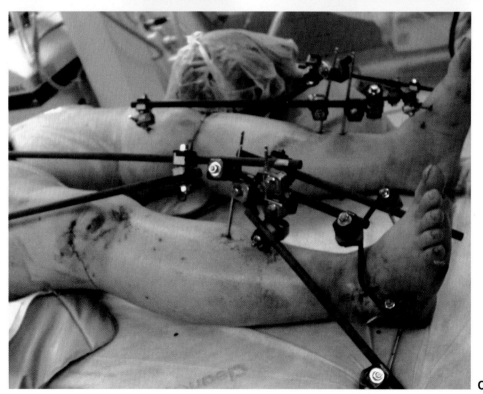

C

Figure 26.15. A. A high-energy fracture with bicondylar and shaft involvement. **B.** Immediate application of a temporary external fixator via ligamentotaxis realigns the metaphyseal condylar fragments as well as the shaft dissociation. **C,D.** Bilateral high-energy plateau fractures are shown in a polytrauma patient who has spanning external fixators bridging both knees to allow soft-tissue recovery. Definitive fixation was accomplished with a limited lateral approach to reconstruct the lateral condyle. The shaft extension was spanned successfully through use of percutaneous application of a locking plate that also supported the medial condyle. (*continues*)

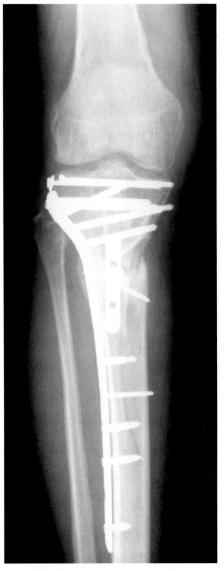

D

Figure 26.15. (*continued*)

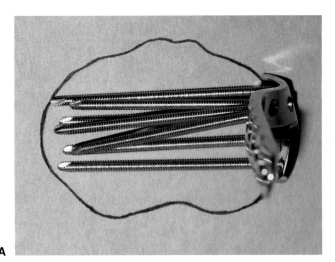

A

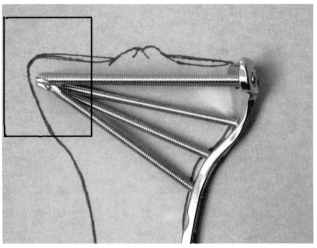

B

Figure 26.16. A,B. Locking plates perform the raft function by supporting the subchondral reconstruction with multiple parallel screws spanning the fracture from lateral plate to medial cortex. Because of the locking function and orientation of all metaphyseal screws, potential varus deformity of the medial condyle is decreased (*square*). Many of these plates have outriggers that allow shaft screws to be applied in a percutaneous manner. (*continues*)

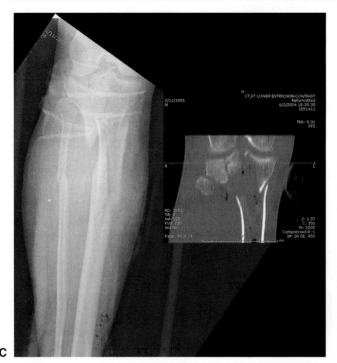

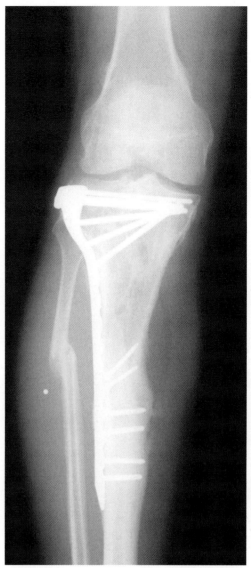

Figure 26.16. (*continued*) **C,D.** Complex Schatzker VI fracture treated with a long peri-articular locking plate healed without varus deformation. The shaft extension was stabilized without direct exposure because the surgeon placed the distal screws via a percutaneous approach with an outrigger device.

be placed with the use of unicortical locking screws. The implant is placed at the apex of the medial tibial condyle as determined by preoperative CT scan. Care should be taken to limit dissection through the second incision and to avoid creation of large skin flaps (Fig. 26.17).

If extensive comminution or soft tissue injury is present, additional incisions are contraindicated to avoid wound problems, and a ring fixator is indicated for stabilization of these complex injuries. It cannot be overemphasized that when extreme soft-tissue compromise is present, formal or even limited open reduction and plate osteosynthesis should be abandoned in favor of small tension wire or hybrid external-fixation techniques.

POSTOPERATIVE MANAGEMENT

Postoperatively the limb is placed into a bulky Jones dressing from the toes to groin. A cephalosporin is administered for 24 to 48 hours after surgery. A suction drain is maintained for at least 24 hours or until drainage is less then 30 mL per 8 hour interval.

If the soft-tissue envelope was not significantly damaged at the time of injury and wound closure was achieved without tension, a continuous passive motion (CPM) machine is recommended. If significant swelling or tension on the suture line is present the CPM is delayed until the swelling has subsided. The bulky dressing is removed at 48 hours and a hinged knee brace that allows gradual increase in range of motion is applied. If a meniscal

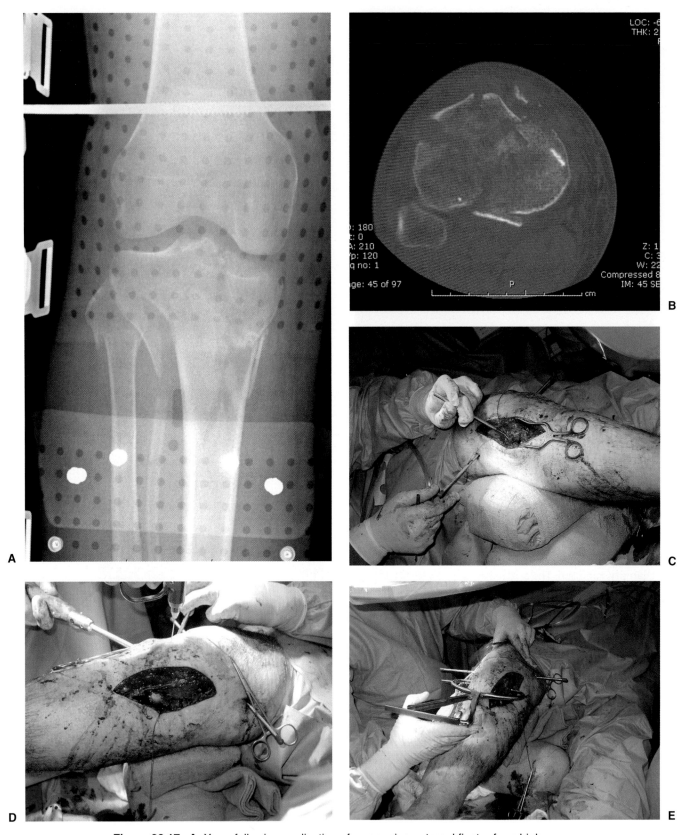

Figure 26.17. A. X-ray following application of a spanning external fixator for a high-energy plateau fracture with bicondylar involvement. **B.** Distraction CT demonstrating bicondylar involvement. The scan also helps localize proposed incision for medial condylar fixation. **C.** The lateral condyle is approached through a standard lateral approach, allowing reduction and elevation of the depressed joint surface through this incision. **D.** The medial incision is located based on CT data. The plate is located between the pes anserine and medial gastrocnemius. Although the incision is sizable, soft-tissue stripping is minimized. **E.** Large reduction forceps are used to manipulate the bicondylar fracture line and to compress the plates to bone for secure fixation. (*continues*)

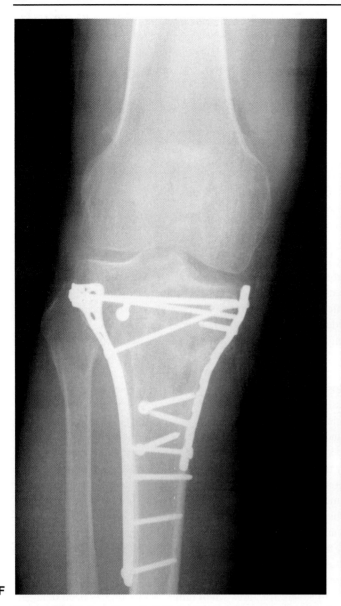
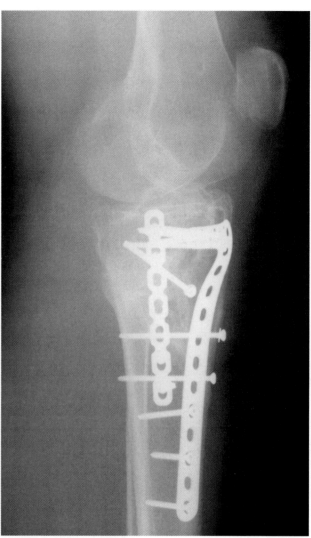

F   G

Figure 26.17. (*continued*) **F,G.** A lateral contoured plate is advanced in submuscular fashion with distal screws placed in percutaneous fashion. The medial condyle was stabilized with a small reconstruction plate and unicortical locking screws.

tear was present and repaired, the range of motion is usually limited for the first 3 weeks with flexion stops at 60 degrees. This protects the peripheral meniscal rim and allows early healing prior to initiation of full, unrestricted range of motion.

Physical therapy is initiated early to begin quadriceps strengthening as well as non–weight-bearing gait training with crutches or a walker. Patients are seen at 2 weeks for suture removal and at monthly intervals thereafter. Once the wound is healed, active and active-assisted range of motion is initiated. The goal is to achieve at least 90 degrees of knee flexion by the 4th week after surgery. Weight bearing of up to 50% of body weight is initiated at 8 to 12 weeks if radiographic evidence show subchondral healing, metaphyseal consolidation, and incorporation of the subchondral void; this evidence is especially important when bone graft or bone graft substitutes have been utilized to fill the subchondral defect.

In the high-energy type V and IV injuries, weight bearing must be delayed for 10 to 12 weeks. In low-energy injuries, patients can usually bear full weight by 12 to 14 weeks. Most patients can expect to resume most simple activities between 4 to 6 months. Running and vigorous athletic activities are often delayed up to 1 year after injury. The patient and surgeon alike can expect a good, functional outcome for most type I, II, and III injuries.

Because of comminution and soft-tissue compromise at the metaphyseal-diaphyseal junction in the type V and VI injuries, the fracture is often slow to consolidate. If union is not progressing, the area should be bone grafted before initiation of weight bearing. The timing of the bone graft is based on the status of the soft tissues. Grafting at 8 to 12 weeks is usually safe. Patients with Schatzker V or VI injuries often need 12 to 18 months before they are able to resume many of their routine daily activities. Functional outcomes in these severe injuries are guarded, and patients rarely resume competitive athletics. Functional range of motion with painless ambulation, normal alignment of mechanical axis, and the resumption of daily activities remain the goal.

COMPLICATIONS

Poorly timed surgical incisions with extensive dissection through traumatized soft tissues often contribute to early wound breakdown and infection. Spanning fixation techniques and delayed surgery can minimize these complications. If wound breakdown occurs, aggressive irrigation and debridement of all devitalized skin, muscle, and bone is mandatory. If the wound can be closed without tension, then closure over suction drains is recommended. If a deep infection with purulence is encountered, the wound should be packed opened and re-débrided every 48 hours. A vacuum-assisted closure (VAC) sponge system is helpful in managing large open wounds. Once a culture-negative wound has been obtained, secondary wound closure should be accomplished. In many cases, especially if a wound VAC system has been utilized, delayed primary closure can be completed. However, in some cases, closure will require a lateral or medial gastrocnemius rotational flap. Occasionally, a free tissue transfer is necessary.

Hardware should be retained if it provides stability at the fracture site. If the hardware is loose, it should be removed and the limb stabilized with a joint-spanning external fixator. This often results in compromised knee function or even a knee fusion as severe intra-articular sepsis combined with instability results in rapid chondrolysis with destruction of the knee joint.

Aseptic nonunion occasionally occurs in the Schatzker type V and VI fractures, specifically at the diaphyseal-metaphyseal junction. These injuries should be bone grafted. Revision fixation may also be necessary. Occasionally, nonunion occurs with late collapse of the articular surface or varus deformity of the metaphyseal-diaphyseal junction. If the mechanical axis is affected, then a corrective osteotomy may be required. If the patient is older and the articular mal-alignment results in significant shift of the mechanical axis, revision to a total knee arthroplasty may be appropriate.

Knee stiffness is common in severe fractures when range of motion has been delayed. Arthroscopic lysis of adhesions combined with gentle manipulation under anesthesia may be helpful for patients who failed to achieve 90 degrees of knee flexion in the first 4 weeks after surgery. Heterotopic ossification rarely occurs in tibial plateau fractures but does occur in concert with coexistent fracture-dislocations of the knee. In these cases, the heterotopic bone should be monitored until obvious maturity has occurred and no other bone formation is visible. CT scans help to delineate the orientation and location of heterotopic bone.

Surgical removal of heterotopic bone can be performed in concert with knee manipulations. Although results are encouraging, patients usually end up with some degree of residual knee stiffness.

ILLUSTRATIVE CASE FOR TECHNIQUE

A 21-year-old man was struck by a moving car. He sustained multiple injuries including a closed, Schatzker VI, bicondylar, tibial-plateau fracture with significant swelling, soft-tissue contusion, and a compartment syndrome (Fig. 26.18). The patient was taken emergently for spanning external fixation and 4 compartment fasciotomies thru lateral and medial incisions. A postoperative, distraction, CT scan demonstrated comminution at the base of the medial condylar fracture with the apex directed posteromedially. Minimal impaction of

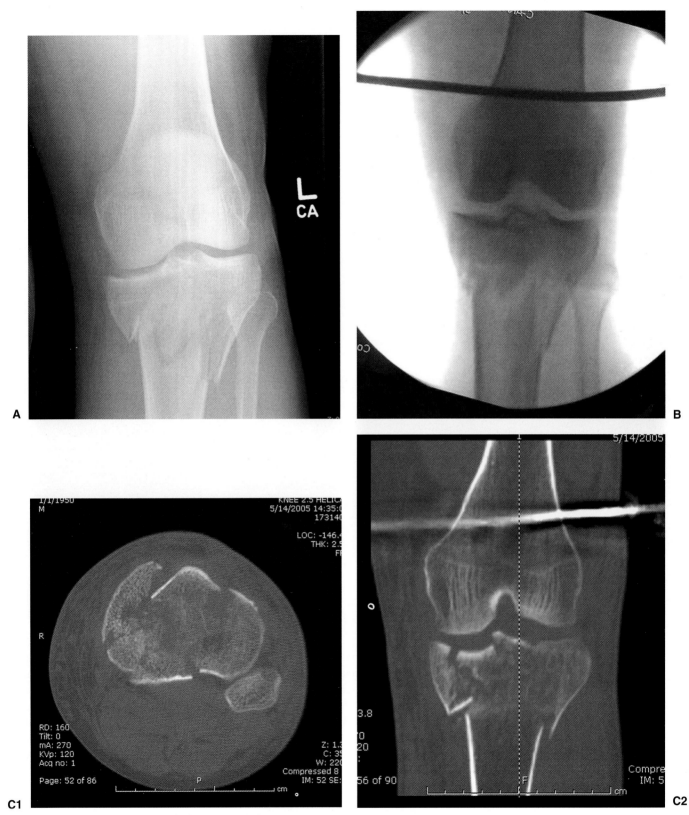

Figure 26.18. A,B. Initial injury film reveals a Schatzker V/VI fracture with associated compartment syndrome. The patient was taken to the operating room for spanning external fixation and fasciotomies. Intraoperative imaging demonstrates ligamentotaxis reduction and shaft realignment. **C1,2.** Distraction CT scan demonstrates bicondylar fracture with medial condylar comminution and coronal split. (*continues*)

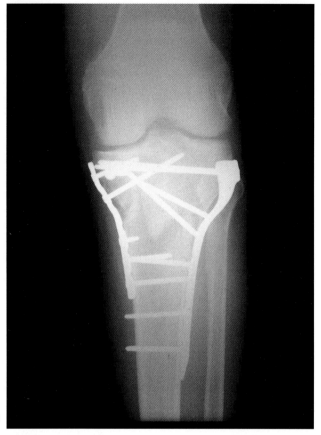

D

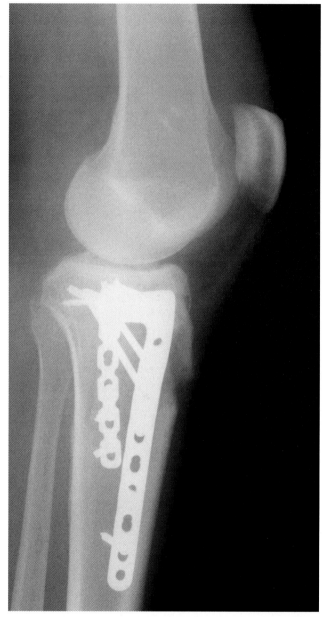

E

Figure 26.18. (*continued*) **D,E.** Follow-up at 1 year demonstrates condylar healing and maintenance of the mechanical axis without varus deformity. Intra-articular congruency has been maintained.

the lateral joint surface is visualized, and overall metaphyseal and shaft reduction has been accomplished with the spanning frame. Seventeen days after injury, a lateral exposure was used to expose the lateral condyle. Using percutaneous joysticks and large reduction forceps, the intracondylar fracture was reduced and held temporarily with K wires.

The preoperative CT scan demonstrated a coronal plane fracture through the medial condyle; this was reduced and compressed with a small tenaculum forceps placed percutaneously. This fracture was stabilized with a front-to-back lag screw. A lateral, periarticular, locking plate was then advanced down the proximal shaft in a submuscular fashion. The proximal raft screws were placed across both the lateral and medial condyles. The distal screws were placed via small percutaneous stab wounds to limit the lateral exposure. Because the distraction CT demonstrated extensive comminution at the base of the medial condyle, a posteromedial locking plate was positioned at the apex of the medial fracture line. The medial plate was located posteriorly to the pes along the posteromedial border of the proximal tibia.

Follow-up films demonstrated no varus deformity with excellent joint congruency maintained at 1 year follow-up. The patient was able to resume daily activities and continue his occupation as a student.

RECOMMENDED READINGS

1. Apley AG. Fractures of the tibial plateau. *Orthop Clin North Am* 1979;10:61–74.
2. Lansinger O, Bergman B, Courmner L, et al. Tibial condylar fractures: a 20 year followup. *J Bone Joint Surg* 1986;68A:13–18.
3. Rasmussen, P. Tibial condylar fractures: impairment of knee joint stability as an indicator for surgical treatment. *J Bone Joint Surg* 1973;55A:1331–1350.
4. Benirschke SK, Agner SG, Mayo KA, et al. Open reduction internal fixation of complex proximal tibial fractures. *J Orthop Trauma* 1991;5:236.
5. Mills WJ, Nork SE. Open reduction and internal fixation of high-energy tibial plateau fractures. *Orthop Clin North Am* January 2002;33(1):177–198, ix.
6. Schatzker J, McBroom R. Tibial plateau fractures: the Toronto experience 1968–1975. *Clin Orthop* 1979;138:94–104.
7. Tejwani NC, Achan P. Staged management of high-energy proximal tibia fractures. *Bull Hosp Joint Dis* 2004;62(1–2):62–66.
8. Watson JT. High energy fractures of the tibial plateau. *Orthop Clin North Am* 1994;25:728–752.
9. Shepherd L, Abdollahi K, Lee J, et al. The prevalence of soft tissue injuries in non operative tibial plateau fractures: *J Orthop Trauma* October 2002;16(9):628–631.
10. Yacoubian SV, Nevins RT, Sallis JG, et al. Impact of MRI on treatment plan and fracture classification of tibial plateau fractures. *J Orthop Trauma* October 2002;16(9):632–637.
11. Galla M, Lobenhoffer P. The direct, dorsal approach to the treatment of unstable tibial posteromedial fracture-dislocations. *Unfallchirurg* March 2003;106(3):241–247.
12. Simpson D, Keating JF. Outcome of tibial plateau fractures managed with calcium phosphate cement. *Injury* September 2004;35(9):913–918.
13. Watson JT. The use of an injectable bone graft substitute in tibial metaphyseal fractures. *Orthopedics* January 2004;27[Suppl 1]:s103–s107.
14. Chan YS, Yuan LJ, Hung SS, et al. Arthroscopic-assisted reduction with bilateral buttress plate fixation of complex tibial plateau fractures. *Arthroscopy* November 2003;19(9):974–984.
15. Hung SS, Chao EK, Chan YS, et al. Arthroscopically assisted osteosynthesis for tibial plateau fractures. *J Trauma* February 2003;54(2):356–563.
16. Cole PA, Zlowodzki M, Kregor PJ. Treatment of proximal tibia fractures using the less invasive stabilization system: surgical experience and early clinical results in 77 fractures. *J Orthop Trauma* September 2004; 18(8):528–535.

27

Proximal Tibia Fractures: Locked Plating

James P. Stannard

INDICATIONS/CONTRAINDICATIONS

The indications for surgical treatment of proximal tibia fractures are somewhat variable and must be individualized for each fracture and patient. The decision for surgery involves an evaluation of the patient, the fracture, and the surgeon. Patient factors include age, activity level, type of employment, associated injuries, and medical co-morbidities. Issues to consider regarding the fracture include pattern, degree of comminution, bone quality, displacement, articular impaction, mechanism of injury, condition of soft tissue around the fracture, and stability of the knee. Surgeon factors that must be considered when deciding whether to treat a fracture surgically include surgeon experience, surgical team experience, and available equipment.

There are three absolute indications for surgical treatment of proximal tibia fractures: open injuries, compartment syndromes, and fractures associated with vascular injuries. Although these are absolute indications for surgery, they are not absolute indications for open reduction and internal fixation (ORIF). In many fractures associated with these three absolute indications for surgery, temporary, spanning, external fixation is the initial treatment of choice (Fig. 27.1). Relative indications for surgical treatment of proximal tibia fractures include most displaced bicondylar and medial condyle tibial-plateau fractures; lateral tibial-plateau fractures that result in knee instability; condylar widening that exceeds 5 mm; fracture dislocations of the knee; nonarticular, proximal, tibia fractures that are displaced or unstable; and any fracture associated with patient or injury factors that will prevent early mobilization of the knee joint if treated nonoperatively (1–5).

After the decision has been made to treat a proximal tibia fracture surgically, the surgeon must decide between conventional osteosynthesis and locked plating. Specific indications for locked plating include bicondylar tibial-plateau fractures, marked comminution, osteopenia or poor bone quality, and a bone gap secondary to loss of bone along one or both columns of the proximal tibia.

Contraindications for locking plate osteosynthesis of the proximal tibia are identical to those for conventional compression plating of the proximal tibia. The primary contraindi-

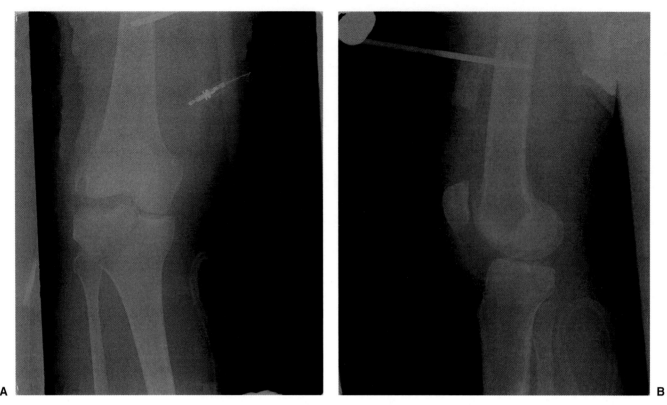

A   B

Figure 27.1. A,B. Spanning external fixator placed for temporary stabilization following a tibial plateau fracture.

cation is a severely damaged soft-tissue envelope (Fig. 27.2) that makes preceding with surgery a dangerous and high-risk proposal. In many cases, soft-tissue and skin damage will be a temporary contraindication for surgery. Delaying surgical treatment for a period of a few days to a few weeks, until optimal soft-tissue conditions exist, minimizes complications (3). Additional contraindications for ORIF include patients with serious medical co-morbidities that make them poor surgical candidates, and stable fractures with minimal displacement. Finally, a contraindication for locked plating is any fracture that can be treated equally well with a conventional compression plate. Plates designed with fixed-angle locking screws are expensive compared to compression plates and should be reserved for fractures that will benefit from locked plating.

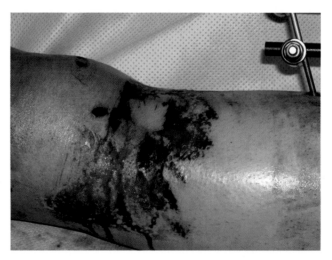

Figure 27.2. Contusions, abrasions, and soft-tissue injury following a high-energy tibial plateau fracture.

PREOPERATIVE PLANNING

The initial step in preoperative planning is a good history and physical examination. One of the crucial steps in developing a treatment plan is determining whether the fracture occurred as a result of high- or low-energy trauma. Locked plating will be used more frequently following high-energy trauma. In cases of proximal tibia fractures that result from high-energy trauma, great care must be taken to assess the skin and soft tissues, the compartments of the leg, the patient's neurological status, and the vascular supply to the distal leg. Careful evaluation of the skin is important. Deep abrasions, contusions, or small open wounds are important to document and consider when determining the location of surgical incisions. I classify closed fractures according to the system proposed by Tscherne (4), highlighting the importance of the soft-tissue envelope in both closed and open fractures. Proximal tibia fractures following high-energy trauma may be associated with a knee dislocation. The surgeon should assume that the patient may have sustained a fracture dislocation and document carefully the neurological and vascular status as well as the fullness of the compartments.

The second step in preoperative planning involves obtaining appropriate imaging studies. Initial radiographs should include a good quality anteroposterior (AP) and lateral view of the knee and proximal tibia. If the fracture demonstrates substantial distal extension, the same views of the tibia should be obtained. Oblique radiographs may also be helpful. Finally, traction views are helpful to determine the quality of reduction that can be obtained using indirect reduction and ligamentotaxis. I frequently obtain these preoperatively using the fluoroscope prior to beginning the surgical procedure. Computed tomography (CT) scanning is frequently used to allow a detailed analysis of the fracture, including the exact location of any impacted articular segments. Advantages of CT include its relatively low cost and availability at most hospitals and medical centers. A major disadvantage is that CT does not provide information regarding the ligaments, menisci, and other structures of the knee.

Magnetic resonance imaging (MRI) is an additional study that provides valuable information regarding both the skeletal and soft-tissue (ligaments, menisci) injuries around the knee. Numerous studies have been published in the last decade or so that establish the role of MRI with tibial plateau fractures. Yacoubian et al (6) found that obtaining MRI in addition to plain radiographs and CT scanning in 52 patients led to a change in the fracture classification in 21% and in the treatment plan in 23% of cases. Holt et al (7) reported that MRI led to a change in fracture classification in 48% and in the treatment plan in 19% of their patients. They also reported a 48% incidence of previously unrecognized injuries in the knee, including two spontaneously reduced knee dislocations.

The protocol over the past 3 years at my institution include MRI rather than CT for tibial plateau fractures that occur as a result of a high-energy mechanism of injury (Fig. 27.3). We have evaluated 103 patients using MRI following tibial-plateau fractures at our institution. Numerous soft-tissue injuries of the knee have been detected, including 25 medial meniscus tears, 35 lateral meniscus tears, 45 anterior cruciate-ligament tears, 41 posterior cruciate-ligament tears, 16 posteromedial corner or medial collateral-ligament tears, and 46 posterolateral corner (PLC) tears. Seventy-one percent of our patients studied had at least one torn ligament associated with their tibial plateau fracture. Fifty-five percent of our patients had two or more ligaments torn, and 26% had injuries to both the anterior and posterior cruciate ligaments (Fig. 27.4) or a fracture dislocation of the knee. Published data demonstrate that between 48% and 90% of patients with tibial plateau fractures have significant associated soft-tissue injuries of the knee. Our data on 103 patients are similar with an incidence of 71% soft-tissue injuries involving the knee following tibial plateau fracture. As noted, MRI scans frequently lead to a change in the treatment plan for patients following tibial plateau fractures (6–11); therefore, because of the difficulty in accurately diagnosing knee injuries associated with tibial plateau fractures, consideration should be given to obtaining an MRI scan for fractures that result from high-energy trauma.

The final step in preoperative planning is the development of the surgical plan. Complex proximal tibia and tibial plateau fractures can be very challenging. Depending on the experience of the surgeon, it may be wise to write a formal surgical plan. Key factors to consider include the location of surgical incisions as determined by fracture displacement and

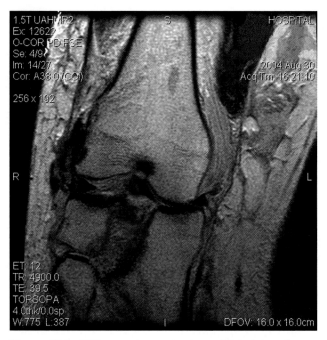

Figure 27.3. MRI scan demonstrating a tibial plateau fracture with a tear of the PLC.

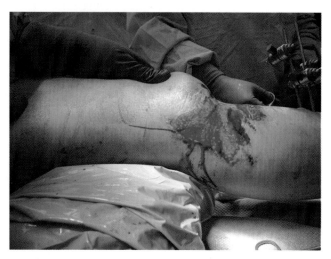

Figure 27.4. Patient with a positive sag sign indicating a torn posterior cruciate ligament in addition to his tibial-plateau fracture.

the condition of the skin, additional instruments (such as the femoral distractor) needed to assist with reduction, the type of implant to treat the fracture, and whether bone graft or a synthetic substitute will be needed.

SURGERY

There are two major types of locked plating systems, each with a unique surgical technique. Each system has its benefits and liabilities, and the surgeon must understand the differences and employ the locked plate that is most suited for the individual fracture.

Standard Locked Plating with an Open Surgical Approach

Numerous orthopedic implant manufacturers have developed locking plates that combine holes allowing standard screws with holes that accept locking screws. The patient should be placed on a radiolucent operating table in the supine position. A roll of sheets is placed under the knee, flexing it approximately 25 degrees (Fig. 27.5). The most

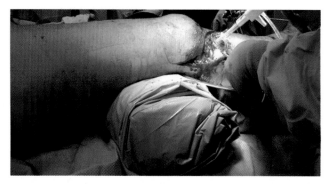

Figure 27.5. Reduction is improved by placing a roll under the distal femur and thus flexing the knee 20 to 30 degrees.

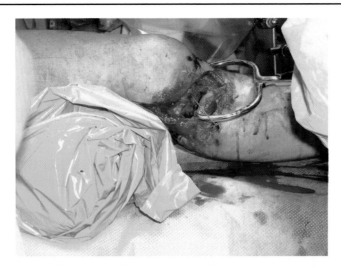

Figure 27.6. Reduction of the condyles using a large tenaculum clamp.

commonly employed surgical approach is a midline or an extended, lateral, parapatellar approach. The length of the incision will be dictated by the distal extent of the fracture. Great care should be taken in handling the soft tissues to minimize trauma inflicted by the surgeon.

Following exposure of the fracture, the first step is reduction of the articular surface. The techniques used are identical to those used with conventional ORIF. Impacted fragments must be manually disimpacted, reduced, and stabilized with Kirschner (K) wires initially and screws definitively. It is critical to evaluate the fracture for widening of the articular condyles. If the widening is present, then great care must be taken to reduce them in addition to reducing the articular surface. The use of a large tenaculum or articular clamps can be very helpful in reducing the condyles (Fig. 27.6). We usually use multiple, long, 3.5-mm screws in a subchondral position to stabilize the articular reduction via the rafting technique. Bone grafting using autograft, allograft, or synthetics may be necessary after any impacted fragments have been elevated.

Following successful reduction and stabilization of the articular portion of the fracture, the locking plate is applied to the tibia. Most of these plates are designed to be applied to the lateral side of the tibia. If the fracture pattern requires a medial-based plate, a plate designed for lateral application on the left tibia will often fit surprisingly well on the medial side of the right tibia. The plate is pinned or clamped to the bone and then affixed to the proximal segment. Both conventional nonlocking screws and locking screws can be used.

Some basic rules for application of these plates are listed in Table 27.1. The surgeon should be familiar with these rules prior to attempting osteosynthesis with a locked plating system. Conventional screws can be used to reduce the proximal fragment to the plate as well as to lag fragments together (such as a butterfly does) proximally. After initial

Table 27.1. *Rules for Screw Placement in Locked Plating*

Number	Rule
1	Conventional screws are usually placed before locking screws.
2	Conventional screws can reduce the bone to the plate.
3	Conventional screws can be used to lag fracture fragments together through the plate.
4	Locking screws will not reduce the bone to the plate.
5	Locking screws form a fixed-angle construct with the plate analogous to a blade plate, remarkably increasing stability in poor quality bone.
6	Lag before you lock. After placing locking screws, no additional compression or reduction of fragments is possible.
7	Locking screws should be placed as the final step of osteosynthesis.

stabilization of the proximal fragment to the plate, the tibia distal to the fracture is reduced and stabilized to the plate using temporary wires or conventional screws. Again, screws are placed using the rules for screw placement with locking plates.

Following this initial stabilization, the surgeon carefully assesses the quality of reduction in all planes. If the reduction is satisfactory, locking screws are placed proximally and distally to increase the stability of the construct.

The exact details of locking screw placement depend on the system that is being used. Most of the systems use drill guides that thread into the threaded plate holes. The drill is used to drill both cortices, and then the locking screws are initially implanted by power with the last few turns made via a manual screwdriver. Absolute data are not available regarding the number and combination of screws that are required for stability using locked plating systems. A minimum of four or five screws should be placed proximally and distally.

Minimally Invasive Locking-Plate Osteosynthesis Using the Less Invasive Stabilization System

The Less Invasive Stabilization System (LISS) (Synthes, Paoli, PA) for internal fixation is unique among locking plate systems because it combines locked plating with a minimally invasive surgical approach. Use of the LISS internal fixator requires a different technique than does conventional plate osteosynthesis. It is critical for the surgeon to remember that the screws will not pull the bone to the implant, and therefore the fixator cannot normally be used as a reduction tool. The pull reduction instrument (commonly referred to as the "whirlybird") has been developed to allow the bone to be pulled to the plate prior to placement of locking screws. No screws should be placed through the fixator prior to restoring length and reduction in the sagittal and coronal planes. After the surgeon has begun placing fixed-angle screws, additional reduction will not be possible.

The patient should be placed in a supine position on a radiolucent operating table. A roll of sheets is placed under the knee to relax the gastrocnemius muscles and assist in the reduction. Generally, a roll that places the knee in approximately 25 to 30 degrees of flexion provides the maximum benefit. However, I recommend evaluating the impact of ligamentotaxis and varying the size and location of the roll to assess the impact on the reduction of the fracture. This process of "learning" the fracture prior to placing the plate can improve the final reduction and save significant time when the implant has been placed in the submuscular plane.

The surgical approach can be accomplished with either a lateral parapatellar or a hockey stick incision. The hockey stick approach (Fig. 27.7) allows posterior and proximal extension if the patient has sustained a tear of the PLC of the knee that requires surgical reconstruction (Fig. 27.8). A relatively small incision is all that is required for implanting the LISS fixator. The articular component of the fracture requires reduction and stabilization

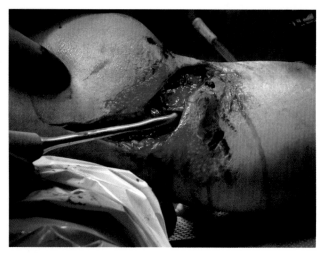

Figure 27.7. Extended hockey stick approach.

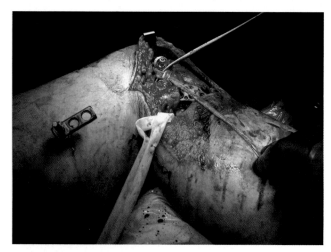

Figure 27.8. Reconstruction of the PLC after ORIF of the tibial plateau.

through techniques that are identical to those used with conventional plating. It is critical for the surgeon to plan the location of any screws utilized to stabilize the articular reduction, while keeping in mind the location of the LISS fixator and screws. One disadvantage of locking screws is that the surgeon cannot vary the angle of implantation in order to avoid other screws. Initially, the articular reduction is stabilized with K wires (Fig. 27.9).

Following satisfactory temporary stabilization, I usually complete fixation of the articular component using a rafting technique with a few 3.5-mm screws. When a satisfactory reduction of the articular surface has been achieved, electrocautery is used to release part of the origin of the anterior compartment muscles to expose the submuscular plane. The submuscular plane is then developed using either a large periosteal elevator or the end of the LISS plate. The submuscular plane is usually not difficult to develop.

The LISS fixator is then slid into the submuscular plane using the aiming handle (Fig. 27.10). An important tip is to keep a finger along the anterior crest of the tibia and feel the tip of the fixator pass distally. This allows a clear understanding of the tibial plate position in the sagittal plane. The implant must be located in the middle of the diaphysis of the distal tibia. If the LISS fixator is not kept in the middle of the diaphysis, the unicortical screws will not have sufficient pull-out strength. The plate should be slid slightly farther distally than the anticipated final position, and then slid back proximally to achieve the best fit to the osseous contour of the proximal tibia (Fig. 27.11).

After placement has been confirmed through fluoroscopy, a threaded wire is utilized to pin the internal fixator to the proximal tibia. Longitudinal traction is then used to obtain length and reduction in the sagittal plane. The time spent learning the appropriate reduction maneuver while learning the fracture at the beginning of the case remarkably eases the process of obtaining a good reduction. A distal skin incision, correlating with the location of the distal hole on the plate, is made. The insertion sleeve and trocar are placed and then the handle is connected to the distal hole on the plate by a threaded stabilization bolt. Another threaded wire is then utilized to pin the LISS fixator to the midlateral portion of the tibial diaphysis.

A lateral view of the tibia using fluoroscopy should be obtained to confirm placement of the plate in the midlateral plane (Fig. 27.12). If it is not located in the middle of the tibial diaphysis, the threaded wire should be removed and the location of the plate adjusted appropriately. An ideal LISS construct involves placing two bicortical whirlybirds, one just proximal and one just distal to the metaphyseal or diaphyseal component of the fracture (Fig. 27.13). Some fractures will only require one whirlybird. The whirlybird is placed

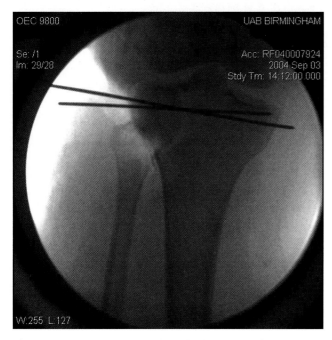

Figure 27.9. Initial stabilization of tibial plateau fracture using K wires.

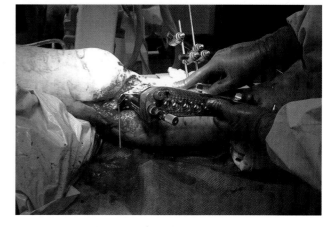

Figure 27.10. Sliding the LISS into place using the aiming handle.

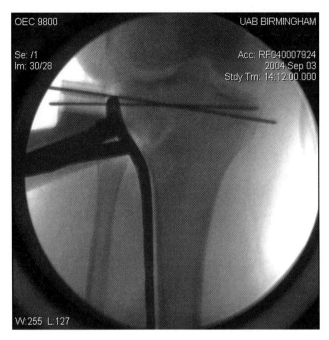

Figure 27.11. Sliding LISS plate back proximally to obtain the best possible fit.

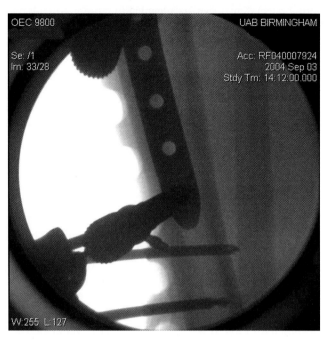

Figure 27.12. Confirming location of the plate in the midlateral plane of the tibia via fluoroscopy.

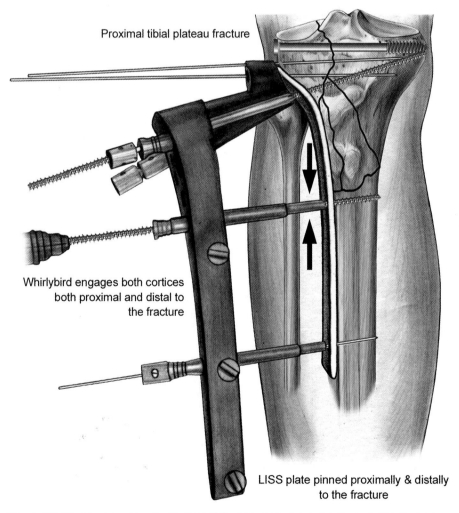

Proximal tibial plateau fracture

Whirlybird engages both cortices both proximal and distal to the fracture

LISS plate pinned proximally & distally to the fracture

Figure 27.13. Ideal construct with the LISS plate pinned proximally and distally and a whirlybird placed just proximal and distal to the fracture.

through a stab incision corresponding to the desired hole on the internal fixator, followed by blunt spreading and placement of the drill guide and trocar. The whirlybird is then drilled into the tibia while the irrigation system is used and then tightened to stabilize and reduce any varus mal-alignment of the fracture.

No screws should be placed into the LISS fixator until a reduction is obtained and the plate is pinned in place with threaded wires proximally and distally and stabilized near the fracture with whirlybirds as needed. The LISS fixator does not have a perfect fit with the proximal tibia in most individuals due to the anatomic variability between patients. Because the locked screws do not pull the fixator to the bone, this can lead to a prominent plate and associated hardware-related pain. An important surgical tip to help reduce this possibility should be employed at this point in the case. Prior to placing the proximal screws, a large reduction forceps should be placed through a stab incision medially and also attached to the small wire hole in the proximal anterior portion of the plate. The forceps is tightened to snug the plate against the tibia prior to the placement of the proximal screws, minimizing the problem of prominent hardware. As soon as one or two locking screws have been placed, the forceps should be removed.

The final stage of osteosynthesis with a LISS internal fixator involves placing the locked screws. The C, D, and E holes should be used with the vast majority of fracture patterns. These screws provide excellent fixation with divergence from one another in three dimensions. A drill guide and cannulated trocar are placed in the E hole (Fig. 27.14). A guide wire is then drilled through the trocar to the desired position for the screw tip. The length of the screw is measured using the depth gauge provided, and the wire and cannulated trocar are then removed. A LISS screw is then drilled into the proximal tibia while irrigation is used. Power drilling should be discontinued just prior to the screw head locking into the holes of the internal fixator. The screw should be locked into the LISS fixator using the torque screwdriver, tightening it until two clicks are heard. If power is used to drive the screw all the way into the locked position, the surgeon runs the risk of creating a cold weld with the screw, which makes removal extremely difficult if not impossible. This procedure is repeated for the D and C screws (Fig. 27.15).

The surgeon must be aware that the D screw diverges posteriorly. Because the screws are powered in and are threaded, it may be difficult to feel if the posterior cortex is perforated. This screw should be placed with the knee flexed to keep the popliteal vessels away from the posterior tibial cortex. The length of the D screw should be adjusted if necessary after a lateral fluoroscopic view is obtained and the location of the D screw is carefully scrutinized (Fig. 27.16). The significance of this screw is easily remembered if the surgeon realizes that "D is for danger" (to the popliteal vessels). Paying attention to this small technique point allows consistent safe placement of this important screw. A fourth screw placed prox-

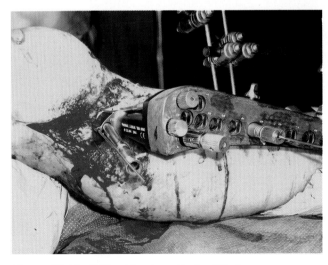

Figure 27.14. Drill guide placed in the E hole.

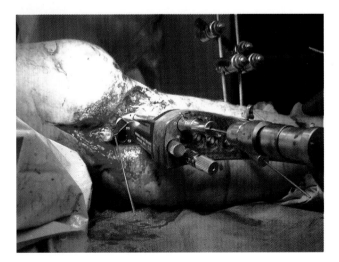

Figure 27.15. Guide wire placed into the C hole to allow measurement of screw length.

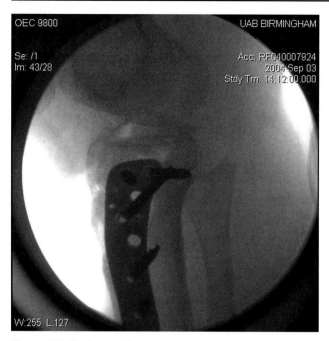

Figure 27.16. Lateral fluoroscopy view to allow assessment of D screw location.

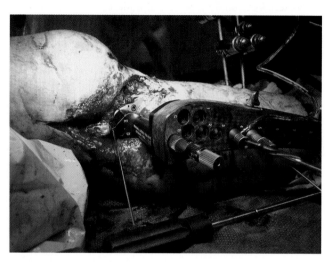

Figure 27.17. Placing screw through the fourth hole by use of the power screwdriver and the irrigation system.

imally usually replaces the proximal whirlybird. Additional screws should be placed based on the fracture pattern and surgeon's judgment. A minimum of four screws should be placed proximally as well as distally.

The remainder of the case involves placing the distal locking screws. The technique is similar to that used for the proximal screws, except that the distal screws are not measured. These screws are either 18- or 26-mm long. Important technique points include using irrigation, finalizing placement using a screwdriver, and placing at least four screws distally (Fig. 27.17). As noted previously, the plate should be in the midlateral plane of the bone to avoid transcortical screw placement. I recommend placing two screws near the fracture site and two screws near the distal end of the plate for maximum stability (Fig. 27.18).

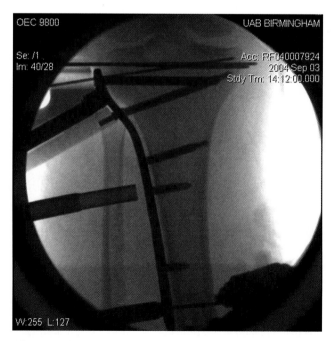

Figure 27.18. AP view showing three of four distal screws in place. The final screw will replace the distal wire.

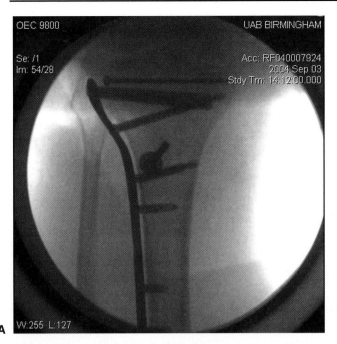
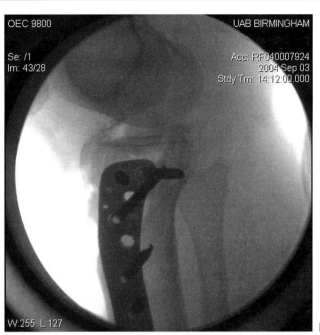

Figure 27.19. A,B. Final fixation of fracture using LISS.

The principles involved in screw location are similar to those involved with placing pins for external fixators. The ideal construct is two screws near the fracture sight and two near the end of the plate (Fig. 27.19). Another important point for the surgeon to remember is that the risk of damage to neurovascular structures increases with more distally placed screws. If the 13-hole plate is being used, great care should be used to spread down bluntly to the bone and place the trocar system for holes 11–13 (12). Alternatively, a small incision may be used to expose directly the distal three holes on the long LISS plate (13).

RESULTS

Locked plating is a new technique with limited published data available to date. Most of the published data relates to the LISS, which was the first commercially available, locked-plating system. Three recently published papers provided results on a total of 149 complex tibial-plateau fractures. Two of the papers reported no problems with loss of articular reduction or alignment (14,15), and the third reported 97% stable fixation in the fractures studied (16). These clinical results substantiate the expected improved stability as a result of the fixed angles formed by the locked screws. A recent biomechanical study demonstrated that there was no difference between a laterally based LISS plate and ORIF with two conventional compression plates (17). The three clinical studies also reported only two deep infections, an incidence of only 1.3%. These results are far better than previously published reports on conventional ORIF of tibial plateau fractures.

The papers reported similarly impressive results in terms of final knee motion and rate of union. Hardware-related pain near the knee joint appears to be one relatively minor problem with the LISS (14–16). It is not clear from the data available whether these early and impressive results are due to the locked plating or to the minimally invasive surgical approach. It is probable that the low infection rate is at least partially related to the minimally invasive surgical approach. The relative contribution of each of these factors will be clarified as additional publications offer results from using locked plating through a conventional open approach. Although the early results using LISS are extraordinarily encouraging, the technique can be challenging and the surgeon can expect to experience a learning curve before mastering minimally invasive locked plating.

Table 27.2. *Complications Associated with Locked Plating Combined with a Minimally Invasive Surgical Approach*

Complication	Incidence (%)
Deep infection	1.3
Superficial infection	2.0
Malunion >10 degrees	1.3
Malunion >5 degrees	8.7
Nonunion	1.3
Loss of reduction	0.0
Hardware failure	1.3
Implant related pain	8.0
Peroneal nerve injury	0.7
Seroma	2.0

POSTOPERATIVE MANAGEMENT

It is difficult to draw clear-cut conclusions regarding postoperative management from the sparse published literature regarding locked plating. Our protocol is to begin early knee motion on the first postoperative day if the soft-tissue injuries will allow. The patient is placed in a continuous passive motion (CPM) machine with an initial range of motion of 0 to 10 degrees. Knee motion is increased by approximately 10 degrees per day as tolerated by the patient. Advancing motion at a rate faster than 10 degrees per day can lead to wound dehiscence and is best avoided. We delay the knee motion for approximately a week if necessary to allow soft-tissue inflammation to subside.

Initially, patients are allowed try toe-touch weight bearing only. We advance to 50% weightbearing as soon as callus is appreciated on radiographs. Callus is usually noted between 4 and 6 weeks following surgical stabilization. Patients are generally advanced to 75% weightbearing after an additional 3 weeks and to full weight bearing by 11 to 12 weeks following surgery. Resistance exercises, athletic activities, and heavy work are avoided until 4 to 6 months following locked plating.

COMPLICATIONS

The complications associated with locked plating are very similar to those associated with ORIF with conventional compression plates. Infection, wound dehiscence, knee instability, loss of knee motion, hardware failure, nonunion, malunion, and hardware-related pain have all been reported. Table 27.2 documents the combined incidence of complications from the three recently published clinical series in which locked plating with a minimally invasive surgical approach was used (14–16). Although the authors reported a variety of complications, the number of incidences is remarkably lower than reports for either conventional ORIF or for stabilization with small-wire external fixators.

Complex tibial-plateau fractures are injuries associated with an exceptionally high risk of complications. The early results for locked plating combined with a minimally invasive surgical approach are very encouraging. There is not sufficient published data to determine the complication rate for locked plating using conventional surgical approaches.

RECOMMENDED READINGS

1. Honkonen SE. Indications for surgical treatment of tibial condyle fractures. *Clin Orthop* 1994;302:199–205.
2. Koval KJ, Helfet DL. Tibial plateau fractures: evaluation and treatment. *J Am Acad Orthop Surg* 1995;3:86–94.
3. Mills WJ, Nork SE. Open reduction and internal fixation of high-energy tibial plateau fractures. *Orthop Clin North Am* 2002;33(1):177–198.

4. Tscherne H, Lobenhoffer P. Tibial plateau fractures: management and expected results. *Clin Orthop* 1993;292:87–100.
5. Wiss, DA. Tibial plateau fractures. In: Wiss DA, ed. *Fractures* [Master techniques in orthopaedic surgery on CD ROM]. Philadelphia: Lippincott Williams & Wilkins; 2000.
6. Yacoubian SV, Nevins RT, Sallis JG, et al. Impact of MRI on treatment plan and fracture classification of tibial plateau fractures. *J Orthop Trauma* 2002;16(9):632–637.
7. Holt MD, Williams LA, Dent CM. MRI in the management of tibial plateau fractures. *Injury* 1995;26(9):595–599.
8. Barrow BA, Fajman WA, Parker LM, et al. Tibial plateau fractures: evaluation with MR imaging. *Radiographics* 1994;14(3):553–559.
9. Brophy DP, O'Malley M, Lui D, et al. MR imaging of tibial plateau fractures. *Clin Radiol* 1996;51(12):873–878.
10. Kode L, Lieberman JM, Motta AO, et al. Evaluation of tibial plateau fractures: efficacy of MR imaging compared with CT. *AJR Am J Roentgenol* 1994;163(1):141–147.
11. Shepherd L, Abdollahi K, Lee J, et al. The prevalence of soft tissue injuries in nonoperative tibial plateau fractures as determined by magnetic resonance imaging. *J Orthop Trauma* 2002;16(9):628–631.
12. DeAngelis JP, DeAngelis NA, Anderson R. Anatomy of the superficial peroneal nerve in relation to fixation of tibia fractures with the Less Invasive Stabilization System. *J Orthop Trauma* 2004;18(8):536–539.
13. Kregor PJ, Stannard JP, Cole PA, et al. Prospective clinical trial of the Less Invasive Stabilization (L.I.S.S.) for supracondylar femur fractures. *J Orthop Trauma* 2000;14(2):133–134.
14. Ricci WM, Rudzki JR, Borrelli J Jr. Treatment of complex proximal tibia fractures with the Less Invasive Skeletal Stabilization System. *J Orthop Trauma* 2004;18(8):521–527.
15. Stannard JP, Wilson TC, Volgas DA, et al. The Less Invasive Stabilization System in the treatment of complex fractures of the tibial plateau: short-term results. *J Orthop Trauma* 2004;18(8):552–558.
16. Cole PA, Zlowodzki M, Kregor PJ. Treatment of proximal tibia fractures using the Less Invasive Stabilization System: surgical experience and early clinical results in 77 fractures. *J Orthop Trauma* 2004;18(8):528–535.
17. Gösling T, Schandelmaier P, Marti A, et al. Less invasive stabilization of complex tibial plateau fractures: a biomechanical evaluation of a unilateral locked screw plate and double plating. *J Orthop Trauma* 2004;18(8):546–551.

28

Tibial Shaft Fractures: Open Reduction Internal Fixation

Brett R. Bolhofner

INDICATIONS/CONTRAINDICATIONS

Open reduction internal fixation (ORIF) through use of plates and screws may be carried out for any fracture of the tibia in which soft-tissue conditions are satisfactory. Although intramedullary interlocking nails have become popular for the treatment of many tibial-shaft fractures, plating remains a viable alternative (1). Compared with an intramedullary implant, plating of the tibia requires greater attention to the condition of the soft tissues, more preoperative planning, and greater attention to surgical detail during the procedure.

Strong indications for plate osteosynthesis of tibial-shaft fractures are the presence of compartment syndrome, neurovascular injury, compromised medullary canal, or compromised access to the medullary canal due to associated injury (2,3).

Relative indications for ORIF include the following conditions: polytraumatized patients, open fractures, late loss of reduction with closed treatment, segmental injury, fractures that extend into either the knee or ankle joint, fractures of the proximal and distal one third of the shaft, and fractures in patients whose livelihood or recreational habits demand perfect restoration of length and rotation (2,3). Certain fracture patterns may be better anatomically restored by plating. For example, a distal, spiral, oblique fracture or a simple oblique fracture with a relatively steep fracture plane may be best treated with a plate as will fractures that extend to the ankle joint.

Relative contraindications to plate osteosynthesis include isolated, displaced, diaphyseal fractures, which may be better treated with a locked intramedullary nail. Grossly contaminated open fractures, which will require serial débridements, are best treated with an external fixator.

A careful assessment of the soft-tissue envelope at the time of injury and at the time of surgery is essential because its condition influences the timing of the surgical procedure. The Tscherne classification may be helpful in evaluating and assessing the soft-tissue injury associated with a particular fracture pattern (4). In patients whose soft tissue does not permit early internal fixation because of swelling, abrasions, or blisters, may benefit from a 10 to 14 day waiting period. The skin should have a very fine wrinkled texture or appearance before plate osteosynthesis is undertaken.

When soft-tissue conditions are satisfactory, the tibia is well suited to plate fixation. It has a large subcutaneous surface that may be used for stabilization without the muscles being stripped (5). Because no muscle needs to be stripped from it, the medial face of the tibia is, in fact, an ideal plating surface. Most of the poor results and subsequent criticisms of tibial plating were due to poor soft-tissue technique, inappropriate implant use, and poor reductions.

PREOPERATIVE PLANNING

The initial assessment of the soft tissues and the radiographic pattern of the fracture is carried out immediately. Attention to the neurovascular status as well as the status of the muscle compartments is mandatory. The presence of soft-tissue contusion, skin necrosis, swelling, compartment syndrome, skin abrasion, or any wounds is carefully documented. Anteroposterior (AP) and lateral views of the tibia, to include both knee and ankle joint, must be obtained (Fig. 28.1).

The timing of the internal fixation is based primarily on the condition of the soft tissues. ORIF of the tibia should only be carried out when satisfactory skin and wound conditions permit a tension-free soft-tissue closure at the conclusion of the procedure. If these conditions do not exist, then internal fixation should be postponed. The extremity should be splinted, casted, or a temporary, spanning, external fixator applied until more favorable conditions exist. If surgery is delayed, the limb should be elevated to help resolve any swelling. Necrotic soft tissue should be well demarcated and excised at the time of surgery. A gastrocnemius, rotational, muscle flap will be required for proximal tibia fractures. In the distal tibia, a free tissue transfer or a fasciocutaneous rotational flap may be needed. When satisfactory soft-tissue conditions are present, the procedure may be carried out with a well-conceived preoperative plan and a surgical tactic.

AP and lateral radiographs of the injured extremity should be obtained. If the fracture is complex or if deformity is significant, an AP and lateral radiograph of the unaffected side or an AP and lateral radiograph of the affected extremity in traction may help the surgeon better conceptualize the fracture pattern. The preoperative drawings, which need not be of artistic quality, should be fashioned so that a step-by-step procedure from start to finish is outlined in a simple fashion (Fig. 28.2). Because the preoperative plans are displayed in the operating room at the time of the surgery, they should list any equipment that might be required. The steps of the procedure are indicated directly on the preoperative plan in numeric order.

The equipment required to carry out the procedure will be AO/ASIF screws and plates including the limited-contact dynamic compression (LCDC) plate with combination holes (Synthes, Paoli, PA). Basic instruments, an AO drill, bone forceps, and associated small soft-tissue retractors and elevators are also required.

Locking the screws to a plate may be an advantage when bone quality is poor due to osteoporosis or when the distal fragment is relatively short. Using a locked construct will allow the creation of a fixed angle device, and when applied to one or the other major fragments, it will allow the plate to be used to facilitate the reduction (i.e., indirect technique). Precontoured plates are available for some fracture patterns and applications. A locked plate must be accurately contoured if it is to be used as a reduction tool because a locked screw will not pull the plate and bone together. In some instances, a more stable construct can be created with locking screws. Preoperative planning may be more difficult because of the uncertainty of the locked screw projections after plate contouring.

Assumption of basic AO technique as well as the use of locking screws is assumed. A complete discussion of locking technique is beyond the scope of this chapter.

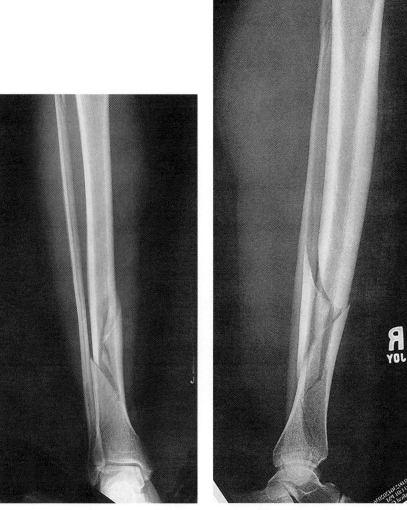

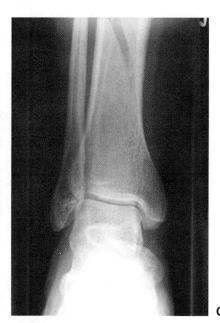

A,B   C

Figure 28.1. AP **(A)** and lateral **(B)** radiographs of the tibia and fibula showing an oblique fracture pattern with butterfly fragments that are mildly displaced. Nondisplaced fracture lines extend toward the ankle joint. **C.** A nondisplaced, medial, malleolar fracture is shown.

SURGERY

When the soft tissues are satisfactory for surgery and a preoperative plan has been established, the procedure may be initiated (Fig. 28.3). Intraoperative findings (such as nondisplaced fracture lines or unrecognized comminution) may contradict the preoperative plan for trauma reconstruction (such as for an osteotomy). In such cases, the order of the preoperative plan may need to be altered.

The patient is placed in the supine position on a regular operating-room table. A tourniquet is not required for the procedure but may be used if desired. Use of either general or spinal anesthesia is satisfactory. The entire leg is prepped from the toes to the groin. Prophylactic intravenous antibiotics, usually a single preoperative dose of cephalosporin, is

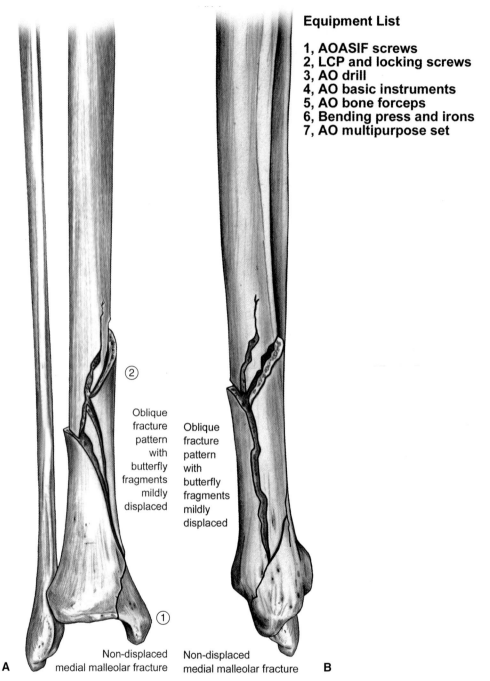

Equipment List

1, AOASIF screws
2, LCP and locking screws
3, AO drill
4, AO basic instruments
5, AO bone forceps
6, Bending press and irons
7, AO multipurpose set

② Oblique fracture pattern with butterfly fragments mildly displaced

Oblique fracture pattern with butterfly fragments mildly displaced

① Non-displaced medial malleolar fracture

Non-displaced medial malleolar fracture

A

B

Figure 28.2. A–D. AP and lateral preoperative drawings illustrate the fracture pattern and subsequent definitive fixation. This is helpful in selecting a plate of proper length to contour. The plate may be used to achieve reduction followed by lag screw fixation or vice versa. The articulating tension device may be used to load the construct if the pattern allows. Preoperative plan: Step 1: Indicate joint axis. Step 2: Reduce and secure butterfly fragments. Step 3: Precontour plate and apply to distal fragment. Step 4: Not shown; push/pull screw may be inserted proximally. Step 5: Adjust reduction. Step 6: Additional lag screws if necessary. Step 7: Additional plate screws to balance fixation. (*continues*)

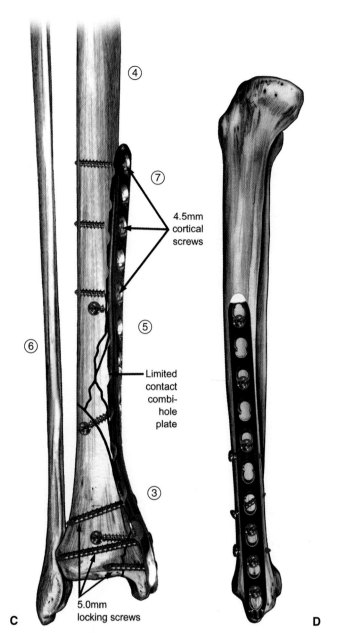

4.5mm
cortical
screws

Limited
contact
combi-
hole
plate

5.0mm
locking screws

C

D

Figure 28.2. A–D. (*continued*)

recommended. The location and length of the incision is drawn on the skin before application of an adhesive iodine-impregnated drape (Fig. 28.4). I prefer to carry out the procedure in the seated position at the foot of the table with the surgical assistant also seated.

Surgical Approach

A long anterior incision is placed 1 cm lateral to the tibial crest and corresponding to Langer's lines (Fig. 28.5) (1). The incision is curved gently at its distal portion at the level of the metaphyseal flare in the supramalleolar region. A long surgical incision is preferred because it allows satisfactory exposure of the tibia and allows the surgeon to avoid unnecessary, vigorous, skin retraction, particularly on the medial skin flap (Fig. 28.6A) (6). The saphenous vein or nerves need not be sacrificed in the distal portion of the incision because the plate may be placed beneath these structures, leaving them completely intact (see Fig. 28.6B). They should be dissected only enough to allow passage

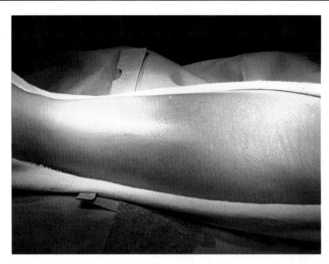

Figure 28.3. The condition of the skin is ascertained before undertaking ORIF. In this case, no ecchymosis or fracture blisters are found. A minimal amount of edema is present and a fine wrinkle pattern can be noted on the skin 10 days after the initial injury.

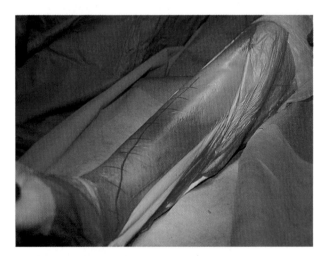

Figure 28.4. Planned surgical incision is indicated on the skin with a marker to assist in the surgical approach as well as wound closure. The operative area is draped with adhesive iodine.

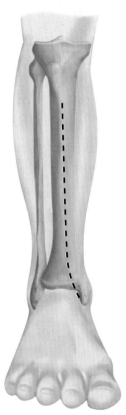

Figure 28.5. The surgical incision is anterior and curvilinear. It begins 1 cm lateral to the tibial crest and curves medially in the distal portion.

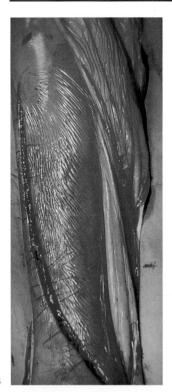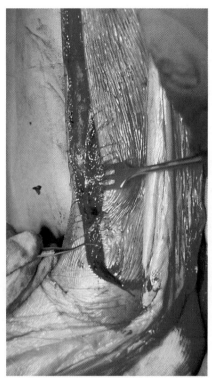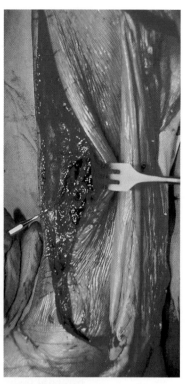

A, B   C

Figure 28.6. A. The surgical incision is carried through the skin and subcutaneous tissue.
B. The small dental instrument indicates the location of the distal saphenous structures,
which are preserved during the surgical approach and the procedure. **C.** The small dental
instrument indicates the presence of fracture hematoma, which is removed for exposure of
the fracture.

of the plate beneath them. In addition, the sheath of the tibialis anterior tendon need not
be entered.

The skin and subcutaneous flap are raised in a medial direction just enough to allow
exposure of the posteromedial border of the tibia and the butterfly fragment, which are seen
after removal of the fracture hematoma. The dissection remains extraperiosteal. The
periosteum is frequently noted to be stripped at the fracture edges as a result of fracture
displacement. If any additional periosteal elevation is necessary to evaluate reduction, then
not more than 1 or 2 mm at the immediate fracture edge should be elevated. The remainder
of the procedure should be carried out entirely extraperiosteally (Fig. 28.7) (1).

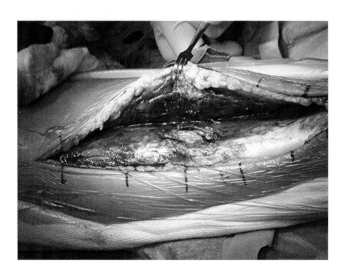

Figure 28.7. After evacuation of the fracture hematoma, the
fracture, including the minimally displaced posteromedial butterfly, can be seen. The edges of the fracture are compared to
the surrounding hemorrhagic periosteum and are noted to be
white. This indicates the amount of periosteum that was
stripped by the injury itself. The stripping done by the injury
allows for sufficient visualization of the fracture edges and subsequent reduction. No further periosteal stripping should be
necessary for reduction and fixation of this fracture. The periosteum is hemorrhagic because of the injury and also because no tourniquet is used.

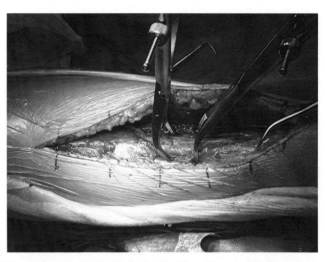

Figure 28.8. The posteromedial butterfly is directly reduced with bone forceps. Even though the butterfly is directly reduced, the bone forceps is applied extraperiosteally; no soft-tissue stripping is necessary to accomplish the reduction. The small elevator indicates the location of the posteromedial butterfly fragment.

Internal Fixation

Once the surgical approach has been completed and satisfactory exposure of the fracture site and the medial surface of the tibia has been achieved, then the preoperative plan is followed in order for reduction and fixation of the fracture (see Fig. 28.2).

The ankle-joint axis is initially marked with a reference Kirschner (K) wire placed by hand in the soft tissues at the level of the ankle joint (step1, Fig. 28.2B). The butterfly fragment in the nondisplaced fracture lines are reduced and secured with bone forceps placed without stripping additional periosteum. If significant displacement of the butterfly fragment exists, an indirect reduction technique is preferable to manual manipulations, which generate risk of soft-tissue stripping and devascularization of the fragment (Fig. 28.8). The butterfly fragment in nondisplaced fracture lines is then secured with lag screws (Fig. 28.9); this is the direct reduction portion of the case.

The remainder of the fixation is achieved using a 4.5-mm combination-hole plate. Because locked screws will not pull the plate to the bone, a locked place should be contoured anatomically (Fig. 28.10). The plate is secured to the distal fragment with locking screws. The bone or undersurface of this particular plate has small undulations so that the plate contacts the bone or periosteum only at intermittent alternating points, allowing (as much as possible) preservation of the periosteal circulation. However, standard stainless-steel plates without the limited-contact feature and without the locking feature are also satisfactory choices. An experienced surgeon can bend and twist the plate during the procedure. Less experienced surgeons can precontour the plate by using a bone model or skeleton before the procedure and then sterilizing it (step 3).

In an alternate procedure, the locking plate may be applied initially on the distal fragment with a standard 4.5-mm cortical screw, which will pull the plate to the bone. Then a second locking screw can be placed to protect the initial screw. Any of the distal fragment holes can be used for the preliminary screw insertion.

A push-pull screw is then inserted 1 or 2 cm proximal to the plate. The AO articulating tension device is then applied at the proximal end of the plate and distracted (step 4, Fig. 28.2C). If the plate is properly contoured, the plate need not be clamped to the shaft proximally. However, if necessary, the surgeon can carefully apply a bone clamp by making a small incision and laterally placing it with minimal stripping of soft tissue.

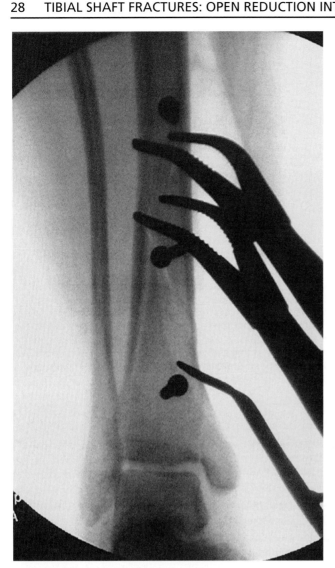

Figure 28.9. An intraoperative image demonstrates lag screw fixation of the butterfly and nondisplaced fracture fragments. The lag screws are placed through the periosteum with care not to strip additional bone. They should be placed so that they do interfere with plate placement. Note the nondisplaced, medial, malleolar fragment that will be secured with the plate.

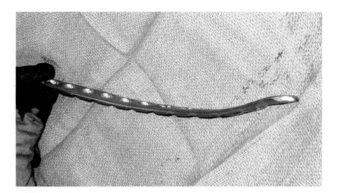

Figure 28.10. A 4.5-mm tibial LCDC plate with combination holes is contoured for the distal-tibial medial surface with a distal bend and a proximal medial twist.

The fracture is then distracted (step 5, Fig. 28.2D), and reduction is adjusted for angulation and rotation with small position changes in the extremity or with reduction clamps placed extraperiosteally (Fig. 28.11). This is the indirect reduction portion of the case (5).

Once the fracture has been reduced, the articulating tension device is placed in the compression mode and compressed to approximately 60 kPa (step 6, Fig. 28.2D) (7). This construct, with only one screw and the articulating tension device, is usually quite stable. This is a good time to obtain intraoperative radiographs for assessing fracture reduction and alignment. Standard overhead films or c-Arm images are obtained to assess the overall axial alignment and preliminary fixation (Fig. 28.12). At this point in the procedure, any step is easily reversed.

If the reduction is satisfactory, then the major fragments should be secured with lag screws placed through or outside the plate. Additional screws are inserted into the plate to enhance stability (Fig. 28.13) (step 7, Fig. 28.2D). The exact number of screws is cannot be precisely predicted, but the surgeon should balance the fixation by dispersing the screws

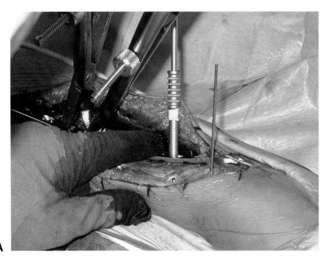
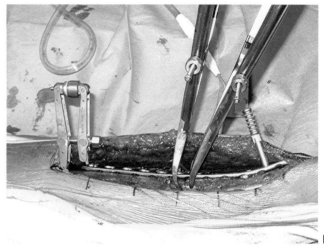

A   B

Figure 28.11. A. The contoured plate is slipped beneath the distal neurovascular structures and applied to the distal fragment with a single locked screw to create a fixed-angle plate. **B.** The ATD is then placed off a proximal push-pull screw and can be used to achieve distraction if necessary and to fine-tune the reduction. Clamps are used extraperiosteally to secure and fine-tune the reduction as well as to protect the lag screws during distraction and compression. Note the distal drill sleeve for insertion of a second, more distal, locking screw. The ATD creates a load-sharing construct between the implant and bone.

equally on either side of the plate. Intraoperative radiographs are obtained and final fixation adjustments are carried out (Fig. 28.14). The final radiograph should correspond closely with the preoperative drawing.

The wound is irrigated with antibiotic solution and closed over a small drain. The skin itself is approximated with interrupted, horizontal, mattress sutures of 4-0 nylon. No tension should be present at the skin edges at the time of closure (Fig. 28.15). If tension-free closure cannot be obtained after osteosynthesis, then I prefer to make multiple, small, relaxing incisions with a no.10 blade on both sides of the surgical incision; this pie-crusting technique frequently allows closure without tension. If wound closure without tension is not possible, then only the portion of the wound that can be closed without tension is carried out, and the remainder of the wound is left open. The patient may then be returned to the operating room in several days for delayed primary closure or flap coverage if necessary.

A sterile nonadhesive dressing is applied over the wound, followed by application of a bulky Jones-type dressing. A splint may be incorporated into the Jones dressing if desired, particularly if more distal injuries are present (Fig. 28.16); the splint also helps to prevent equinus deformity. Postoperatively, the limb is elevated on a Bohler-Braun frame for 1 to 3 days.

Diaphyseal tibial fractures are frequently accompanied by an associated fibular fracture, which usually does not require repair. However, if the tibia fracture is proximal or distal, plate osteosynthesis may be carried out at the time of tibial stabilization to enhance fracture stability. If the fracture results in excessive shortening, fibular osteosynthesis carried out before the tibial osteosynthesis may be additionally helpful. Care must be taken in preoperative planning to allow for satisfactory skin bridges between the tibial and fibular incisions, which should be kept to a minimum of 8 cm.

POSTOPERATIVE CARE

If his/her condition permits, the patient is mobilized on the first postoperative day with partial weight bearing (20 kg) on the affected side. The use of locking screws does not affect the weight-bearing capability of the construct, and full weight bearing on the plate should not be permitted merely because the screws are locked.

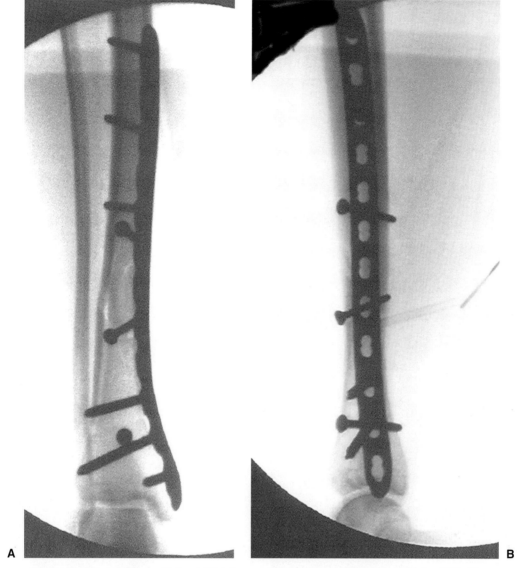

A   B

Figure 28.12. AP **(A)** and lateral **(B)** intraoperative images after removal of the ATD. The proximal screws are standard, 4.5-mm, cortical screws and the distal screws are 5.0-mm locked screws. Due to fracture configuration, additional lag screws through or outside the plate were not necessary.

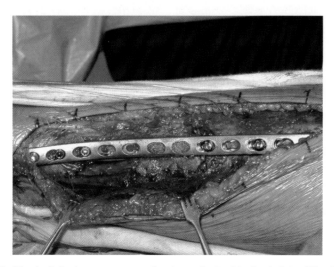

Figure 28.13. Final clinical appearance of extraperiosteal locked plate. Distally (*left*) the plate is beneath the saphenous structures.

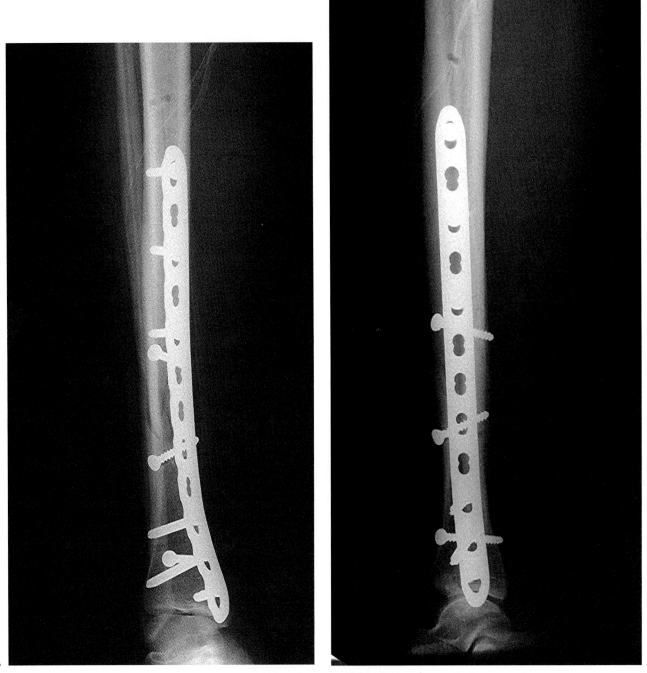

A

B

Figure 28.14. AP **(A)** and lateral **(B)** radiographs of the final osteosynthesis are made at the conclusion of the case.

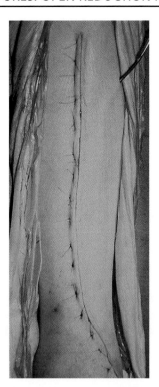

Figure 28.15. Skin closure is carried out with interrupted, horizontal, mattress sutures of 4-0 nylon. No tension should be present in the skin at the time of closure.

The drain is usually removed between 2 and 4 days after surgery, followed by removal of the surgical dressing the next day. Active and active-assisted range of motion of the ankle, hip, and knee is then initiated. A light dry dressing may be required for several days for any subsequent wound drainage. Depending on the clinical situation, any portion of the postoperative regimen may be carried out on an outpatient basis.

The patient is followed up at 4-week intervals with clinical examination and radiographs. Weight bearing is advanced based on the clinical examination of discomfort or localized tenderness and the radiographic appearance of the fracture at follow-up. Typically, weight bearing will be advanced to partial (50 kg) by 6 to 8 weeks and to full by 8 to 12 weeks.

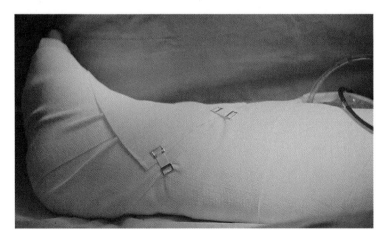

Figure 28.16. Bulky soft-tissue dressing is applied at the conclusion of the operation.

COMPLICATIONS

Of primary concern after ORIF of a tibial fracture is that the incision heals uneventfully. Even with the utmost care, minimal skin and wound-edge necrosis of 1 to 2 mm may be found on occasion; it usually requires nothing more than observation. More extended skin and wound-edge necrosis may require surgical excision with irrigation, debridement, and reclosure of the wound (occasionally with flap advancement). Significant loss of skin and soft tissue in the postoperative period may require flap coverage.

Deep infection, occurring in the first 6 to 8 weeks after ORIF, should be treated with wound irrigation and reclosure over drains with or without antibiotic beads if the fixation remains intact and secure. Late infection in the presence of loosened hardware will require irrigation, debridement, removal of the hardware, and external fixation of the tibia until satisfactory wound and soft-tissue conditions can be obtained.

Treatment of delayed union and nonunion of a tibial shaft fracture after ORIF depends on whether the hardware remains intact or has failed, either by loosening or breakage. If the fixation remains intact and the soft-tissue conditions are satisfactory, then delayed union or nonunion may be treated with bone grafting and maintenance of protected weight bearing. If the internal fixation shows signs of failure, then the hardware must be removed and the internal fixation repeated with the addition of bone graft and an additional period of protected weight-bearing ambulation. Locking plates are not more difficult to revise than standard plates, and old locking holes can be reused for new locking screws.

RECOMMENDED READINGS

1. Perren SM. Physical and biological aspects of fracture healing with special reference to internal fixation. *Clin Orthop* 1979;138:175–196.
2. Muller MR, Allgower M, Schneider R, et al. *Manual of internal fixation.* 2nd ed. New York: Springer-Verlag; 1979.
3. Ruedi T, Webb JK, Allgower M. *Experience with the dynamic compression plate (DCP) in 418 recent fractures of the tibial shaft. Injury* 1976;7:265.
4. Oestern HJ, Tscherne H. Pathophysiology and classification of soft tissue injuries associated with fractures. In: Tscherne H, Gotzen L, eds. *Fractures with soft tissue injuries.* Berlin: Springer-Verlag; 1984.
5. Borrelli J Jr, Prickett W, Song E, et al. Extraosseous blood supply of the tibia and the effects of different plating techniques: a human cadaveric study. *J Orthop Trauma* 2002;16(10): 691–695.
6. Ruedi T, Webb JK, Algower M. Experience with the dynamic compression plate (DCP) in 418 recent fractures of the tibial shaft. *Injury* 1976;7:265.
7. Mast J, Jakob R, Ganz R. *Planning and reduction technique in fracture surgery.* Berlin: Springer-Verlag; 1989.

29

Tibial Shaft Fractures: Intramedullary Nailing

Robert A. Winquist, Kenneth Johnson,*
and Donald A. Wiss

INDICATIONS/CONTRAINDICATIONS

Intramedullary nailing of tibial shaft fractures gained widespread acceptance with the introduction of nails with locking capabilities. A large body of literature supports the use of intramedullary nailing in both closed and open fractures. Nevertheless, controversies abound with regard to the role of reaming in high-energy and open fractures, the timing of surgery, and its application in very proximal and distal fractures. Because the spectrum of injuries to the tibia is so broad, no single method of treatment is applicable to all fractures.

Nonoperative treatment with casts or braces, while minimizing the risk of infection, often results in unacceptable shortening, malrotation, or angulation in high-energy injuries. Although the better choice for improving alignment and function, operative treatment is associated with increased risks of infection and nonunion. Recent advantages in plate osteosynthesis with peri-articular and locked plating have lowered complication rates but are less applicable for diaphyseal tibial fractures. Another alternative, stabilization with an external fixator, while decreasing risk of infection, is associated with poor patient acceptance, repeated surgeries, and angulation after fixator removal. To improve overall outcome, locked intramedullary nailing for unstable, displaced, closed and open, tibial fractures is a useful treatment alternative.

Intramedullary nailing of high-energy tibial fractures, while mechanically sound, may be biologically less attractive. Studies on reamed intramedullary nails have shown substantial endosteal vascular damage incurred by multiple passes of the reamer, thermal necrosis of bone, impaction of the haversian canals with the products of reaming, and an increased risk of infection. Nevertheless, the advantages of intramedullary reaming

*deceased.

include placement of a larger nail and screws, which improves alignment and reduces hardware failure. Despite the risks of reaming, the literature strongly supports the use of a reamed intramedullary nail as the implant of choice for most unstable, closed, tibial-shaft fractures. However, multiple studies also support the use of both reamed and non-reamed nails for Gustillo grade I, II, and IIIA open tibial fractures. For grade IIIB and IIIC fractures, we favor temporary or definitive external fixation or on occasion a non-reamed, small-diameter, statically locked nail.

Intramedullary stabilization of the tibia is indicated in patients with multiple injuries; an ipsilateral fracture of the femur, ankle, or foot; a vascular injury; compartment syndrome; and bilateral fractures. Fractures located in the middle two thirds of the tibia that are amenable to nailing include transverse, short oblique, spiral, comminuted, and segmental fractures (Figs. 29.1 to 29.4). Indications for nailing may extend proximally or distally, particularly in segmental fractures. Unstable fractures with high-grade soft-tissue injury, whether closed or open, require operative stabilization. Unacceptable fracture position after closed reduction and casting is also an indication for nailing. Those with shortening more than 1.5 to 2.0 cm and angulation in excess of 5 degrees of varus or valgus or 10 degrees of anterior or posterior angulation may be candidates for intramedullary nailing. Tibial fractures with an intact fibula should only be stabilized if the tibial fracture is displaced or in angulation (Figs. 29.5 and 29.6). For a minimally or nondisplaced oblique or spiral fracture, nonoperative treatment is satisfactory. Nearly all open fractures require stabilization to allow improved management of the soft tissue.

Contraindications to nailing include immature patients with open epiphyses and a tibial tubercle apophysis. Patients with damage to the apophysis may experience hyperextension. A lateral radiograph should be carefully inspected because very small medullary canals may present a hazard during nailing (Fig. 29.7). If the surgeon elects to proceed with nailing in patients with small canals, a small-diameter Ender nail can be placed, or 5-mm-diameter reamers must be used to start a careful reaming process that will not burn the bone. A tourniquet should not be used for reaming in any patient during tibial nailing.

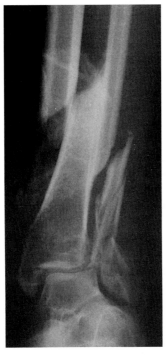

Figure 29.1. AP radiograph of grade I, open, distal-tibial fracture and ankle fracture.

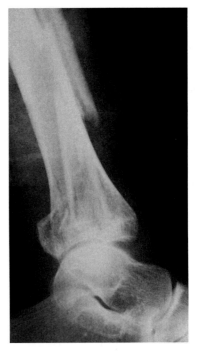

Figure 29.2. Lateral radiograph showing posterior malleolar fracture.

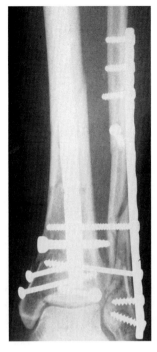

Figure 29.3. Postoperative AP radiograph showing lag screws for ankle fracture and interlocking nail for tibial fracture.

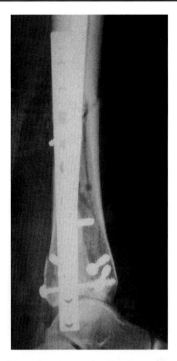

Figure 29.4. Lateral radiograph showing reduction of posterior malleolus.

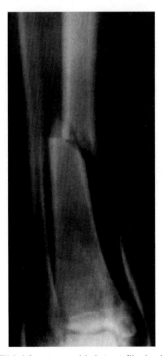

Figure 29.5. Tibial fracture with intact fibula. Varus angulation and translation indicate operative treatment.

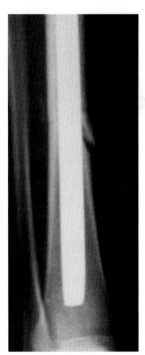

Figure 29.6. Postoperative AP radiograph with nonlocked intramedullary nail in a stable fracture.

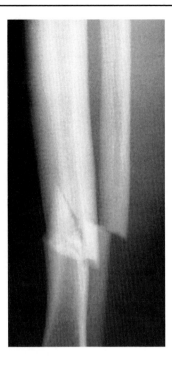

Figure 29.7. Lateral radiograph demonstrating an extremely small medullary canal. Reaming should be avoided or carried out with very small reamers (starting at 5 mm).

Another contraindication is infection. Nailing in an area of infection carries a high risk for chronic osteomyelitis and decreased union. Infected injuries are best handled with debridement and external fixators.

PREOPERATIVE PLANNING

In a careful physical examination of the patient, the physician should look for other injuries. Examination for neurovascular compromise is important. The degree of swelling and any fracture blisters, whether serous or sanguineous, should be recorded. Palpation of the compartment at the fracture site is an important means of determining the tightness of the compartment. Active motion of the toes, pain on passive stretch, and hypesthesia should be noted. If compartment syndrome is suspected, then pressure measurements are valuable. With careful monitoring, any patient who develops a preoperative or postoperative compartment syndrome requires release of the compartments and stabilization with a nail. Open fractures should be carefully evaluated and the fracture wound classified according to Gustillo and Anderson. Patients with both closed and open fractures should be placed in a long-leg splint during the interval between injury and intramedullary nailing.

Patients with closed fractures should be given a cephalosporin one hour before and 24 hours after the nailing procedure. Patients with open fractures should also be treated with cephalosporin for 48 to 72 hours, and if the fractures are contaminated, they should also concomitantly receive aminoglycosides.

A preoperative anteroposterior (AP) and lateral radiograph of the fractured extremity, including both the knee and the ankle, is critical for defining the fracture and geometry of the tibia and the injury. The lateral radiograph should be carefully inspected, and the size of the intramedullary canal should be measured. An ossimeter is used to measure the tibia so that the length and diameter of the nail can be established. Positive nail-design features include static and dynamic interlocking holes, oblique holes for proximal fractures, clustered distal holes for distal fractures, and cannulation for ease of placement over a guide wire as well as for removal of any broken nail.

SURGERY

Anesthesia

General anesthesia is preferred for tibial nailing. If a spinal is used, it should be very short-acting because evaluation of the neurologic status and pain level is very important after surgery. A continuous epidural should be avoided in the treatment of tibial fractures: Although it may provide pain relief for the patient, it makes clinical compartment monitoring difficult.

Prep and Drape

A tourniquet is placed on the thigh but rarely inflated. The entire limb is prepped and draped. If the fracture is open, the traumatic wounds are irrigated and débrided. The traumatic wound is commonly extended to improve exposure and visualization. All nonviable cortical fragments are removed as are foreign bodies or necrotic tissue. The debridement must be orderly, sequential, and complete to render the wound surgically sterile in preparation for the nailing. The fracture ends are carefully inspected and cleaned to ensure that the proximal and distal intramedullary canal is free from debris. If the degree of contamination is high and the wound cannot be reliably rendered clean and sterile, external fixation may be preferable to nailing. The traumatic wound is irrigated, via pulsed lavage, with 9 to 12 L of normal saline.

After the irrigation and debridement, the surgeon's attention is turned to skeletal stabilization. All instruments used for the washout are removed from the field. The surgeon, assistants, and nurse change into clean gowns and gloves. Then clean, dry, sterile drapes are applied to the patient.

Fracture Reduction

Tibial reduction and nailing can be achieved through the surgeon's use of a fracture table, a sterile bolster or triangle under the knee, or a distractor. A sterile radiolucent triangle under the knee is the simplest technique and is particularly useful in the treatment of open fractures that require debridement and re-prep before nailing (Figs. 29.8 and 29.9).

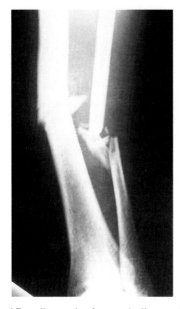

Figure 29.8. AP radiograph of a grade II open fracture with tibial and fibular fracture at same level.

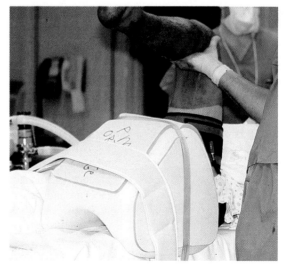

Figure 29.9. Foam shoulder immobilizer used for a bolster under the knee.

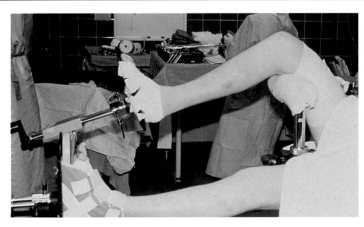

Figure 29.10. Fracture table. Knee is flexed 90 degrees and peroneal post is against distal thigh rather than popliteal fossa.

The knee is flexed over the triangle, which permits access to the proximal tibia as well as visualization of the starting point.

The triangle method presents difficulty for obtaining and maintaining fracture length as well as for controlling angulation and rotation. The assistant also will have difficulty holding the leg perfectly still during distal interlocking. This technique works best with stable fracture patterns.

A fracture table is more complex to set up but is effective in maintaining leg length and rotation during the procedure. It is particularly helpful in nonteaching hospitals where a scrubbed assistant may not be available. With the fracture table, the knee is flexed 90 degrees over a post, which is placed proximal to the popliteal fossa to prevent compression of the vessels or peroneal nerve (Fig. 29.10). Tape is placed around the leg to prevent external rotation of the extremity. A fracture table works best in treating patients with isolated closed injuries of the tibia and is more difficult to use for patients with multiple trauma or open fractures.

A distractor can be used with a pin placed proximally in the posterior tibia and distally just above the ankle joint. In acute fractures, a unilateral frame is usually adequate. After 10 to 14 days, length is more difficult to restore, and a unilateral frame may lead to angulation. Therefore, through-and-through proximal and distal tibial pins are used with a bilateral frame in conjunction with simultaneous medial and lateral distraction. Compared with a bolster or triangle, this method takes longer and is more complex, but it provides good alignment and stability during nailing and interlocking.

Incision and Starting Point

The joint is palpated and marked on the knee. The incision starts at the joint line and extends proximally (Fig. 29.11). The incision need not go distally down to the tibial tubercle. For fractures of the midshaft or below, the incision and starting point is just medial to the patellar tendon. The joint is palpated, and the awl is inserted where the anterior tibia reaches the joint (Fig. 29.12). The surgeon must stay in the extra-articular area because back out of the nail may impinge on the femoral condyle. He/she must not enter distally at the tibial tubercle, as this leads to a more oblique anterior-to-posterior starting angle, which causes greater risk of nail penetration into the posterior cortex. In proximal third fractures, the incision and starting point is just lateral to the patellar tendon (Figs. 29.13 and 29.14). A sharp, curved, tibial awl is used, and its position is checked in both the AP and lateral planes with an image intensifier before portal placement. On the lateral radiograph, the point of the awl should be on top of the bone (Fig. 29.15). On the AP view, it should be in line with the long axis of the tibia (Fig. 29.16). When treating proximal fractures, the surgeon may find that staying more lateral helps prevent both translation and angulation. The Synthes (Synthes, Paoli, PA) unreamed nail has been a particular problem in proximal tib-

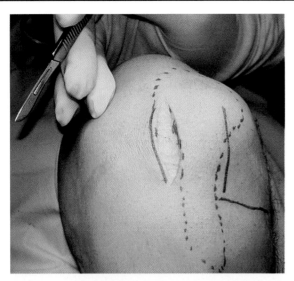

Figure 29.11. Skin marking with patella and patellar tendon outlined. The horizontal mark is on the lateral joint line, and a longitudinal mark is on the lateral border of the patellar tendon. A medial incision is seen over the medial border of the patellar tendon. The incision is started at the joint line and is continued proximally.

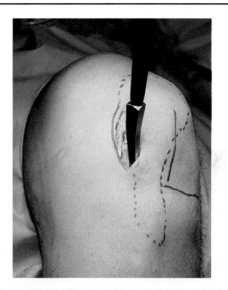

Figure 29.12. Sharp awl inserted in the incision.

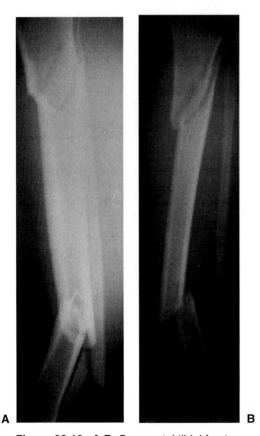

A   **B**

Figure 29.13. A,B. Segmental tibial fracture.

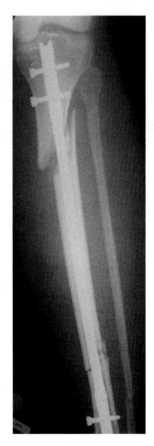

Figure 29.14. Mal-alignment of the proximal component of a segmental fracture with surgical starting point too far medial.

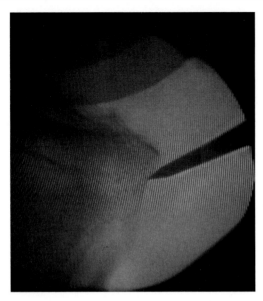

Figure 29.15. Lateral radiograph with awl slightly inferior to correct starting point.

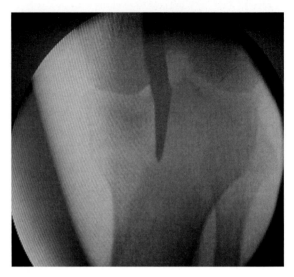

Figure 29.16. AP radiograph showing that the awl is slightly medial.

ial fractures because of its long and distal curve, which can lead to both translation and angulation of the fracture site (Fig. 29.17). In proximal fractures, temporary stabilization with a clamp or small plate is sometimes necessary. To prevent angulation or translation, blocking screws are another option in proximal fracture treatment.

Bulb-Tip Guide

A bulb-tip guide wire is inserted down the canal. A small bend in the guide wire made 2 cm from the tip can be helpful because it can facilitate passage of the wire across the fracture site. A T handle, which is used to control the bulb-tip guide, is placed in the midportion of the guide. The bulb tip is initially aimed posteriorly, and after it has entered the tibia, it is immediately turned anteriorly and passed down to the fracture site; the surgeon must avoid penetration of the posterior cortex proximally and exiting through the fracture site posteriorly. The guide wire is advanced to the fracture site, and under biplanar image intensification, is passed into the distal fragment (Fig. 29.18). It is impacted into the subchondral bone above the ankle to stabilize the bulb tip and to aid in determining length (Fig. 29.19). A second bulb tip, of identical length to the first, is placed at the joint line, and a long ruler is used to determine nail length. In another method of determining nail length, the tibia is measured externally with a long ruler, hatch marks are made, and the measurements are confirmed with an image intensifier. Many manufacturers provide a cannulated depth guide that allows a direct measurement of nail length.

Reaming

Based on the preoperative plan and the personality of the fracture, the surgeon determines whether to use a reamed or nonreamed technique. If reaming is selected, it must be done properly so that complications are avoided (Figs. 29.20 and 29.21). Because the risk of heat necrosis increases during reaming, it should be carried out at a low torque with sharp reamers that dissipate heat and pressure (Fig. 29.22). A tourniquet should be avoided. To prevent soft-tissue damage around the incision, a skin protector should be used. The surgeon should start with a small-diameter reamer and increase in one-half millimeter increments until cortical contact is reached. For closed fractures, reaming one additional millimeter is usually sufficient. The fracture must be reduced as the reamer passes (aided by the bulb-tip guide).

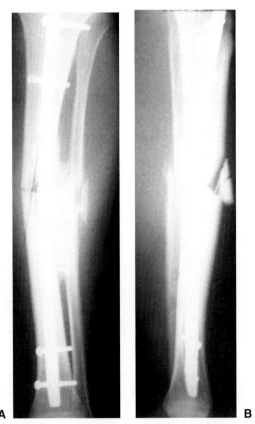

Figure 29.17. A,B. Postoperative radiograph of comminuted proximal-tibial fracture with AO nail. The long Herzog curve with some external rotation of the nail has created a deformity.

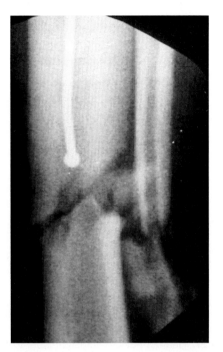

Figure 29.18. Bulb tip approaching fracture site.

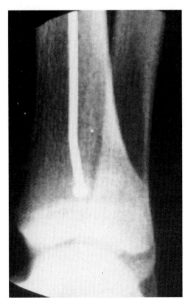

Figure 29.19. Bulb tip down to subchondral bone.

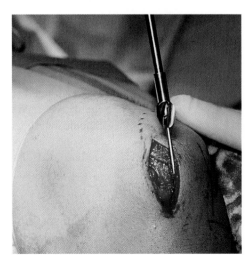

Figure 29.20. Reamer inserted over bulb tip.

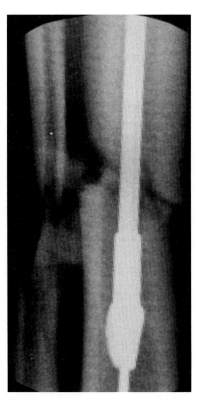

Figure 29.21. Reamer passed across fracture to metaphyseal flare. Minimal reaming in grade I open fracture.

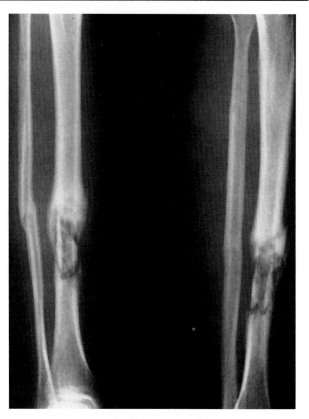

Figure 29.22. Heat necrosis of tibia.

If the canal diameter permits, placement of a nail of 10 mm or greater diameter is mechanically beneficial. Excessive reaming should not be done to achieve this, particularly in open fractures. If necessary, an 8- or 9-mm nail may be used. However, with smaller nails, the patient's postoperative management must be modified. The patient should be kept from weight bearing until healing is evident, and if healing is slow, the surgeon should consider dynamization or nail exchange.

Several investigators have suggested that reaming may increase the possibility of a compartment syndrome. At the conclusion of nailing, the compartments should be palpated, and if any concern exists, the compartment pressure can be measured.

Exchange Tube

Before nail insertion, a plastic exchange tube is passed over the bulb tip and across the fracture site (Figs. 29.23 and 29.24). Once the bulb tip is removed, a nail-driving guide without bulb tip is inserted, and the plastic tube is removed. The nail is driven over this guide wire. Because the reduction can be maintained with this guide, cannulated nails should be used. Rarely does the fracture site need to be opened to pass the nail. Solid nails offer no mechanical advantage nor do they decrease the risk of infection more than do cannulated nails. Furthermore, in our experience, solid nails make the passage of the nail less predictable and the removal of a broken nail extremely difficult.

Nail Insertion

The nail is inserted over the guide wire with the surgeon pushing posteriorly on the proximal end of the nail to minimize penetration of the posterior cortex (Fig. 29.25). A lateral

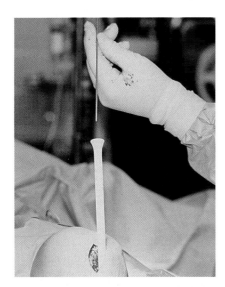

Figure 29.23. Exchange tube with nail-driving guide.

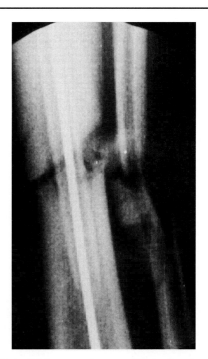

Figure 29.24. Exchange tube on radiograph seen crossing the fracture site.

image should be used while driving the nail in the upper third of the tibia. As the nail approaches the fracture site, the fracture must be aligned in two planes (Fig. 29.26). The nail must be inserted in slight external rotation. If the nail is allowed to rotate internally, interlocking will take place on the posteromedial cortex proximally and distally, which is much more difficult to complete than is interlocking carried out on the flat surface of the tibia. Therefore, to make targeting an easier process, the nail should be externally rotated approximately 10 degrees in relation to the long axis of the tibia.

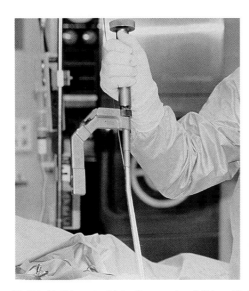

Figure 29.25. Nail inserted into the proximal tibia with hand pulling the nail posteriorly to push the tip of the nail anteriorly.

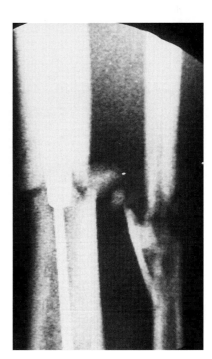

Figure 29.26. Fracture must be aligned prior to passage of the nail.

As the nail crosses the fracture site, the surgeon must avoid distraction. Overreaming by 1 mm is helpful. In stable fracture patterns, traction should be released when the tip of the nail is 1 cm past the fracture. This should then allow impaction and avoid distraction. To prevent distraction, the surgeon may need to apply distal counterpressure as the nail crosses the fracture. Because tibial nails are small and the screw diameters are similarly small, the application of a distal screw with the back-slap technique carries a risk of early fatigue of the distal locking screws. As the nail is driven down the tibia, the surgeon should reassess the accuracy of its length. The tibia should be inspected proximally and distally. If the nail is too short or too long, then it should be removed and replaced with another nail. In distal fractures, the nail should reach the subchondral bone. The nail should not be countersunk into the proximal tibia for greater than 2 to 3 mm or later extraction will be difficult. Several manufacturers have nail extenders, which can be beneficial for making small adjustments in length.

Insertion of Proximal Screws

Targeting devices that attach to the intramedullary nail are very successful in placing the proximal-tibial locking screws (Fig. 29.27). Use of anterior-to-posterior screws introduce a slight risk of injury to vascular structures and should be avoided if possible (Fig. 29.28). Oblique screws for proximal fractures are safer. Only one proximal screw is necessary for fractures in the midshaft and below (Fig. 29.29). For proximal fractures, two or three screws are necessary in the proximal end of the nail. Blocking screws can also be helpful to control angulation or translation. For stable transverse or short, oblique, tibial fractures, the use of the dynamic slot at the proximal end of the nail allows for impaction of the fracture. If comminution or a spiral component is found in conjunction with the fracture, the nail should be statically locked.

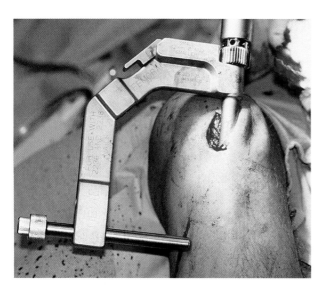

Figure 29.27. Proximal targeting jig.

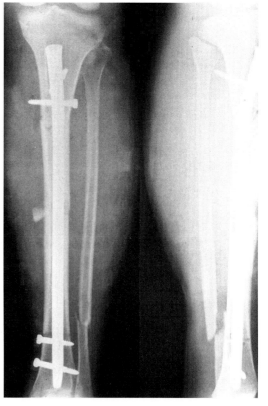

Figure 29.28. Use of anterior-to-posterior screw increases risk of vascular injury.

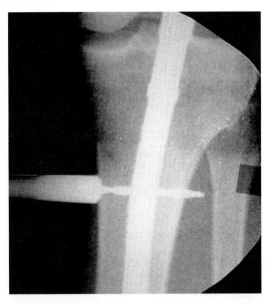

Figure 29.29. Depth gauge used to measure screw length.

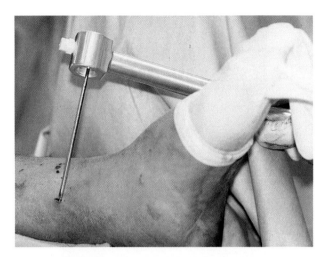

Figure 29.30. Sharp trocar to mark skin incision.

Distal Screw Insertion

We prefer the freehand technique of distal screw insertion because none of the external guides is consistently helpful. For length-stable fractures in the middle to the proximal half of the tibia, only a single distal screw is necessary, whereas in distal fractures, two or three screws should be used with or without blocking screws. A medial-to-lateral screw and an anterior-to-posterior screw can be used, but if using the latter, the surgeon must pay close attention to both the anterior tibial tendon and posterior vascular structures.

The nail should be externally rotated 10 degrees to allow targeting on a flat surface. Via the freehand technique, the first step is targeting of the skin incision. The image intensifier is lined up with the nail and tilted and rotated until a perfectly round hole is visualized. An image intensifier that can magnify the hole twice its normal size is the best choice. Also, the C-arm head should be moved away from the tibia to increase the working space and aid in magnification of the hole. The sharp point of the trocar-tipped pin is placed on the skin until it is centered in the hole (Fig. 29.30). A 1-cm stab wound is made directly over the hole on the medial aspect of the tibia. Because the saphenous vein is very close to the targeted area, laceration is possible. The sharp point guide is again placed on the bone until it is centered in the hole (Fig. 29.31). It is brought into the longitudinal axis and checked with fluoroscopy to ensure that it is centered in all planes (Fig. 29.32); a halo should be evident around the guide (Fig. 29.33). The sharp point is then passed into the tibia with a mallet and then removed. The drill bit is then placed freehand through the hole and through the nail. The AP view is checked, and the lateral tibia is drilled and measured for placement of the screw. The screw should be 5 mm longer than the measurement so it will be easier to remove if it breaks (Fig. 29.34). The screw should protrude through the cortex; if the screw is not prominent, then it will be very difficult to retrieve if breakage occurs (Fig. 29.35). A lateral radiograph should be checked again to be absolutely certain the screw is in the nail and that it has not moved anteriorly or posteriorly (Fig. 29.36).

Wound Closure

A long-acting local anesthetic is injected into all the wounds. The wounds are then irrigated and closed. If necessary, the patient is checked for increased compartmental pressure. Most grade I and II open wounds and some grade IIIA fractures are closed primarily, while

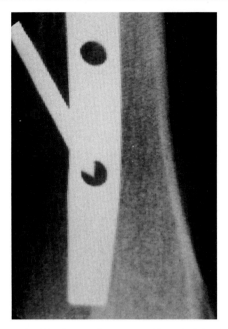

Figure 29.31. Trocar in center of interlocking hole.

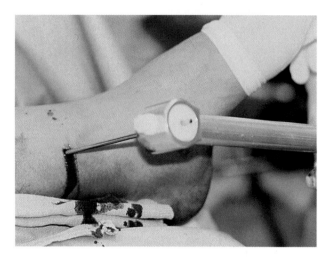

Figure 29.32. Trocar brought in axis of the hole.

contaminated IIIA fractures are left open and closed after a delay. Grade IIIB fractures are scheduled for return to the operating room for repeated debridements and early flap coverage.

POSTOPERATIVE MANAGEMENT

The patient is placed in a posterior splint with the ankle neutral or in slight dorsiflexion to prevent an equinus deformity. The patient remains in a splint until the swelling decreases.

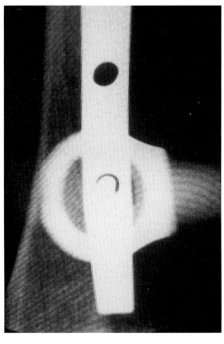

Figure 29.33. Fluoroscopy is used to ensure that trocar is centered.

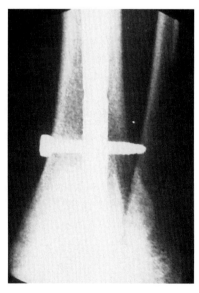

Figure 29.34. The screw tip should extend 5 mm past the cortex to allow for removal if the screw breaks.

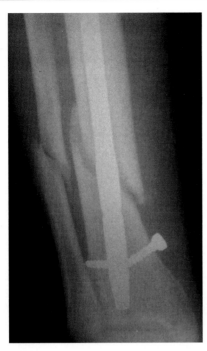

Figure 29.35. Broken screw. Inadequate fixation in a distal one-third fracture.

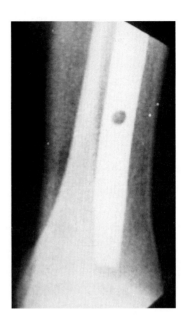

Figure 29.36. Lateral radiograph is used to ensure that distal screw is centered in the hole.

This may take as little as 1 week or as long as 6 weeks. If the cast is removed too early, the patient tends to be more uncomfortable, and the foot drops into equinus. In a reliable patient with a stable fracture pattern and a dynamic locking construct, partial weight bearing is desirable with progressive weight bearing over the first 4 weeks. In an unstable pattern or an unreliable patient, weight bearing is not recommended for at least 6 to 8 weeks. Mild swelling of the leg can be controlled by use of a thick elastic stocking.

For open fractures, continued wound monitoring is necessary, and the frequency is dictated by the severity of the wound. The first postoperative office visit is in 1 to 2 postoperative weeks for a change of the splint and inspection of all wounds. After that, patients are followed at 4 to 6 week intervals, with AP and lateral radiographs obtained until the fracture is healed. If after 2 to 4 months the healing is questionable, oblique radiographs may be necessary to ascertain fracture healing. Weight bearing is usually started at 2 months if callus is forming.

In addition to callus formation, the surgeon should look for broken screws, which signify instability and a possible change in treatment. If a screw is broken in a fairly stable fracture pattern, healing may continue and no further treatment will be necessary. If screw breakage occurs in an unstable fracture pattern, shortening will result and the risk of a nonunion is increased.

Healing is slow in the tibia, and patients should be informed of the length of the process. Patients rarely have realistic expectations because of lack of knowledge. Postoperative knee pain is almost universal and calms down over 4 to 6 months. Physical therapy is required for gait training, and quad sets with straight-leg lifts and active range of motion of the ankle are necessary postoperative treatments. Passive range of motion exercises of the knee or ankle do not appear to be beneficial, and resistive range of motion of the knee only increases the patellofemoral pain.

Most patients require crutch support for 2 to 4 months. Walking without support gradually increases over 4 to 6 months after injury with a very gradual loss of limp. Patients usually return to running after 6 to 12 months. Full recovery often takes 1.5 to 2.0 years. Patients may return to activity according to their comfort levels. Bicycling and swimming are gentle forms of exercise to build up muscle and strength before moving into more active sports.

COMPLICATIONS

Delayed Union and Nonunion

Delayed union and nonunion of the tibia are common complications of intramedullary nailing. A nonoptimal outcome is related to the poor soft-tissue envelope around the tibia, which is further compromised by the injury. Implant failure is common. Therefore careful postoperative monitoring is important, and further surgical procedures are expected in comminuted high-energy fractures.

Dynamization is an excellent choice of treatment for stable-pattern fractures that are slow to heal at 2 or 3 months and will not be excessively shortened or rotated. If callus is not evident at 2 to 3 months in this group, then removal of screws at the end of the nail farthest from the fracture is beneficial. Bone grafting is used in patients with a skeletal defect. This treatment is most effective when delayed: a 6 to 8 week interval appears to be appropriate. Because these are unstable fractures and will shorten, a static nail should be left in place.

Exchange nailing also is used for slow-healing stable fractures. It is ideal for patients who were initially stabilized with small-diameter nails and screws. Two to 3 months after injury, when the soft tissues are well healed, a larger nail is placed; the fracture pattern will dictate whether it is to be statically locked.

Hardware Failure

Screw failure occurs in 10% to 40% of statically locked tibial nails. Weaker screws include those with small diameters and those made of titanium. If screw failure occurs in a stable fracture pattern, then surgery is not required, and the fracture will usually heal. In unstable fracture patterns, including distal fractures, screw breakage is frequently a precursor to a nonunion. In these patients, the broken screws should be removed, and larger nails should be inserted with larger screws in either a static or dynamic mode.

Nail breakage occurs in 3% to 5% of fractures, generally after 4 to 6 months. Broken nails should be exchanged. For cannulated nails with a large diameter, a hook can be used for removal. For small-diameter cannulated nails, a bulb-tip guide with a smooth guide rod alongside it can be used to remove the distal fragment. Removal of the distal fragment is extremely difficult when solid nails are employed, and we advise against using them.

Infection

Infection after nailing may be subclassified as acute or chronic. In acute infections found within a week of surgery, debridement and drainage is the treatment of choice. The nail can be left in place, and for 6 weeks parenteral antibiotics are used. If the infection resolves, the nail is left in place, and the patient is followed until healing. If healing is slow, a posterolateral bone graft may be necessary.

A chronic infection may indicate a possible segmental sequestrum. In these patients, the nail and a segment of tibia must be removed to eradicate the infection. These patients are then placed in external fixators and require cancellous bone grafting for small defects and segmental transport for large defects. Intravenous antibiotics are necessary and should be administered for at least 6 weeks.

Compartment Syndrome

Compartment syndromes can be difficult to diagnose. They generally occur within the first 24 to 48 hours after injury but can be seen as late as 5 days following fracture. Frequent physical examinations in an awake patient constitute the most reliable diagnostic technique, and pressure measurements in the comatose or uncooperative patient are the safest diagnostic techniques. Multiple pressure measurements are particularly beneficial to determine a trend. In institutions with frequent monitoring capabilities, the compartment pressure can increase to within 30 mm Hg of diastolic pressure before a compartment release is done. In situations in which monitoring is not optimal at night or on the weekends, release of compartment at lower pressure and with suggestive signs is advised. A four compartment fasciotomy can be performed through either a single lateral incision or a lateral and posteromedial incision. The posteromedial incision is the best choice for distal injuries.

ILLUSTRATIVE CASE FOR TECHNIQUE

A 38-year-old man was involved in a ski accident. He suffered a high, proximal, oblique, metaphyseal-tibial fracture and an oblique, distal-tibial fracture at the junction of the middle and distal thirds (Fig. 29.37). The distal fracture was classified as a Gustillo grade IIIA open, which did not require a flap. The patient was treated with primary debridement of the open fracture with temporary stabilization via use of an external fixator and a primary plate and screw fixation of the proximal tibial fracture (Fig. 29.38). The wound was allowed to heal and the soft-tissue swelling decreased.

Five weeks after injury, the external fixator was removed, and after a week (to minimize the risk of infection) the tibia was nailed. The proximal plate was then removed, and both

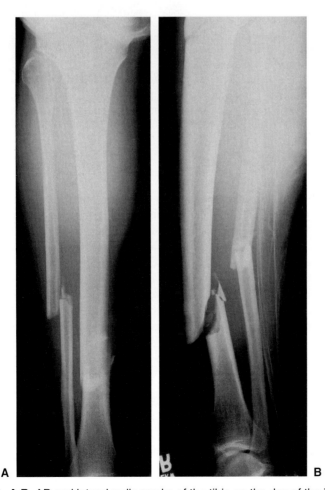

Figure 29.37. A,B. AP and lateral radiographs of the tibia on the day of the injury. These images show displacement of the distal fracture with distinct soft-tissue injury and a very high, slightly oblique, proximal fracture.

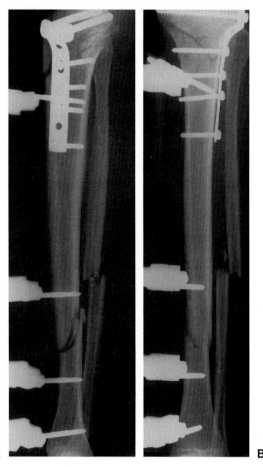

Figure 29.38. A,B. Postoperative AP and lateral radiographs on the day of injury. A proximal tibial T-plate is in position with an external fixator for the distal open fracture.

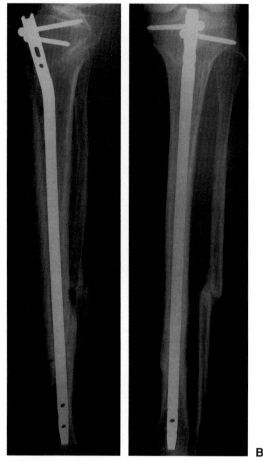

Figure 29.39. A,B. Six months after injury, the AP radiograph shows complete healing and the lateral radiograph shows partial healing. The nail has stabilized both fractures.

the proximal and distal fractures were fixed by using a metaphyseal-diaphyseal (MD) nail without distal interlocking. At the time of plate removal, shortening and rotation was not considered to be a future problem. The proximal fracture, however, was stabilized with two oblique proximal screws that fit high in the tibia and are ideal for this fracture (Fig. 29.39). Both fractures healed excellently without infection, and the patient has a full range of motion of the ankle and knee with only minimal aching in the tibia.

Another treatment option would have involved primary nailing on the day of the injury. Proper reduction of the proximal fracture is always difficult, and reamed versus unreamed nailing of the distal-tibial open fracture remains controversial.

RECOMMENDED READING

Blick SS, Brumback RJ, Lakatos R, et al. Early prophylactic bone grafting of high-energy tibial fractures. *Clin Orthop* 1989;240(3):21–41.

Bone LB, Johnson KD. Treatment of tibia fractures by reaming and intramedullary nailing. *J Bone Joint Surg Am* 1986;68(6):877–887.

Browner BD. Pitfalls, errors and complications in the use of locking Kuntscher nails. *Clin Orthop* 1986;212:192–208.

Carr JB. Use of the reamed nail in tibial shaft fractures. In: Cardea JA, ed. *Operative techniques in orthopaedics.* Philadelphia: WB Saunders; 1991:319–325.

Collins DN, Pearce CE, McAndrew MP. Successful use of reaming and intramedullary nailing of the tibia. *J Orthop Trauma* 1990;4:315–322.

Court-Brown DM. The clinical results of reamed intramedullary nailing. *Tech Ortho* 1996;11(1):79–85.

Gustillo RB, Mendoza RM, Williams DN. Problems in the management of type III (severe) open fractures: a new classification of type III open fractures. *J Trauma* 1984;24:742.

Henley MB. Intramedullary devices for tibial fracture stabilization. *Clin Orthop* 1989;240:87–96.

Henley MB, Champman JR, Agel J, et al. Treatment of type II, IIIA and IIIB open fractures of the tibial shaft: a randomized prospective comparison of unreamed interlocking nails and half-pin external fixators. *J Orthop Trauma* 1998;12:1–7.

Leunig M, Hertel R. Thermal necrosis after tibial reaming for intramedullary nail fixation. *J Bone Joint Surg Br* 1996;78(4):584–587.

McQueen MM. Intramedullary reaming and compartment pressure. *Tech Ortho* 1996;11(1):41–44.

Muller C, McIff T, Rahn BA, et al. Intramedullary pressure strain on the diaphysis and increase in cortical temperature when reaming. *Injury* 1993;3[suppl]:31.

Rhinelander FW. Tibial blood supply in relation to fracture healing. *Clin Orthop* 1974;105:34.

Schendelmaier P, Kettek P, Tscherne H. Biomechanical study of nine different tibial locking nails. *J Orthop Trauma* 1996;10(1):37–44.

Swiontkowski MF. Tibial shaft fractures. In: Hansen ST, Swiontkowski MF, eds. *Orthopaedic trauma protocols.* New York: Raven Press; 1993.

Tornetta P III, Berman M, Watnik N, et al. Treatment of grade IIIB open tibial fractures. *J Bone Joint Surg Br* 1994;76(1):13–19.

Trafton PG. Tibial shaft fractures. In: Browner BD, Jupiter JB, Levine AM, et al, eds. *Skeletal trauma.* Philadelphia: WB Saunders; 1992:1809–1821.

Whittle AP, Russell TA, Taylor JC, et al. Treatment of open fractures of the tibial shaft with the use of interlocking nailing without reaming. *J Bone Joint Surg Am* 1992;74(8):1162–1171.

Wiss DA. Flexible medullary nailing of acute tibial shaft fractures. *Clin Orthop* 1986;212:122–132.

30

Tibial Shaft Fractures: Spatial Frame

J. Charles Taylor

INDICATIONS / CONTRAINDICATIONS

Tibial shaft fractures are relatively common injuries in adults and adolescents. Because of its subcutaneous location and because it is frequently the site of direct injury, tibial fractures are open more often than other long bone fractures. Even in closed fractures, severe soft-tissue injury may be evident or initially suspected. Swelling, fracture blisters, and even subsequent full-thickness skin loss may complicate an initially closed fracture. Compartment syndrome may be present in open as well as closed fractures. In addition to injuries caused by direct trauma, the tibia and fibula may fracture as a result of torsional and bending forces. This usually occurs at the junction of the distal 1/4 tibia where there is the lowest section modulus.

Indications for treatment with Spatial Frame include (a) open fractures with bone loss, (b) fractures with compartment syndrome, (c) open fractures, (d) unstable closed fractures, and (e) fractures with subsequent loss of reduction following initial casting. Although not addressed specifically in this chapter, delayed union, nonunion, and malunion of the tibia can also be treated with the Spatial Frame.

Because external fixation historically has been reserved for the worst clinical situations, there is no contraindication for its use as the primary definitive method for acute shaft fractures.

PREOPERATIVE PLANNING

The initial exam should include a thorough inspection of the limb and complete neurovascular assessment, which must be repeated regularly to detect impending compartment syndrome. In the conscious patient, increasing pain and decreasing sensation are the earliest signs and symptoms of compartment syndrome. The limb must be inspected for open wounds and hemarthrosis of the knee or ankle. The entire lower extremity is then splinted in a well-padded, long, leg splint to achieve at least gross realignment of the fragments.

Proximal or distal shaft fractures may include extension into the joint. If the initial antero-posterior (AP) and lateral radiographs of the tibia and fibula from knee to ankle are suspicious but inconclusive for intra-articular extension, a computed tomography (CT) scan including the joint should be obtained to help aid diagnosis and treatment.

The Spatial Frame may be used in two modes, acute reduction or gradual reduction. In the simplest mode, after fracture fragments are fixed, the frame can be acutely manipulated to reduce the fracture under direct vision for open fractures and c-arm control for closed and open fractures. The frame is then locked in position. No computer is necessary for this type of acute reduction. In the most versatile mode, any frame may be gradually adjusted to reduce the fracture. This reduction is done daily and gradually usually over 1 to 2 weeks. Additional anesthetics are unnecessary. This gradual reduction can be used for the entire reduction process or after an initial acute reduction.

INTRODUCTION TO SPATIAL FRAME

The Taylor Spatial Frame fixator consists of two rings or partial rings connected by six telescopic struts with special universal joints (Fig. 30.1). By adjusting only strut lengths, one ring can be repositioned with respect to the other. Special FastFx struts have two modes of adjustment. In the unlocked position, they are free to slide like a piston for an initial reduction in surgery (Fig. 30.2). In the locked mode, the struts can be gradually adjusted allowing further reduction of the residual skeletal deformity in the clinic or patient's home (Fig. 30.3). The Spatial Frame fixator is capable of correcting all six axes of the deformity, three translations, two angulations, and rotation by adjusting lengths of struts only.

The ability to make gradual adjustments to the frame after the surgical application allows the surgeon to divorce fracture fixation from reduction. The surgeon can concentrate on a stable fix of major fragments during surgery with relative disregard of reduction. After stable fixation, the fragments can be acutely reduced with the FastFx struts in their unlocked

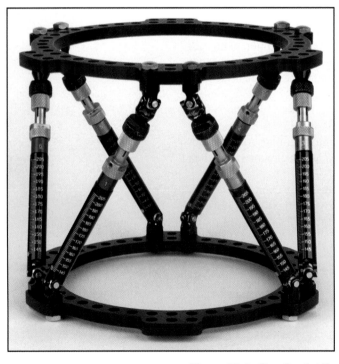
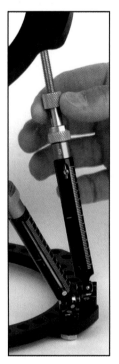
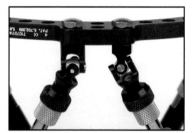
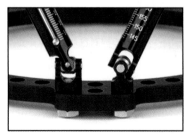

Figure 30.1. One Spatial Frame ring can be repositioned with respect to the other by adjusting strut lengths. (Copyright © J. Charles Taylor.)

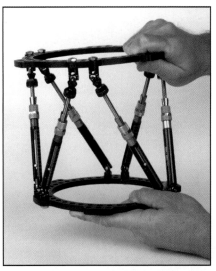
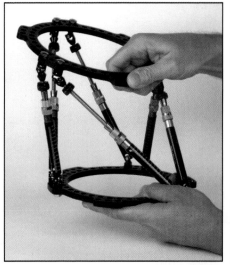
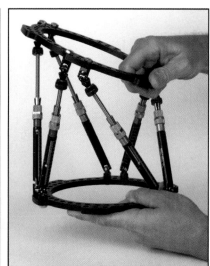

Figure 30.2. A Spatial Frame may be acutely adjusted by hand with all struts in the un-locked position. (Copyright © J. Charles Taylor.)

position or gradually reduced in the locked position. This ability to achieve delayed near anatomic reductions is the greatest strength of the Spatial Frame technique.

Frames can be tapered by using rings of different sizes to make them less cumbersome and safer while descending stairs. Generally 1 to 2 fingerbreadths clearance anterior between the ring and skin and 2 to 3 fingerbreadths posteriorly are adequate (Fig. 30.4). To allow full knee flexion, a 2/3 ring with open posterior is frequently used for proximal tibial fractures. Complete and 2/3 rings range in size from 80- to 300-mm internal diameter and are available in 25-mm increments. Accessory rings and partial rings may be attached to extend the levels of fixation (Fig. 30.5). Standard and short foot plates are available in 155- and 180-mm internal diameters. U plates are also used for foot fixation (Fig. 30.6).

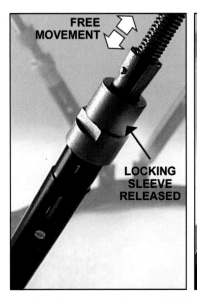
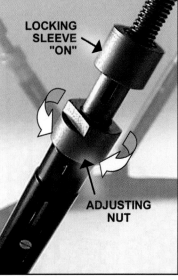

Figure 30.3. Fast Fx struts are free to slide in the unlocked position for acute fracture reduction. The locking sleeve is advanced to lock the strut. The locked strut can still be gradually adjusted by rotation of the nosepiece. (Copyright © J. Charles Taylor.)

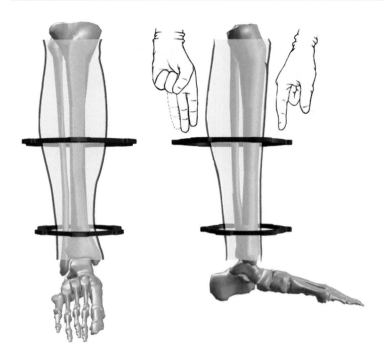

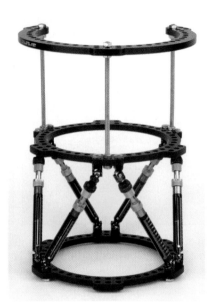

Figure 30.4. Spatial Frames may be tapered and eccentric. Sufficient soft-tissue clearance should be allowed to prevent frame impingement. (Copyright © J. Charles Taylor.)

Figure 30.5. A tapered frame consisting of a 180-mm diameter 2/3 ring proximally connected to a 155-mm Spatial Frame, distally, Ilizarov threaded rods. The proximal 2/3 ring with the opening positioned posteriorly allows full knee flexion. (Copyright © J. Charles Taylor.)

The assembly drawing is shown in Figure 30.7. The open area of a 2/3 ring can be positioned based on surgeon's choice. Six identifier clips, uniquely colored and numbered 1 through 6, are provided with each frame. Each numbered/colored clip is applied to a strut beginning with strut 1 (which is attached to a tab directly anterior on the proximal ring) and progressing counterclockwise as viewed from the proximal end of the frame.

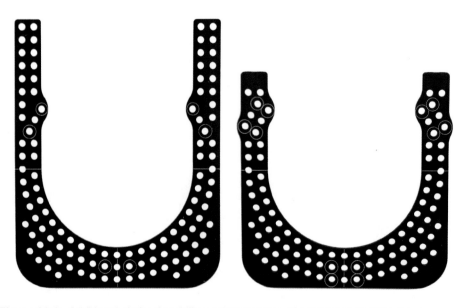

Figure 30.6. Additional skeletal stability and prevention of equinus deformity may be gained by fixing the foot to a foot plate or U plate. (Copyright © J. Charles Taylor.)

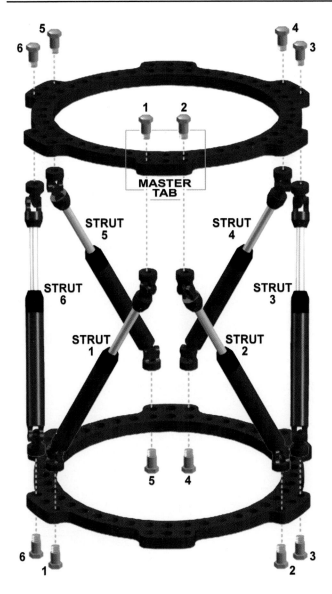

Figure 30.7. Each numbered and colored clip is applied to a strut beginning with strut no. 1 (which is attached anteriorly to the designated master tab) and progressing counterclockwise as viewed from the proximal end of the frame. The computer program assumes the universal joints connecting strut no. 1 and no. 2 to the proximal ring are aligned directly anterior with respect to the reference fragment. Different rotational alignments, especially for more proximal femoral and humeral applications, can be accommodated by changing rotary frame offset. (Copyright © J. Charles Taylor.)

Adequate Fixation

Threaded, titanium, half pins and/or tensioned 1.8-mm diameter stainless-steel wires were designed to be used with the Spatial Frame. To minimize the number of pins and wires, their placement should be optimized to provide the greatest stability within anatomic constraints. The entire length of the anterior/medial tibia is available for half pin fixation. Four millimeter and 5-mm titanium half pins are used for adolescents and small adults. Usually 6-mm half pins are used in large children and adults.

Long fragments are fixed with at least two and often three half pins in different planes. Pins should be spread longitudinally along a significant portion of each fragment but out of the zone of soft-tissue injury (Fig. 30.8). Obviously this is not always possible.

Shorter peri-articular fragments are fixed with at least two multiplanar half pins at approximately 70 degrees to each other. Adding a single olive wire in the coronal plane adds significant stability to a short fragment.

Alternatively, three 1.8-mm olive wires can be used to stabilize a short proximal or distal fragment (Fig. 30.9). The crossing angle of these wires must be optimized within anatomic limits. Olives should block the fragment from each side and the third olive wire should be blocking the fracture obliquity. Stability for a very short proximal tibial fragment

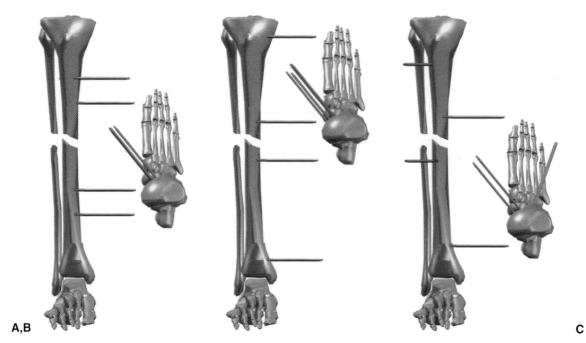

Figure 30.8. A. The surgeon should not limit mechanical stability by two sets of parallel pins. **B.** Fracture stability is significantly improved by extending the working length in each fragment. **C.** Stability is further increased by inserting pins in different planes, achieving multiplanar fixation. (Copyright © J. Charles Taylor.)

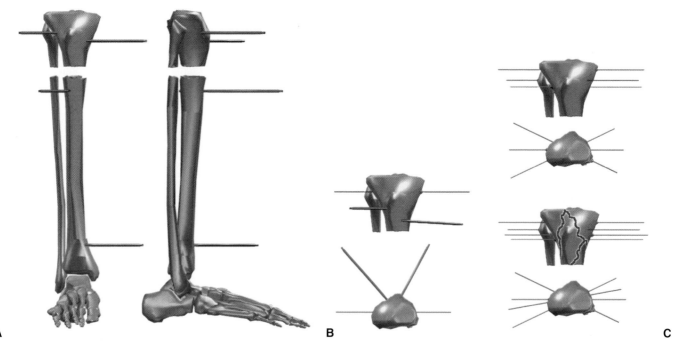

Figure 30.9. A. Short peri-articular fragments can be stabilized with two or three multiplanar half pins. **B.** Stability is improved significantly by at least one tension wire. **C.** For short extra-articular fragments, good stability is provided by three multiplanar tension wires. Four multiplanar wires are used for intra-articular fractures such as a bicondylar tibial-plateau fracture. (Copyright © J. Charles Taylor.)

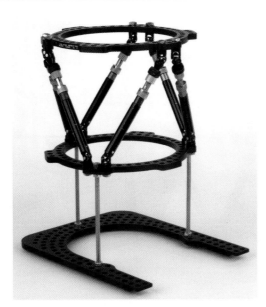

Figure 30.10. The accessory foot plate or U plate is attached to the Spatial Frame with threaded rods. (Copyright © J. Charles Taylor.)

can be increased by transfixing the tibia and fibula at the level of the fibular head with a tension wire.

For very short, distal, tibial fragments, transosseous wires can be used as needed in the syndesmotic region. Intermediate length fragments may be fixed with a combination of wires and half pins.

The foot may also be included at least temporarily for fracture stability, soft tissue immobilization, and prevention of equinus contracture. A distal shaft fracture with significant soft-tissue injury and especially with peripheral nerve injury or closed head injury should have the fixation extended to the foot at least temporarily (Fig. 30.10). The foot plate is attached to the distal ring of the Spatial Frame with threaded rods. Usually a combination of olive wires and half pins are placed in the calcaneus and two wires are placed in the metatarsals (Fig. 30.11). Shorter frames may be constructed with short body struts. Tapered

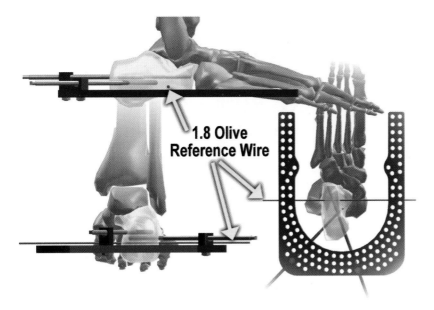

Figure 30.11. Angled wires and/or pins are used in the calcaneus. Usually two wires are used in the forefoot (not shown) at the level of the metatarsal necks. (Copyright © J. Charles Taylor.)

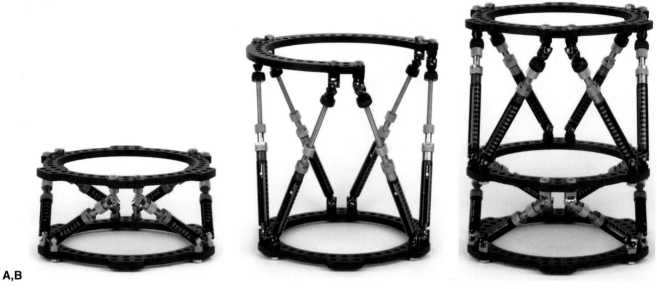

A,B

C

Figure 30.12. A. Shorter struts allow more stable fixation when indicated. Accessory rings could be added to extend level of fixation. **B.** The component system permits custom frames such as this tapered open-section frame for distal femoral application. **C.** Each ring has six tabs and can serve as the intermediate ring for a segmental application. Spatial Frames come preassembled or can be assembled from components. (Copyright © J. Charles Taylor.)

and open-section frames may be applied. Segmental fractures are usually treated with a ring or 2/3 ring for each major fragment (Fig. 30.12).

Steerage Pin

Oblique fracture stability can be improved by using steerage pins on either side of the fracture (1). These pins should be angled 15 to 20 degrees from the transverse plane along the plane of the fracture (Fig. 30.13). These pins will cause dynamic interfragmentary com-

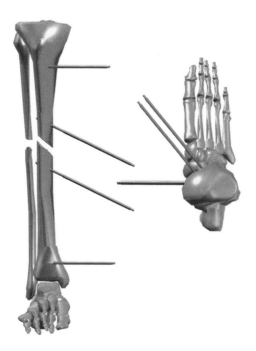

Figure 30.13. Steerage pins are angled 15 to 20 degrees, approximating the major oblique-fracture plane. They are placed on each side of the fracture and are used with other pins and/or wires. Steerage pins increase interfragmentary compression and reduce shear at the fracture site during ambulation. (Copyright © J. Charles Taylor.)

pression with weight bearing and minimize fracture shear. It is still beneficial if only one steerage pin is used.

SURGERY

Positioning

General, spinal, or continuous epidural anesthetics may be used as indicated. The patient is positioned supine on a padded radiolucent table top. The most user-friendly tables contain no metal rails (even peripherally) to interfere with visualization with the image intensifier. The image intensifier should be positioned on the opposite side of the injury. A well-padded tourniquet is placed about the proximal thigh but generally is only used during debridement of open fractures. Even if used for debridement, the tourniquet should be deflated prior to pin and wire insertion. Longitudinal traction through a calcaneal wire may be used to improve overall alignment, but it is rarely used. A few folded towels are used to elevate the leg segments as needed as the frame is applied.

Pin and Wire Technique

Pin and wire location and insertion technique are some of the most important factors for patient tolerance, frame longevity, and minimization of need for additional surgery. Bayonet point wires with cutting relief are the safest for metaphyseal and especially diaphyseal bone (Fig. 30.14). Wires are inserted percutaneously to the near cortex, then slowly drilled across both cortices with frequent pauses to prevent overheating, and tapped through the far soft tissue. The wire is bathed in saline for additional cooling. The surgeon should strive to achieve bicortical purchase with wires and pins to enhance mechanical purchase and decrease thermal necrosis. If burned bone is in the flutes of the predrill for half pins or on the tip of the emerging bayonet tipped wire, do not use that pin or wire. The small incision to insert the drill sleeve or release the skin for the olive is closed with a simple suture.

Frame Application

The Spatial Frame is assembled with two rings and six medium FastFx struts in their unlocked position (see Fig. 30.7). After choosing the approximate level for one ring, the surgeon marks the skin. Then the surgeon marks the skin 18 cm away for the position of the second ring (Fig. 30.15). The surgeon then slides the frame onto the leg (Fig. 30.16). The frame need not be centered longitudinally over the fracture. Make a short longitudinal in-

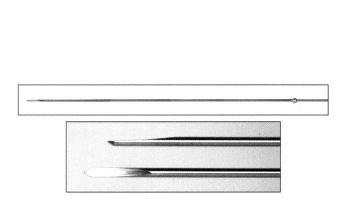

Figure 30.14. Olive wire with close-up of cutting tip. (Copyright © J. Charles Taylor.)

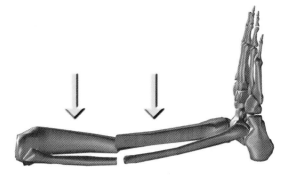

Figure 30.15. Determine the approximate position of one ring, usually on the shorter fragment, and mark the skin. Place a second mark 18 cm from the first for FastFx struts or 15 cm for standard struts. These marks are the approximate positions for the rings. (Copyright © J. Charles Taylor.)

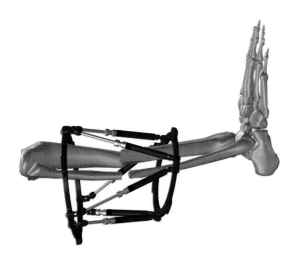

Figure 30.16. The frame is slid over the leg. (Copyright © J. Charles Taylor.)

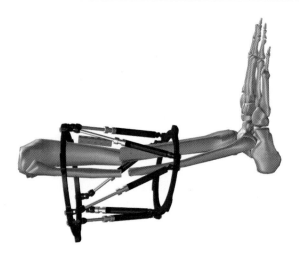

Figure 30.17. Lay a long Rancho Cube along the tibial crest for a sagittal pin. (Copyright © J. Charles Taylor.)

cision for a sagittal-plane half pin. Using a five-hole Rancho Cube as a drill guide (Fig. 30.17), the surgeon drills a pilot hole for the half pin. After inserting the half pin (Fig. 30.18), the surgeon attaches it to an appropriate length Rancho Cube while maintaining the desired soft-tissue clearance (Fig. 30.19). The Rancho Cube is attached to the Spatial Ring via the inner tier of holes at the anterior position (Fig. 30.20) on the master tab, the junction of the no. 1 and no. 2 struts. Using as long a Rancho Cube as possible, the surgeon inserts a half pin in the anterior-medial plane off the proximal face of the proximal ring (Fig. 30.21). Using a Rancho Cube as a drill guide (Fig. 30.22), the surgeon inserts a half pin in the sagittal plane on the proximal portion of the distal fragment (Fig. 30.23). Maintaining 1 to 2 fingerbreadths of soft-tissue clearance, the surgeon then attaches the Rancho Cube to the pin in the distal fragment (Fig. 30.24). The Rancho Cube is attached to the distal ring in the anterior hole (Fig. 30.25).

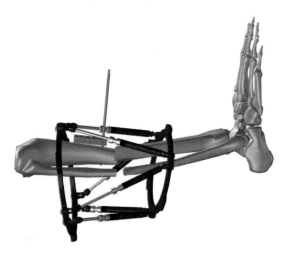

Figure 30.18. Using the Rancho Cube as a drill sleeve guide, the surgeon drills the appropriate pilot hole and inserts a half pin by hand. (Copyright © J. Charles Taylor.)

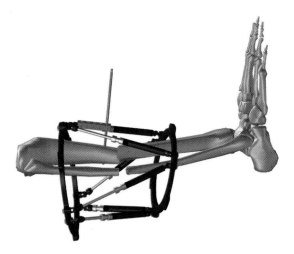

Figure 30.19. The Rancho Cube is slid along the pin to adjust anterior/posterior soft-tissue clearance, and the pin is tightened to the cube with a set screw or short bolt. (Copyright © J. Charles Taylor.)

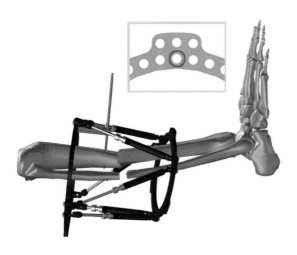

Figure 30.20. The Rancho Cube is attached to the anterior hole of the ring via the inner tier of holes. See inset. (Copyright © J. Charles Taylor.)

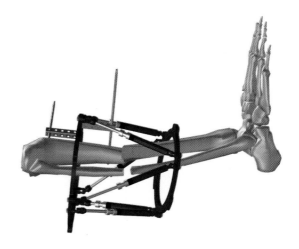

Figure 30.21. With as long a Rancho Cube as possible, a second half pin is inserted in the anterior medial plane. (Copyright © J. Charles Taylor.)

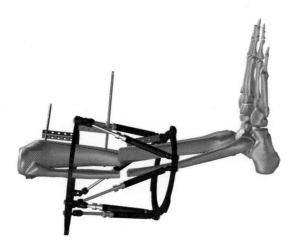

Figure 30.22. A long Rancho Cube is laid along the tibial crest of the second fragment for a sagittal pin. (Copyright © J. Charles Taylor.)

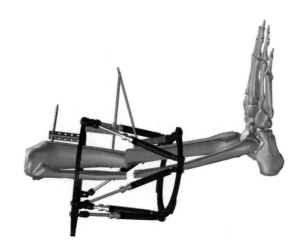

Figure 30.23. Using the Rancho Cube as a drill sleeve guide, the surgeon drills the appropriate pilot hole and inserts a half pin by hand. (Copyright © J. Charles Taylor.)

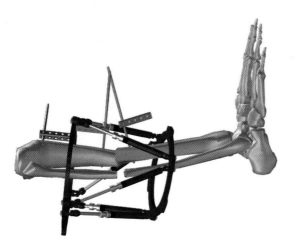

Figure 30.24. The Rancho Cube is slid along the pin to adjust anterior/posterior soft-tissue clearance, and the pin is tightened to the Rancho Cube with a set screw or short bolt. (Copyright © J. Charles Taylor.)

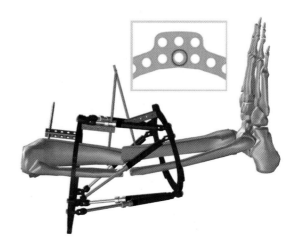

Figure 30.25. The Rancho Cube is attached to the anterior hole of the ring via the inner tier of holes. See inset. (Copyright © J. Charles Taylor.)

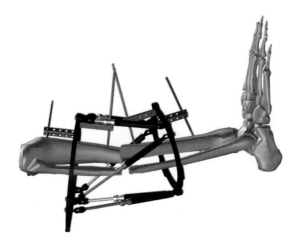

Figure 30.26. With as long a Rancho Cube as possible, a second half pin is inserted in the anterior medial plane. (Copyright © J. Charles Taylor.)

A second half pin is inserted in the distal fragment in the anterior-medial plane through use of as long a half pin as possible (Fig. 30.26). Usually a third half pin is inserted in each fragment in a different plane and attached to their respective rings with a one- or two- hole Rancho Cube (Fig. 30.27). Stability can be increased on longer fragments by extending the spread of fixation with an accessory ring connected to one of the primary rings with threaded rods or posts (see Fig. 30.5).

With all struts unlocked, the distal ring is repositioned with respect to the proximal ring thereby reducing the fracture (Figs. 30.28 and 30.29). While the reduction is maintained, the struts are locked (see Figure 30.3). After a simple suture is placed to close the short in-

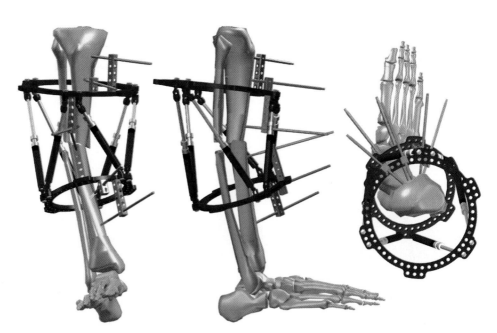

Figure 30.27. Usually a third half pin is inserted in each fragment in an intermediate plane. This third pin is usually attached to the ring with a one- or two-hole Rancho Cube. (Copyright © J. Charles Taylor.)

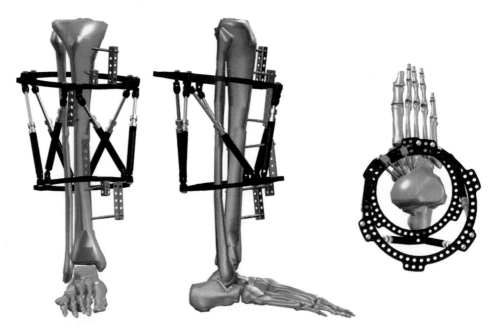

Figure 30.28. With struts unlocked, the frame is manipulated to reduce the fracture. Struts are then locked. (Copyright © J. Charles Taylor.)

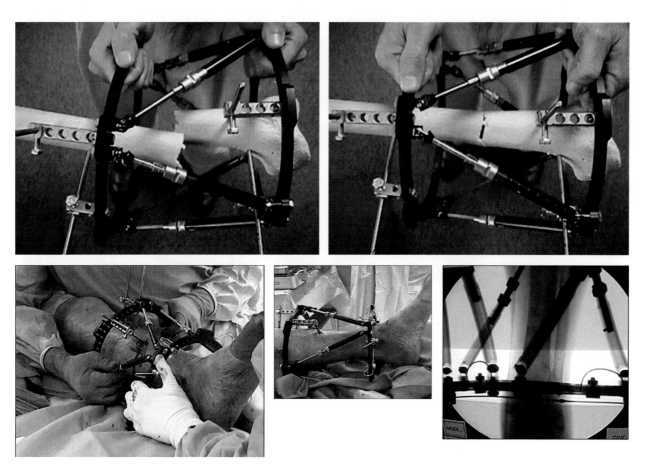

Figure 30.29. After pin and wire fixation of each major fragment, with all struts unlocked, the fracture is reduced under c-arm control or direct vision for open fractures. Each strut is then locked, thereby securing the reduction. (Copyright © J. Charles Taylor.)

cision, each pin or wire entry is covered by a piece of Xeroform or Adaptic dressing and a gauze sponge. The leg is wrapped with a roll gauze dressing. The foot, if not included in the frame, is supported in plantigrade position with a sling or postoperative shoe tied to the Spatial Frame.

Creating Temporary Deformity to Close Soft-Tissue Defects

It may be possible to minimize or eliminate the soft-tissue defect sometimes present in open fractures. After initial stabilization, rather than trying to achieve anatomic reduction, the surgeon can position fragments with a certain amount of shortening and angulation, allowing the muscle and skin to be apposed. This malreduction can be held for weeks if necessary, allowing the soft tissues to heal without tension. The fragments can then be gradually reduced obviating the need for more complex plastic coverage (Fig. 30.30).

Bone Transport for Open Fractures with Segmental Bone Loss

The open fracture with segmental bone loss is a good indication for external fixation, remote osteotomy, and bone transport into the defect. The Spatial Frame allows the transported fragment to be positioned accurately on the docking site without reoperation (Fig. 30.31).

Spatial Frame–Specific Postoperative Management

By fully characterizing postoperative skeletal deformity, recording the proximal and distal ring diameters and the six strut lengths, and measuring the position of the frame on the limb, the surgeon can gradually reduce fractures utilizing the total residual deformity correction method.

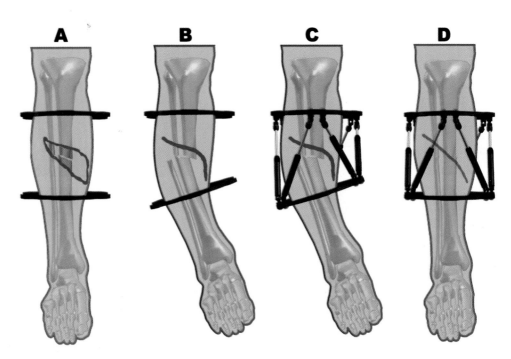

Figure 30.30. A. Open fractures may have a soft-tissue defect if anatomically reduced. **B.** With overriding and angulation, the soft tissue gap might be eliminated or at least significantly reduced. The vascular status must be closely monitored. **C.** Struts are applied in the malreduced position and the soft tissues are allowed to heal over 2 to 4 weeks. **D.** The fracture is gradually reduced. (Copyright © J. Charles Taylor.)

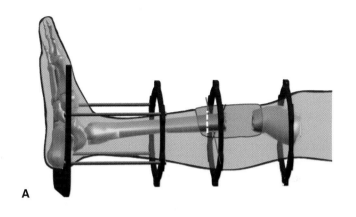
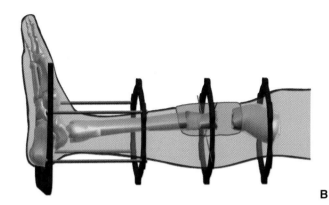

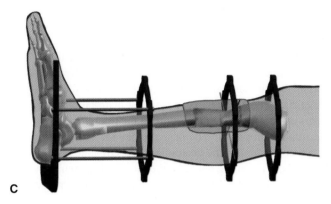

Figure 30.31. The Spatial Frame can be used for bone transport. Usually the Spatial struts are used at the docking site. Regular threaded rods or Spatial struts can be used for the osteotomy site. The foot may be included for additional soft-tissue and boney stability. Antegrade or retrograde transport may be performed. (Copyright © J. Charles Taylor.)

Skeletal deformity is completely characterized by measuring six deformity parameters: the three projected angles (rotations) and three projected translations between major fragments. The frame parameters consist of proximal and distal ring diameters and the strut lengths. Four mounting parameters are measured radiographically and clinically after surgery for acute fractures: AP view, lateral view, axial, and rotary frame offsets.

These parameters are input to a computer program that determines new strut lengths for the Spatial Frame fixator, which will completely correct the skeletal deformity. "Structure at risk" and a "safe velocity" options may be selected to control precisely a gradual reduction.

Choosing a Reference Fragment and the Origin

Orthopedic convention characterizes the deformity of the distal fragment with respect to the proximal fragment. The proximal fragment is the reference fragment; the distal fragment is the moving or deformed fragment.

Deformities can also be measured where the proximal fragment is characterized with respect to a reference distal fragment. This characterization of the deformity by describing abnormal position of the proximal fragment is especially useful in distal fractures with a short distal fragment. The location of the attachment of the distal ring (using the joint surface as a landmark) will be more exactly determined in surgery and postoperative measurement than the level of attachment of the proximal ring on the longer proximal fragment. It also allows the surgeon to fully characterize the deformity even though the radiographs are too short to include the level of attachment of the proximal ring. The distal fragment is the reference fragment; the proximal fragment is the moving fragment.

Either fragment could be the reference fragment. In ideal situations, the reference fragment should satisfy two criteria:

1. The reference fragment should be one with anatomic planes that most closely match the planes of the AP and lateral radiographs.
2. AP and lateral radiographs include the level of attachment of a ring to the reference fragment.

The patella provides a prominent landmark for distal femoral or proximal tibial fractures. The foot provides a prominent landmark for distal tibial fractures. Frequently, the best choice for the reference fragment is the short fragment in conjunction with the prominent landmark. The x-ray technician is more likely to align successfully with the landmark (criterion 1) and if the joint line is included in the radiographs (as it should), then the level of attachment of a ring to that fragment is also included (criterion 2).

The actual deformity is the same whether the physician characterizes the distal fragment with respect to the proximal fragment or alternatively characterizes the proximal fragment with respect to the distal fragment. However, the working measurements of even an oblique, plane, angular deformity will be different depending upon which fragment is chosen as the reference fragment. The final external fixation frames for these different deformity characterizations (based on alternative reference fragments) are identical and will effect the same complete correction. It is important that the same fragment be maintained as reference fragment for AP and lateral radiographs as well as the clinical exam for malrotation.

Translation between fragments is measured from an origin on the reference fragment to its corresponding point on the moving fragment. The best choices for origin and corresponding point are points that are coincident in the anatomic (reduced) state. The tip of a spike on the reference fragment and the matching notch on the moving fragment would be reasonable choices in posttraumatic deformity if these points are easily discerned on AP and lateral radiographs. (Fig. 30.32).

However, the mechanical axis at the fracture site of the reference fragment and the mechanical axis at the fracture site on the moving fragment are the most commonly used choices for origin and corresponding Point (Fig. 30.33). The implied coordinate system on which these translational and rotational measurements are made is the coordinate system of the reference fragment. The AP view translation, lateral view translation, and axial translation are measured along grid lines that can be envisioned to align with the mechanical axes of the reference fragment.

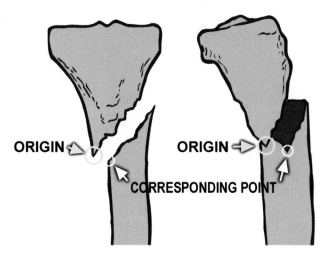

Figure 30.32. A spike and its matching notch, if discernible on AP and lateral films, is one possible choice for the origin and corresponding point, which are used to measure translations at the fracture site. (Copyright © J. Charles Taylor.)

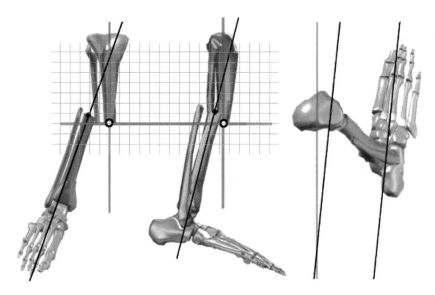

Figure 30.33. Measurements of translation and rotation are made along an imaginary grid aligned to the reference fragment. (Copyright © J. Charles Taylor.)

Frame Parameters

Proximal and Distal Ring Internal Diameters The internal diameter is printed on each ring, partial ring, or foot plate (Fig. 30.34).

Strut Lengths FastFx struts are available in xx-short, x-short, short, medium, and long sizes ranging in functional length from 75 to 284 mm. For any size, the strut has a specific range from its shortest to longest length and a midposition marked on each strut. Struts are marked with millimeter graduations with the actual strut length printed every 10 mm. The achievable strut length overlaps by a few millimeters at each transition from one body to the next (Fig. 30.35). The strut length is read at the indicator (Fig. 30.36).

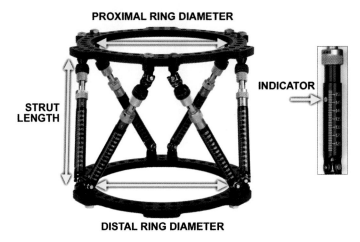

Figure 30.34. The frame parameters, the description of the frame, consist of the internal diameters of the ring that are printed on the rings and the strut lengths that are read at the indicator of each strut. (Copyright © J. Charles Taylor.)

REGULAR STRUTS   **FASTFX™ STRUTS**

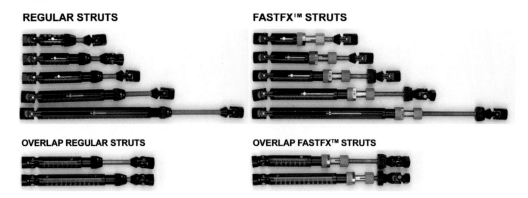

OVERLAP REGULAR STRUTS   **OVERLAP FASTFX™ STRUTS**

Figure 30.35. Struts are available in xx-short, x-short, short, medium, and long bodies. The achievable length of struts overlap by 5 to 10 mm from one body to the next in the series. (Copyright © J. Charles Taylor.)

Deformity Parameters

For a limb segment in anatomic position (Fig. 30.37A), the two fragments adjoin at the origin. With fracture or deformity (see Fig. 30.37B), the two fragments are angulated and translated. The translations are measured as the separation of the adjacent (or corresponding) point from the origin. Translations are measured along the coordinate axes of the reference fragment (actually the reference ring).

Select one fragment as the reference fragment. (Fig. 30.38). Translation is measured between the origin and its corresponding point on AP and lateral views. Axial translation can be measured on either radiograph as the distance between the interior ends of fragments measured along the reference fragment centerline. AP and lateral angulations are measured as the angles between respective centerlines; the axial angle is measured clinically.

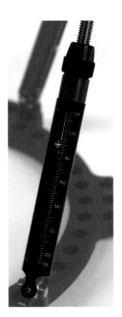

Figure 30.36. Strut length is read directly at the indicator pin. (Copyright © J. Charles Taylor.)

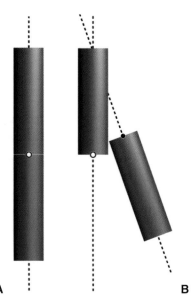

A   B

Figure 30.37. A. When anatomically reduced, the origin and corresponding point are coincident and there is no angulation or rotation between the fragments. **B.** In general, there could be a six axes deformity, consisting of three translations and three angulations, after initial fracture reduction. (Copyright © J. Charles Taylor.)

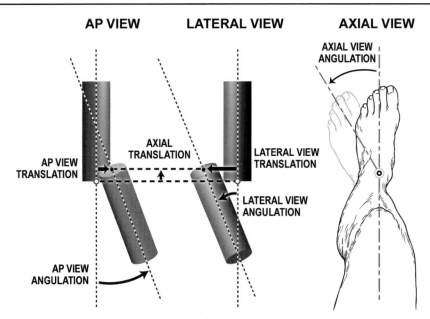

Figure 30.38. Translation (displacement) is the perpendicular distance from the reference fragment to its corresponding point on the moving fragment. To measure translations, the surgeon determines where the corresponding point is with respect to the origin. (If a distal reference is chosen, the AP view and lateral view translations will generally be opposite those of proximal reference.) Note that angulation and rotation are determined based on a view of the deformity from the reference fragment. For example, if a proximal reference is chosen and the AP view along the reference fragment shows a varus deformity, then it is a varus deformity. If a distal reference is chosen and an axial view taken along the axis of the distal fragment (usually in a clinical exam) shows that the distal fragment is internally rotated with respect to the proximal fragment, then it is an internal rotation deformity. (Copyright © J. Charles Taylor.)

Mounting Parameters

There are four mounting parameters that describe the position of the reference ring with respect to the origin: axial frame offset, AP-view frame offset, lateral-view frame offset, which are measured on postoperative films, and rotary frame offset. The latter is generally assessed by clinical inspection.

Axial Frame Offset Axial frame offset is the measurement of length parallel to the frame centerline from the origin to the reference ring (Fig. 30.39). This can generally be measured on AP or lateral films. This measurement in millimeters partially specifies the orientation of the frame with respect to the origin.

AP-View and Lateral-View Frame Offset If the tibia is significantly shifted from center on the AP view, the distance from the origin to the centerline of the rings should be measured. This distance is the AP-view frame offset. (Figs. 30.40A and 30.41). In most tibial mountings with circular fixators, the tibia is located anterior to the geometric center of the ring. The distance from the origin to the centerline of the frame should be measured. This distance in millimeters is the lateral-view frame offset (see Figs. 30.40B and 30.41).

Rotary Frame Offset The preferred (reference) rotational orientation of the Taylor Spatial Frame is with the proximal-ring universal joints (master universal joints) for Strut 1 and Strut 2 located exactly anterior on the proximal fragment (Fig. 30.42). When used for fractures, the frame may be inadvertently malrotated when applied. To correct the malrotation, the surgeon enters the angular position of the sagittal plane of the reference ring with respect to the reference fragment in rotary frame offset (see Figs. 30.7 and 30.43).

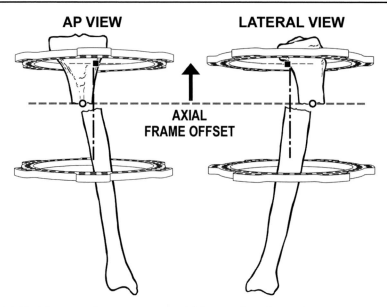

Figure 30.39. The mounting parameter, axial frame offset, is used to measure the axial distance from the origin to the reference ring. (Copyright © J. Charles Taylor.)

Structure at Risk and Rate of Correction

It is incumbent upon the surgeon to be aware of the structures at risk on the concavity of the deformity. When dealing with rotation about the longitudinal axis in addition to conventional angular correction, the risks may be fewer or greater depending on direction of axial rotation. For example, when correcting a flexion-valgus external-rotation deformity of the proximal tibia, the peroneal nerve is at increased risk. However, when correcting a flexion- valgus internal-rotation deformity, the axial rotation will tend to offset the stretch on the peroneal nerve created during the correction of the flexion valgus.

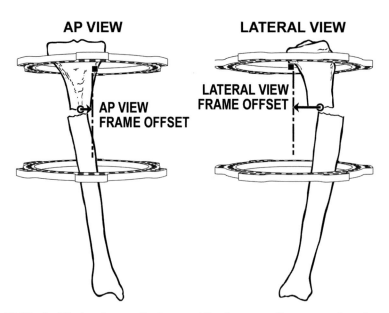

Figure 30.40. A. AP-view frame offset, one of the four mounting parameters, is measured from the origin to the centerline of the frame on AP view. **B.** Lateral-view frame offset, measured from a lateral view, describes the distance from the origin to the centerline of the frame. (Copyright © J. Charles Taylor.)

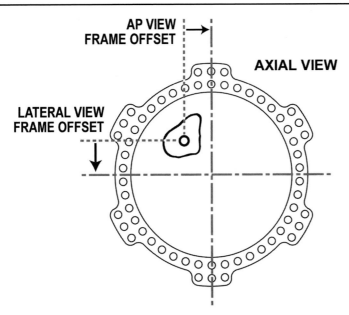

Figure 30.41. The AP- and lateral-view frame offsets describe how the center of the reference ring is positioned in a transverse plane with respect to the origin. (Copyright © J. Charles Taylor.)

The computer program allows the surgeon to input the coordinates of the structure at risk with respect to the origin and set the maximum daily displacement of the structure at risk. The program creates a daily adjustment schedule moving the structure at risk the prescribed amount each day until the deformity is eliminated (fracture is reduced).

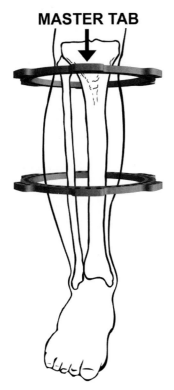

Figure 30.42. The Spatial Frame computer program assumes the master tab is always directly anterior on the proximal ring. (Copyright © J. Charles Taylor.)

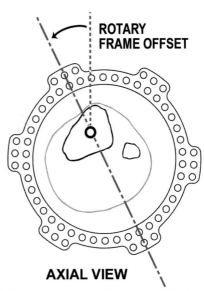

Figure 30.43. Rotary frame offset, one of the four mounting parameters, is measured clinically as rotation of the sagittal plane of the reference ring with respect to the sagittal plane of the reference fragment. (Copyright © J. Charles Taylor.)

A Second Chance for Correction

Because of nonorthogonal initial radiographs, error in measuring radiographs, or excessive preload and bending of wires and pins, there may still be residual skeletal deformity when the struts have reached their target lengths at the completion of a total residual deformity correction. By measuring the radiographs to determine new deformity parameters and making a clinical exam for malrotation, the surgeon can determine new strut lengths to correct the residual deformity through the Total Residual Deformity Correction Program. New mounting parameters can be entered if the original parameters were in error. Alternatively, during any gradual correction a total residual-deformity correction may be undertaken by measuring current parameters and noting current strut settings.

Internet-Based Software for Gradual Reduction of Fractures

A powerful Web-based tool, Total Residual Correction Program, prepares an adjustment schedule to correct any residual skeletal deformity after a Spatial Frame is applied (Fig. 30.44). The surgeon can progress from tab to tab in the program only if sufficient information has been submitted at each step. The program will prompt the surgeon for all necessary information.

Patient and file information, as well as specific case notes, can be saved to a secure, international, Internet server. Saved cases can be reopened and modified, then saved again as a different case or scenario.

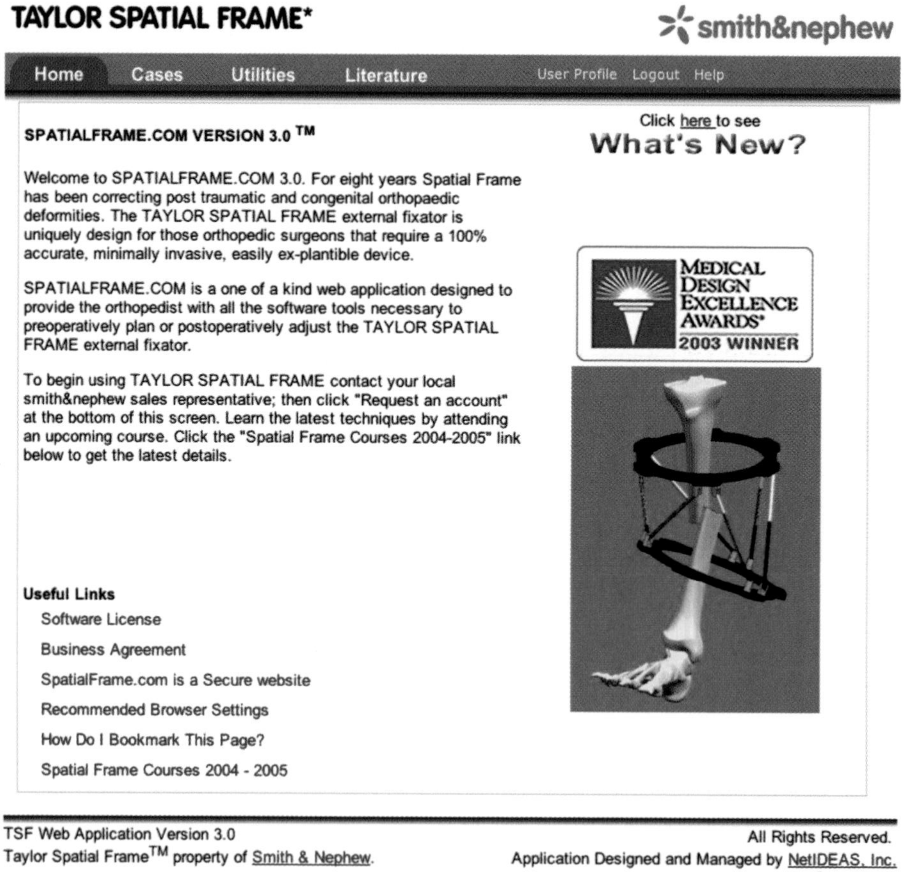

Figure 30.44. *Home Section* for Web-based software used to prepare gradual schedule for deformity correction, including residual skeletal deformity after fracture application. (Copyright © J. Charles Taylor.)

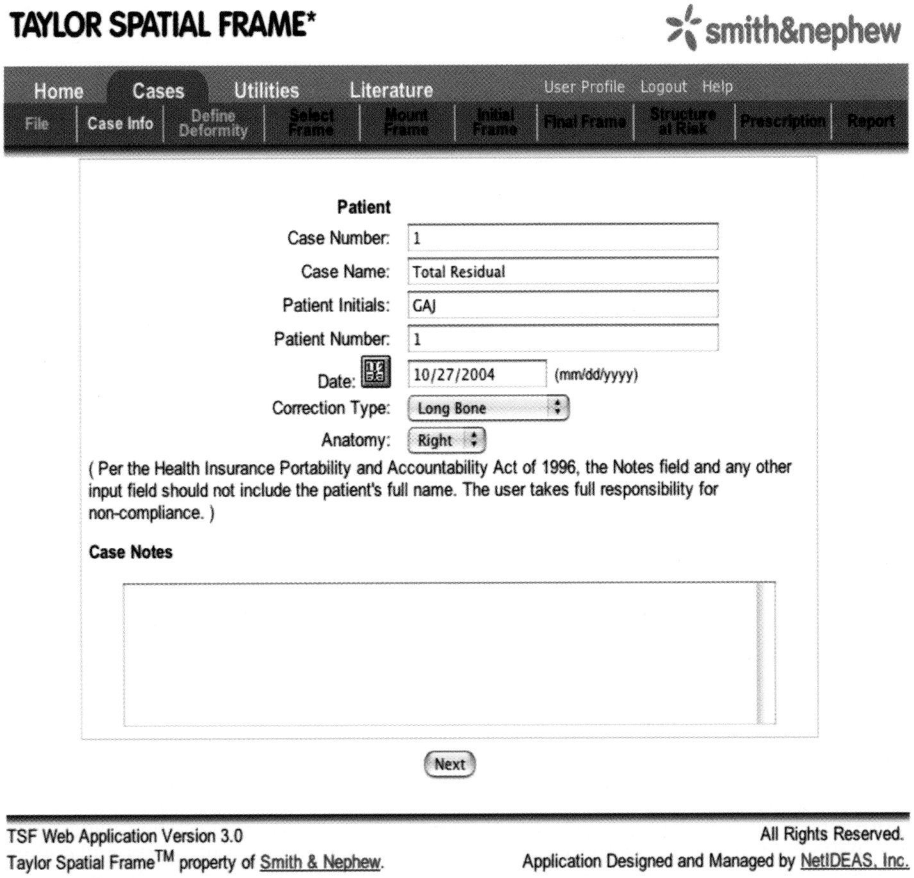

TAYLOR SPATIAL FRAME*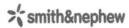

File | Case Info | Define Deformity | Select Frame | Mount Frame | Initial Frame | Final Frame | Structure at Risk | Prescription | Report

Patient

Case Number: 1

Case Name: Total Residual

Patient Initials: GAJ

Patient Number: 1

Date: 10/27/2004 (mm/dd/yyyy)

Correction Type: Long Bone

Anatomy: Right

(Per the Health Insurance Portability and Accountability Act of 1996, the Notes field and any other input field should not include the patient's full name. The user takes full responsibility for non-compliance.)

Case Notes

Next

Figure 30.45. *Cases Section, Case Info* must include at least "Long Bone" as the *Correction Type* and "Right" or "Left" as *Anatomy*. (Copyright © J. Charles Taylor.)

To begin, the surgeon enters patient information and the side ("Left" or "Right"). For tibial fractures, he/she selects "Long Bone" as the *Correction Type* (Fig. 30.45). *Case Name* will appear as the default title of the case when the case is finally saved.

In the next window (Fig. 30.46), the surgeon selects the proximal or distal reference fragment and inputs the six skeletal-deformity parameters. When *Regenerate Views* is then selected, the software provides the surgeon with updated AP, lateral, and axial views of the skeletal deformity. The pointed end of the blue rod is the origin and the pointed end of the green rod is the corresponding point. Using the pull-down menu in the next window, the surgeon selects the "Proximal Ring Diameter," "Distal Ring Diameter," and "Strut Body Type" (Fig. 30.47).

Next, the surgeon selects the *Operative Mode*, which for fractures, usually corresponds with the "Total Residual" button (Fig. 30.48). The position of the reference ring with respect to the origin is input into the *Mounting Parameters*. The regenerated views confirm the relation of the reference ring on the reference fragment.

Each of the six strut lengths is entered in the next window (Fig. 30.49). The computer then provides a graphical representation of the initial crooked frame on crooked bone.

In the *Final Frame* window, the computer solves for the necessary strut lengths to correct the skeletal deformity and presents it graphically (Fig. 30.50).

In the next window, the coordinates of the *Structure at Risk* and the *Maximum Safe Velocity* are entered (Fig. 30.51). The computer determines the number of days required for the correction. The surgeon may also override the number of days.

In the report window (Fig. 30.52), surgeon and patient information is reiterated. The mounting parameters, initial and final strut settings, the coordinates of the structure at risk, as well as the safe velocity are shown in table form. The daily adjustment schedule is also

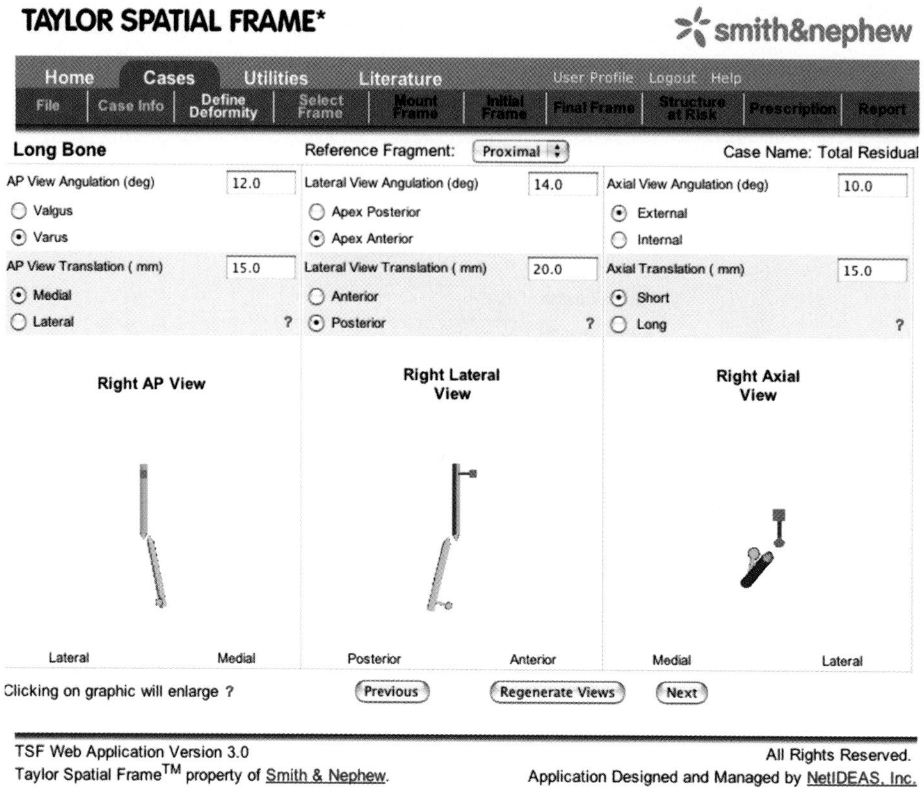

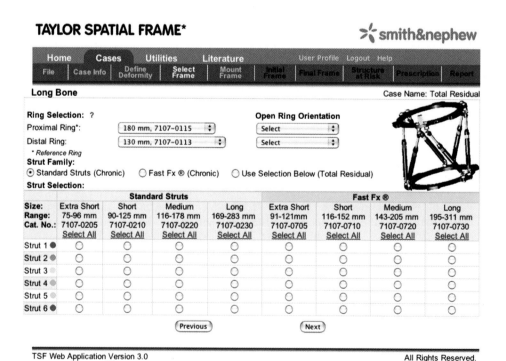

Figure 30.46. *Define Deformity* provides for the selection of the *Reference Fragment* and input of the deformity parameters. After deformity parameters are input, a schematic representation of the deformity appears after the "Regenerate Views" button is selected. (Copyright © J. Charles Taylor.)

Figure 30.47. *Select Frame* identifies the diameter of the rings used as well as the location of the open section of the ring for 2/3 rings and foot plates. Also, the type of strut and body size are input for each of the six struts. (Copyright © J. Charles Taylor.)

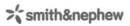

Home | Cases | Utilities | Literature | User Profile | Logout | Help

File | Case Info | Define Deformity | Select Frame | Mount Frame | Initial Frame | Final Frame | Structure at Risk | Prescription | Report

Long Bone   Case Name: Total Residual

Operative Mode ?

⊙ Total Residual   ○ Chronic   ○ Residual

Mounting Parameters

| AP View Frame Offset (mm) | 10.0 | Lateral View Frame Offset (mm) | 15.0 | Axial Frame Offset (mm) | 40.0 |

○ Medial to Origin   ○ Anterior to Origin   ⊙ Proximal to Origin

⊙ Lateral to Origin   ⊙ Posterior to Origin   ○ Distal to Origin

Rotary Frame Angle (deg) [   ]

○ Frame Externally Rotated

○ Frame Internally Rotated   ?

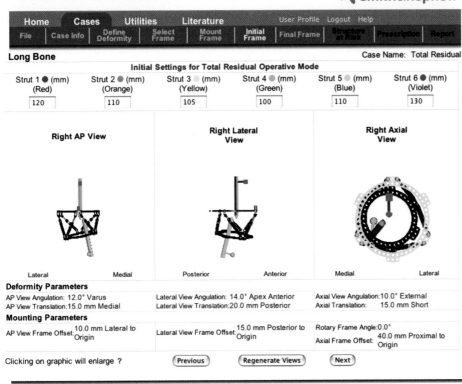

Right AP View   **Right Lateral View**   **Right Axial View**

Lateral   Medial   Posterior   Anterior   Medial   Lateral

Clicking on graphic will enlarge ?   (Previous)   (Regenerate Views)   (Next)

Figure 30.48. *Mount Frame* is used to select the operative mode being utilized, which is almost always the "Total Residual" for fractures. Also, the mounting parameters are input in this section. (Copyright © J. Charles Taylor.)

Home | Cases | Utilities | Literature | User Profile | Logout | Help

File | Case Info | Define Deformity | Select Frame | Mount Frame | Initial Frame | Final Frame | Structure at Risk | Prescription | Report

Long Bone   Case Name: Total Residual

Initial Settings for Total Residual Operative Mode

Strut 1 ● (mm) (Red)	Strut 2 ● (mm) (Orange)	Strut 3 ○ (mm) (Yellow)	Strut 4 ● (mm) (Green)	Strut 5 ○ (mm) (Blue)	Strut 6 ● (mm) (Violet)
120	110	105	100	110	130

Right AP View   **Right Lateral View**   **Right Axial View**

Lateral   Medial   Posterior   Anterior   Medial   Lateral

Deformity Parameters

AP View Angulation: 12.0° Varus | Lateral View Angulation: 14.0° Apex Anterior | Axial View Angulation:10.0° External
AP View Translation:15.0 mm Medial | Lateral View Translation:20.0 mm Posterior | Axial Translation: 15.0 mm Short

Mounting Parameters

AP View Frame Offset: 10.0 mm Lateral to Origin | Lateral View Frame Offset: 15.0 mm Posterior to Origin | Rotary Frame Angle:0.0°
Axial Frame Offset: 40.0 mm Proximal to Origin

Clicking on graphic will enlarge ?   (Previous)   (Regenerate Views)   (Next)

Figure 30.49. *Initial Frame* for fractures is used to input each of the six strut lengths after the acute fracture reduction. (Copyright © J. Charles Taylor.)

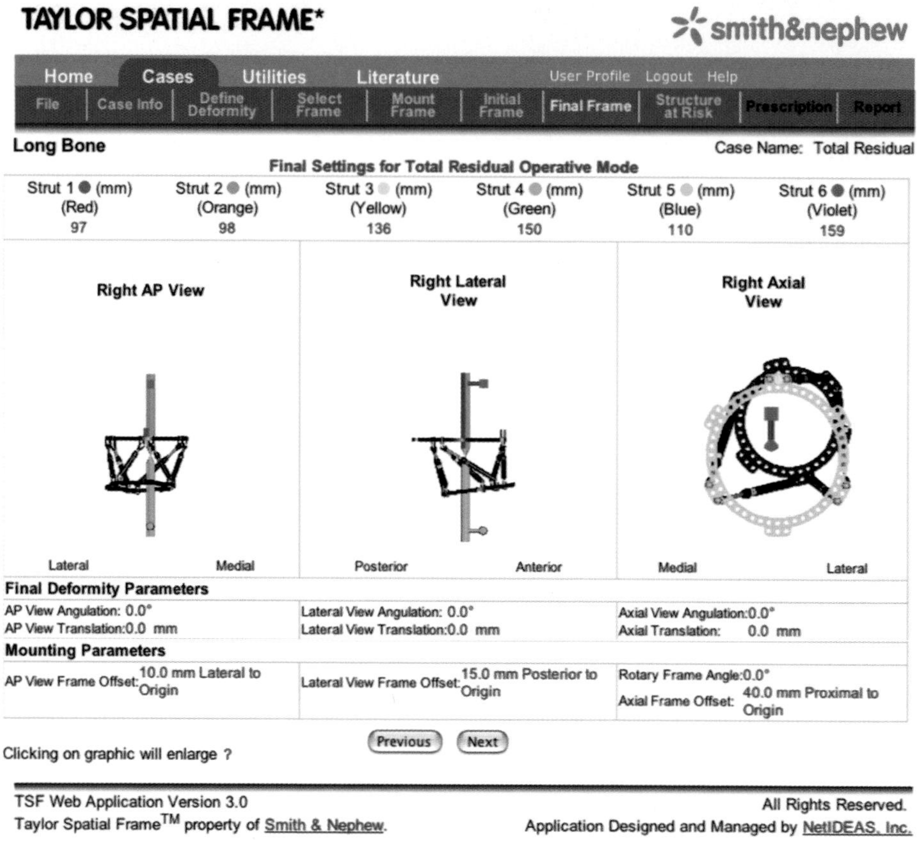

TAYLOR SPATIAL FRAME*   ✳ smith&nephew

Home	Cases	Utilities	Literature	User Profile	Logout	Help		
File	Case Info	Define Deformity	Select Frame	Mount Frame	Initial Frame	Final Frame	Structure at Risk	**Prescription**	**Report**

Long Bone   Case Name: Total Residual

Final Settings for Total Residual Operative Mode

Strut 1 ● (mm) (Red) 97	Strut 2 ● (mm) (Orange) 98	Strut 3 ○ (mm) (Yellow) 136	Strut 4 ● (mm) (Green) 150	Strut 5 ○ (mm) (Blue) 110	Strut 6 ● (mm) (Violet) 159

Right AP View   Right Lateral View   Right Axial View

Lateral   Medial   Posterior   Anterior   Medial   Lateral

Final Deformity Parameters

AP View Angulation: 0.0° AP View Translation:0.0 mm	Lateral View Angulation: 0.0° Lateral View Translation:0.0 mm	Axial View Angulation:0.0° Axial Translation: 0.0 mm

Mounting Parameters

AP View Frame Offset:10.0 mm Lateral to Origin	Lateral View Frame Offset:15.0 mm Posterior to Origin	Rotary Frame Angle:0.0° Axial Frame Offset: 40.0 mm Proximal to Origin

Clicking on graphic will enlarge ?   (Previous) (Next)

Figure 30.50. *Final Frame* is an output area for the six new strut lengths that will correct the residual skeletal deformity. Also, a graphic of the corrected frame appears. (Copyright © J. Charles Taylor.)

TAYLOR SPATIAL FRAME*   ✳ smith&nephew

Home	Cases	Utilities	Literature	User Profile	Logout	Help		
File	Case Info	Define Deformity	Select Frame	Mount Frame	Initial Frame	Final Frame	**Structure at Risk**	Prescription	**Report**

Long Bone   Case Name: Total Residual

AP View SAR Offset (mm)   0.0   Lateral View SAR Offset (mm)   0.0

○ Medial to Origin   ○ Anterior to Origin
◉ Lateral to Origin   ◉ Posterior to Origin

Axial SAR Offset (mm)   0.0   Max Safe Distraction Rate (mm/day)   2

○ Proximal to Origin
○ Distal to Origin

Minimum Correction Time (days): ____   (Calculate Minimum Correction Time)

Enter Correction Time (days): 15

(Previous) (Next)

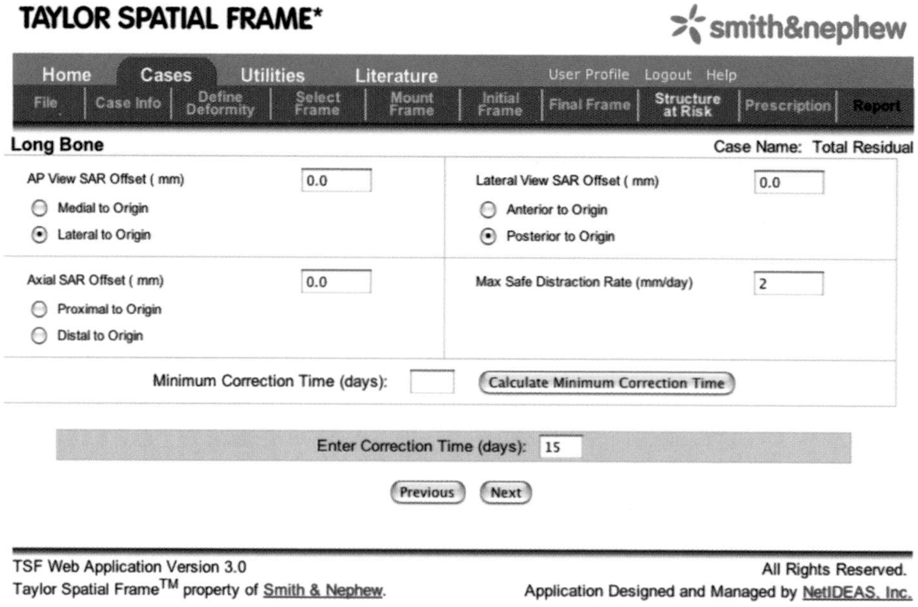

Figure 30.51. *Structure at Risk* is used to input the location of the structure on the concavity of the deformity that is to be protected by controlling the rate of correction. Also, the *Max Safe Distraction Rate* can be selected. Alternatively the *Correction Time* may be arbitrarily set. (Copyright © J. Charles Taylor.)

TAYLOR SPATIAL FRAME*

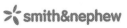 smith&nephew

🖶 Open a printable version of this page in a new window

Dr. J. Charles Taylor , Office Phone: Date: 10/27/2004
Patient Initials: GAJ , Case Name: Total Residual , Case Number: 1
Correction Type : Long Bone

Deformity Parameters

AP View Angulation: 12.0° Varus   Lateral View Angulation: 14.0° Apex Anterior   Axial View Angulation:10.0° External
AP View Translation:15.0 mm Medial   Lateral View Translation:20.0 mm Posterior   Axial Translation: 15.0 mm Short

Anatomy: Right   **Operative Mode:** Total Residual

Frame Parameters

Proximal Ring:180mm Ring (7107-0115)   Reference:Proximal
Distal Ring: 130mm Ring (7107-0113)
Strut 1: Short Strut (7107-0210)   Strut 4: Short Strut (7107-0210)
Strut 2: Short Strut (7107-0210)   Strut 5: Short Strut (7107-0210)
Strut 3: Short Strut (7107-0210)   Strut 6: Medium Strut (7107-0220)

Mounting Parameters

AP View Frame Offset: 10.0 mm Lateral to Origin   Lateral View Frame Offset: 15.0 mm Posterior to Origin   Rotary Frame Angle:0.0°
                                                                                         Axial Frame Offset: 40.0 mm Proximal to Origin

Initial Strut Settings

Strut 1 (Red)	Strut 2 (Orange)	Strut 3 (Yellow)	Strut 4 (Green)	Strut 5 (Blue)	Strut 6 (Violet)
120	110	105	100	110	130

Final Strut Settings

Strut 1 (Red)	Strut 2 (Orange)	Strut 3 (Yellow)	Strut 4 (Green)	Strut 5 (Blue)	Strut 6 (Violet)
97	98	136	150	110	159

Structure at Risk

AP View SAR Offset: 0.0 mm   Lateral View SAR Offset: 0.0 mm
Axial SAR Offset: 0.0 mm   Max Safe Distraction Rate (mm/day) :2.0
Correction Time (days):15

Prescription

Date	Day	Strut 1 (Red)	Strut 2 (Orange)	Strut 3 (Yellow)	Strut 4 (Green)	Strut 5 (Blue)	Strut 6 (Violet)	View
10/27/04	0	120	110	105	100	110	130	View
10/28/04	1	118	109	107	103	110	132	View
10/29/04	2	117	108	109	107	110	134	View
10/30/04	3	115	108	111	110	110	136	View
10/31/04	4	114	107	113	113	110	138	View
11/1/04	5	112	106	115	117 [a]	110	140	View
11/2/04	6	111	105	117 [b]	120 [a]	110	142	View
11/3/04	7	109	104	119 [b]	123 [a]	110	144	View
11/4/04	8	108	104	122 [b]	127	110	145	View
11/5/04	9	106	103	124 [b]	130	110	147	View
11/6/04	10	105	102	126	133	110	149	View
11/7/04	11	103	101	128	137	110	151	View
11/8/04	12	102	100	130	140	110	153	View
11/9/04	13	100	100	132	143	110	155	View
11/10/04	14	99	99	134	147	110	157	View
11/11/04	15	97	98	136	150	110	159	View

Strut Change-Outs

Change-Out	Strut	Overlap Interval First Day	Overlap Interval Last Day	Strut Change From	Strut Change To
a	4 (Green)	5 (11/1/04)	7 (11/3/04)	7107-0210 Short Standard	7107-0220 Medium Standard
b	3 (Yellow)	6 (11/2/04)	9 (11/5/04)	7107-0210 Short Standard	7107-0220 Medium Standard

Parts List

Part	Quantity
180mm Ring (7107-0115)	1
130mm Ring (7107-0113)	1
Standard Identification Band Kit (7107-0320)	1
Short Strut (7107-0210)	5
Medium Strut (7107-0220)	3

Case Notes

(Previous)

Figure 30.52. *Report* reiterates all surgeon inputs, and it outputs a frame adjustment *Prescription,* a *Strut Change-out Schedule,* and a *Parts List.* (Copyright © J. Charles Taylor.)

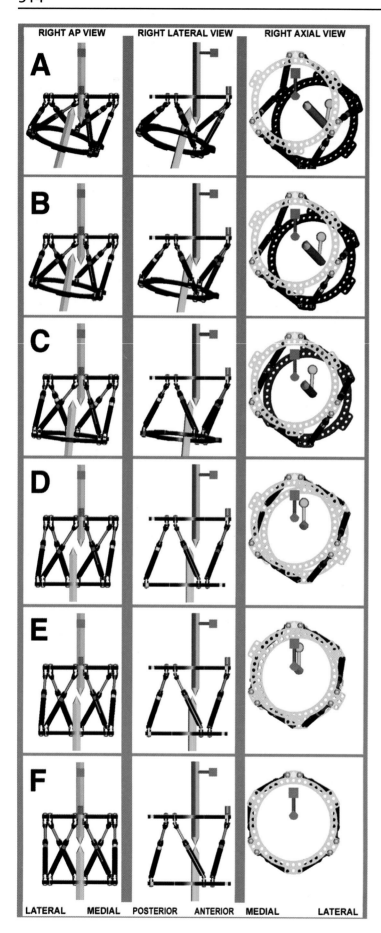

RIGHT AP VIEW   **RIGHT LATERAL VIEW**   **RIGHT AXIAL VIEW**

A

B

C

D

E

F

LATERAL   MEDIAL   POSTERIOR   ANTERIOR   MEDIAL   LATERAL

Figure 30.53. **A–D.** A *Waypoint Reduction*, though rarely needed, may be performed by inputting the deformity parameters in two separate steps. A first *Total Residual Correction* is run with "AP View Angulation," "Lateral View Angulation," "Rotation," and "Length" as the deformity parameters to get the fragments to the way point position. **D–F.** Next, a second *Total Residual Correction* is run with "AP View Translation" and "Lateral View Translation" as the deformity parameters to get the fragments to anatomic position. (Copyright © J. Charles Taylor.)

provided. Critical days when struts need to be exchanged are highlighted, color coded, and identified with a letter. The strut exchanges are listed and explained in chronological order, and a list of necessary Spatial Frame parts is also given.

The Total Residual Correction Program can be used to prepare a daily schedule to reduce a fracture that is significantly overlapped by using a *Waypoint*. In the case shown in Figure 30.53, angulation, rotation, and length are corrected in the first step (see Fig. 30.53 rows A, B, C, and D), and translation is corrected in a second step (see Fig. 30.53 rows D, E, and F). In the first step, only the deformity parameters pertaining to angulation, rotation, and length are input to achieve the corresponding strut lengths to get to the *Waypoint*. Next, to take the fragments from the waypoint to anatomic position, AP- and lateral-view translation are entered as the only deformity parameters.

GENERAL POSTOPERATIVE MANAGEMENT

Patients are allowed to practice partial weight bearing when their general condition allows. Cleaning of the pin-skin interface is usually commenced 5 to 7 days postoperatively, often in the outpatient clinic. If good AP and lateral radiographs were not obtained in the hospital, they are taken at this first postoperative visit. These initial radiographs need to be wide enough to include the full diameter of the ring so that mounting parameters can be accurately measured. The patient is seen at 1 to 2 week intervals, especially while the frame is being gradually adjusted. Adjustments are usually performed over 1 to 2 weeks for fracture reductions. As many adjustments as necessary can be performed. Usually one or two adjustment schedules are run for fractures.

PO antibiotics are used as needed during treatment. Fracture healing time averages 18 weeks and ranges from 7 to 24 weeks depending on a number of factors. Wires that suddenly become painful may have lost tension and should be retensioned in the office.

As the fracture heals, the patient will increase weight bearing on the injured leg. Patients usually will go to a single crutch by 8 to 10 weeks and fully weight bearing by 12 weeks. When the patient is fully weight bearing and if radiographs show that the fracture appears healed, one or two struts are removed in the office and the patient walks around the office for 30 minutes. If the patient experiences no pain, he or she walks at home for a week with only four struts in place. If subsequent radiographs show no change in position of the fragments, the fracture still appears healed, and the patient reports no increase in pain, the frame is removed. Most frames are removed in the office with local anesthetic. More complex frames are removed in surgery under general anesthetic or IV sedation. A prefabricated short-leg walking brace is used for a few weeks in most cases.

COMPLICATIONS

Most complications are avoided by applying a mechanically stable frame with pins and wires cautiously inserted. The surgeon should be vigilant and perform Total residual deformity corrections of any skeletal deformity remaining after initial operative reduction. Precautions should be taken to prevent equinus contracture, including, sometimes, foot fixation. Patients should strive for to be fully weight bearing.

An arterial Doppler is used preoperatively and postoperatively to assess the arterial supply to the foot. An acute arterial injury in surgery might be picked up by an absent pulse or continued bleeding from a pin or wire site. Late bleeding from a pin or wire is usually from arterial erosion and often requires emergent surgical treatment.

Plantigrade position of the foot should be sought aggressively. If the patient is able to actively extend the ankle above neutral, a padded night splint or sling may be used to prevent equinus contracture. If the patient is unable to actively dorsiflex the ankle to neutral because of swelling or pain, then the foot should be placed in a sling or post operative shoe with straps to the Spatial Frame. Alternatively, a Dynasplint may be used to prevent progression of the equinus and to bring the foot to neutral slowly as swelling and pain subside postoperatively. As stated earlier, patients with fractures that are distal, open, with associated peroneal nerve injury, or those found in conjunction with closed head injury or compartment syndrome are at greater risk for developing a contracture and probably should have the foot included in the frame even though fracture stability is satisfactory with only the tibial fragments fixed. Frequent periods of at least partial weight bearing are beneficial to fracture healing and the prevention of contracture.

Some equinus contractures existing at time of fracture healing, especially if multiple transfixion wires were used, will resolve with weight bearing and physical therapy. Persistent contracture can be treated with application of a spanning Spatial Frame across the ankle, gradual correction of the equinus, and 4 to 5 mm of distraction across the ankle.

Persistent symptomatic contractures can be addressed with the Spatial Frame still on the tibial shaft fracture by applying a foot plate and connecting it to the most distal tibial ring with Ilizarov hinges placed along the ankle axis, or if space permits, applying Spatial Frame struts between the distal tibial plate and the foot plate and performing a deformity correction.

Pin or wire skin interfaces should be cleaned daily with antibacterial soap and water beginning at approximately day 5 if soft-tissue wounds allow. A light-pressure gauze sleeve about wires emerging through muscles will decrease soft-tissue motion along the pin. Antibiotics by mouth are frequently but not always needed in the 4.5 months average healing time of adult fractures treated with external fixation. A wire that suddenly becomes painful is usually loose and can be retensioned in the office, usually with immediate relief of pain. Pins or wires that develop redness or drainage are treated by initiating PO antibiotics, increasing dose, or (rarely) IV antibiotics. Pin or wire sites that do not respond should be treated with pin removal, curettage if sequestrum is suspected, and additional pin insertion if the removed pin was mechanically essential.

A spectrum of callus patterns is seen with external fixation from healing that looks like primary bone to that with a more fusiform appearance. In several series the average time to healing for adult tibial fractures treated with primary external fixation is approximately 4.5 months. Varus/valgus or flexion/extension stress views with the struts removed, or a CT scan can be performed to assess healing. If fragments are well reduced and there are no signs of healing at 3 months, an autogenous bone graft should be considered. Also, the mechanical stability of the construct should be questioned. The frame may need to be revised by adding pins, wires, or even an accessory ring to extend the level of fixation.

Failure of the method is uncommon. Each case should be closely analyzed to determine a best course for subsequent treatment. Treatment options include cast or brace, repeat external fixation, intramedullary nail, or plate fixation with or without autogenous bone grafting.

RESULTS

Results with Spatial Frame compare favorably to the results with other external fixation, intramedullary nails, and plating of tibial fractures. During its development, the Spatial system was thoroughly tested for theoretical accuracy of the computer program, combined mechanical accuracy in correcting severe six-axis deformities, and frame stiffness. The computer program is mathematically accurate to within $1/10^6$ of an inch and a $1/10^4$ of a degree. The combined mechanical accuracy of the program, as applied to the frame by hand, is 1 mm translation and 0.6-degree angulation. The Spatial Frame is as stiff as the Ilizarov in axial loading and twice as stiff in bending and torsion.

The Spatial Frame has been used since approximately 1996. Although initially reported for fractures and deformity correction (2), its early acceptance was for deformity correction and nonunions (3–8) and has gradually gained acceptance for primary treatment of fractures (5,9–14). Historically, malunion was the leading complication of external fixation, which reflects the difficulty in making adjustments to other frames after the initial surgery and the reluctance to return to surgery. Not only does repeat surgery pose a risk to the patient, but an effort to improve one aspect of fracture reduction another could result in a complication for another aspect of it.

The ability to make prescribed gradual adjustments to the Spatial Frame in the postoperative period is the greatest strength of the system. The program provides a daily adjustment schedule for the struts, which are easy to adjust using the direct read indicator for each strut. McFadyen and Atkins (10) demonstrated a 100% compliance of their patients adjusting the frame as prescribed. Near anatomic realignment and repositioning of the externally fixed, major fragments has been routinely achieved. Binski and Hutchinson (9), McFadyen and Atkins (10) as well as Whately (14) report a 95 to 100% rate of anatomic or near anatomic restoration of alignment and position. Likewise, these same authors report a 96 to 100% rate of primary union and remarkably low rates of reoperation (approximately 5%) for delayed union.

RECOMMENDED READINGS

1. Taylor JC. Dynamic interfragmentary compression in oblique fractures stabilized with half pin external fixation: the steerage pin. Poster presented at: Annual Meeting of the American Academy of Orthopaedic Surgeons. New Orleans, LA; February 1994.
2. Taylor JC. Complete characterization of a 6-axes deformity; complete correction with a new external fixator, "The Spatial Frame." Presented at: The Annual Meeting of Association for the Study and Application of the Method of Ilizarov; North America 1997.
3. Rozbruch SR, Helfet DL, Blyakher A. Distraction of hypertrophic nonunion of tibia with deformity using Ilizarov/ Taylor Spatial Frame. *Arch Orthop Trauma Surg* 2002;122:295–298.
4. Taylor JC. The Taylor Spatial Frame. Presented at: The Annual Meeting of Association for the Study and Application of the Method of Ilizarov; New Orleans, LA; 1998.
5. Taylor JC. The Rings First Method for Fractures and Deformity Correction. Presented at: The Annual Meeting of Association for the Study and Application of the Method of Ilizarov; North America; 1999.
6. Taylor JC. The Spatial Frame as a reconstructive hinge: theoretical and practical considerations. Presented at the Annual Meeting of Association for the Study and Application of the Method of Ilizarov; North America; 2000.
7. Taylor JC. 6, 6 + 6, and 6 × 6 correction of ankle and foot deformities with the spatial frame. Presented at: The Annual Meeting of Association for the Study and Application of the Method of Ilizarov; North America; 2003.
8. Taylor JC. Reconciliation of CORA and Origin/Corresponding Point Methods of Deformity Characterization. Presented at: The Annual Meeting of Association for the Study and Application of the Method of Ilizarov; North America; 2004; Toronto, Ontario, Canada.
9. Binski JA, Hutchinson B. Treatment of tibial shaft fractures with the Taylor Spatial Frame. Paper presented at: The International Society for Fracture Repair; Novermber 2–6, 2004; Bologna, Italy.
10. McFadyen I, Atkins R. The Taylor Spatial Frame in limb reconstruction; review of 100 cases. Presented at: The British Orthopaedic Association Annual Congress. September 15–17, 2004; Manchester, England.
11. Taylor JC. The last malunion with primary external fixation of fractures: the power of residual deformity correction with the Spatial Frame. Presented at: The Annual Meeting of Association for the Study and Application of the Method of Ilizarov North America; 2000.
12. Taylor JC. Skew parameters and the total residual deformity correction: a geometric method. Presented at: The Annual Meeting of Association for the Study and Application of the Method of Ilizarov; North America; 2001.
13. Taylor JC. Complete correction of residual deformity following chronic deformity correction or fracture external fixation: the total residual deformity correction. Presented at: The Annual Meeting of Association for the Study and Application of the Method of Ilizarov; North America; 2002.
14. Whately C. The Taylor Spatial Frame for acute tibial fractures. Presented at: the Annual Meeting of As sociation for the Study and Application of the Method of Ilizarov; North America; 2004; Toronto, Ontario, Canada.

31

Tibial Pilon Fractures: Open Reduction Internal Fixation

Joseph Borrelli, Jr.

INDICATIONS/CONTRAINDICATIONS

Intra-articular fractures of the distal tibial articular surface (pilon fractures) represent approximately 1% of all fractures, and approximately 3% to 9% of all tibia fractures (1). Generally, two types of tibial pilon fractures have been recognized. Rotational type fractures usually arise from a relatively low-energy, rotational force, similar to that which may occur during recreational skiing. These fractures typically are spiral in nature and are generally associated with little articular comminution and limited surrounding soft-tissue injury. The more problematic type of pilon fracture is the high-energy, axial compression-type fracture. These fractures typically occur in high-energy motor-vehicle crashes, falls from a considerable height, and crush injuries like those incurred in industrial accidents. This fracture is commonly associated with articular and metaphyseal comminution and significant soft-tissue injury (2). In either case, the fibula may or may not be fractured. It is important that the treating physician recognize the difference between these two fractures types, for although the indications for operative treatment are the same, the timing for definitive treatment, the patient's prognosis, and the outcome, will differ.

Surgical indications for tibial pilon fractures include the following: (a) articular fracture displacement of ≥2 mm, (b) unstable fractures of the tibial metaphysis, and (c) open pilon fractures. Contraindications to formal open reduction and internal fixation (ORIF) include severe soft- tissue injury where blistering and skin necrosis or persistent swelling precludes safe surgical intervention, and severe articular comminution, which would make satisfactory articular reduction and stabilization extremely difficult or impossible. Relative contraindications to formal ORIF include infirmity of the patient; advanced patient age and osteopenia; prior local surgery or previous soft-tissue transfers; advanced, peripheral, vascular disease (associated with a history of smoking, and/or diabetes); and other comorbidities that would make surgical intervention too risky. Also, patients who would be unable or unwilling to cooperate in postoperative weight bearing restrictions (i.e., those with generalized weakness, dementia, or neurologic deficit) are also felt to have relative contraindications for surgery.

PREOPERATIVE PLANNING

Preoperative planning is essential for a successful outcome following treatment of a pilon fracture. Thorough preoperative planning is dependent upon the surgeon developing a complete understanding of the fracture pattern, surgical approaches, blood supply to the fracture fragments, and awareness of the availability, applicability, and limitations of the various surgical implants. A thorough history and physical examination of the patient and the limb is essential. Particular attention is paid to the condition of the soft tissues in the lower leg and ankle. A detailed neurovascular exam and evaluation of the compartments of the leg must be documented. Fracture blisters are common and may influence the timing and method of treatment.

To gain a complete understanding of the fracture pattern, a detailed study of the radiographic images is necessary. Routine radiographic assessment of pilon fractures includes anteroposterior (AP), mortise, and lateral views of the ankle (Fig. 31.1). In case of fracture displacement or shortening, traction radiographs may be extremely helpful. These are often obtained following application of a spanning external fixator. Axial computed tomography (CT) scans are necessary for understanding the fracture pattern in general and the articular injury in particular. The CT scan of the distal tibia and ankle is most helpful when performed after a preliminary reduction and application of the spanning external fixator. Axial, sagittal, and coronal reconstructions of the CT scans are recommended (Fig. 31.2). Plain radiographs of the contralateral ankle can be helpful for preoperative planning as they serve as a template for the fractured side.

The preoperative plan should include a thorough step-by-step description of how the surgery is to be carried out and a diagram of the fractured distal tibia and of the desired final fixation construct. In general, the plan begins with patient positioning, site(s) to be prepared for surgery, a description of the approach(es) to be used, the steps necessary to restore articular congruity, and the restoration of length, alignment, and rotation of the limb. It also includes the creation of a stable fixation construct that will allow early mobilization of the patient and the ankle.

SURGERY

Surgery is performed under general or spinal anesthesia. A first-generation cephalosporin is administered and continued for 24 to 48 hours postoperatively. The use of a tourniquet is

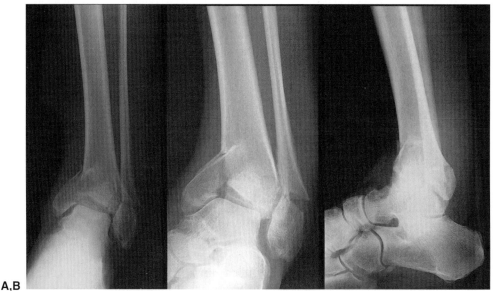

A,B	C

Figure 31.1. A. AP, **(B)** lateral, and **(C)** mortice plain radiographs of a high-energy tibial-plafond fracture. The fibular fracture is relatively transverse, and the articular surface of the tibia is comminuted with a portion of the cartilage impacted into the distal tibia.

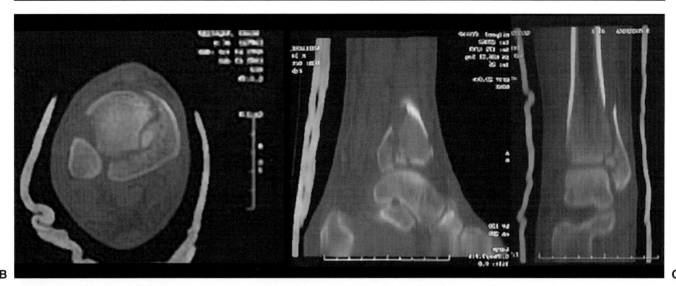

A,B   **C**

Figure 31.2. A. Axial, **(B)** sagittal, and **(C)** coronal reconstructions of a CT scan demonstrate clearly the fracture pattern and the presence of an impacted articular fragment.

left to the discretion of the surgeon. Formal ORIF of displaced pilon fractures should be carried out in two stages to minimize the risk of surgical complications. For each of these two stages, the patient is positioned supine with a padded bump beneath the ipsilateral greater trochanter and hip to help maintain the operative leg in neutral rotation. The first stage, which includes application of a spanning external fixator and internal fixation of the fibula, should be performed within 24 to 36 hours of the fracture, when possible. The fibula is approached through a slightly more posterolateral incision than usual and the fracture is reduced and plated with either a one-third tubular plate (metaphyseal fracture) or a 3.5 limited-contact dynamic-compression (LCDC) plate (diaphyseal fracture). When appropriate for the fracture pattern, the construct should be supplemented with a lag screw placed across the fracture. Occasionally the fibula can be stabilized with a single, partially threaded, cancellous screw placed from distal to proximal within the medullary canal of the fibula as an intramedullary splint. This method is particularly effective when the fracture is transverse and helpful when it is associated with lateral soft-tissue compromise.

The role of the spanning external fixator is to reapproximate the tibial fracture fragments through ligamentotaxis, provide pain relief, prevent further soft-tissue injury, and allow mobilization of the patient (Fig. 31.3). When the fixator is applied, barring any other serious injuries, the patient can be mobilized with crutches and subsequently discharged to home. This treatment strategy is reflected in the term "traveling traction," which has been used to refer to the use of this simple spanning external fixator.

The spanning external fixator is generally applied with two 16-mm carbon-fiber rods, two 4.5-mm or 5.0-mm half pins, and a 5.0-mm transfixation pin, a multiple pin clamp, and several pin-to-bar clamps (Fig. 31.4). Occasionally, this frame is supplemented with a 4.0-mm half pin placed into the first metatarsal and an additional pin-to-bar and bar-to-bar clamp and short carbon-fiber rod. Using the multipin clamp as a guide, the two half pins are placed in the midsagittal plane of the tibial diaphysis. The Schanz screws should be placed proximal to the zone of injury to avoid the fracture hematoma and the path of subsequent incisions. These Schanz screws should gain purchase in both the anterior and posterior cortices and therefore should be started one-half fingerbreadth medial to the tibial crest. The calcaneal transfixation pin should be placed from medial to lateral through the posterior-plantar aspect of the calcaneal tuberosity. Manual traction is applied on the transfixation pin to restore limb length and reapproximate the fracture fragments while maintaining the talus beneath the tibial plafond. When the limb is brought to length, the carbon fiber rods are attached to the multipin clamp proximally (1 bar medially and 1 bar laterally) and the transfixation pin is added distally. If the talus is unstable beneath the plafond, ORIF of the fibula or modification of the frame will be necessary.

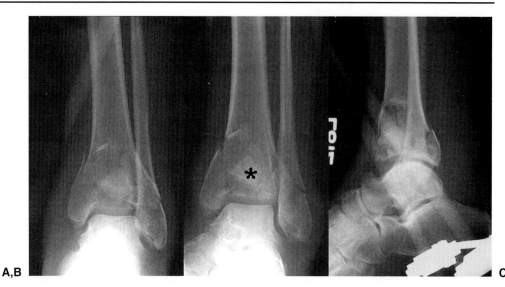

A,B   C

Figure 31.3. A. AP, **(B)** mortice, and **(C)** lateral plain radiographs after application of a spanning external fixator. The limb has been realigned, fracture fragments reapproximated, and the limb brought out to length. Note that the impacted fragment (*) with no soft tissue attachments remains impacted in the metaphysis.

In this situation, where the talus is unstable, modification of the frame includes the placement of a 4.0-mm half pin into the base of the first metatarsal and the attachment of this pin to the medial carbon-fiber rod with a third rod and a bar-to-bar clamp. This pin will improve stability of the talus as well as help avoid the development of an equinus contracture of the ankle, but it is not routinely necessary. It is important when applying this spanning external fixator that the hind foot and mid foot be positioned in neutral or slight valgus alignment.

When the swelling about the ankle has resolved and the soft tissues have recovered, generally 14 to 21 days after injury, it is possible to embark on the second stage, internal fixation of the distal tibia.

A nonsterile tourniquet is typically applied to the proximal thigh, and the leg is prepped and draped in the usual sterile fashion. Although using a tourniquet during the surgery will provide a bloodless field, its use may lead to increased postoperative swelling and should be limited to 2 to 2½ hours at 250 to 300 mmHg. Several approaches to the distal tibia have been described: The anteromedial approach is most consistently used, with the anterolat-

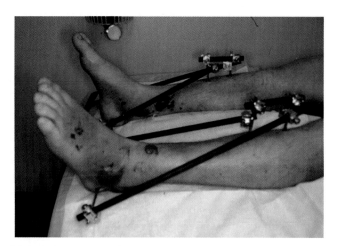

Figure 31.4. Clinical photograph of a patient with bilateral pilon fractures treated initially with spanning external fixators.

eral approach used for selected fracture patterns. A direct medial incision to the distal tibia should be *avoided at all costs* because of the high rate of soft-tissue complications.

The anteromedial approach is started proximally at, or just above, the proximal extent of the fracture, one-half fingerbreadth lateral to the tibial crest. It is extended distally, curving gently toward the talonavicular joint, paralleling the path of the anterior tibialis tendon. Leaving the periosteum attached to the underlying bone and bone fragments, the anterior tibialis, extensor hallucis longus, and the extensor digitorum tendons, along with the dorsalis pedis artery and venae, and the superficial peroneal nerve are retracted laterally, and an arthrotomy performed. With gentle retraction of the skin and tendons, the articular fragments of the distal tibia are reconstructed. In general, the largest and least displaced fracture fragments are reduced first and then the smaller, more displaced fragments are addressed.

Using image intensification in the AP, lateral, and oblique views will aid in assessing the reduction of the articular fragments. Assessment of the reduction can also be performed under direct visualization by looking into the joint from below. It is important to keep in mind that if the very distal aspect of the fibula has been plated, then the plate will obscure the articular surface when the fluoroscope is in the true lateral position. If recognized in advance, temporary stabilization of the fibula can be performed with pointed reduction forceps, and then definitive fixation performed after the tibial plafond has been reduced and stabilized. If the fibula has been previously reduced and plated, oblique images of the distal tibia can be used to assess the adequacy of the reduction. Temporary stabilization of the reduced articular fragments is obtained with Kirschner (K) wires (either 1.6 mm or 2.0 mm) and pointed reduction forceps, and these are subsequently replaced with interfragmentary small-fragment lag screws. When these fragments are stabilized, the articular block is then reduced to the tibial shaft and again held with pointed reduction forceps and/or K wires while length, alignment, and rotation are restored.

Definitive fixation of the distal tibia should be carried out with small fragment implants. Generally, plates are placed along the medial aspect of the tibia to secure the articular block to the shaft and buttress the distal tibia, which will help avoid varus mal-alignment. Often a small fragment plate is needed anteriorly to buttress the anterior articular and metaphyseal fragments. Again, small-fragment low-profile plates are best for this area (Fig. 31.5). If respect for the soft-tissue attachments is maintained during the surgery, large metaphyseal fragments will heal relatively quickly, and large fragment plates are not needed for strength. Because of their size, the large fragment plates can become quite bothersome to the overlying soft tissues.

On occasion, stable reduction and temporary stabilization of the articular fragments is not possible or large articular fragment may only be minimally displaced from the diaphysis. In these situations, it is often better to anatomically reduce these fragment(s) to the intact diaphysis initially and then build the remaining articular fragments back to them. If this method is employed, it is essential that the large fragments are anatomically reduced to the shaft because any malreduction at the metaphyseal level will lead to an even greater malreduction at the articular level.

Small supplemental incisions may also be necessary to address displaced articular fragments, including a limited anterolateral incision to address and fix displaced, anterolateral, Chaput tubercle fragments.

To support the articular fragments and the healing process as well as to fill metaphyseal voids, the use of bone grafts has been advocated in the past. A variety of bone graft materials are currently available. Cost, morbidity, and proven efficacy should be taken into consideration before deciding on whether to harvest an iliac-crest bone graft or use a bone graft substitute. In general, only large metaphyseal defects resulting from impaction of the cancellous bone are routinely bone grafted. Bone grafts should not be placed in acute, open, distal, tibia fractures. In the setting of an open fracture, use of a bone graft to improve the chances of distal tibia healing following bone loss should be performed only after the soft tissues have completely healed or soft tissue coverage has matured. Typically, this is done approximately 3 to 6 weeks after soft tissue closure.

Wound closure after osteosynthesis should be performed meticulously to avoid further soft-tissue injury. After closure of the deep tissues, the skin is closed with nylon sutures

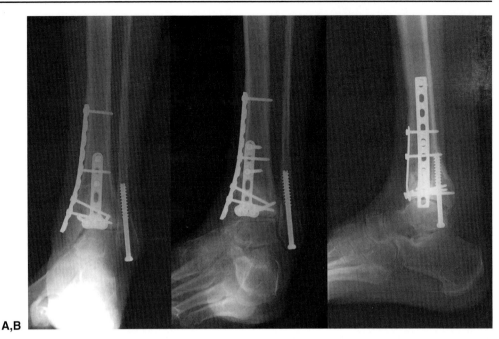

A,B   C

Figure 31.5. A. AP, **(B)** mortice, and **(C)** lateral plain radiographs 15 months after ORIF of a high-energy tibial-plafond fracture.

through the use of Allgöwer's modification of the Donati stitch. In the operating room, final plain radiographs are made to assure articular reduction. Also, a well-padded short-leg splint, with the ankle in neutral position, is applied.

POSTOPERATIVE MANAGEMENT

Patients are discharged to home approximately 24 to 48 hours after surgery. They are released in their postoperative splint and maintaining toe-touch weight bearing. At approximately 8 to 12 postoperative days, the patient is brought back to the clinic where the splint is removed and the incisions are inspected. If the incisions are each clean and dry and without evidence of skin necrosis, the sutures are removed and Steri-Strips applied. It is not uncommon to find small areas of superficial skin necrosis at the central portion of the tibial incision. In these cases, the sutures are generally left in place and a sterile dressing (Xeroform) is reapplied, and the ankle is immobilized again in a short-leg splint.

The patient is seen weekly until this area has healed, and when the sutures are removed, the patient is placed in a removable boot and active-assisted range of motion of the ankle, subtalar joint, and foot/toes is initiated. Patients are encouraged to perform these exercises three to four times each day for 20 minutes each session. Radiographs are routinely taken at 2, 6, and 12 weeks after surgery. If at the 6-week postoperation exam there is no change in the fracture fragments, alignment, and fixation construct, the patients are advanced to partial weight bearing and begin a formal physical therapist–directed program. This program should include aggressive active-assisted range of motion of the ankle as well as active-assisted and passive range of motion of the subtler join and foot. Muscle strengthening and pro-preconception training can also be initiated at this time if motion has improved. At 12 postoperative weeks, as long as there is evidence of further healing and no evidence of fracture instability, the patients are advanced to full weight bearing and weaned from the boot and crutches. In ideal situations, physical therapy is continued until near normal muscle strength and ankle, subtalar, and foot range of motion is recovered. Often laborers require a period of work hardening to regain labor-specific function and strength.

RESULTS

In an effort to decrease the incidence of soft-tissue complications associated with the treatment of pilon fractures, a two-staged approach has been proposed. Although this treatment protocol appears to have its roots in the late 1980s, it was not until the late 1990s that the benefits of this protocol were published (3,4).

Wyrsch et al (5) performed a randomized prospective study of two methods of fixation of tibial plafond fractures. Two groups of patients were studied including those who underwent ORIF of the tibia and fibula ($n = 18$) and a second group of patients ($n = 20$) who were managed with external fixation with or without limited internal fixation. Attesting to the high energy nature of these fractures, 26 were open fractures and 44% were Rüedi and Allgöwer type III fractures (6,7). They reported 15 operative complications in 7 patients who had been managed with ORIF and four complications in 4 patients who had been managed with external fixation. At an average follow-up of 39 months (range, 25 to 51 months) they concluded that external fixation of tibial plafond fractures was associated with fewer complications than was internal fixation. However, the patients who underwent ORIF were typically operated on within 48 hours of the injury, "unless severe swelling or fracture blisters were present" (average time of 5 days [range of 3 hours to 17 days]). It is quite possible that the many complications and adverse outcomes following formal ORIF was related to the fact that these fractures were treated before the soft tissues had fully recovered. Internal fixation of high-energy tibial-plafond fractures should only be performed after the soft tissues have recovered, generally in 14 to 21 days.

In 1999, Sirkin et al (4) reported their experience using this two-staged protocol in the treatment of 46 Orthopedic Trauma Association (OTA) type C fractures. Twenty-nine of these fractures were closed and 17 fractures were open. This entire group was made up of patients with particularly high-energy, distal, tibial fractures. In all cases, a temporary, spanning, external fixator was applied within 24 hours of the injury, and the fibula was plated. Open fractures were treated with serial debridement and soft-tissue closure or flap coverage, generally within 5 to 7 days of injury. Definitive fixation of the closed tibia fractures was performed on an average of 12.7 days (range of 4 to 30 days), whereas the average time to definitive fixation in the open pilon group was 14 days (range of 4 to 31 days). At a minimum follow-up of 12 months, one patient in the closed-fracture group had a deep infection (5%). In the open fracture group, three patients had a deep infection that resulted in a below knee amputation (BKA) in one patient and resolution of the infection in the others. In general, the authors felt that the patients in these groups who had been treated with this two-step protocol had an overall good result and an acceptably low complication rate (4).

Patterson and Cole (3) reported their experience with the treatment of 22 patients also with OTA type C fractures. Each patient was treated with a spanning external fixator and internal fixation of the fibula shortly after injury. Definitive fixation of the tibia was performed at an average of 24 days (range, 15 to 49 days) postinjury. At the 24-month follow-up, they reported no infections or soft-tissue complications, and their clinical results were similar to other studies reporting on ORIF of pilon fractures. They too concluded that patients with high-energy, distal tibial fractures are best treated with a two-staged protocol.

More recently, to assess midterm health, function, and impairment after pilon fractures and to determine which patient, injury, or treatment characteristic influence outcome most, Pollak et al (8) reported on 80 patients at 3.2 years after injury. Patients were recruited from two separate trauma centers, one that generally treats these injuries with formal internal fixation, and the other where most patients are treated with external fixation. They found that patients treated with external fixation, with or without limited-internal fixation, had greater loss of ankle motion and reported more pain and ambulatory dysfunction than did patients treated with internal fixation ($p < 0.05$). Although the general physical health of patients the two treatment groups was not significantly different, the average Sickness Impact Profile ambulation subscale score was 19.8 points higher (poorer) for patients treated with external fixation with or without limited- internal fixation. Based on these data, the authors concluded that patients who sustain a pilon fracture continue to experience major physical and psychosocial health problems long after the initial injury and that well-controlled prospective studies are needed to identify the best way to treat these injuries.

COMPLICATIONS

Infection and soft tissue complications are the most feared complications following fixation of high-energy tibial plafond fractures (9–14). When deep infections occur they commonly follow soft tissue complications, but occasionally the deep infections develop without postoperative wound complications. Aggressive treatment of soft-tissue complications and infections should be initiated when recognized. For full-thickness skin loss or deep infection, management includes aggressive surgical debridement of the dead and/or infected skin, subcutaneous tissue, and free bone fragments as well as the administration of culture-specific intravenous antibiotics. In addition, consideration is given for placement of a vascularized muscle flap for the residual soft-tissue defect. If the fracture remains well fixed and the implants are stable, efforts should be made to leave the implants in place until the fracture has healed; this strategy is an attempt to prevent the development of an infected nonunion. If the fracture or implants are unstable, serious consideration must be given to removal or exchange of the implants and application of a spanning or nonspanning external fixator.

Nonunions are not uncommon in these fractures and most commonly involve the metaphyseal portion of the tibia. Signs and symptoms of a nonunion include persistent pain and swelling about the ankle, progression of deformity, and at times, gross motion at the fracture site and failed screws and/or plates. Intraoperatively, soft tissue–friendly techniques, which include preservation of the soft-tissue attachments to the fracture fragments, and infection avoidance, are probably the best ways to minimize the development of a nonunion. When nonunion is diagnosed, measures (including the use of laboratory tests and occasionally open biopsy) should be taken to make sure an occult infection is not present. Treatment for nonunions is typically operative and includes the correction of limb alignment, revision internal fixation, and bone grafting.

Malunions typically develop after a delayed union or nonunion and usually involve varus mal-alignment of the distal tibia. Premature removal of the implants, particularly the medial buttress plate, has been associated with the development of a malunion, and therefore, the implants should not be removed until the fracture has completely healed. Fractures are considered completely healed when the fracture lines are absent, bridging bone across the fractures line is present on the plain radiographs, and weight bearing activities are tolerated. Treatment for the malunion includes the correction of alignment and revision internal fixation of the tibia and fibula. Typically this requires an osteotomy at the site of the malunion, correction of alignment, and the insertion of a tricortical bone-graft wedge prior to fixation. This technique has been very effective for correcting the alignment of the limb while maintaining limb length.

Posttraumatic osteoarthritis commonly occurs following pilon fractures and is felt to be related to primary cartilage injury, residual articular incongruity, and joint instability. Although little can be done at this time to reverse the primary cartilage injury, many feel that at least cartilage nutrition, which is dependent on joint motion, can be maximized by fracture stabilization and early joint motion. Articular incongruity should be minimized by paying particular attention to the reduction of the articular fragments during surgery. The hallmarks of treatment remain accurate articular reduction, stable internal fixation, early range of motion exercises, and delayed weight bearing. Only after sufficient time has elapsed to allow healing of the articular fragments can protected weight bearing be initiated.

Gross ankle instability is not commonly seen after fixation and healing, but there is experimental evidence that alteration in joint stability may occur after fracture, particularly if articular incongruity is present. Therefore, all efforts should be made to restore the tibial plafond and stability of the joint.

Treatment of posttraumatic arthritis involves the use of nonsteroidal anti-inflammatory agents, ankle bracing, and shoe and activity modification. Intermediate and end-stage posttraumatic osteoarthritis can be treated with a solid ankle-foot orthosis and cane. If these measures provide comfort for patients with advanced posttraumatic osteoarthritis, then only in the elderly or very low-demand individuals should total ankle arthroplasty be considered. In physiologically young patients with symptomatic disabling arthritis, an ankle fusion remains the gold standard.

SUMMARY

High-energy tibial-plafond fractures are difficult to treat and their treatment is associated with considerable risks. To minimize the risks of complications, a two-staged protocol has been developed. In the initial stage, shortly after injury, a spanning external fixator should be applied and the fibular fracture plated. When the surrounding soft tissues have recovered (marked by wrinkling of the skin about the foot and ankle) and the fracture blisters have resolved, internal fixation of the distal tibia can be performed and the spanning external fixator removed.

Postoperatively, the surgeon must remain vigilant and treat wound complications aggressively. The typical postoperative protocol includes 6 weeks of touch-toe weight bearing and 6 weeks of partial weight bearing before full weight bearing is allowed and formal physical therapy initiated. As a result of the severe nature of these injuries, some loss of ankle and hind foot motion occurs, and some patients have pain, which requires shoe and lifestyle modifications.

RECOMMENDED READINGS

1. Tornetta P III, Weiner L, Bergman M, et al. Pilon fractures: treatment with combined internal and external fixation. *J Orthop Trauma* 1993;7:489–496.
2. Kellam JF, Waddell JP. Fractures of the distal tibial metaphysis with intra-articular extension: the distal tibial explosion fracture. *J Trauma* 1979;19:593–601.
3. Patterson MJ, Cole JD. Two-staged delayed open reduction and internal fixation of severe pilon fractures. *J Orthop Trauma* 1999;13:85–91.
4. Sirkin M, Sanders R, DiPasquale T, et al. A staged protocol for soft tissue management in the treatment of complex pilon fractures. *J Orthop Trauma* 1999;13:78–84.
5. Wyrsch B, McFerran MA, McAndrew M, et al. Operative treatment of fractures of the tibial plafond: a randomized, prospective study. *J Bone Joint Surg Am* 1996;78:1646–1657.
6. Ruedi T. Fractures of the lower end of the tibia into the ankle joint: results 9 years after open reduction and internal fixation. *Injury* 1973;5:130–134.
7. Rüedi TP, Allgöwer M. The operative treatment of intra-articular fractures of the lower end of the tibia. *Clin Orthop* 1979:105–110.
8. Pollak AN, McCarthy ML, Bess RS, et al. Outcomes after treatment of high-energy tibial- plafond fractures. *J Bone Joint Surg Am* 2003;85:1893–1900.
9. Dillin L, Slabaugh P. Delayed wound healing, infection, and nonunion following open reduction and internal fixation of tibial plafond fractures. *J Trauma* 1986;26:1116–1119.
10. Helfet DL, Koval K, Pappas J, et al. Intraarticular "pilon" fracture of the tibia. *Clin Orthop* 1994:221–228.
11. McFerran MA, Smith SW, Boulas HJ, et al. Complications encountered in the treatment of pilon fractures. *J Orthop Trauma* 1992;6:195–200.
12. Teeny SM, Wiss DA. Open reduction and internal fixation of tibial plafond fractures: variables contributing to poor results and complications. *Clin Orthop* 1993:108–117.
13. Thordarson DB. Complications after treatment of tibial pilon fractures: prevention and management strategies. *J Am Acad Orthop Surg* 2000;8:253–265.
14. Trumble TE, Benirschke SK, Vedder NB. Use of radial forearm flaps to treat complications of closed pilon fractures. *J Orthop Trauma* 1992;6:358–365.

32

The Treatment of Distal Tibia Peri-articular Fractures with Circular Ring Fixators

James J. Hutson, Jr.

INDICATIONS/CONTRAINDICATIONS

Circular tensioned-wire fixators are dynamic devices that provide the surgeon with the ability to fabricate a customized external fixator to treat complex, distal tibia, peri-articular fractures. The fixators are constructed based on the position and quality of the fracture fragments and the severity of injury to the soft tissues. Basic principles are applied in sequence resulting in alignment and fixation of the fractures.

Type B fractures have an intact column of bone maintaining length and are ideal for buttress plating with low profile plates and fibula fixation. Type A and C fractures with moderate soft-tissue injury are treated with internal fixation or half-pin bridging frames with limited internal fixation. As soft-tissue damage and bone comminution worsen, the indication to use circular tensioned wires to treat these complex injuries increases (1). Extension of the fracture pattern proximally to the midshaft compromises the ability to use limited plating, but the stiffness of circular fixators allows fixation using the entire shaft of the tibia with fixation pins and wires to treat these extensile fractures. Pilon fractures combined with complex foot injuries are an indication for circular tensioned-wire fixation.

Patients with ischemic vascular disease or diabetes who would have difficulty healing wounds over plates and screws or who are not candidates for local and free flaps are well treated with tensioned-wire fixation. Open wounds can be treated with local wound-healing methods, resulting in closure by secondary intention, or delayed split-thickness skin grafting. The local wound-healing modalities include hyperbaric oxygen treatment, saline wet-to-dry dressing changes, and vacuum sponge dressings. A relative indication is the need for early ambulation. Patients treated with circular fixators can apply partial weight early after fixation, whereas limited low-profile plating must be protected for 3 or more months. The patient with multiple extremity fractures or morbid obesity will be able to use his or her externally stabilized pilon fracture for transfer assistance or partial weight gait, reducing their dependency on a wheel-chair.

PREOPERATIVE EVALUATION AND PLANNING

Distal tibia peri-articular fractures often occur in patients with multiple trauma. The patient is evaluated for life-threatening injuries. Once stable, the extremity is evaluated, and the dorsalis pedis and posterior tibial pulse are palpated. If undetectable, a Doppler evaluation is conducted. The lower leg and foot is evaluated for compartment syndrome. The extremity is stabilized and a careful physical examination is performed. A detailed neurologic exam with specific testing of deep and superficial peroneal, medial, lateral and calcaneal plantar, saphenous, and sural nerve function is recorded. Open wounds are observed for size and location. Intravenous cephalosporin antibiotics are started immediately in patients with open fractures. With sterile gloves, the wound may be lavaged with normal saline and a sterile dressing applied. Exploration of the wound in the emergency room should be avoided. The lower extremity is splinted with a bulky dressing and plaster splints.

Full length films of the tibia and fibula, as well as anteroposterior (AP), lateral, and mortise views of the ankle should be obtained.

Lower-energy fractures are maintained in the splint. Open fractures and fractures with compartment syndrome require emergent operative intervention. Following debridement and compartment release, the fracture is temporarily stabilized with bridging half-pin fixation and a transverse calcaneal pin (Fig. 32.1). Closed fractures with comminution and displacement also are stabilized with bridging half-pin fixation. If these comminuted fractures are not stabilized and reduced, massive edema and fracture blisters will occur. Calcaneal traction on a Bohler-Braun frame, or traveling traction, is an alternative if the patient cannot be taken to surgery (Fig. 32.2).

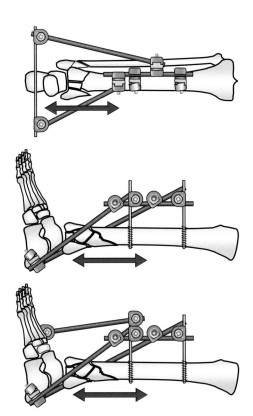

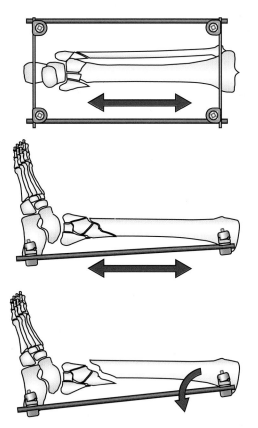

Figure 32.1. Basic distraction frame. A horizontal half pin is distracted by two connecting rods to a two-pin fixation block. The foot is controlled with a pin to the first metatarsal to prevent equinus. This frame in lower-energy fractures is combined with limited internal fixation for definitive treatment. It is removed if circular fixation will be used as definitive treatment. (Copyright © James J. Hutson, Jr., MD.)

Figure 32.2. Traveling traction described by Tracy Watson. A horizontal pin is placed through the proximal tibial metaphysis and calcaneus. Distraction is placed with connecting rods. The pilon can displace posteriorly if the heel is not supported. (Copyright © James J. Hutson, Jr., MD.)

The goal of initial bridging fixation is to bring the fracture out to anatomic length and to align the dome of the talus with the central axis of the tibial shaft on the AP and lateral view. The second toe of the foot must be aligned with tibial tubercle at the knee for the surgeon to align correctly the rotation of the extremity. The forefoot is controlled with a first metatarsal pin and the foot is aligned in plantar neutral position. It is essential that excellent alignment be established with this initial trauma resuscitation frame. Failure to achieve these goals will compromise subsequent reconstruction. Repeat debridement and antibiotic bead pouches are indicated for severe open fractures with gross contamination.

Serial examination of the extremity during the first week is critical. A small number of patients will have further soft-tissue compromise requiring a return to the operating room for further debridement. A small subset of patients will have a fragment of the posterior plafond rotated and displaced against the tibial nerve (Fig. 32.3). These patients have paresthesia or anesthesia of the plantar surface of their foot. Reduction of this fragment is indicated urgently, even if the soft-tissue envelope is not in ideal condition. In a small subset of patients with grade IIIB or grade IIIC fractures, early amputation may be indicated (2).

The majority of closed and simple open fractures will show improvement in the soft-tissue envelope during the first 7 to 14 days. The skin condition determines the timing of the reconstruction of the pilon fracture. When the edema has resolved and the fracture blisters healed, definitive fixation of the pilon fracture can be performed.

The plain films and computed tomography (CT) scan are carefully evaluated. The fibula fracture is observed for level of fracture, comminution, and separation of the fibula from the tibia. The proximal extension of the tibia fracture and comminution of the plafond is evaluated. The CT scan helps the surgeon plan the location of incisions when an open approach is needed. Pilon fractures can be approached through the anterior medial, anterior lateral, or posterior medial exposures. The condition of the soft tissues will be compared to the fracture pattern to avoid dissection through soft tissues with extensive damage. At this time, the decision will be made about the treatment approach: (a) open reduction and internal fixation (ORIF), (b) bridging fixation with limited internal fixation, or (c) circular tensioned-wire fixation. The following sections will describe the treatment strategies for tensioned wire fixation.

The technical goals of treatment are to align the fracture axially with correct rotation, reduce the joint surface to match the contour of the dome of the talus, reconstruct the mortise, and reconstruct metaphyseal bone loss and comminution. These goals are approached with cautious handling of the soft tissues. Distraction is the key to reduction. Because of the terminal location of pilon fractures, the mid tibial shaft is used as a fixation base to reduce the fracture. When circular fixators are used, a fixation block is applied with two half

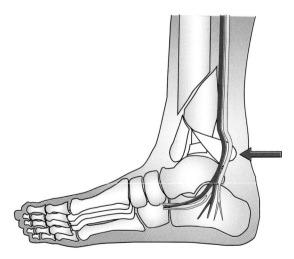

Figure 32.3. A posterior fragment can be forced into the neurovascular bundle compromising blood flow and plantar sensation. This fragment requires early reduction to prevent permanent damage to these essential structures. (Copyright © James J. Hutson, Jr., MD.)

pins in the AP plane in an orthogonal position. This fixation block is used as a base to support the distal fixation rings, which are placed at the level of the plafond or calcaneus to distract the fracture. If the plafond or calcaneus (hind foot) is distracted axially with correct rotation, the distal tibia fracture will be spatially reduced with correct rotation, alignment, and length. This initial reduction will facilitate the local alignment of the joint surface and the metaphysis by percutaneous or open techniques. The better the alignment gained by accurate distraction, the easier the reduction of the joint and metaphysis. It is almost impossible in complex pilon fractures to reduce the plafond if the dome of the talus is malaligned, shortened, and rotated. This fact pertains to any type of external fixator used to treat pilon fractures (monolateral, clamp and rods, and circular tensioned fixators). The dome of the talus must be aligned correctly in distraction before beginning the reduction of the fracture fragments.

REDUCTION TECHNIQUE FOR TYPE A, C1, AND C2 FRACTURES

The level of the horizontal reference-wire placement is determined by the fracture pattern being treated. In type A distal tibia fractures, the joint surface is intact. In C1 and C2 fracture patterns of the joint, there is a simple fracture plane with two large fragments. A limited open reduction and fixation with subchondral lag screws will reduce the joint surface anatomically creating a unified bone block. This reconstructed metaphysis can be treated as a type A fracture (Fig. 32.4).

The proximal ring block is aligned on the tibial shaft with two anterior posterior 5- or 6-mm half pins. The half pins should be spread apart 10 cm or more to increase stiffness of the fixator. Mounting these pins with universal fixation cubes facilitates alignment of the frame. The distal half pin is placed 3 cm above the proximal extent of the fracture. Placing the half pins far superior to the fracture increases the working length and thus leads to frame instability. It is important to align the fixation block in an orthogonal position. The frame should be parallel to the tibia on the AP and lateral views, and the tibia should be placed

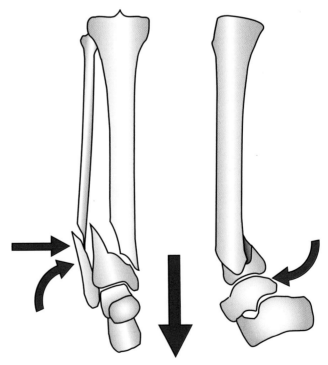

Figure 32.4. Type A distal tibia fracture. Reduction is gained by distraction to length, correction of rotation, and axial alignment of the plafond with the proximal shaft. (Copyright © James J. Hutson, Jr., MD.)

into the rings to provide clearance for the soft tissues. The ring over the plafond must clear the anterior soft tissues of the ankle, and the superior ring of the fixator block must not impinge on the posterior leg where the gastrocnemius and soleus muscles bulge posteriorly. See Figures 32.5 and 32.6.

If the fixation block on the tibia is orthogonal, then the joint surface of the plafond will be in anatomic alignment when the joint forms a 90-degree angle with the axis of the shaft and orthogonal, ring, stable base. The plafond on the AP view forms an angle of 90 degrees to the axis of the tibia. This anatomic fact allows the surgeon to align distal tibia fractures accurately by placing a horizontal reference wire parallel to the joint surface. The plane of the carbon-fiber fracture-reduction ring, which is connected to the orthogonal stable base, is 90 degrees to the shaft. The horizontal reference wire in the plafond is placed onto the distal surface of the carbon-fiber fracture ring and manipulated with fluoroscopic guidance so that the plafond aligns axially and with correct rotation. The horizontal reference wire may need to be loosened and repositioned several times until excellent alignment is obtained. Small angular corrections are done with washers on one side of the ring to improve alignment if needed. Once the wire is tensioned, distraction is placed across the fracture to reduce the metaphysis. See Figures 32.7 to 32.9.

The alignment in the lateral view is examined. Often the foot can be manipulated into dorsi flexion to rotate the plafond around the horizontal reference wire. Arc wire technique and manipulation with half pins are used to correct apex anterior and posterior malalignment. Occasionally, during this phase of the reduction, it will become obvious that the

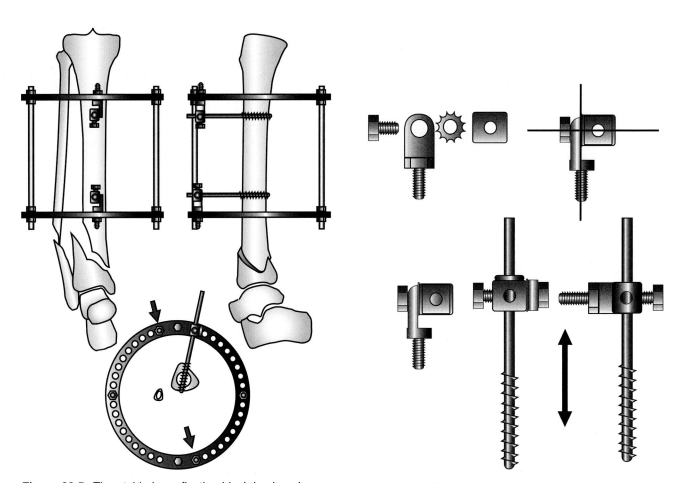

Figure 32.5. The stable-base fixation block is placed proximal to the fracture by 2 to 3 cm. The fixation block is orthogonal to the tibia. Accurate alignment of the stable base facilitates fracture reduction. (Copyright © James J. Hutson, Jr., MD.)

Figure 32.6. The half pins are connected to the rings on the stable base with universal fixation cubes. An 8-mm bolt connects the Rancho Cube (Smith-Nephew) to a male hinge or post. These universal attachments allow fine-tuning of the stable base and small corrections of the tibial shaft alignment with the plafond. (Copyright © James J. Hutson, Jr., MD.)

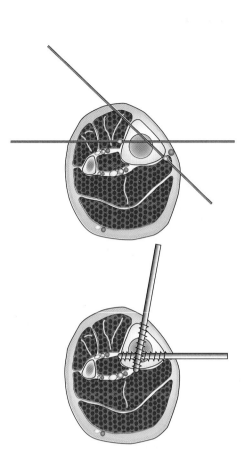

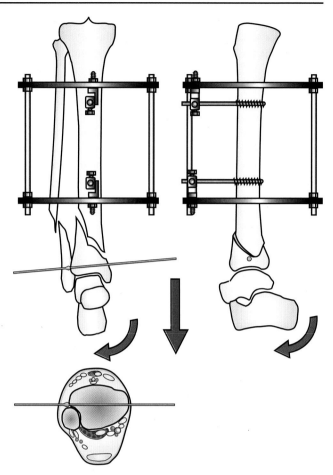

Figure 32.7. Half pins are placed with 90-degree divergence at the mid tibia. Over drilling the half pins can damage the anterior and posterior nerves and arteries. Olive wires are used if half pins are not available. (Copyright © James J. Hutson, Jr., MD.)

Figure 32.8. A horizontal reference wire is placed parallel to the anterior joint. The wire is placed approximately 8 to 12 mm above the joint. (Copyright © James J. Hutson, Jr., MD.)

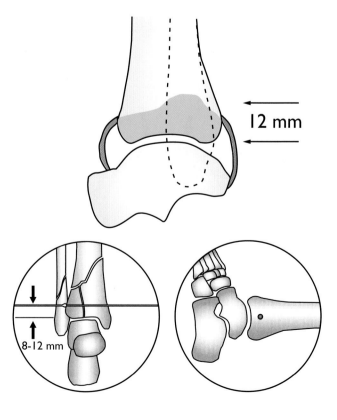

Figure 32.9. The joint may extend superior adjacent to the fibula. Fibular fixation is always placed on the superior side of the ring to avoid this area of the joint. (Copyright © James J. Hutson, Jr., MD.)

horizontal reference wire needs to be adjusted anterior or posterior on the ring to align the plafond anatomically. Once the plafond is aligned, at least two additional divergent olive wires are placed across the fracture in the 60-degree safe zone of wire pathways. A fourth wire is placed if space is available. Two wires are never adequate fixation. At least three olive wires should be placed. A medial-face half pin is added to the stable base. A minimum of two AP half pins and a medial-face half pin are necessary on the stable base. A fourth medial face pin is placed in large patients. See Figures 32.10 through 32.19.

A sequential guide to type A and C1-2 distal tibia fractures is as follows:

1. The simple fracture of the C1-2 fracture is reduced and fixated with a 3.5- or 4.5-mm subchondral screw.
2. A stable base is fixated to the mid tibia with the rings aligned orthogonal on the tibia with two AP half pins on universal mountings.
3. A horizontal reference wire is placed 8- to 12-mm above the plafond, and the plafond bone block is adjusted and aligned on the carbon fracture ring; thus the fracture axially aligned and with correct rotation (3,4).
4. The fracture is aligned in the lateral view with apex anterior and posterior mal-alignment corrected using manipulation of the foot and reduction techniques to reduce the fracture.
5. The plafond is fixated with three or four divergent olive wires in the 60-degree arc of safe wire placement. A third medial-face half pin is added to the fixation block.
6. The fracture is compressed.

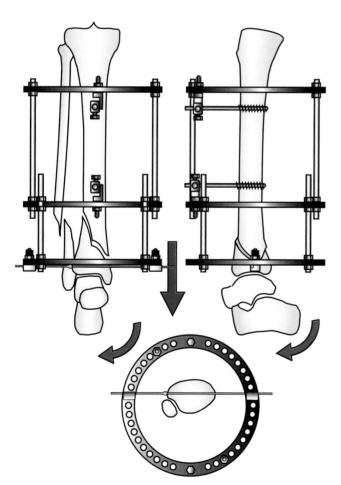

Figure 32.10. The plafond is centered in the distal ring in alignment with the tibia shaft. Once the ring is aligned, the wire is tensioned and the distal ring distracted. Rotating the foot into dorsiflexion will align the lateral fluoroscopic image. (Copyright © James J. Hutson, Jr., MD.)

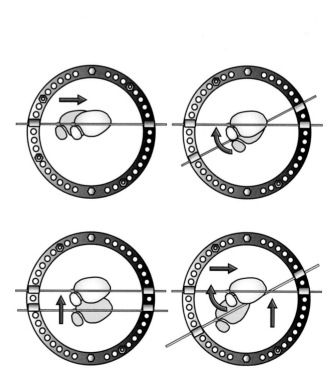

Figure 32.11. The plafond and horizontal reference wire is manipulated to correct rotation and translation. The second toe is aligned with the tibial tubercle. (Copyright © James J. Hutson, Jr., MD.)

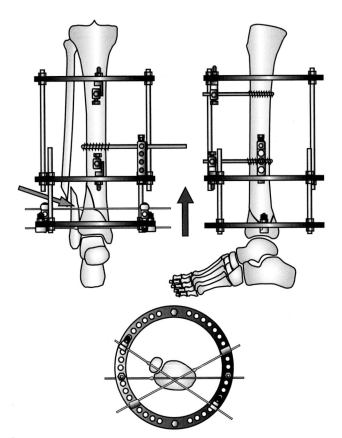

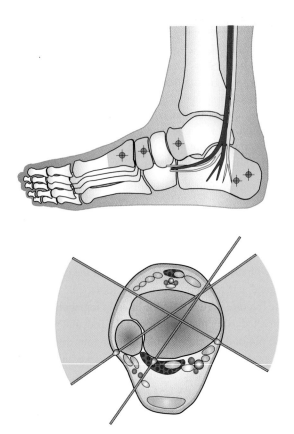

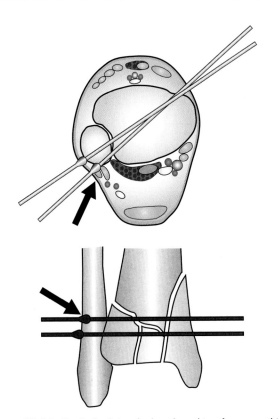

Figure 32.12. At least two additional, divergent, olive wires are added to the ring. Oblique fractures are fixated with olive wires placed to improve fixation (orange arrow). The fracture is compressed. A third medial-face half pin is added to the stable base. (Copyright © James J. Hutson, Jr., MD.)

Figure 32.13. Safe wire pathways. Wires may be placed in the posterior calcaneus, talar head, or cuneiform and metatarsal bases. Green 60-degree arc of safe wire placement at level of plafond. The wire posterior lateral to anterior medial can be used to secure posterior malleolar fragment. (Copyright © James J. Hutson, Jr., MD.)

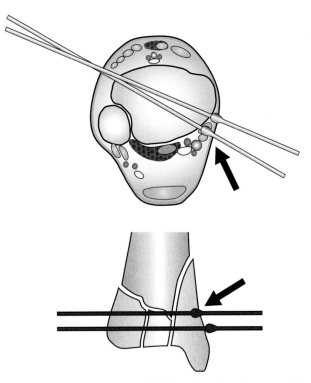

Figure 32.14. Posterior lateral wire placed too far around the lateral malleolus (black arrow) will penetrate the peroneal tendons. In the fluoroscopic view, the olive is behind the lateral malleolus. (Copyright © James J. Hutson, Jr., MD.)

Figure 32.15. Posterior medial wire placed too far around plafond will penetrate the posterior tibial and long flexor tendons. The AP fluoroscopic view will show the olive behind the plafond (black arrow). (Copyright © James J. Hutson, Jr., MD.)

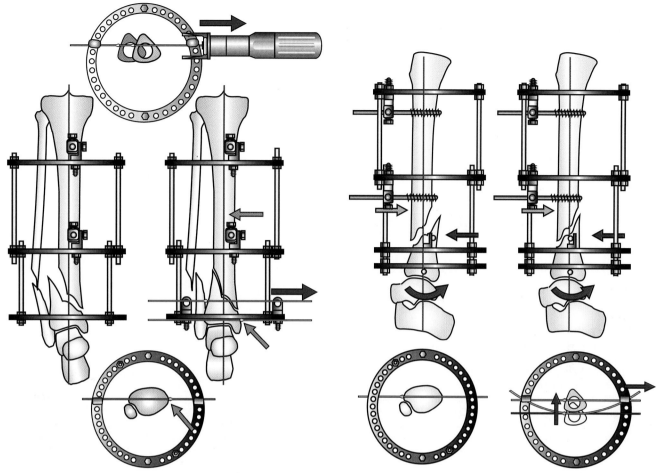

Figure 32.16. Draw wire technique to reduce sagittal plane fracture. The olive wire bolt is not tightened. The tensioner tool pulls the olive toward the tensioner. The bolt is tightened and the wire tensioned. (Copyright © James J. Hutson, Jr., MD.)

Figure 32.17. Arc wire technique. A wire is arced to the fixation bolt on either side of the ring. When tensioned, the arc flattens, reducing the posterior fragment. The AP half pin resists the force of the reduction (orange arrow). The metaphyseal bone block rotates around the tensioned, horizontal, reference wire (red arrow). (Copyright © James J. Hutson, Jr., MD.)

An alternative method available to reduce distal tibia fractures is the application of universal connecting rods between a fixation block on the tibia and plafond (Fig. 32.20). Orthogonal rings are placed on the tibia and plafond. The tibial block has two AP half pins and medial face pin. The plafond has at least three divergent olive wires on the ring and the ring is placed orthogonal to the joint. The fixation blocks are connected by universal rods. The fracture is manipulated manually and the rods tightened. This technique appears to be simple, but often results in poor reduction because the surgeon cannot generate enough leverage to distract and reduce the fracture. This technique has been greatly improved by the concept of the Spatial Frame (Smith-Nephew, Andover, MA). This technique uses the concept of slow reduction. The fracture is reduced by defining fracture parameters on x-rays and generating a computer print-out to reduce the tibial-shaft fixation block to the plafond fixation block in small incremental steps by adjusting six connecting rods. The technique is especially indicated when a late reduction of a distal tibia fracture is required 3 or more weeks after the injury. The early callus can be slowly distracted and the fracture reduced over 2 to 3 weeks avoiding the risk of aggressive reduction maneuvers.

REDUCTION TECHNIQUE OF C3 PILON FRACTURES

Pilon fractures with comminution of the joint surface cannot be reduced without distraction across the joint (Fig. 32.21). The reduction technique with circular fixators uses

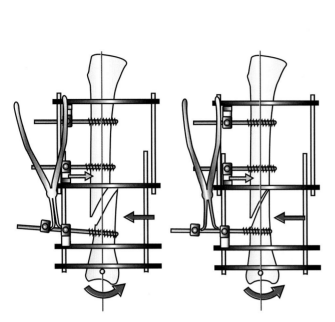

Figure 32.18. Laminar spreader technique. A second cube is added to the half pin and tightened. The ring cube is loosened. The laminar spreader is opened, powerfully reducing the oblique fragment of a longer type-A fragment. (Orange arrow shows resisting-fixation half pin.) The metaphysis rotates around the horizontal reference wire. (Copyright © James J. Hutson, Jr., MD.)

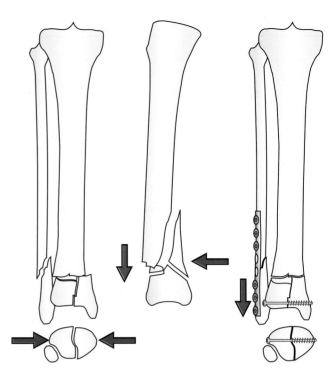

Figure 32.19. C2 distal tibia fracture. A lag screw and fibula plate convert this to a type A fracture. Depending on the soft-tissue condition, the fracture is treated with internal or external fixation. (Copyright © James J. Hutson, Jr., MD.)

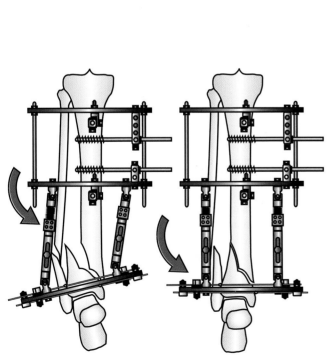

Figure 32.20. Universal connecting rods. The surgeon uses physical manipulation to reduce the two fragments connected by universal connecting rods. This technique often leads to less than satisfactory reduction. (Copyright © James J. Hutson, Jr., MD.)

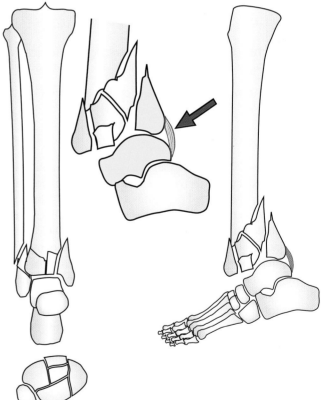

Figure 32.21. C3 distal tibia pilon fracture. There is comminution of the joint, and the plafond is dissociated from the shaft. Observe the dense posterior capsule that controls the position of the posterior malleolar fragment. Wherever the talus resides, the posterior fragment displaces. The talar dome must be aligned to reduce this essential fragment. (Copyright © James J. Hutson, Jr., MD.)

distraction between a stable orthogonal base and a horizontal reference wire placed into the calcaneus and tensioned on a foot plate. The dome of the talus must be distracted and aligned anatomically to reduce the joint surface. If the limb is shortened, the talus will physically occupy the space where the joint fragments need to be positioned to reduce the plafond. If the talus is malpositioned posterior or anterior, the soft-tissue attachment across the joint will tether the fragments and prevent reduction. The posterior fragment that is attached to the talus by the posterior capsule is impossible to reduce unless the talus is axially aligned with the shaft (Figs. 32-22 to 32-24).

The strategy of reduction is to apply distraction through a calcaneal, horizontal, reference wire to align the talus axially with correct rotation (Figs. 32-25 and 32-26). The talar dome is used as template to align the crushed fragments of the plafond. Reduction of the posterior fragment is the key to reduction. Distraction will reduce the fragment in many fractures. Some fractures will have persistent posterior displacement or the posterior malleolus will be rotated and incarcerated in the posterior capsule. The fragment is gently freed with a smooth edged elevator. A threaded Steinman pin is placed into the fragment. The fragment is rotated and pulled anteriorly over the dome until it is in anatomic position. It is pinned in place and used as a guide to reduce the mid and anterior joint fragments. In low-energy fractures, there will be large fragments to assemble with small screws and wires. In high-energy fractures there will be fragments of crushed cartilage, morselized subchondral bone, and deformation of larger joint fragments from crushing of the cancellous bone. These fragments will not have anatomic contours. It is possible to have the cortex reduced anatomically, but the joint is angulated because of the crushing of the subchondral bone. These fragments may require small osteotomies and local bone grafting to regain alignment matching the talar dome. A level of joint crushing will be encountered in which there are not fragments that can be reassembled, and small Steinman pins are used to corral the fragments into a salvage joint, which will provide support to the talus but ankle joint motion will be lost. See Figures 32.27 to 32.30.

When crushing of the cancellous bone of the plafond superior to the joint fragment occurs, there will be a void that needs to be filled with cancellous bone graft or a bone graft substitute. The graft is placed as a spacer to prevent the joint fragments from displacing superior into the metaphysis.

Small spring plates are also used locally to control anterior fragments that are difficult to control with tensioned wires. The combined use of Steinman pins, small screws, bone graft, and local plates reduces the plafond. The fixation only needs to align the joint surface. The bridging external fixation maintains axial alignment. This is the essential strategy difference

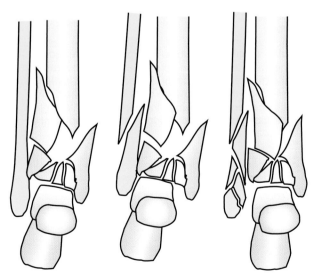

Figure 32.22. The three possible lateral malleolus fracture patterns: intact, simple, and comminuted. The fracture pattern of the fibula will influence the strategy for plafond reduction. (Copyright © James J. Hutson, Jr., MD.)

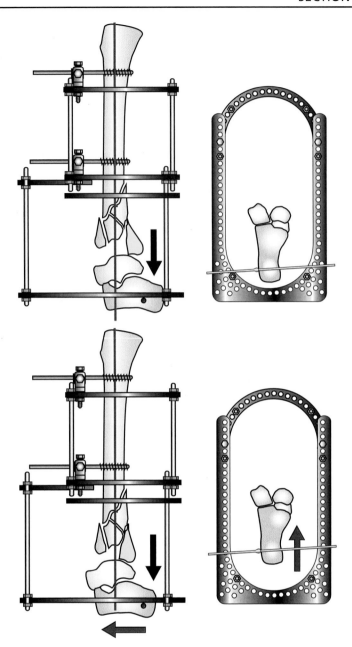

Figure 32.23. A stable orthogonal base is applied to the tibia. Two, posterior, threaded rods are connected to the foot plate. The fracture reduction ring is placed into the frame in a proximal position to be used later in the reduction. A horizontal reference wire is placed in the calcaneus. The foot is positioned to align the dome of the talus with the shaft. The posterior displacement of the foot must be corrected to reduce the joint fragments. Notice how the posterior malleolus (yellow) is reduced by moving the foot anterior. (Copyright © James J. Hutson, Jr., MD.)

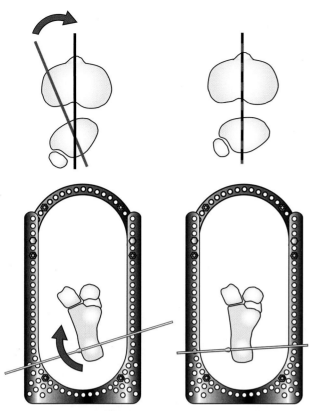

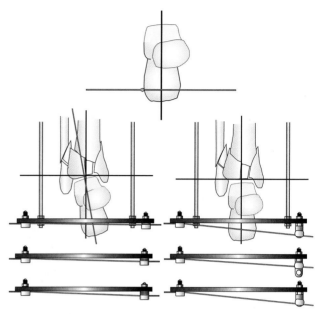

Figure 32.24. The foot is rotated on the foot plate until the second toe aligns with the tibial tubercle. Rotational alignment must be established at this point of the reduction. (Copyright © James J. Hutson, Jr., MD.)

Figure 32.25. The horizontal reference wire in the calcaneus is placed 90 degrees to the axis of the ankle joint. If the wire is placed in valgus or varus, or the talus does note reduce with traction, the wire can be adjusted away from the foot plate on washers, hinges, and post. Rarely, distraction will reveal an occult hind foot dislocation. The joint is reduced and pinned, and the reduction continues. (Copyright © James J. Hutson, Jr., MD.)

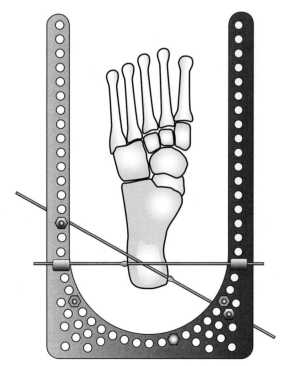

Figure 32.26. The foot is positioned in plantar neutral position. A second, opposed, olive wire is placed superior to the foot plate from posterior medial to anterior lateral. The threaded rods are placed posteriorly, connecting the stable base to the foot plate (orange nuts). Notice that the medial calcaneus has no wires placed anteriorly where they could injure the posterior tibial nerve branches or artery. (Copyright © James J. Hutson, Jr., MD.)

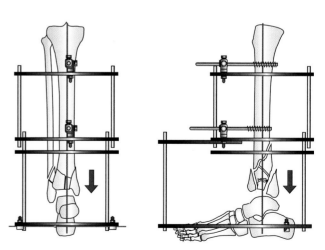

Figure 32.27. With the two AP pins tightened, the foot plate is distracted until the dome of the talus pulls away from the impacted plafond. Distraction of 10 to 15 mm is applied by moving the nuts connecting the foot plate rods to the stable base. (Copyright © James J. Hutson, Jr., MD.)

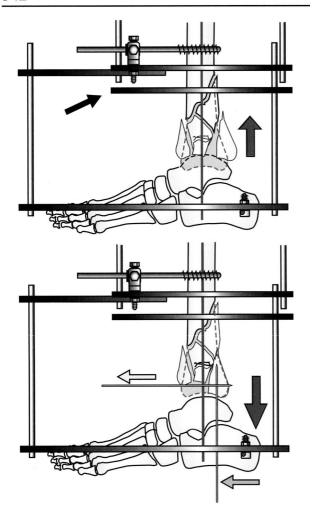

Figure 32.28. Over distraction is the key to reduction. Without distraction, the dome of the talus occupies the space (green), which the plafond joint fragments occupy when reduced. If the posterior malleolar fragment does not reduce with distraction, a threaded Steinman pin (yellow arrow), small bone hook, or pulling device is used to pull the fragment anteriorly over the dome of the talus. The posterior malleolus is pinned in place (blue arrow) and the anterior fragments reduced. The fracture reduction ring is positioned superior and will be moved inferior after the joint reduction (black arrow). (Copyright © James J. Hutson, Jr., MD.)

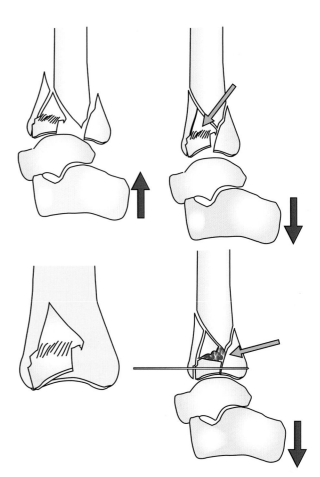

Figure 32.29. High-energy pilon fractures have impaction of the osteocartilagenous fragments. Dense white areas on the lateral view of the x-ray indicate crushed trabecular bone. The cortical fragments can be aligned anatomically (yellow outline), but the joint fragments are still not reduced and are crushed into the metaphysis (blue arrow). These fragments are dislodged and reduced onto the dome of the talus and held in place with local bone graft and small wire or screw fixation. (Copyright © James J. Hutson, Jr., MD.)

with plating and tensioned wire fixation. Plating technique requires that the axial alignment is maintained by the plates and screws and the plates must traverse the comminuted metaphysis to the shaft. Circular tensioned wire technique requires that the internal fixation only align the joint. Axial stability and alignment is maintained by the external fixator and no hardware traverses the comminuted metaphyseal zone of injury. This strategy is valuable in treating patients with compromised soft tissues (1,5). See Figures 32.31 to 32.35.

Following reduction of the joint, an assessment is made of metaphyseal comminution. If there are larger fragments, the metaphysis is fixated with a cluster of three to four divergent olive wires after closure of the approach for the open reduction. The fracture reduction ring is initially placed in the frame but located superior to the ankle. After open reduction, the ring is moved over the plafond to fixate the fracture. If there is severe comminution of the plafond and local fixation would have few intact bone fragments to purchase, the fracture fixation ring is not moved down over the plafond. The frame is used as a bypass bridging frame and maintained until the fracture heals. The downside to this

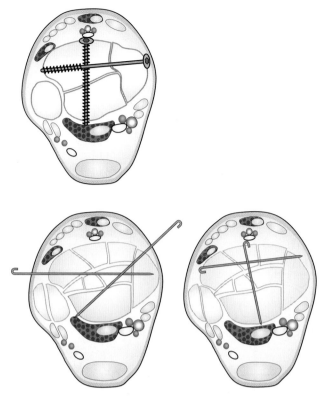

Figure 32.30. Small screws and wires are used to fixate the fragments. Free wires protrude through the skin and are removed at 6 weeks in patients with bridging distraction. Brad wires are bent over 180 degrees and tamped into the bone. This prevents the pin from migrating. The anterior-to-posterior lag screw is used to control the posterior malleolus when the anterior plafond is not crushed. (Copyright © James J. Hutson, Jr., MD.)

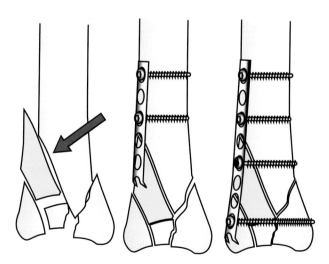

Figure 32.31. Spring plates are useful to control unstable anterior fragments. In some fracture patterns, a plate or multiple plates can be extended to the joint, and the circular fixator can be used as a bridging frame for 3 to 4 months (tensioned-wire fixation converted to external fixation with limited internal fixation). (Copyright © James J. Hutson, Jr., MD.)

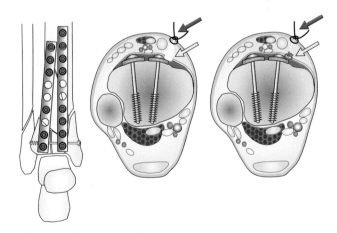

Figure 32.32. Internal fixation must be low profile. The retinaculum and capsule of the joint need to be closed (yellow arrow). If there is swelling and large plates, the skin will be closed over a hematoma, which will lead directly to the hardware and fracture. Early wound dehiscence and infection may result from this tenuous closure. (Copyright © James J. Hutson, Jr., MD.)

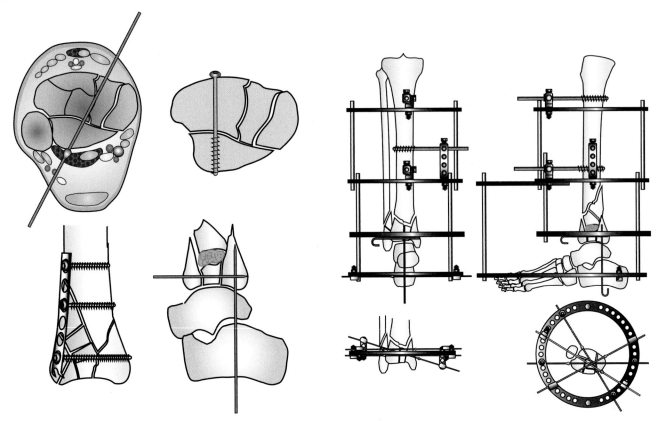

Figure 32.33. The posterior malleolus can be fixated with the following techniques: An olive wire is placed though the interval between the peroneal and Achilles tendon; an anterior to posterior screw is placed if the cortex is not comminuted anteriorly; an anterior buttress plate is placed and the posterior malleolus is lagged into the comminution; or a Steinman pin (0.062 or 0.094 in) can be drilled through the calcaneus and talus to pin the fragment to the dome and left in place for 6 weeks with the hind foot fixated by a distraction foot plate. The talar calcaneal pin is very useful to hold the initial reduction during limited open reduction. It is removed after screw fixation. (Copyright © James J. Hutson, Jr., MD.)

Figure 32.34. After the open reduction with limited internal fixation (the fixation only maintains the alignment of the joint), the carbon-fiber fracture-reduction ring is moved down the threaded rods and three to four olive wires are placed. The olive wires are positioned to reinforce the limited internal fixation. Two threaded rods are added anteriorly between the stable base and fracture reduction ring. A medial-face half pin is added to the stable base. (Copyright © James J. Hutson, Jr., MD.)

technique is that the fracture in this frame configuration requires 4 to 6 months to heal. Subtalar joint stiffness will occur and require prolonged physical therapy. Patients can walk with 50% weight with this frame in place. This is not possible with half pin cantilever frames. See Figures 32.36 and 32.37.

The initial step when using internal fixation of pilon fractures is reduction and fixation of the fibula (Fig. 32.38). Axial length on the lateral side of the pilon is reestablished. Fixation of the fibula to anatomic length requires that the plafond also must be reconstructed to anatomic length (Figs. 32.39 and 32.40). Slight shortening of the medial column will result in varus or a fibula plus mortise. If there is metaphyseal comminution, bone grafting is indicated to reconstruct the gap (Fig. 32.41). When using circular tensioned-wire fixation, the fixator distracts the fracture to length and fixation of the fibula becomes elective. Pilon fractures with moderate comminution are reconstructed to anatomic length, and the fibula should be aligned and fixated with a plate or an intramedullary pin (Fig. 32.42). If there is severe crushing, the surgeon has the option to shorten through the zone of comminution and compressing the fragments to encourage union (see Fig. 32.42). Patients with ischemic vascular disease, osteopenic bone, or diabetes can have salvage reconstruction with acute shortening. The tibial shaft can be compressed into the soft mushy bone, which is molded

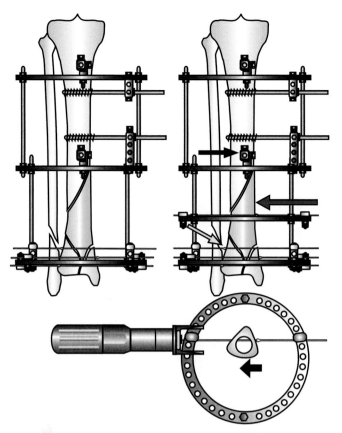

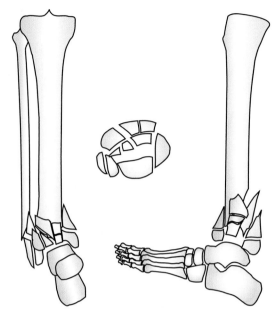

Figure 32.35. Working length ring. Pilon fractures can have proximal extension. A ring is placed in the fixator to place proximal wires or pins. The placement of this ring is determined during preoperative planning. In this example, a draw wire technique is used to compress (red arrow) the shaft. A half pin proximal (black arrow) and olive wire distal (yellow arrow) are placed to resist the force of the reduction. (Copyright © James J. Hutson, Jr., MD.)

Figure 32.36. C3 pilon fractures that have severe comminution will be encountered. The fragments are not amendable to tensioned wire or internal plating. (Copyright © James J. Hutson, Jr., MD.)

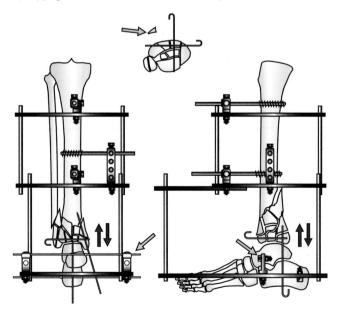

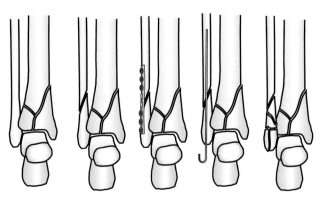

Figure 32.37. The circular fixator is applied as a distraction frame aligning the joint. A medial to lateral olive wire is placed through the talar neck to stabilize the hind foot in neutral plantar flexion. Small brad and free wires are used to align the crushed joint with the dome of the talus used as a mold. Once the joint is aligned, the talus is mildly shortened to improve bone contact of the fragments. (Copyright © James J. Hutson, Jr., MD.)

Figure 32.38. The lateral malleolus will have five possible configurations when pilon fractures are treated: intact, no fixation, plate fixation, intramedullary fixation, and comminuted. (Copyright © James J. Hutson, Jr., MD.)

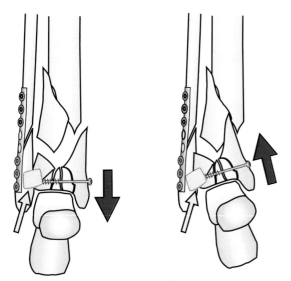

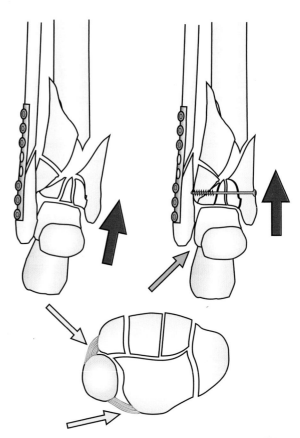

Figure 32.39. By plating the fibula to length, the surgeon must also reconstruct the plafond to length. If the plafond is not reconstructed and held distracted, a nonunion will occur. If the tibia-fibula ligaments (yellow arrow) are intact, the classic varus collapse will occur after frame removal. (Copyright © James J. Hutson, Jr., MD.)

Figure 32.40. If the fibula is plated and the tibia-fibula ligaments are disrupted (yellow arrow), the entire plafond can shorten, creating a fibula plus outcome where the lateral malleolus impinges on the calcaneus (green arrow). Both columns must always be reconstructed to the same length. (Copyright © James J. Hutson, Jr., MD.)

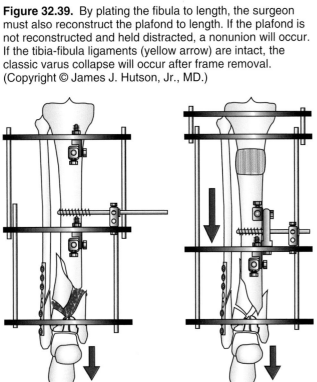

BONE GRAFTING   BONE TRANSPORT

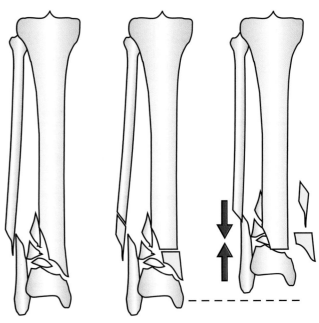

Figure 32.41. If the soft-tissue envelope is stable, metaphyseal bone loss and crushing is reconstructed with local bone graft. When soft tissue is compromised, bone loss is reconstructed with an intercalary bone transport. Living bone is transported into the zone of injury and new bone is created proximally away from the injury. (Copyright © James J. Hutson, Jr., MD.)

Figure 32.42. Acute bone shortening is a salvage technique to gain bone-on-bone contact in distal tibia fractures with bone loss and poor soft-tissue condition. The fracture ends are cut back as needed to allow stable bone-on-bone contact. The fibula also will have a bone resection so the columns are equal length. Acute shortening should not be greater than 2 to 3 cm. (Copyright © James J. Hutson, Jr., MD.)

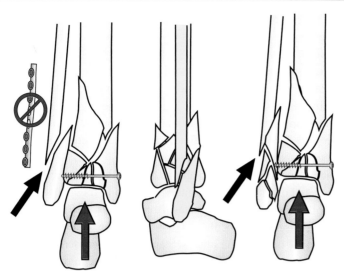

Figure 32.43. Oblique fractures without fixation can shorten but tend to displace (yellow). A lateral malleolus with comminution may shorten with less displacement. If the plafond is comminuted and mild shortening will be accepted, then oblique, lateral, malleolus fractures will need to have a section removed to allow shortening without fibular malalignment. (Copyright © James J. Hutson, Jr., MD.)

over the dome of the talus. Distortion of the lateral malleolus will occur with 2- to 3-cm of shortening (Fig. 32.43). This can be improved by removing a small segment of the fibula shaft to recreate a new mortise. This technique also improves soft-tissue coverage when patients have open wounds and are not candidates for free flaps. A proximal lengthening to equalize leg length is combined with shortening when patients have appropriate physiologic status (Fig. 32.44).

The technical sequence for C3 pilon fractures is as follows:

1. The stable base is applied to the midshaft with two AP half pins or universal mounting cubes. The base is orthogonal.

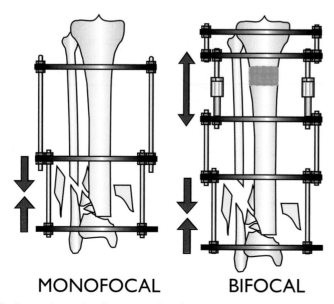

MONOFOCAL   BIFOCAL

Figure 32.44. Acute shortening is accepted as leg length in patients who are not candidates for lengthening. An elevated shoe is prescribed. A proximal corticotomy with lengthening is used to regain length in patients who are physiologically capable of bone transport. (Copyright © James J. Hutson, Jr., MD.)

2. A horizontal reference wire is placed in the calcaneus. The hind foot is aligned on the foot plate to center the dome of the talus with the axis of the tibia on AP and lateral fluoroscopic images.

3. The fracture is distracted. If the fracture can be reconstructed to length, the fibula is fixated with a plate or pin. When shortening of the comminuted metaphysis will be used to facilitate healing, the fibula is not fixated.

4. Distraction may produce anatomic alignment of the joint surface. Percutaneous screws and pins are placed to fixate the plafond. Percutaneous screws are also used to align proximal metaphyseal and shaft fragments.

5. If distraction does not produce acceptable reduction, the fracture is approached through the anterior medial or anterior lateral interval. The joint fragments are reduced and fixated with small screws, wires, and plates. Bone graft is used to support crushed fragments. The deep fascia and reticulum is closed over the ankle joint. The skin is closed with interrupted 3-0 or 2-0 nylon sutures. Staples are never used for pilon fractures. Surgical wounds after open reduction of pilon fractures can require 3 to 4 weeks before the sutures can be removed.

6. The carbon-fiber fracture ring is moved over the metaphysis, and at least three opposed divergent olive wires are placed. An opposed olive wire is added to the foot fixation.

7. Olive wires will not be placed at the metaphysis when one of two fracture patterns are presented: (a) The comminution is so severe that there are literally no fragments large enough for fixation, or (b) the technique of bridging distraction with limited internal fixation will be accepted as the definitive technique. The foot fixation will add a second opposed olive wire in the calcaneus and a medial to lateral talar-neck wire.

8. A medial-face half pin is placed on the stable base.

9. A bulky compressive dressing is placed around the ankle.

POSTOPERATIVE CARE

Maintenance of the pin/wire interface with the skin is essential to reduce inflammation and subsequent pin/wire infections. Once the surgical wounds are healed, the leg is washed in the shower with soap, removing all blood and secretions where the pin/wire enters the skin. Skin that is tenting over wires is released under local anesthesia. Gauze sponges are applied to skin that is over wires and develops inflammation. Oral antibiotics (cephalexin, tetracycline, ciprofloxacin hydrochloride, and trimethoprim-sulfa methoxazole) are prescribed if inflammation worsens. Rarely, a patient will have purulent drainage and require wire removal and intravenous antibiotics.

Depending on the frame configuration, active-assisted range of motion of the ankle and hind foot, or/and forefoot and toe therapy is started. The patients are encouraged to place partial weight on the leg using a sandal and increase weight as tolerated. Patients should be placing 50% weight by the sixth week and some will be on their full weight before frame removal.

If the patient had bridging distraction with wire fixation through the plafond/metaphysis, the foot plate and calcaneal wires are removed in clinic 4 to 6 weeks after surgery. If the patient had bridging distraction without wire fixation, the frame has to be maintained for at least 4 to 6 months (the significant drawback of this technique).

Frame removal is indicated when callus has bridged the multiple fragments and the patient can place 50% or more of his/her weight on the extremity. If the patient is not bearing weight at 3 to 4 months, the fracture is not united. Average frame time is 4 to 6 months for pilon fractures (Fig. 32.45). A local bone graft is indicated if there is no callus formation after 3 to 4 months. Outpatient frame removal with deep monitored sedation or general anesthesia is recommended. The ankle is casted for 2 weeks and the patient is encouraged to bear full weight in the cast. The cast is removed in the office and a hinged ankle orthosis is placed,

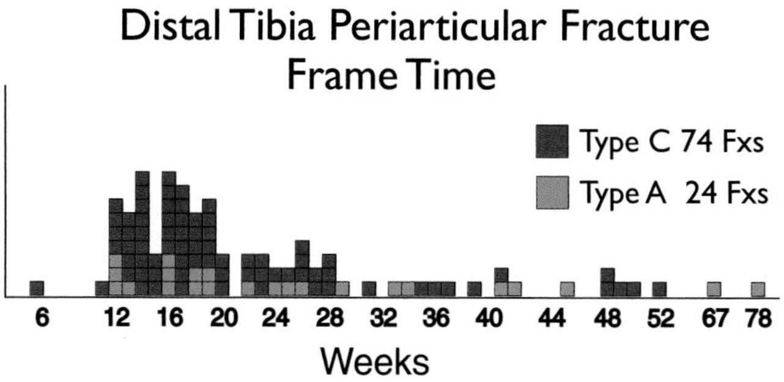

Figure 32.45. Frame removal time on 98 distal tibia type A and C fractures (F × s). Most fractures heal between 3 and 6 months. More complex fractures may need additional reconstructive procedures and may require many more months in the fixator. (Copyright © James J. Hutson, Jr., MD.)

which the patient uses until mature callus is observed at the fracture site. Physical therapy continues for an additional 6 months if funds are available. The functional result at 1 year postinjury will be the extent of recovery.

RECOMMENDED READINGS

1. Watson JT, Moed BR, Karges DE, Cramer KE. Pilon fracture treatment protocol based on severity of soft tissue injury. *Clin Orthop* 2000;375:78–90.
2. Pollak AN, McCarthy ML, Shay BR, Agel J, Swiontkowski MF. Outcomes after treatment of high-energy tibial plafond fractures. *J Bone and Joint Surg Am* 2003;85A:1893–1900.
3. Vora AM, Haddad SL, Kadakia A, Lazarus ML, Merk BR. Extracapsular placement of distal tibia transfixation wires. *J Bone and Joint Surg Am* 2004;86A:988–993.
4. De Coster TA, Stevens MS, Robinson B. Safe extracapsular placement of proximal and distal tibial external fixation pins. Poster Presented at: The Annual Meeting of The Orthopedic Trauma Association; 1997.
5. Watson JT. Tibial pilon fractures. *Tech Ortho* 1996;11:150–159.

33

Ankle Fractures: Open Reduction Internal Fixation

David J. Hak and Mark A. Lee

INDICATIONS/CONTRAINDICATIONS

Ankle fractures are among the most common orthopedic injuries. Nondisplaced fractures can almost always be successfully treated nonoperatively with close follow-up. Most displaced bimalleolar fractures benefit from operative reduction and fixation if no surgical contraindications exist.

Certain displaced-ankle fractures can be treated with closed reduction, and if successful, carefully followed to union with nonoperative treatment. Isolated, distal, fibula fractures without mortise widening or talar shift can usually be successfully managed nonoperatively if the fibular displacement is less than 2 mm. These patients must be differentiated from individuals who also have an obvious or occult injury to the medial side of the ankle. While the decision for operative versus nonoperative treatment is frequently clear, for a group of patients, the treatment decision is more difficult; for these patients, reduction may be borderline acceptable or follow-up x-rays suggest some loss of reduction.

Two classification systems of ankle fractures are commonly used. Lauge-Hansen described a classification based on the foot position (supination or pronation) at the time of injury and the direction of the injury force (external rotation, adduction, or abduction) on the foot (Fig. 33.1). The Danis-Weber classification is based on the location of the fibula fracture with respect to the ankle joint. In Danis-Weber injuries, the fibula fracture is distal to the ankle joint and is usually the equivalent to Lauge-Hansen supination-adduction injuries. In Danis-Weber B injuries, the fibula fracture is at the level of the ankle joint and can be either a supination–external rotation or pronation-abduction injury. Type C Danis-Weber fractures are characterized by a fibula fracture proximal to the ankle joint and are usually the equivalent of the Lauge-Hansen pronation–external rotation injury.

Supination–external rotation injuries are thought to be the most common fracture pattern. In this injury, the supinated foot is subjected to an external rotation force that may cause a varying degree of soft-tissue and bony damage. The first structure to be injured is the anterior tibiofibular ligament (stage I). As the external rotation force continues, the

DANIS-WEBER

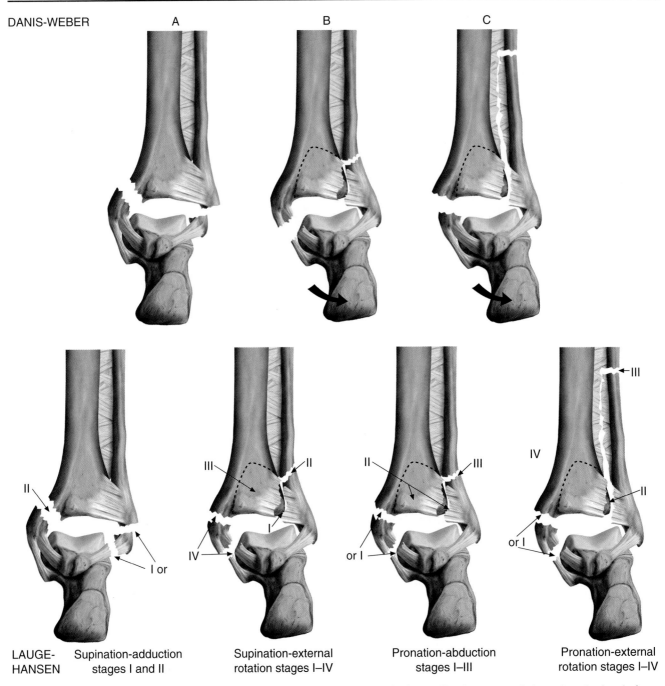

Figure 33.1. The Danis-Weber (AO/ASIF) classification system is based on the level of the fibula fracture. The Lauge-Hansen system is based on experimentally verified injury mechanisms. Type A Danis-Weber injuries are usually Lauge-Hansen supination-adduction injuries. Type B can be either supination–external rotation or pronation-abduction injuries. Type C injuries are usually pronation–external rotation injuries.

fibula is fractured (stage II). Further force results in rupture of the posterior tibiofibular ligament or a fracture of the posterior malleolus (stage III). Finally, the deltoid ligament is ruptured or the medial malleolus is fractured (stage IV). Because of their clinical significance, stage II injuries must be differentiated from stage IV supination–external rotation injuries. Stage II injuries can be managed nonoperatively because the deltoid ligament is intact, stabilizing the talus in the mortise. However, in stage IV injuries, the ankle is unstable, and surgical management is usually recommended (1).

Traditionally, medial ecchymosis and tenderness when the ankle is palpated have been used as clinical indicators for occult injury to the medial deltoid ligament. Recent studies have shown that these traditional signs are not sensitive for predicting deltoid ligament incompetence (1,2). Stress radiographs should routinely be obtained in patients with isolated fibula fractures that are classified as supination–external rotation injuries (Danis-Weber type B) so the physician can identify occult injury to the deltoid ligament. Several different methods for obtaining stress radiographs have been described and include the use of gravity, valgus stress, or external rotation (2,3).

We prefer a careful evaluation of high-quality plain x-rays in the absence of plaster, which may obscure important findings. Occasionally, contralateral radiographs are useful to evaluate unusual abnormalities. The physician must understand the normal radiographic landmarks and relationship of the fibula with the distal tibia. Equal medial, lateral, and superior joint space should be seen surrounding the talus on the mortise view. The position of the distal fibula with respect to the incisura should be carefully evaluated. This is measured 1 cm proximal to the tibial plafond. Specific measurements may vary depending on the ankle rotation and angle of the x-ray beam. The distance between the medial border of the fibula and the incisura should be less than 6 mm on both the anteroposterior (AP) and mortise view. On the AP view, the fibula should overlap the tibia by 6 mm, or 42 % of the fibular width, and there should be at least 1 mm of overlap between the fibula and tibia on the mortise view. Finally, the length of the fibula is assessed by evaluating the talocrural angle, which on average should measure 83 ±4 degrees and can be compared with the contralateral ankle (Fig. 33.2). In addition, fibular shortening will lead to incongruity in a line drawn along the tibial plafond and the medial border of the distal fibula (Fig. 33.3).

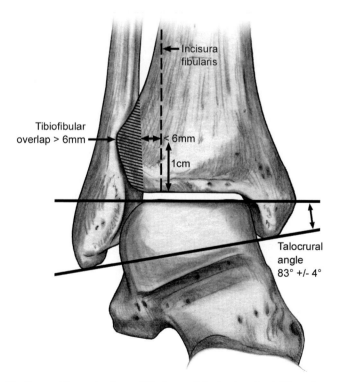

Figure 33.2. Radiographic projection of fibula on tibia in standard AP radiograph. When measured 1-cm proximal to the ankle joint, the distance between the medial border of the fibula and the incisura should be less than 6 mm on any view. On the AP view, the fibula should generally overlap the tibia (*shaded area*) by greater than 6 mm or more than 42% of the fibular width; however, individual variation and beam angle may effect individual measurements. There should be more than 1 mm of overlap of the tibia and fibula on any view.

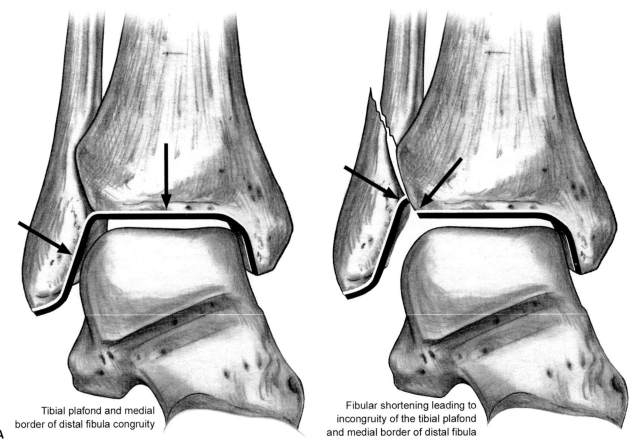

Tibial plafond and medial
border of distal fibula congruity

A

Fibular shortening leading to
incongruity of the tibial plafond
and medial border of distal fibula

B

Figure 33.3. Normally, there is congruity in a line drawn along the tibial plafond and the medial border of the fibula. When the fibula is shorted, incongruity is observed at the junction of the tibia and fibula.

One of the major goals of ankle fracture management, whether operative or nonoperative, is to maintain anatomic reduction of the tibiotalar joint. Lateral displacement of the talus will reduce ankle joint contact, resulting in joint-contact stress alterations that may predispose the patient to posttraumatic osteoarthritis (4–6).

Closed reduction and splinting are the first step in fracture management. The majority of rotational ankle fractures will require little more than longitudinal traction and internal rotation reduction to be achieved. A well-padded, posterior, plaster splint with the ankle at neutral dorsiflexion will provide comfort and immobilization and allow for soft-tissue swelling. In general, immediate circumferential casting should be avoided, even if this is eventually chosen as the definitive treatment method, as ongoing swelling can lead to dangerous constriction and exacerbation of the soft-tissue injury. Edema control with judicious elevation is a well-accepted approach to early management if compromised vascular inflow is not an issue. Cryotherapy may reduce swelling and may have analgesic benefit. More recently, intermittent compression devices have been utilized to help control swelling both preoperatively and postoperatively (7,8).

Occasionally, when managing fractures with significant soft-tissue injuries or those with large, posterior, malleolar fractures that cause persistent talar subluxation, the surgeon may find that temporary external fixation is required. External fixation provides fracture and soft-tissue stability, allows for free access and easy evaluation of the soft tissues, and optimizes patient mobilization.

Many ankle fractures requiring open reduction and internal fixation can be addressed with immediate surgery. However if soft-tissue swelling is a concern, the operation is delayed and the limb is immobilized and elevated. Examination of the skin should be performed preoperatively to insure that the soft tissues can safely permit operative treatment. This requires removal of the splint or cast prior to the induction of anesthesia. The "wrinkle sign" is often used to assess the readiness of soft tissues for surgical intervention. The ankle is dorsiflexed to the neutral position and the anterior ankle skin is observed for the presence of wrinkles. Absence of wrinkles suggests excessive soft-tissue swelling and edema.

PREOPERATIVE PLANNING

While open reduction and internal fixation (ORIF) of most ankle fractures is straightforward, care should be exercised to avoid unexpected findings. A careful review of high-quality plain radiographs (without obscuring plaster) should be performed. A preoperative plan or surgical tactic, while often neglected for this "simple" fracture, may provide mental preparation and avoid unnecessary mistakes. Forging ahead, assuming the case is a simple straightforward ankle fracture, can lead to suboptimal outcomes when unusual fracture variations are encountered.

SURGERY

Patient Positioning

Patients are generally positioned supine, and a general or spinal anesthetic is administered. Prophylactic intravenous antibiotics are administered prior to surgery. A first-generation cephalosporin is used unless there is an allergic contraindication, in which case an alternative antibiotic is chosen. A towel roll is placed beneath the ipsilateral buttock to provide easier access to the fibula (Fig. 33.4). As is routine, a pneumatic tourniquet is applied to the upper thigh. The leg is sterilely prepped. A sterile sheet is then placed beneath the leg to prevent inadvertent contamination of surgical gowns during the draping process. A stockinette is applied to the leg, and the leg is draped free. The toes are sealed with a plastic adhesive drape and the stockinette is removed to the midcalf.

Prone positioning may occasionally be indicated for trimalleolar ankle fractures with a large, displaced, posterior, malleolar fragment that will be fixed through a posterolateral approach. Reduction and fixation of the medial malleolus in the prone position may be easiest performed after the knee is flexed.

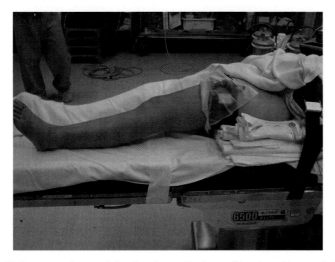

Figure 33.4. Before prepping and draping the patient, a roll is placed beneath the ipsilateral buttock to facilitate easier access to the fibula. A tourniquet and occlusive drape may be placed around the upper thigh.

Technique

Bony landmarks are palpated and marked. The location of the fracture can also be marked based on palpation and radiographic review. We generally perform surgery under tourniquet control to minimize blood loss, to maximize visualization, and to speed the surgical procedure. After confirming that preoperative prophylactic antibiotics have been administered, we exsanguinate the extremity with an elastic (Esmarch) bandage and inflate the tourniquet to the appropriate level.

In bimalleolar fractures, the surgeon's preference dictates whether the medial malleolus or the fibula is fixed first. In cases of osteopenia, we prefer to fix the medial malleolus first because it may aid the subsequent reduction of the fibula. Care must be exercised when using reduction clamps on osteopenic bone. Excessive pressure with reduction clamps may easily cause iatrogenic comminution of the fibula. In addition, the ankle joint can usually be visualized through the medial malleolar fracture site in most circumstances. This allows inspection of the articular surface and removal of any intra-articular debris. While joint inspection and irrigation can be performed either before or after fixation of the fibula, we often do this prior to rigid fixation of the fibula.

Medial Malleolar Fixation. Our preferred medial incision is straight and aligned with the long axis of the tibia. This incision should also be placed slightly anterior to the midcoronal axis to allow inspection of the anterior aspect of the ankle joint. Other surgeons prefer a slightly angled incision, but too much, distal, anterior angulation may make difficult the access to the screw insertion site. The saphenous vein and its accompanying saphenous nerve branches should be preserved whenever possible (Fig. 33.5).

Adequate exposure is required to ensure an anatomic reduction. This can best be confirmed by visualizing the anterior aspect of the fracture. Because of the orientation of the fracture plane, anterior or posterior malreduction may not always be appreciated when looking at the lateral surface.

Distal retraction of the medial malleolus allows irrigation and thorough inspection of the articular surface of the tibia and talus (Fig. 33.6). Any osteocartilaginous debris should be removed. Articular damage to either the tibia or talus should be noted in the operative report.

Approximately 2 mm of periosteum is excised along the edges of the fracture. A 2.5-mm drill is used to perforate the medial tibial cortex to allow anchorage of a bone tenaculum. A small, pointed, bone tenaculum can be placed on the medial malleolar-fracture fragment from anterior to posterior and used to guide the reduction. A second small or large, pointed, bone tenaculum is then used to achieve compression of the reduction. One tine is placed in the tibial metaphyseal drill hole and the other is placed around the distal aspect of the medial malleolus. (Fig. 33.7).

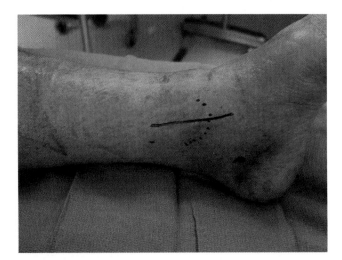

Figure 33.5. A relatively straight incision is used for the medial malleolus. Excessive, distal, anterior angulation may interfere with the necessary screw-insertion angle. The saphenous vein and nerve should be visualized and protected during the medial approach to the ankle.

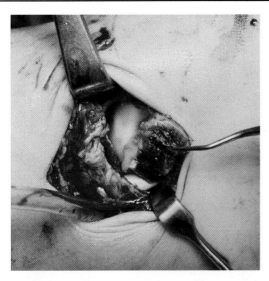

Figure 33.6. Retraction of the medial malleolar fragment distally allows inspection and irrigation of the ankle joint.

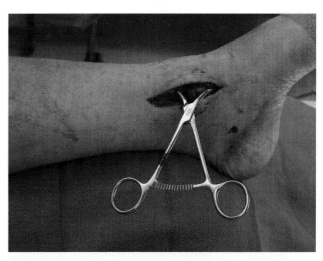

Figure 33.7. A pointed reduction tenaculum is used to provide provisional reduction of the medial malleolus. One tine is placed in a drill hole placed in the medial tibial metaphysis and the other tine is placed around the distal aspect of the medial malleolus. Partially threaded, cancellous, lag screws are inserted anterior and posterior to the tenaculum.

Large, one-piece, medial, malleolar fractures are usually secured with two 4.0-mm, partially threaded, cancellous screws. With the tenaculum centered on the fragment, one screw is placed anteriorly and one is placed posteriorly to the tenaculum. A scalpel is used to split the superficial deltoid ligament in line with the fibers to facilitate placement of the drill against bone. With the hind foot slightly everted, a 2.5-mm drill bit is then drilled across the fracture site in line with the long axis of the tibia. A second drill bit or Kirschner (K) wire may be placed to avoid rotational forces during the screw insertion. We routinely use a 40-mm cancellous screw because the nonthreaded portion is usually long enough so that the threads are positioned beyond the fracture site and engage the denser, distal-tibial, cancellous bone. For optimal results, the threads should be placed in the denser distal-tibial metaphysis, especially in patients with osteoporosis. A second 4.0-mm cancellous screw is then inserted parallel to the first screw.

The surgeon must match the implant size to the fracture fragment size to avoid iatrogenic comminution and malreduction. The use of 4.0-mm cancellous screws may not be advisable if the medial malleolus-fracture fragment is very small or comminuted. Other options for small-fragment fixation include the use of a single lag screw with a K wire, small diameter screws, or tension band wiring. Extra-long 2.0- and 2.7-mm screws are available; although they may not be stocked on standard sets, they are useful for very small medial-malleolar fragments. Tension band fixation is performed by inserting 1.6-mm K wires in a direction similar to the standard screw fixation. Eighteen-gauge wire or no. 5 suture is then passed around the K wires and crossed in figure-of-eight fashion around a screw placed in the tibial metaphysis. The ends of the K wires are then bent and impacted.

Vertical malleolar fractures, as occur in supination-adduction type injuries should be fixed either with horizontal screws (placed at right angles to the fracture) or with a short, low-profile, medial, buttress plate. Washers may be required in osteoporotic patients to prevent the screw from sinking through the thin metaphyseal cortex. This fracture pattern may also be associated with marginal impaction of the tibial plafond. Reduction of the tibial plafond and support with bone graft or bone graft substitute may be required prior to medial malleolar reduction (Fig. 33.8).

Fibular Fixation. The fibular incision is based on the location of the fracture and the planned position of fixation. Adjustments may be needed due to associated soft-tissue abrasions or healed blisters. The fibula is generally approached through a relatively straight

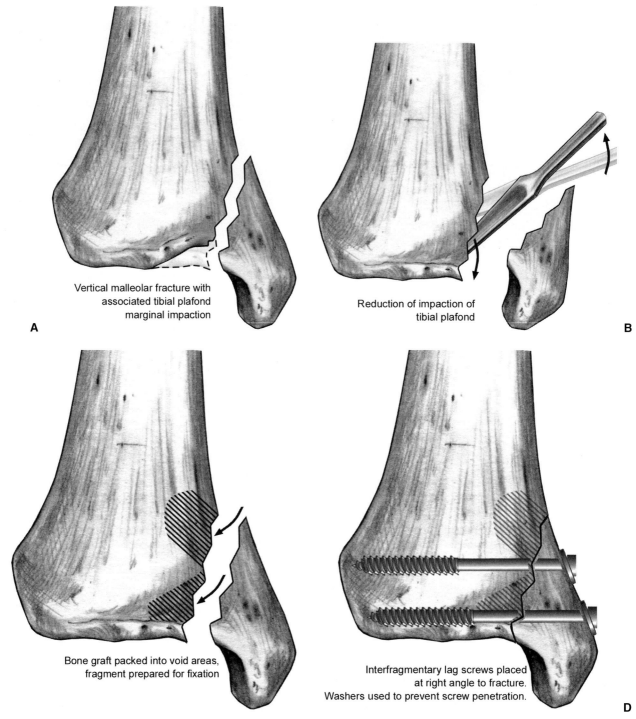

Figure 33.8. Impaction of the medial, distal, tibial-articular surface may be seen in supination-adduction injuries. Following reduction, this segment may be buttressed with either local metaphyseal bone, allograft bone, or bone graft substitutes. Because of the vertical orientation of the fracture plane, the interfragmentary lag screws are usually placed parallel to the ankle joint.

incision (Fig. 33.9). Angling the distal portion of this incision slightly anteriorly will allow access to the anterolateral corner of the ankle. This will allow access to the anterolateral aspect of the ankle joint and permit fixation of a Chaput-Tillaux fragment, which is an avulsion of the anterior, inferior, tibiofibular ligament. A more posterior incision may be used if a posterior antiglide plate is planned. Care should be taken to preserve the

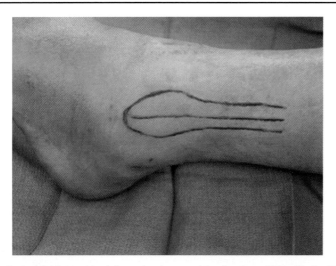

Figure 33.9. A straight lateral incision may be used for fixation of the fibula. The incision may be adjusted anteriorly or posteriorly depending on the fracture patterns and the planned fixation.

superficial peroneal nerve, which may cross the surgical approach at a subcutaneous or fascial level, to avoid painful neuroma formation.

The periosteum at the edges of the fracture should be elevated, but further periosteal stripping is kept to a minimum, especially in comminuted fractures. Care must be exercised when reducing the fibular fracture to avoid iatrogenic comminution. This precaution is especially critical in older patients with osteoporosis. Fracture reduction can be achieved by using one or more of the following techniques: Traction and rotation can be applied to the hind foot to assist with fracture reduction; a bone tenaculum may be attached to the distal fragment and used to manually reduce the distal fragment; the tines of a bone tenaculum may be placed at right angles to the fracture plane and used to obtain and secure the fracture reduction. Fracture reduction is usually fairly easy immediately after injury but may be more difficult in delayed cases with fibular shortening.

Simple, oblique, fibula fractures are usually reduced and fixed with an interfragmentary lag screw and a neutralization plate. Occasionally, long oblique fractures can be adequately fixed with only interfragmentary lag screws (9). While we usually use a 3.5-mm cortical screw for the lag screw fixation, in smaller fragments it is occasionally advantageous to use a smaller diameter screw, such as a 2.7-mm or 2.0-mm cortical screw (Fig. 33.10).

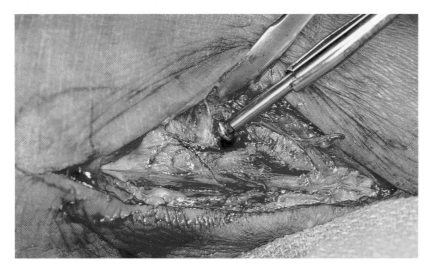

Figure 33.10. For oblique fibular fractures, a 3.5-mm cortical screw is placed in lag fashion perpendicular to the fracture plane.

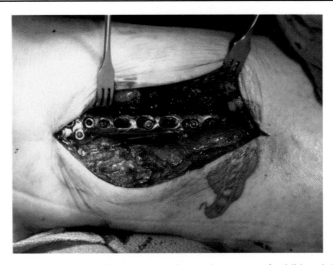

Figure 33.11. This fibular peri-articular plate allows placement of additional distal-screw fixation, which may be particularly useful for obtaining additional screw fixation in very distal fractures.

For comminuted fibular fractures in which lag screw fixation is not feasible, plate fixation is applied in a bridging mode such that the comminuted fracture area is bypassed. For many fractures, simple one-third tibular plates are adequate, but for very distal fractures we prefer to use a bone-specific, custom, fibula plate (Zimmer, Warsaw, IN) that allows a larger number of distal screws (Fig. 33.11). As an alternative approach, a small-fragment locking plate could also be used to provide improved fixation stability in a small, distal, fracture fragment. When no bony keys are available to determine reduction, the distal fragment may be reduced to the talus provisionally with K wires. After visual and radiographic confirmation of the reduction, the surgeon can apply a plate in a bridging mode.

We usually examine and irrigate the ankle joint through the medial incision. However, in selected circumstances, visualization of the anterior ankle joint can also be performed by dissecting anterior to the fibular and retracting the soft tissues with a small right-ankle retractor (Fig. 33.12). This exposure may also be used to reduce and internally fix avulsion fractures involving the anterior tibiofibular ligament (Chaput-Tillaux fragments).

Soft tissues are handled as gently as possible throughout the procedure, especially during wound closure when excessive skin-edge manipulation with forceps can traumatize the tissue. We typically close incisions in an interrupted fashion with no. 3-0 or 4-0 nylon

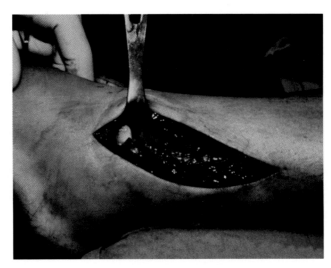

Figure 33.12. Exposure of the anterolateral ankle joint may be performed by dissecting anterior to the fibula and retracting soft tissues with a small right-angle retractor.

sutures via an Allgöwer-Donnatti technique. Because of the limited deep tissue, a two-layer closure is usually not feasible; however, deep absorbable sutures may help align the incision and relieve tension for the skin closure.

Posterior Malleolus Fixation. Clinical studies have shown that ankle fractures with posterior malleolar involvement have a higher incidence of posttraumatic osteoarthritis than do bimalleolar ankle fractures. Simulated, posterior, malleolar fractures have shown a modest increase in ankle contact stresses in static mechanical-loading studies. Development of arthrosis may also be due to associated chondral damage and joint instability. Rather than significantly increasing contact joint stress, a pronounced anterior shift in the location of the articular contact area was found in a recent study in which dynamic ankle motion was examined in a simulated, posterior, malleolus fracture (4). The authors postulated that this shift in location produced substantial loading of articular cartilage not accustomed to bearing stress and thus initiated the arthrosis.

Posterior, malleolar, fracture fragments may vary greatly in their size. Small fragments are often extra-articular. These small fragments are attached to the posterior, inferior, tibiofibular ligament and are usually adequately reduced with anatomic reduction of the fibula. However, larger, posterior, malleolar fragments may comprise a significant portion of the articular surface, and anatomic reduction is probably essential for good long-term function.

Evaluation of posterior, malleolar, fracture-fragment size is limited with plain radiographs and is better evaluated with a computed tomography (CT) scan (10). If a CT scan is unavailable, then a 50-degree external-rotation view may better allow assessment of the posterior fragment size (11,12).

The decision that the posterior malleolus needs to be fixed should ideally be made preoperatively based on the size of the fragment. Most authors recommend fixation of posterior malleolar fractures that comprise more than 25% of the articular surface. Closed reduction with dorsiflexion of the ankle and percutaneous anterior-to-posterior fixation has been described as an alternative treatment for nondisplaced or minimally displaced, posterior, malleolar fractures. However, the accuracy of this method may not always result in an anatomic position. Our preference for treatment of large, posterior, malleolar fractures requiring fixation is to reduce and stabilize these fractures prior to fixation of the fibula because the application of a plate on the fibula usually obscures lateral radiographic visualization of the articular surface. A large pointed tenaculum may be inserted posteriorly through the fibular incision. A small incision is made over the anterior tibia and blunt dissection carried down to the bone to allow placement of the anterior tine (Fig. 33.13). Minor manipulation of the fragment can be achieved with dorsiflexion of the ankle and

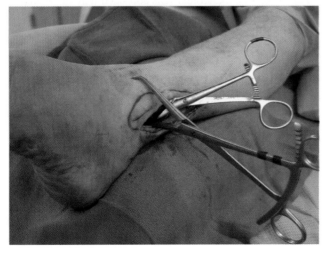

Figure 33.13. A large bone tenaculum is placed around the fibula and can be used to manipulate and reduce the posterior malleolus. The small tenaculum in this photo is maintaining reduction of the fibula fracture.

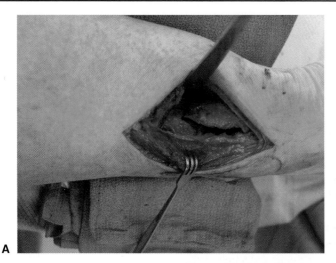

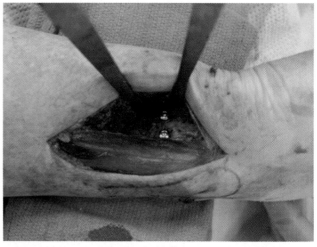

A   B

Figure 33.14. **A.** This large, posterior, malleolus fragment was exposed through a posterolateral approach along the lateral border of the Achilles tendon. **B.** Following direct
reduction of the fracture fragment, posterior-to-anterior lag-screw fixation with 4.0-mm
cancellous screws and washers. After posterior malleolus fixation, fibula fixation can be
achieved using a posteriorly placed antiglide plate.

rotational torque of the tenaculum. Anterior to posterior fixation of the fragment is then
achieved with either standard screws or cannulated screws placed through one or more
percutaneous incisions.

For large, noncomminuted, posterior, malleolar fragments, fixation may be achieved
through an open posterior approach. The patient is positioned prone and a posterolateral
approach to the fragment is performed along the lateral border of the Achilles tendon
(Fig. 33.14). This allows accurate fragment reduction via visualization of the fragment at
the posterior tibial metaphysis. The fracture fragment is internally fixed with two or three
posterior-to-anterior screws. Washers are often used to prevent penetration of the screw
heads through the thin tibial cortex. In an alternative, a short, two- or three-hole, one-third,
tubular plate may be applied in an antiglide mode to the posterior tibia.

For fractures in which the posterior malleolus is more medially based, or in which there
is metaphyseal cortical comminution that may not provide an adequate reduction key,
reduction of the posterior malleolar fragment may be obtained through the medial approach
prior to reduction of the medial malleolus. This approach will allow direct visualization of
the articular surface. The flexor tendons are retracted posteriorly with a small Homan
retractor, and a small bone hook or pointed tenaculum is used to obtain fragment reduction.
Fixation is then achieved with anterior-to-posterior lag screws inserted through small stab
incisions.

Syndesmotic Assessment and Fixation. Disruption of the tibiofibular syndesmosis may occur with type-C ankle fractures; however, transsyndesmotic fixation may not be
required in all cases. Anatomic reduction and stable fracture fixation may restore adequate
syndesmotic stability. More distal fibula fractures secured with rigid plate fixation may
offer sufficient stability to obviate the need for transsyndesmotic fixation (13,14). If the
deep deltoid ligament is intact, rigid fixation of the medial malleolus will also provide an
additional stabilizing force that prevents talar subluxation.

Regardless of the location of the fibula fracture and the rigidity of the fracture fixation,
we recommend careful assessment of the syndesmosis in all ankle fractures. Traditionally,
syndesmotic stability in ankle fractures has been assessed by pulling the fibula laterally in
the coronal plane either with a clamp or bone hook (i.e., the "Hook test"). The distal
tibiofibular syndesmosis consists of the anterior tibiofibular, posterior tibiofibular, and the
interosseous ligaments. Additional stability is provided by the interosseous membrane and
the medial deltoid ligament, both of which may have been injured to varying degrees.

Rather than pulling the fibula laterally, we recommend stressing the fibula anteriorly and posteriorly in the sagittal plane. Disruption of the syndesmosis will produce significant instability of the fibula that may be best appreciated in the sagittal plane. The improved sensitivity of this testing method was recently described in a cadaveric study (15).

Several areas of controversy are contended in syndesmotic fracture fixation. These issues include screw diameter, number of screws, number of cortices engaged, timing of weight bearing, and the need and timing of screw removal.

We prefer to use a large-fragment 4.5-mm screw for syndesmotic fixation because of its increased strength and its ease of removal. However, it requires availability of an additional implant set. The larger head can be easily palpated at the time of removal and there is no risk of incorrectly removing one of the small-fragment screws. We generally engage only three cortices except in cases of severe osteopenia, in which case it may be advantageous to place a screw across the far tibial cortex to improve purchase. The use of three cortices allows some angular freedom of the screw and may prevent mechanical screw fracture. Except in cases of very proximal fibular fractures (Maissoneuve injury), we only use a single syndesmotic screw. We generally allow patients to weight bear on their syndesmotic screws after 6 weeks and plan removal of the syndesmotic screw at 3 months. This can usually been done in the office under local anesthesia.

Steps we use during placement of syndesmotic screws include the following:

1. Elevate the heel on a towel roll to allow the surgeon room to position the drill to direct the screw correctly. Because the fibula is located at the posterior border of the tibia, syndesmotic screws should be angled anteriorly approximately 30 degrees from the coronal axis.

2. Position the ankle in neutral dorsiflexion. Because the talar dome is wider anteriorly than posteriorly, fixation with the ankle plantarflexed may, in theory, overtighten the mortise.

3. Reduce the syndesmosis. The syndesmotic reduction can usually be held manually with light pressure, although temporary K-wire fixation may also be used. Caution should be exercised in using any type of clamp because if the clamp is not perfectly centered its use may create unappreciated malrotation or translation of the fibula.

4. A 3.2-mm drill hole is made approximately 2 cm above the ankle joint. This should be parallel to the ankle joint and directed anteriorly approximately 30 degrees (Fig. 33.15).

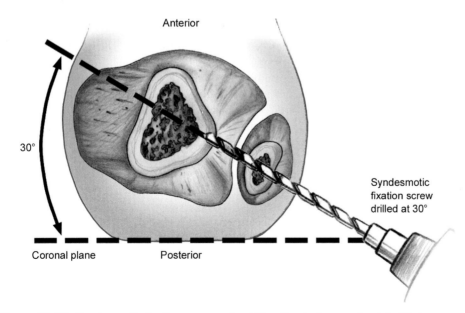

Figure 33.15. Syndesmotic fixation screws should be directed approximately 30 degrees anterior to the coronal plane.

We drill through the opposite cortex and measure the total length with a depth gauge. In most cases, we choose a screw approximately 1 cm shorter than the measured length so the far cortex is not engaged. In cases of severe osteopenia, we choose to engage the far cortex. The fibula and near cortex is then tapped with a 4.5-mm tap and the screw is inserted. Accurate reduction is then confirmed with bi-planar fluoroscopic views of plain radiographs.

In Maissoneuve fractures in which the proximal fibular fracture is not internally fixed, we manually reduce the syndesmosis and secure it provisionally with one or more K wires. After the reduction is confirmed with bi-planar fluoroscopic imaging, we place two 4.5-mm screws as described above.

Postoperative X-Rays. We carefully scrutinize all postoperative ankle x-rays. In addition to evaluation of fracture reduction and hardware position, we look for radiographic parameters of anatomic syndesmotic reduction. With the AP and mortise views, we verify adequate tibiofibular overlap. We also examine the position of the fibula with respect to the incisura. While specific measurements may vary based on the x-ray beam ankle, on the AP view the fibula and tibia should overlap by at least 6 mm, and the distance between the medial border of the fibula and the incisura should be less than 6 mm on any view. Equivocal findings merit comparison to the contralateral-ankle stress radiographs. If there are equivocal findings following syndesmotic ORIF, then we recommend CT to evaluate proper position of the fibula within the tibial incisura. Finally the length of the fibula is assessed by evaluating the talocrural angle, which on average should measure 83 ($\pm$4) degrees (see Fig. 33.2).

RESULTS

In a study of 20 patients with unstable ankle fractures who underwent ORIF, significant improvements in all domains of the SF-36 Health Survey, except for general health, were seen between 4 and 20 months after the operation. However, after 20 months their physical functioning scores remained below those of the US population norm (16).

Similar findings were reported in another study of 30 patients undergoing operative treatment of displaced Danis-Weber type-B ankle fractures. At 24 months, the authors noted significantly lower SF-36 physical function and role physical scores compared to the US norms (17).

POSTOPERATIVE MANAGEMENT

A nonadherent dressing and sterile gauze pads are applied to the wounds and held in position with sterile cast padding. With the ankle held in neutral dorsiflexion, additional cast padding is applied followed by a short-leg, posterior, stirrup splint. The splint is maintained until the patient can comfortably dorsiflex the injured ankle and thus prevent equinus contracture. The leg is elevated postoperatively to minimize swelling. Patients with sufficient home-care assistance may be discharged directly home, but many patients require overnight observation.

Patients are seen in follow-up appointments between 7 and 14 days after surgery. The splint is removed and if adequate wound healing is evident, the sutures are removed. Radiographs are checked to confirm maintenance of reduction. Reliable patients are instructed in active ankle and subtalar range-of-motion exercises. Patients are placed in a removable short-leg orthotic.

We generally restrict weight bearing for 6 weeks postoperatively. Repeat x-rays are obtained at 6 weeks, and patient weight bearing is advanced at this time. If necessary, physical therapy is initiated to assist with regaining range of motion, proprioception, and strengthening.

Persistent dependent swelling may persist for many months and may require use of compression stockings or elastic wraps. Patients are cautioned against returning to sports until they have regained adequate strength and agility. Return to driving is left to the patient's judgment, although a recent study has shown that simulated braking time returned to normal at 9 weeks following internal fixation (1).

COMPLICATIONS

Some preventable complications are due to a failure to appreciate initially the complexity of the ankle fracture pattern. While many ankle fractures are simple standard fractures that can be easily fixed with anticipation of an excellent outcome, other fractures will be more complex and anatomic reduction may be difficult. The physician's failure to appreciate the size of a posterior malleolar fragment, the presence of articular impaction, or intraarticular fragments will likely predispose the patient to a suboptimal outcome (18).

Stiffness

Loss of motion, especially dorsiflexion, can be problematic following ankle fracture. If independent range-of-motion exercises and stretching is not rapidly successful in restoring a functional range of motion, early referral should be made to physical therapy. Rarely, a posterior, soft-tissue, capsular release along with lengthening of the Achilles and other flexor tendons may be indicated to improve severely restricted ankle dorsiflexion.

Loss of Fixation

Screw purchase is often compromised in patients with severe osteopenia. Newly developed locked-screw plate constructs may be considered to improve stability in certain circumstances. The use of injectable one-graft substitute pastes that harden in situ has been shown to improve screw purchase in patients with severe osteopenia. Insertion of intramedullary K wires to cross thread with the fibular plate screws has also been said to improve fixation in both biomechanical and clinical studies (19).

Infection and Wound Complications

Postoperative infection usually presents as wound drainage or wound breakdown with accompanying erythema. Operative debridement and culture-specific antibiotics are usually required. Because of the risk of ankle joint involvement, ankle aspiration through a noncellulitic area is also suggested. Once the infection is under control and the soft tissues are healthy, delayed tension-free closure can be performed. Tension relief using a "piecrust" technique may be helpful to obtain a tension free closure (Fig. 33.16). Small stab wounds are placed in the skin and allowed to heal by secondary intention.

Posttraumatic Arthritis

The incidence of posttraumatic arthritis following ankle fractures is not known. While it is generally thought to be low, few reported long-term follow-up studies are available. A higher percentage of poorer results have been seen with studies reporting relatively long-term follow-up (20). Posttraumatic arthritis can be anticipated in cases where there has been significant articular cartilage damage, such as may seen in supination-adduction fracture patterns, and where malreduction is followed by talar subluxation. Factors reported to be associated with the development of posttraumatic arthritis include a shortened fibula, a widened ankle mortise, and Danis-Weber type-B fractures.

Nonunion/Malunion

Nonunion following ankle fractures are uncommon. Patients with nonunion usually present with persistent pain localized to the fracture site. Shortening and malrotation of the fibula can frequently occur after both operative and nonoperative management of

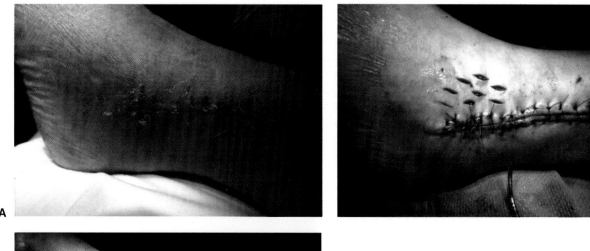

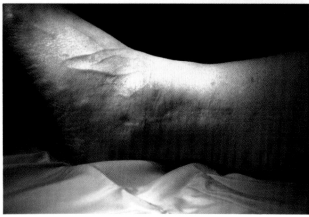

Figure 33.16. A. Breakdown of distal fibula wound with exposed screw head. **B.** After excision of the affected area, the pie-crust technique was used to permit skin closure. **C.** The small pie-crust stab wounds heal by secondary intention.

malleolar fractures (21,22). This can lead to ankle valgus and disruption of talocrural mechanics. Various lengthening osteotomies for the fibula that can restore normal joint mechanics and alleviate clinical symptoms have been described (23).

Hardware Prominence and Pain

Hardware prominence is fairly common in thin individuals following ankle fracture fixation due to the subcutaneous location of the hardware (24). This most commonly involves lateral fibular plates and screws. Symptomatic relief can usually be obtained with outpatient hardware removal after the fracture is adequately healed. We normally encourage patients to wait 1 year from the time of surgery before removing their hardware. Patients are permitted full weight bearing after hardware removal but are cautioned against activities that could cause significant torsional force for 6 to 12 weeks following hardware removal.

In one study of 126 patients, 31% had lateral pain overlying their fracture hardware. Of the 22 patients with hardware-related pain who had undergone hardware removal, only one half had improvement in their lateral ankle pain following hardware removal. In addition, functional outcome scores were poorer for patients with pain overlying lateral-ankle hardware than in those with no pain at this location; this poorer outcome seems to be independent of whether the hardware had been removed.

RECOMMENDED READINGS

1. Egol KA, Amirtharage M, Tejwani NC, et al. Ankle stress test for predicting the need for surgical fixation of isolated fibular fractures. *J Bone Joint Surg* 2004;86:2393–2398.

2. McConnell T, Crevy W, Tornetta P III. Stress examination of supination-external rotation-type fibular fractures. *J Bone Joint Surg* 2004;86:2171–2178.
3. Michelson JD, Varner KE, Checcone M. Diagnosing deltoid injury in ankle fractures: the gravity stress view. *Clin Orthop* 2001; 387:178–182.
4. Fitzpatrick DC, Otto JK, McKinley TO, et al. Kinematic and contact stress analysis of posterior malleolus fractures of the ankle. *J Orthop Trauma* 2004;18:271–278.
5. Thordarson DB, Motamed S, Hedman T, et al. The effect of fibular malreduction on contact pressures in an ankle fracture malunion model. *J Bone Joint Surg Am* 1997;79:1809–1815.
6. Vrahas M, Fu F, Veenis B. Intraarticular contact stresses with simulated ankle malunions. *J Orthop Trauma* 1994;8:159–166.
7. Caschman J, Blagg S, Bishay M. The efficacy of the A-V impulse system in the treatment of posttraumatic swelling following ankle fracture: a prospective randomized controlled study. *J Orthop Trauma* 2004;18:596–601.
8. Thordarson DB, Ghalambor N, Perlman M. Intermittent pneumatic pedal compression and edema resolution after acute ankle fracture: a prospective, randomized study. *Foot Ankle Int* 1997;18:347–350.
9. Tornetta P III, Creevy W. Lag screw only fixation of the lateral malleolus. *J Orthop Trauma* 2001;15: 119–121.
10. Ferries JS, DeCoster TA, Firoozbakhsk KK, et al. Plain radiographic interpretation in trimalleolar ankle fractures poorly assesses posterior fragment size. *J Orthop Trauma* 1994;8:328–331.
11. Ebraheim NA, Mekhail AO, Haman SP. External rotation-lateral view of the ankle in the assessment of the posterior malleolus. *Foot Ankle Int* 1999;20:379–383.
12. Egol KA, Sheikhazadeh A, Mogatederi S, et al. Lower-extremity function for driving an automobile after operative treatment of ankle fracture. *J Bone Joint Surg* 2003;85:1185–1189.
13. Boden SD, Labropoulos PA, McCowin P, et al. Mechanical considerations for the syndesmosis screw. *J Bone Joint Surg* 1989;71:1548–1555.
14. Yamaguchi K, Martin CH, Boden SD, et al. Operative treatment of syndesmotic disruptions without the use of a syndesmotic screw: a prospective clinical study. *Foot Ankle Int* 1994;15:407–414.
15. Candal-Couto JJ, Burrow D, Bromage S, et al. Instability of the tibio-fibular syndesmosis: have we been pulling in the wrong direction? *Injury, Int J Care Injured* 2004;35:814–818.
16. Obremskey WT, Dirschl DR, Crowther JD, et al. Change over time of SF-36 functional outcomes for operatively treated unstable ankle fractures. *J Orthop Trauma* 2002;16:30–33.
17. Bhandari M, Sprague S, Hanson B, et al. Health-related quality of life following operative treatment of unstable ankle fractures: a prospective observational study. *J Orthop Trauma* 2004;18:338–345.
18. Andreassen GS, Hoiness PR, Skraamm I, et al. Use of a synthetic bone void filler to augment screws in osteopenic ankle fracture fixation. *Arch Orthop Trauma Surg* 2004;124:161–165.
19. Koval KJ, Petraco DM, Kummer FJ, et al. A new technique for complex fibula fracture fixation in the elderly: a clinical and biomechanical evaluation. *J Orthop Trauma* 1997;11:28–33.
20. Day GA, Swanson CE, Hulcomble BG. Operative treatment of ankle fractures: a minimum ten-year follow-up. *Foot Ankle Int* 2001;22:102–106.
21. Rukavina A. The role of fibular length and the width of the ankle mortise in post-traumatic osteoarthritis after malleolar fracture. *Int Orthop* 1998; 22:357–360.
22. Walsh EF, DiGiovanni C. Fibular nonunion after closed rotational ankle fractures. *Foot Ankle Int* 2004;25:488–495.
23. Marti RK, Nolte PA. Malunited ankle fractures: the late results of reconstruction. *J Bone Joint Surg Br* 1990;72:709–713.
24. Brown OL, Dirschl DR, Obremskey WT. Incidence of hardware-related pain and its effect on functional outcomes after open reduction and internal fixation of ankle fractures. *J Orthop Trauma* 2001;15:271–274.

34

Talus Fractures: Open Reduction Internal Fixation

Paul T. Fortin and Patrick J. Wiater

INDICATIONS/CONTRAINDICATIONS

Displaced talus fractures are uncommon but devastating injuries. Because they are seen infrequently, most surgeons have limited experience managing these fractures and their sequelae. Two thirds of the talus is covered in articular cartilage, and all fractures are articular injuries affecting one or more of the adjacent joints. Operative treatment is usually necessary to restore hind foot anatomy and mechanics, as well as joint congruity in the majority of these fractures. Disruption of articular congruity and/or loss of talar length, alignment, and rotation are general indications for operative treatment. Even small residual-fracture displacement can result in a significant compromise of subtalar, ankle, or talonavicular joint function.

In general, talar neck and body fractures should be treated operatively if the fracture is displaced more than 1 to 2 mm. Talar neck fractures are classified into one of four types (Fig. 34.1). Hawkins described types I, II, and III and Canale and Kelly described type IV injuries that involve the talonavicular joint. Type I talar neck fractures are nondisplaced injuries and can be managed nonoperatively in cooperative patients who agree to frequent follow-up x-rays. Any displacement should be considered significant and usually warrants surgical intervention. Nondisplaced talar neck fractures that are not visible on plain x-rays but diagnosed with other imaging modalities, such as magnetic resonance imaging (MRI), computed tomography (CT), or bone scans, may be treated nonoperatively. Types II, III, and IV talar neck fractures are, by definition, displaced and require reduction and fixation.

Talar body fractures often involve articular disruption of both the tibiotalar and subtalar joints, and surgical restoration of articular congruity, talar height, and ligamentous stability of the ankle is usually the best option. Talar body fractures can be classified into cleavage, crush, and tubercle or process fractures (Fig. 34.2). Because of the impaction mechanism of many of these injuries, anatomic reduction of the joint surface is not always possible, but restoration of height and stability of the hind foot is indicated to help diminish long-term complications.

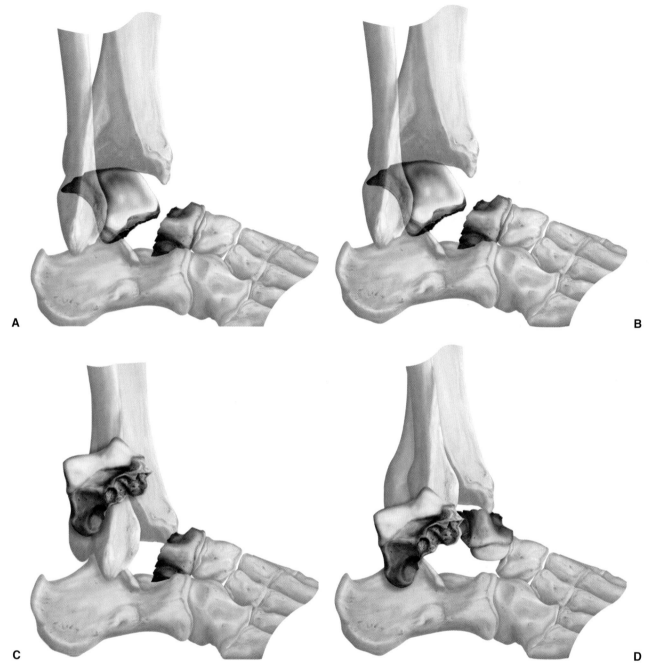

Figure 34.1. Hawkins classification of talar neck fractures. **A.** Type I. **B.** Type II. **C.** Type III. **D.** Type IV.

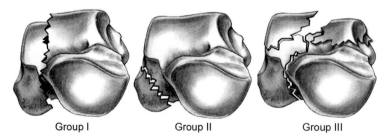

Figure 34.2. Talar body fractures. **A.** Group I cleavage fractures (horizontal, sagittal, coronal). **B.** Group II process or tubercle fractures. **C.** Group III crush with compression/impaction.

Talar neck and body fractures are usually the result of high-energy injuries. However, talar injuries are commonly overlooked and may go unrecognized. This is particularly true in multiply injured patients, and late treatment of the talar injury often results in suboptimal outcomes. Occult foot or ankle injuries should be suspected when foot and ankle swelling or ecchymosis is presented even when obvious radiographic abnormalities are not found.

Significant neuropathy, peripheral vascular disease, soft-tissue compromise, and limited ambulatory capacity are relative contraindications to surgical management. Peripheral neuropathy is highly variable in severity, and many elderly patients have some degree of peripheral neuropathy that should not necessarily preclude operative treatment. Loss of protective sensation, however, as judged by the ability to differentiate a 5.07 monofilament, is a sensitive indicator of significant neuropathy; therefore, failure to differentiate the monofilament should be considered a relative contraindication to surgery. The decision to operate also depends upon the fracture pattern, ankle stability, and presence of dislocation or significant joint subluxation and should be made on a case by case basis. A minimally displaced talar body fracture in a patient with significant neuropathy may be best treated nonoperatively, whereas a Hawkins III talar neck fracture with posteromedial extrusion of the talar body should be treated operatively, even in patients with significant neuropathy, to relieve soft-tissue and/or neurovascular compromise. Elderly patients with limited ambulatory capacity, similarly, may be best treated nonoperatively if the joint is not significantly displaced or dislocated.

On occasion, poor soft-tissue conditions complicate the operative treatment of these fractures. For example, a dual incision approach to a talar neck fracture may be contraindicated in situations where the anterolateral skin is compromised (Fig. 34.3). Extensile exposures may also be contraindicated in patients with marginal perfusion of the extremity.

Preoperative Planning

The urgency of reduction and timing of surgical intervention for talar injuries remains controversial. Initial fracture displacement, rather than the timing of reduction, is thought to be a major factor controlling the development of osteonecrosis following talar neck fractures. Fractures associated with joint subluxation or dislocation, as well as those with soft-tissue compromise due to fracture displacement, necessitate emergent reduction to avoid neurovascular compromise and/or skin necrosis (see Fig. 34.3). Because of the urgency of expedient reduction in these circumstances, preoperative planning is invariably limited. If the peritalar joints are reduced and fracture displacement is not significant, operative fixation can be performed when soft-tissue swelling and bruising are resolving and proper imaging studies have been obtained. In most patients, a well-padded plaster or fiberglass splint provides adequate temporary support and pain relief. Provisional, spanning, external fixation to restore length and stability may occasionally be necessary when the soft-tissue status precludes early open reduction.

The standard radiographic evaluation for talar injuries includes anteroposterior (AP), lateral, and oblique views of the foot and ankle. The Canale oblique view (Fig. 34.4) may be helpful to assess length and alignment of the talar neck. Shortening of the medial column of the talus secondary to impaction is common in talar neck fractures and is well seen on the Canale view. CT scans are also useful in defining the fracture pattern and detecting occult fractures in the ankle and foot (Fig. 34.5). Concomitant osteochondral fractures are common with talar neck fractures and are not well visualized on plain x-rays.

Knowledge of the fracture pattern and classification is very helpful when planning the surgical approach, methods of reduction, and fixation techniques. For example, talar body fractures and type III talar neck fractures with posteromedial extrusion of the talar body often require transmalleolar exposure either through a concomitant medial-malleolar fracture or osteotomy of the medial malleolus. Reduction aids such as a femoral distractor may be necessary to reduce an extruded talar body. Chondral and osteochondral fractures often necessitate small-diameter subarticular screws or bioabsorbable implants. By definition, talus fractures are articular injuries, and having an assortment of small-diameter plates and screws will facilitate anatomic restoration of the joint surface and rigid fracture fixation to allow early motion.

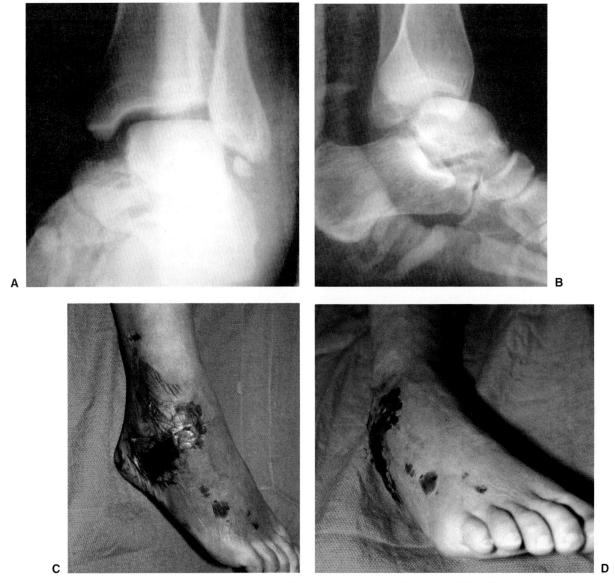

Figure 34.3. A,B. AP and lateral x-rays of a displaced talar neck fracture. **C,D.** Clinical photos of the same patient with soft-tissue compromise and impending full-thickness necrosis because an early reduction was not performed.

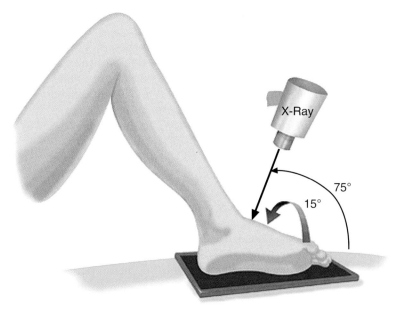

Figure 34.4. Canale view to assess talar neck length and alignment.

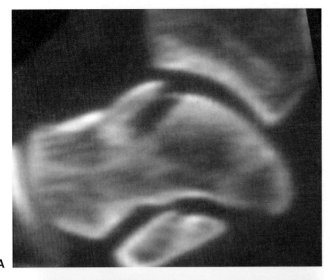

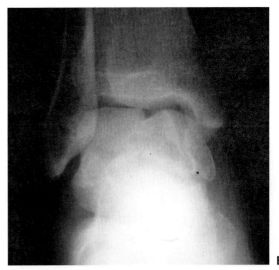

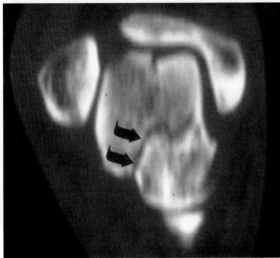

Figure 34.5. CT scanning can be helpful in identifying occult osteochondral fractures **(A)** or fracture lines unrecognized on plain x-rays, such as this talar-neck fracture that occurred concomitant with a talar body fracture **(B,C)**.

Surgical Technique

Access to the talus for fracture surgery is limited, and extensile approaches are not recommended. Fracture pattern and associated soft-tissue disruptions suggest potential avascular zones. The goal of fracture surgery is to gain access to the bone for reduction and fixation without further compromise of the remaining blood supply. Unnecessary dissection should be avoided and ligamentous attachments should be protected.

X-rays are carefully assessed to determine fracture pattern, areas of comminution, medial neck shortening, and associated osteochondral fractures (Fig. 34.6). The patient is positioned supine on a radiolucent operating table with a bolster placed under the affected extremity. A well-padded pneumatic tourniquet is placed on the proximal thigh. General anesthesia with muscle paralysis is preferred to counteract potential muscular-deforming forces in the hind foot. Intraoperative c-arm fluoroscopy is utilized (Fig. 34.7).

For most displaced talar neck fractures, we prefer a dual incision technique in which anteromedial and anterolateral incisions are utilized. Visualization of both the medial and lateral talar neck regions allows for more accurate fracture reduction (Figs. 34.8 and 34.9). Oftentimes the dorsal and medial talar neck is comminuted and the lateral and plantar portion are not or visa versa.

The anteromedial incision extends from the anterior aspect of the medial malleolus to the medial cuneiform and is centered midway between the tibialis anterior and tibialis posterior

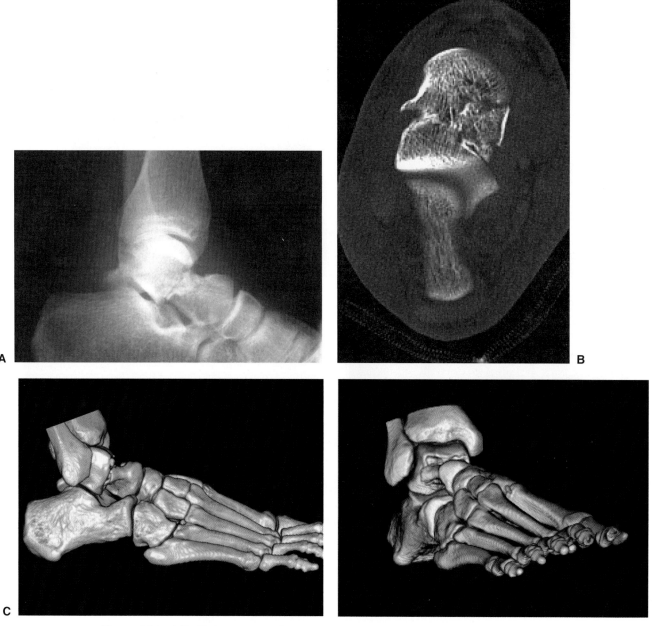

Figure 34.6. A,B. Plain x-ray and CT image of Hawkins II talar neck fracture. **C,D.** Reconstruction images demonstrate medial neck comminution and varus angulation of the talar neck and supination of the foot.

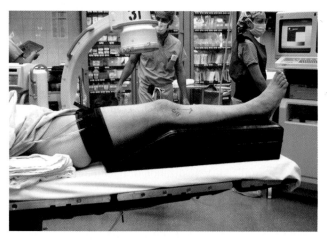

Figure 34.7. Patient positioning.

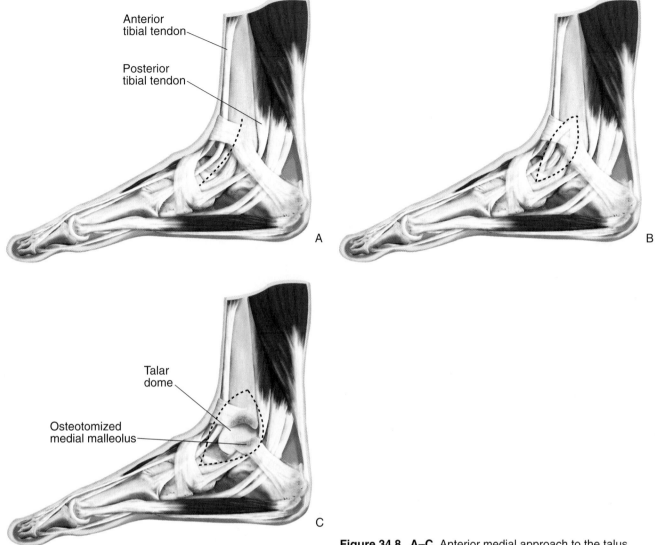

Anterior
tibial tendon

Posterior
tibial tendon

A

B

Talar
dome

Osteotomized
medial malleolus

C

Figure 34.8. A–C. Anterior medial approach to the talus.

tendons (Fig. 34.10). This approach exposes the dorsomedial talar head and neck as well as the anteromedial body. Proximally, the greater saphenous vein and nerve are identified and protected. The tibiotalar and talonavicular joints are exposed.

The remaining blood supply to the talus should be preserved. The posterior, tibial, arterial branches should be protected by avoiding plantar dissection along the medial neck. Similarly, the integrity of the deltoid ligament must not be violated, and extensive dissection of the tibiotalar joint capsule should be avoided. Frequently the dorsal medial talar neck contains comminuted and or impacted segments. The dorsal soft tissues are left intact and attached to these fragments. Only 1 to 2 mm of periosteum around the fracture site is elevated so a cortical reduction can be adequately visualized.

The anterolateral incision parallels the fourth ray and is centered at the ankle (Fig. 34.11A). Proximally, it is midway between the tibia and fibula, and distally it heads for the base of the fourth metatarsal. The intermediate branch of the superficial peroneal nerve may be injured as it resides just superficial to the fascia and extensor retinaculum (see Fig. 34.11B). The nerve should be mobilized and protected. The extensor retinaculum is sharply incised and the tendons retracted for improved visualization.

The anterior compartment contents are left as a unit and can be mobilized from lateral to medial by blunt dissection. The extensor digitorum brevis is elevated and retracted distally and inferiorly. This exposes the anterolateral body, lateral process, and lateral talar neck, as well as the sinus tarsi.

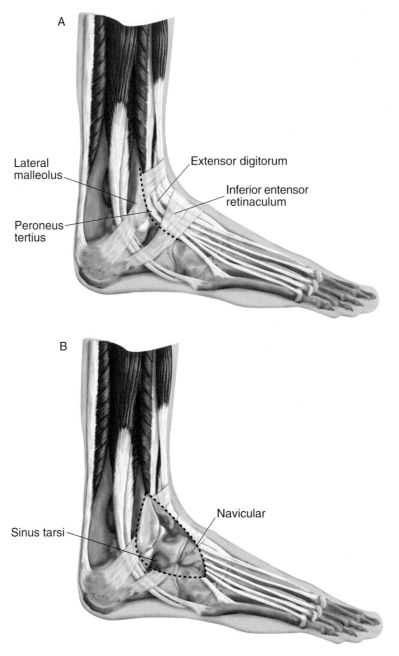

Figure 34.9. A,B. Anterior lateral approach to the talus.

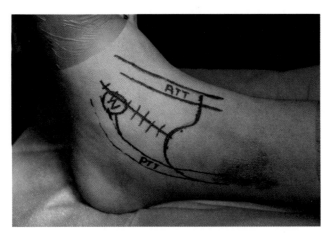

Figure 34.10. Medial approach: incision in the interval between the anterior and posterior tibial tendons from the medial malleolus to the navicular tuberosity. Proximal extension allows exposure for malleolar osteotomy.

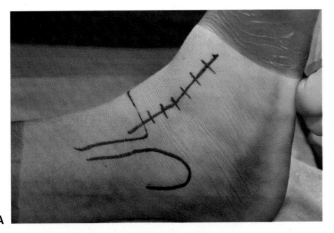
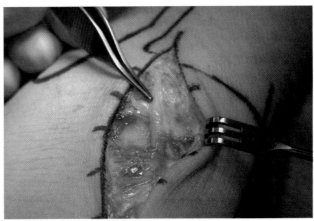

A   B

Figure 34.11. Anterolateral approach. **A.** Incision from the anterolateral ankle joint in line
with the fourth ray. **B.** Superficial peroneal nerve is vulnerable in the superficial dissection.

To decrease the potential for flap necrosis, the skin and soft tissues between the two
incisions should not be undermined. The dorsalis pedis artery supplies this tissue flap, as
well as contributes blood supply to the talus through the dorsal soft-tissues branches. If
more exposure is desired, the anterior joint capsule can be released from the anterior tibia.
The fat pad about the sinus tarsi can be debrided so the lateral neck and lateral process of
the talus can be better visualized. The subtalar joint is accessible through the lateral
incision. Longitudinal traction is then applied through the calcaneus to distract the subtalar
joint, and a pituitary rongeur is used carefully to debride the joint (Figs. 34.12 and 34.13).

The talus is exposed at this point and is ready for reduction and fixation. A Kirschner (K)
wire can be placed across the talar head fragment to act as a joystick and aid in reduction
(Fig. 34.14C). Typically, the lateral talar neck is not comminuted, and an anatomic cortical
reduction is possible. Length, alignment, and rotation are corrected as the surgeon uses both
incisions to judge reduction. Smaller comminuted fragments are first reduced to the larger
intact segments and stabilized with K wires (see Fig. 34.14). Once the gross reduction is
achieved, it is checked with c-arm fluoroscopy. Intraoperative axial alignment of the talar
neck is best evaluated using the Canale view. The tibiotalar reduction is best seen on
mortise and lateral views, and the subtalar joint is best assessed on the lateral and 45-degree
mortise view. The radiographic reduction can be compared to like views of the contralateral side taken preoperatively.

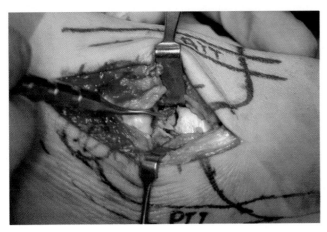

Figure 34.12. Medial exposure showing medial neck com-
minution and shortening. (Copyright © 2001 American
Academy of Orthopaedic Surgeons, Reprinted from the
Journal of the American Academy of Orthopaedic Surgeons,
Volume 9(2), pp. 114–127, with permission.)

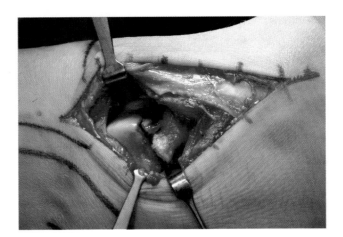

Figure 34.13. Anterolateral exposure showing displacement
of the lateral talar neck.

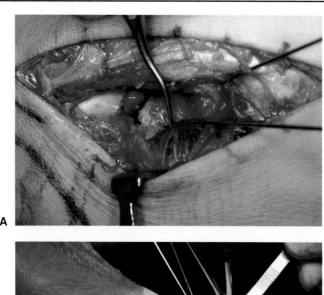

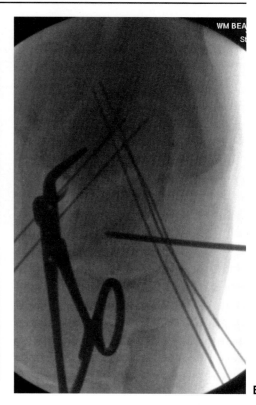

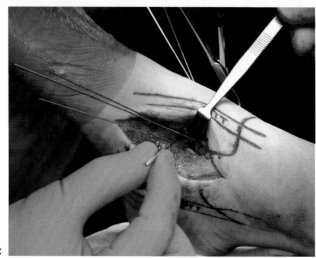

Figure 34.14. A. Provisional K-wire fixation. **B,C.** K wire in the talar head used as a joy stick to correct varus angulation and to restore medial neck length.

Definitive fixation depends on fracture type, comminution, and bone quality. Small-fragment and minifragment implants of adequate strength and variety must be available. For noncomminuted talar neck fractures, longitudinal, 3.5-mm, cortical, lag screws placed from the talar head into the body provide adequate fixation (Fig. 34.15). These screws are placed in both the medial and lateral columns of the talus. The desired orientation of the screws approximates parallel, but this is difficult to achieve because the navicular covers the talar head and the forefoot hinders a longitudinal trajectory. The medial navicular can be recessed using a burr or rongeur to allow a more lateral and longitudinal starting point and trajectory for the medial screw. When placing screws from an articular starting point, the surgeon should countersink the screw head to minimize impingement.

In many high-energy talar neck fractures, there is dorsomedial comminution. Longitudinal lag-screw fixation in these cases results in fracture shortening, angulation, or displacement. For these fractures, to improve fracture stability and prevent talar neck shortening, minifragment plates and screws are necessary; 1.5-, 2.0-, 2.4-mm implants are available (Fig. 34.16).

Lateral neck plating, as described by Benirschke, can be used for both comminuted and noncomminuted fractures. A five-hole 2.0-mm plate is contoured to fit the lateral talar neck and spans from the anterior surface of the lateral process of the talus, along the lateral talar neck, to the head and neck junction. This plate is extra-articular, and the best fit is usually slightly plantar rather than directly lateral. Lateral fixation can be supplemented with a longitudinal, cortical, set screw from the talar head into the body (Fig. 34.17A).

Medial talar neck comminution can also be addressed with plate fixation to prevent varus collapse. However, the medial talar neck and tibiotalar joint anatomy limits options for plate placement. A 2.0-mm blade plate works well. The blade is placed transversely

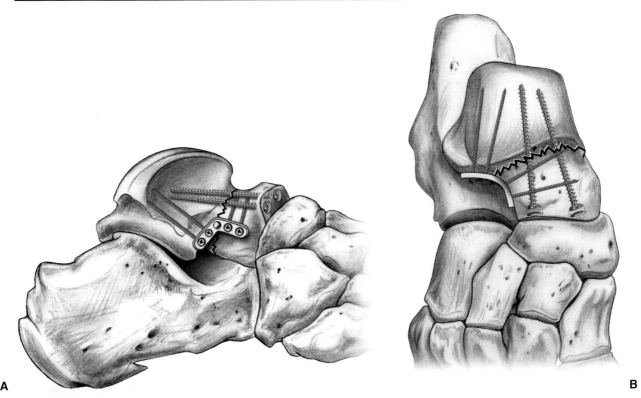

Figure 34.15. Typical construct for talar neck fracture without significant medial comminution showing lateral plating and medial set screw.

across the distal talar neck from medial to lateral, just posterior to the medial talar-head articular surface. The plate is directed posteriorly to sit just plantar to the medial talar-body articular cartilage (see Fig. 34.17B). Care must be taken to insure that the plate and screw heads sit below the level of the articular surface. Final x-rays are assessed to confirm anatomic reduction and to assure that there has not been intra-articular penetration of screws (Fig. 34.18).

Hawkins type-III fracture dislocations are complicated injuries and difficult to treat. The talar body frequently dislocates posteromedially, hinging on the deltoid ligament. Reduction of the dislocation should be done on an urgent basis. A closed reduction can be attempted in the emergency department but is rarely effective. An irreducible dislocation is best addressed by the dual incision technique described.

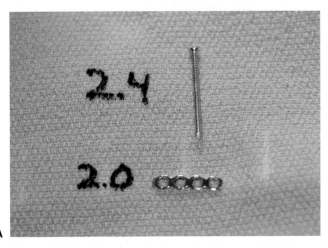

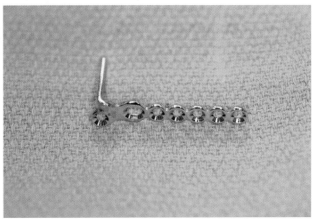

Figure 34.16. A. Implants for lateral plating: no. 2.0 plate and 2.4-mm screws. **B.** Miniblade plate for medial fixation.

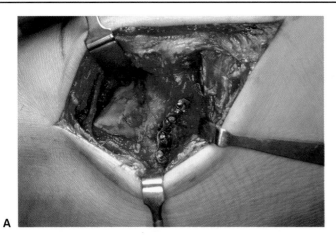
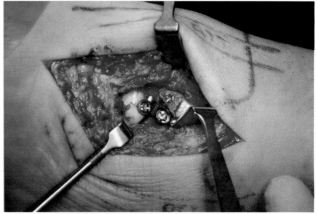

A   B

Figure 34.17. A. Lateral plate fixation. **B.** Medial plate fixation.

The anteromedial incision is opened first. Skeletal muscle paralysis is imperative. The knee is flexed to relax and longitudinal traction is placed through the calcaneus. The femoral distractor can be a useful reduction aid. One Schantz pin is placed into the antero-medial face of the tibia, and the other pin is placed transversely across the calcaneus from medial to lateral. Small osteochondral fragments are removed from the ankle joint. The tendons and neurovascular bundle are carefully retracted, and the talar body is manipulated back into the ankle joint. Usually the only remaining soft-tissue attachment to the talar body is the deltoid ligament. Care should be taken that the deltoid ligament not be cut because this ligament transmits branches of the posterior tibial artery to the talar body.

Closed fractures with deficient bone in the talar neck should be bone grafted. Autologous cancellous bone is readily available from the ipsilateral distal tibia or calcaneal tuberosity. Crushed cancellous allograft is also effective.

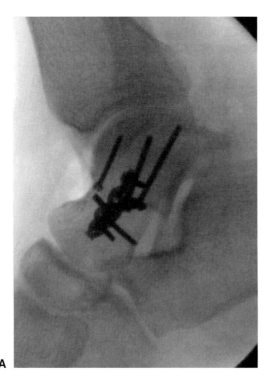
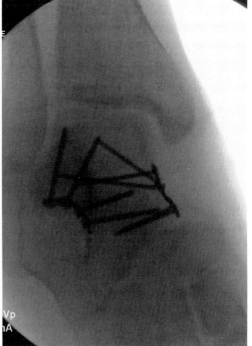

A   B

Figure 34.18. A,B. Final x-rays.

The talar body fracture pattern dictates the surgical approach. A portion of the anterior talar body is accessible through both the anteromedial and anterolateral incisions. Simple sagittal fractures can be treated using a single exposure, and the incision chosen is based on the fracture orientation seen on the CT scan. Joint distraction using the femoral distractor as described can aid in exposure of the talar dome.

More complex talar body fractures including comminuted and coronal plane patterns, as well as associated body and neck fractures, are best addressed using the dual incision technique. The anteromedial and anterolateral exposures can allow access to the anterior one third to one half of the talar body. For fractures that involve the posterior half of the dome, a medial malleolar osteotomy is usually necessary. The anteromedial incision is extended proximally along the mid anteromedial-tibial face. Subperiosteal dissection exposes the medial malleolus. The deltoid ligament is then left intact. Fixation for the malleolar osteotomy should then be planned. Transverse lag screws with an antiglide plate or lag screws directed up the medial malleolus parallel to the medial joint surface are adequate for fixation. Prior to the osteotomy, the fixation implants are placed and then removed so that the screw paths will line up perfectly when the osteotomy is reduced.

The osteotomy is started proximally in the medial tibial metaphysis. It is inclined obliquely to enter the apex of the medial ankle joint between the medial malleolus and the tibial plafond (see Fig. 34.8C). Retractors are placed posterior to the medial malleolus to protect the tendons and neurovascular bundle. The osteotomy path is outlined by creation of multiple, small, drill holes. A microsagittal saw is used to cut through the cancellous bone to the subchondral bone just above the joint. A thin osteotome is used to complete the osteotomy and fracture the cartilage. The osteotomy is displaced distally to expose the medial talar body.

The femoral distractor is used for joint distraction and dome visualization. Indirect reduction techniques are utilized for fracture reduction. Sagittal plane fractures can be fixed using medial to lateral lag screws. Fragment size dictates the implant diameter. When placed across articular cartilage, smaller implants are preferable and include 1.5-, 2.0-, or 2.4-mm, countersunk, cortical, lag screws. Medial to lateral lag screws can also be placed extra-articularly through the deltoid fossa on the medial talar body. These screws should also be countersunk to prevent impingement. As an alternative, headless subarticular screws can be used (Fig. 34.19). Small osteochondral fragments are stabilized with countersunk, minifragment, cortical, lag screws or bioabsorbable implants (Fig. 34.20). Associated neck fractures are reduced and stabilized as described previously.

Lateral process-talus fractures occur either as a solitary fracture or as an associated pattern. The CT scan best details these fractures. Fragment size, amount of comminution, and degree of posterior facet involvement dictate treatment strategy. Large solitary fragments can be approached via the anterolateral exposure. The anterior talofibular ligament inserts on the lateral process and this attachment should be preserved. Fixation depends on fragment size. A 2.0-mm plate and lag screw fixation can be used for large solitary fragments.

POSTOPERATIVE MANAGEMENT

Patients are placed in a bulky dressing with a posterior splint. Prophylactic antibiotics are administered for 24 hours following surgery. Once the wound is healed, patients are placed into a removable boot and begin active range-of-motion exercises of the ankle, subtalar, and midfoot joints. Patients refrain from weight bearing for 10 to 12 weeks or until the fracture is healed; the radiographic presence of osteonecrosis is not a contraindication to weight bearing. Supervised physical therapy is instituted on a case by case basis depending upon the patient's ability to comply and progress with a self-directed home program.

Radiographic evaluation is performed at 6 to 8 week intervals to assess healing and to monitor for signs of osteonecrosis. A "Hawkins sign," which is a subchondral radiolucency of the talar dome, is usually visible between 6 and 8 weeks after the injury. The presence of a Hawkins sign is a reliable indicator that the talus is vascularized and osteonecrosis is

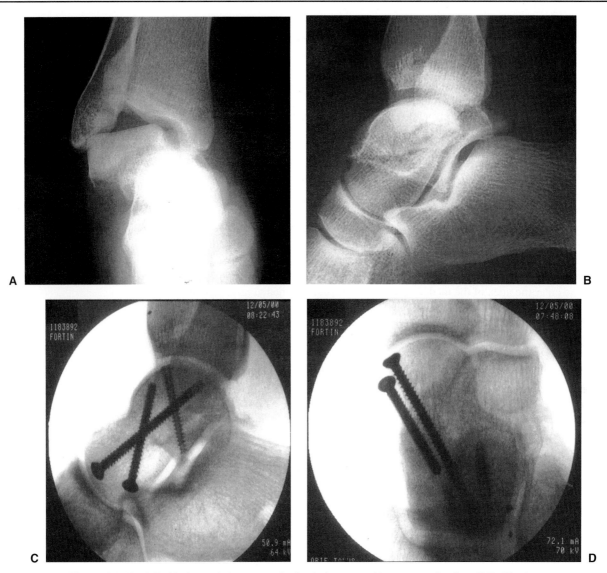

Figure 34.19. A,B. Horizontal-cleavage talar body fracture without comminution. **C,D.** Final fixation with lag and subarticular screws.

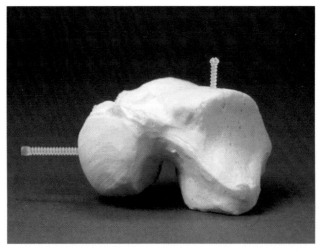

Figure 34.20. Small bioabsorbable screws may be helpful alternatives to screws for small osteochondral fragments.

not likely to occur. The absence of a Hawkins sign does not, however, reliably predict the development of osteonecrosis. The utility of MRI scanning for monitoring of osteonecrosis is controversial. It is not practical or cost effective to perform serial MRI scans on a routine basis. It can occasionally be helpful in determining the extent of avascularity when subsequent reconstructive surgical procedures are contemplated. Titanium implants have been suggested to cause less interference with MRI visualization. CT scanning can be very helpful in assessing healing when plain x-rays are equivocal.

COMPLICATIONS

Soft-Tissue Compromise/Infection

Fracture displacement and/or joint dislocation can lead to excessive skin tension and soft-tissue compromise. Expedient reduction is necessary to avoid the disastrous complication of full-thickness tissue loss (see Fig. 34.3). Delaying operative treatment can be preferable, however, when the fracture is not significantly displaced and significant swelling could compromise wound closure and healing. The dual surgical approach for talar neck and body fractures necessitates careful soft-tissue handling and proper timing to avoid wound edge necrosis. Superficial wound-edge necrosis, although infrequent, can occur, and while it usually responds to local wound care, it delays the initiation of range-of-motion exercises. Open injuries require immediate and serial irrigation and debridement followed by the appropriate coverage or closure to avoid deep infection. Early onset of deep infection necessitates urgent irrigation and culture-specific, intravenous, antibiotic therapy. Deep infection can result in septic destruction of all of the peritalar joints with significant bone loss that can be very difficult to salvage.

Osteonecrosis

Osteonecrosis is largely a consequence of the injury rather than a complication of treatment. The incidence of osteonecrosis following talar neck fractures is related to the initial fracture displacement and the extent of comminution rather than the timing of reduction. Focal osteonecrosis without collapse is common following talar neck and body fractures. It often is asymptomatic and does not necessarily doom the patient to a poor result. Diffuse or global osteonecrosis can result in collapse of the talar dome and progressive posttraumatic arthritis in the ankle and subtalar joints. In the past, the initial period in which weight bearing was suspended was prolonged until revascularization, which was believed to protect the talar dome from collapse, was completed. However, this approach is largely unproven and impractical. Nonsurgical management of symptomatic osteonecrosis includes bracing and shoe wear modification. Surgical salvage typically consists of arthrodesis of the involved joints. As an alternative in circumstances of complete fragmentation and collapse of the talar body, a modified Blair fusion with removal of the nonviable body and fusion of the talar neck and head to the anterior distal tibia, can help control pain. With this procedure, patients retain more motion than with a tibial talocalcaneal fusion.

Posttraumatic Arthritis

Joint stiffness and posttraumatic arthritis are the most frequent consequences of talar body and neck fractures. This often occurs with some degree of focal osteonecrosis. It can be the result of chondral damage at the time of injury or from abnormal joint kinematics caused by malunion. Stable internal fixation that allows early motion may minimize peritalar joint stiffness. When conservative measures are ineffective, arthrodesis of the affected joint(s) is often necessary for pain relief. Proper imaging studies prior to arthrodesis are often necessary to detect areas of osteonecrosis, which may help the surgeon determine the method of fusion or the need for bone grafting.

Malunion or Nonunion

Varus malunion following talar neck fracture has been reported to occur in up to 36% of patients who underwent open reduction and internal fixation. Shortening of the medial neck of the talus caused by comminution or impaction can lead to varus malunion. The dual incision approach facilitates adequate visualization and proper restoration of talar length and alignment and therefore helps minimize this complication.

Apex dorsal malunion can occur when the body of the talus is left plantarflexed relative to the neck and the head fragment remains dorsal to the neck. This often leads to symptomatic impingement of the dorsal talus on the distal tibia with maximal ankle dorsiflexion. Even small amounts of residual displacement or mal-alignment can lead to altered joint mechanics and arthrosis. Treatment of symptomatic talar malunion can be extremely difficult and is dependent upon the integrity of the peritalar joints. Long-standing varus malunion with peritalar joint arthritis typically can only be salvaged by arthrodesis with realignment to obtain a plantigrade foot. Varus malunion typically leads to shortening of the medial column of the foot and needs to be addressed at the time of salvage arthrodesis. Malunion recognized before the onset of significant arthritis can be treated by osteotomy with restoration of length, alignment, and rotation. This may involve structural bone grafting to regain talar neck length.

RECOMMENDED READING

Canale ST, Kelly FB. Fractures of the neck of the talus: long-term evaluation of seventy-one cases. *J Bone Joint Surg* 1978;60:143–156.

Fortin PT, Balazsy JE. Talus fractures: evaluation and treatment. *J Am Acad Orthop Surg* 2001;9:114–127.

Hawkins MD. Fractures of the neck of the talus. *J Bone Joint Surg* 1970;52:991–1002.

Sanders DW, Busam M, Hatwick E, et al. Functional outcome following displaced talar neck fractures. *J Orthop Trauma* 2004;18:265–270.

Vallier HA, Nork SE, Barei DP, et al. Talar neck fractures: results and outcomes. *J Bone Joint Surg* 2004;86:1616–1628.

Vallier HA, Nork SE, Benirschke SK, et al. Surgical treatment of talar body fractures. *J Bone Joint Surg* 2003;85:1716–1724.

35

Open Reduction Internal Fixation Using an Extensile Lateral Approach for a Joint Depression Fracture

Roy W. Sanders and Paul Tornetta, III

INDICATIONS/CONTRAINDICATIONS

The indications for open reduction and internal fixation (ORIF) of the calcaneus remain controversial. Results after surgery are superior to nonoperative management outcomes only if the posterior facet is anatomically reduced and if complications are avoided (1–3). The best indication for internal fixation of the calcaneus is an intra-articular fracture with displacement of the posterior facet in a young active patient with no medical problems. Middle-aged patients should be considered operative candidates based on their lifestyles and fracture patterns. The more active a patient is, the more likely that he/she would bene- fit from properly performed surgery. Even in less active patients, surgery may improve the functional result if the fracture displacement produces significant widening or shortening of the heel, because skeletal distortion increases the chances of a poor result when the frac- ture is treated nonoperatively.

Contraindications to surgery may be related to the patient's overall health, including mental status, the fracture pattern, and/or the surgeon's experience. Relative contraindications to internal fixation include neuropathy, insulin-dependent diabetes, peripheral vascular dis- ease, venous stasis or congestion, lymphedema, immune compromise, and other disorders or behaviors, such as smoking, that might impede healing. Advanced age is a relative con- traindication. Patient compliance is important in obtaining a good functional result after sur- gical intervention and must be considered preoperatively. Patients with a history of jumping from heights must be carefully scrutinized for signs of mental illness or depression. When ap- propriate, these patients should be evaluated by a mental health professional.

Despite improved surgical techniques and implants, a subset of calcaneal fractures with severe comminution of the posterior facet are resistant to anatomic reduction and internal fixation. In these injuries, primary fusion may be a good alternative to internal fixation. Less comminuted but complex injuries with multiple fractures through the posterior facet offer a relative contraindication for surgeons who do not have significant experience in the operative treatment of calcaneal fractures.

Open fractures present difficult management problems. A thorough irrigation and debridement of the traumatic wounds and the fracture constitute the first priority after resuscitation and trauma evaluation. If the wound is lateral and allows reduction of the posterior facet, then it is reduced and fixed with lag screws. This is performed only after re-prepping and redraping after the debridement. If the wound is medial, internal fixation is delayed until the soft-tissue environment has been addressed. Temporary, triangular, external fixation on the lateral side of the foot and ankle can be used to maintain the general alignment of the heel until definitive management is undertaken. The external fixation pins are placed in the tuberosity, the cuboid, and the talus. Definitive ORIF is performed 2 to 3 weeks after wound closure if the soft tissues are in good condition.

PREOPERATIVE PLANNING

Initial Survey

Physical examination of the patient with a calcaneus fracture must include a careful and complete survey of the axial as well as the appendicular skeleton. Spinal fractures are common in patients with calcaneal fractures because the mechanism of injury is often axial loading caused by a fall from a height. X-rays of the affected extremity and spine should be routine.

To rule out open fracture or compartment syndrome, the surgeon begins the physical examination of the foot and ankle with the evaluation of the soft tissues. Compartment syndrome of the foot is difficult to diagnose clinically. Calcaneal fractures are painful but usually respond to splinting, elevation, ice, and analgesics. Severe and unrelenting pain should be considered a compartment syndrome until proven otherwise. Significant swelling in the foot is common after calcaneal fracture, and the region may not feel tense even in the face of compartment syndrome. Sensation is rarely affected, and its absence does not rule out compartment syndrome. Pain on passive extension of the metatarsophalangeal joints is the best method of clinical examination but is not sensitive enough to rule out a compartment syndrome.

Direct, intracompartmental, pressure measurement is the most accurate method of diagnosis. Pressures should be taken in the central (interosseous) and medial compartments. Handheld devices and arterial line monitors are equally effective in measuring compartment pressures. We perform a fasciotomy if the compartment pressure is within 30 mm Hg of the diastolic pressure. If the pressure measurements are borderline and if significant clinical symptoms are absent, then the foot may be observed and pressures rechecked in 30- to 60-minute intervals. If a fasciotomy is required, the calcaneal fracture is not usually fixed at this time because the incisions necessary for the fasciotomy are not useful for reduction and fixation of the calcaneus.

The remainder of the physical examination of the foot and ankle is directed at diagnosing concomitant injuries. Palpation of the entire lower leg, ankle, and foot may help in identifying such injuries. Commonly associated regional injuries include ankle fractures (especially the lateral malleolus), ankle-ligament injury, peroneal tendon dislocation, mid foot fractures, talar fractures, and metatarsal fractures. Radiographic evaluation of symptomatic or suspicious areas is essential.

Specific Radiographs

The specific radiographs that are necessary to evaluate an injury to the hind foot include anteroposterior (AP), lateral, and mortise views of the ankle; AP, lateral, and oblique views of the foot; and an axial view of the calcaneus (Harris view). Contralateral axial and lateral views of the calcaneus and an oblique view of the contralateral foot may be useful in delineating the patient's normal anatomy. The ankle radiographs are necessary so the surgeon can rule out concomitant ankle or talar fractures as well as evaluate the calcaneus, subtalar joint, and calcaneocuboid joint. The lateral view of the calcaneus allows preliminary classification of the fracture and information about the integrity of the posterior facet (Fig. 35.1).

Even in comminuted and displaced fractures, a portion of the posterior facet is usually intact, and the relationship of the subtalar joint can be evaluated. The lateral radiograph may demonstrate a double density when part of the posterior foot is impacted or depressed. This image may be confused with an oblique view of the joint. However, the confusion can be clarified easily because in a true oblique view the posterior facet of the talus will also appear as a double density, and in a calcaneal fracture, it will appear as only one line. The calcaneocuboid joint and anterior calcaneus are best visualized on the foot films. The axial view demonstrates the position of the tuberosity, the status of the medial wall, and the location of the fracture(s) through the facet (Fig. 35.2).

Computed Tomography Scans

To gain a better understanding of the fracture morphology, the surgeon obtains bi-planar computed tomography (CT) scans with 2- or 3-mm cuts. The scan should include images in the plane of the foot as well as in a plane perpendicular to the posterior facet of the talus. The most important of these are the axial images of the hind foot perpendicular to the posterior facet of the talus. The image is described in reference to the talus because the posterior facet of the calcaneus is displaced. This view is obtained with the foot flat on the table, the knee flexed, and the gantry angled 30 degrees forward. The axial images are used to classify the fracture and to evaluate the fracture anatomy. The surgeon should make note of pertinent anatomic points such as the position and integrity of the tuberosity, the location and number of fractures in the posterior facet, displacement of the lateral wall, the location of medial-wall comminution or fracture lines, the size of the sustentacular fragment, fractures in the anterior calcaneus, the presence or absence of an anterolateral fragment, and the position of the peroneal tendons (dislocated or not) (Figs. 35.3 and 35.4).

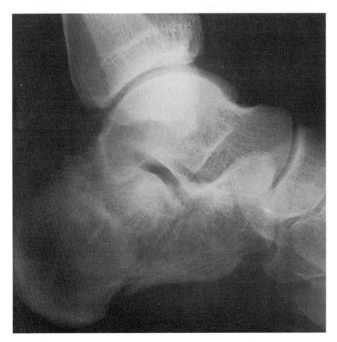

Figure 35.1. The lateral view of the calcaneus demonstrates a joint-depression fracture with a portion of the posterior facet impacted into the cancellous bone of the tuberosity. The sagittal plane rotation of the displaced posterior facet is best seen on this view.

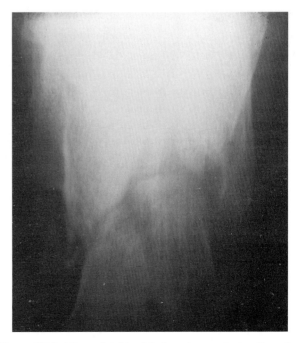

Figure 35.2. The axial (Harris) view demonstrates the primary fracture line, medial comminution, the fractures into the facet, and the varus angulation of the tuberosity.

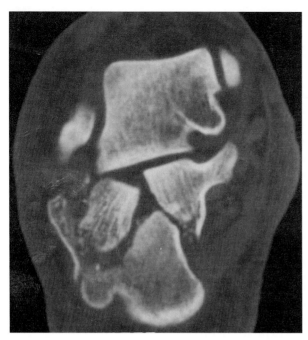

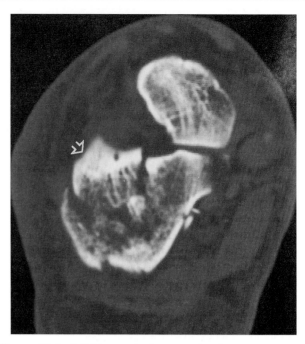

Figure 35.3. The 30-degree semicoronal CT image demonstrates the comminution and degree of depression of the posterior facet. The separation and step-off are easily seen, but the sagittal plane rotation of the fragments is not well visualized. The wedging effect of the tuberosity fragment separating the facet fragments and the lateral wall blowout is well visualized.

Figure 35.4. A CT image farther anterior demonstrates a separate anterolateral fragment (*open arrow*).

The CT images in the plane of the foot are used to evaluate the anterior calcaneus and sustentaculum tali. Fractures of the sustentacular fragment in the coronal plane may decrease the bone available for fixation of the facet. These fractures may not be seen in the other radiographs or axial CT scans but are visible on the CT images of the plane of the foot (Fig. 35.5).

Classification

The fracture is classified by the system of Essex Lopresti (4) by using the plain films and by that of Sanders (5) from the 30-degree, semicoronal, CT scan (Fig. 35.6). By initially classifying the injury into either a joint depression or tongue-type fracture, the surgeon can better plan the reduction tactic. The Sanders classification was devised based on the ease of reduction and fixation via the lateral approach and has been predictive of outcome (2,5). The greater the number of fractures in the facet and the more medial their location, the harder will be the reduction. In the Sanders classification, the fracture lines are designated A through C by their location from lateral to medial, respectively. In a type 2C fracture, the entire facet is displaced from the intact medial calcaneus.

Planning the Reduction and Fixation

Before undertaking the ORIF, the surgeon must thoroughly understand the anatomy of the fracture, not only as it relates to displacement but also as it relates to the tactic for surgical reduction. Two steps are critical in planning the reduction and fixation of a calcaneal fracture. First are references for reduction, which include the anteroinferior margin of the facet (the angle of Gissane), the posterior facet of the talus, the intact posterior facet of the

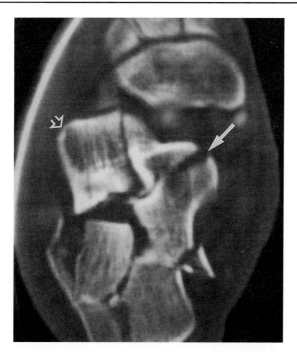

Figure 35.5. The CT scan in the plane of the foot is the best view to evaluate the sustentaculum region. On this CT image, a vertical fracture through the sustentaculum, which is not seen on any other projection, is visible (*solid arrow*). The displaced lateral portion of the posterior facet is seen to be impacted into the tuberosity adjacent to the sustentacular region. The separate anterolateral fragment is seen on this view as well (*open arrow*).

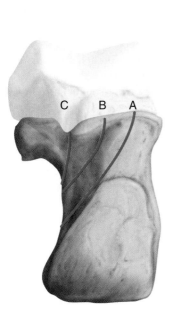
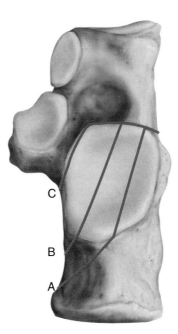

Figure 35.6. The CT classification of Sanders. The fracture is described by the number and location of fracture lines in the posterior facet. Each fracture is given a number and a letter corresponding to the number of fragments of the posterior facet and their location. For example, a 2B fracture has one fracture line in the B location (see Fig. 35.3), and a 3BC has two fracture lines, one in the B position and one in the C position.

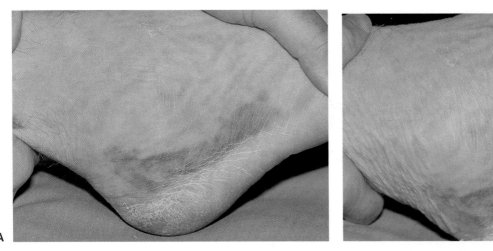

A   B

Figure 35.7. The wrinkle test is done by bringing the foot from the plantarflexed position **(A)** into dorsiflexion and observing the wrinkles **(B)** that form on the lateral side of the ankle and foot.

calcaneus, the calcaneocuboid joint, the tuberosity, and the lateral wall. Second are the standard fixation points used, which include the sustentaculum tali, medial wall, tuberosity, and anterior calcaneus.

Evaluation of the Soft Tissues

So that postoperation wound complications are avoided, the initial postinjury swelling must be resolved. This commonly takes 10 to 21 days to occur but dramatically improves the condition of the soft tissues. The lateral bulge caused by lateral wall displacement can be confused with swelling, so the pliability of the skin is a better characteristic than swelling to test the status of the soft tissues.

Blisters are a contraindication for surgery. If they are blood filled, then they should be allowed to resolve without intervention. Clear blisters are aspirated and then unroofed several days later. In either case, blisters are treated as burns once they are open. Sterile dressings with silver sulfadiazine (Silvadene) cream are used until epithelialization occurs.

If blisters are eliminated, the "wrinkle" test is a good predictor of whether the soft tissue will tolerate surgery. It is performed by bringing the ankle from a plantar-flexed position to neutral. If the skin wrinkles, then it is ready for surgery (Fig. 35.7). Ecchymosis is common and is often distributed along the peroneal tendons. As long as blisters are absent, this is not a contraindication to surgery. The foot is kept in a bulky dressing of soft roll and elevated until the soft tissues will tolerate the surgery. The patient may be discharged home and the foot examined every 5 days until the swelling resolves.

SURGERY

For proper treatment of all patients, high-quality plain radiographs (Figs. 35.8 and 35.9) as well as a CT scan (Fig. 35.10) must be obtained prior to surgery. Once soft-tissue swelling has decreased and skin wrinkling is seen, surgery can be performed. The patient is placed on the operating room table in the lateral decubitus position, and a beanbag or some other device is used to maintain torso stability. The legs are placed apart, in a scissor-like configuration such that the contralateral down limb is straight, and the operative limb is bent at the knee. The operative heel should lie at the corner of the table so that the surgeon can easily access the limb and the fracture. In addition, this positioning will allow the surgeon to use the c-arm without superimposition of the opposite leg. The nonoperative leg

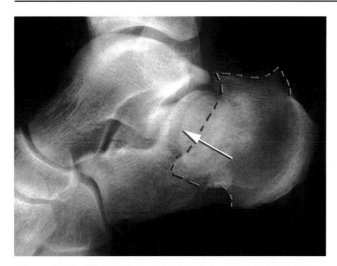

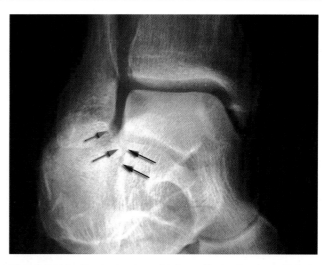

Figure 35.8. Plain radiographs of a joint depression fracture. The depressed joint fragment (*white arrow*) is impacted below the stable medial fragment. This creates a double density. The impaction of the posterior tuberosity is noted by the *dotted red line*.

Figure 35.9. Broden's view of intra-articular fracture. This is a perfect mortise view of the ankle. Primary fracture line is shown by *black arrows*, and the shifted superolateral fragment is indicated by *red arrows*.

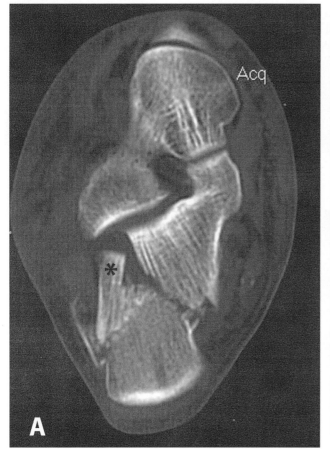

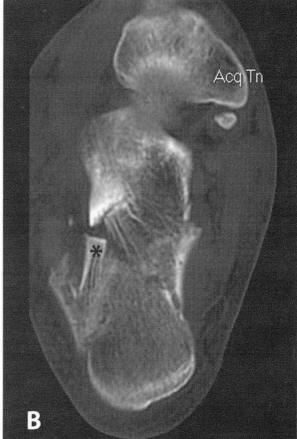

Figure 35.10. CT scan of fracture. The superolateral fragment (*) is seen on both the semicoronal **(A)** and transverse **(B)** projections.

should have padding placed to protect the peroneal nerve as well as any bony prominences, and a pillow is placed between the legs (Fig. 35.11).

The lateral extensile incision is then marked (Fig. 35.12). A drawn line is initiated from 2 cm proximal to the tip of the lateral malleolus, at the lateral edge of the Achilles tendon, and is continued down toward the plantar surface of the heel. As the surgeon's pen approaches the heel pad, the line is curved to parallel the superior edge of the pad. The marking then follows the pad toward the insertion of the peroneus brevis tendon, but it should be angled up so that the surgeon can access the calcaneocuboid joint if needed.

The limb is exsanguinated and a tourniquet is used. The skin incision is made at the proximal part of the vertical limb and extended plantarly. The incision should become full thickness when the calcaneal tuberosity is reached, and the surgeon should avoid beveling the skin when turning the corner with the knife. As the knife parallels the plantar surface of the foot, pressure is again relaxed and a layered incision is developed distally.

A full thickness flap is then developed by raising the corner of the incision subperiosteally (Fig. 35.13). When the periosteal flap is partially developed, retractors may then be used to pull the periosteum upward (Fig. 35.14). Earlier use of retractors will tear the skin away from the periosteum, which could potentially cause late necrosis of the skin.

With continued dissection, the calcaneofibular ligament is encountered and resected from the calcaneus; this will expose the peroneal tendons and their inferior sheath at the level of the peroneal tubercle. The peroneal tendons must be carefully identified and retracted, or one or both tendons will be lacerated during the dissection (Figs. 35.15 to 35.17).

Once the flap is sufficiently developed, the peroneal tendons are slightly subluxed anteriorly, and a 1.6-mm Kirschner (K) wire is then inserted into the fibula to retract the peroneal tendons. A second K wire is placed in the talar neck to retract the midportion of the peroneal tendons and the skin flap, and a third K wire is placed in the cuboid, thereby retracting the distal aspect of the peroneal tendons and the full-thickness skin flap. The exposure of the entire lateral wall can be completed by placing a small retractor into the sinus tarsi over the anterolateral corner of the calcaneus (Fig. 35.18).

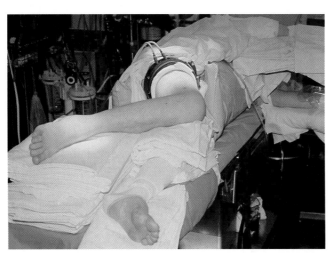

Figure 35.11. Positioning of the patient.

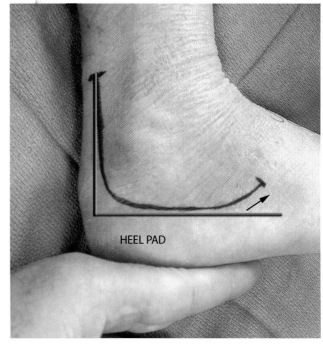

Figure 35.12. Lateral extensile incision (*red line,* landmarks), (*black arrow,* direction of distal end of incision used to access calcaneocuboid joint). Also, the skin has ample wrinkles, indicating that edema is no longer in the skin flap.

HEEL PAD

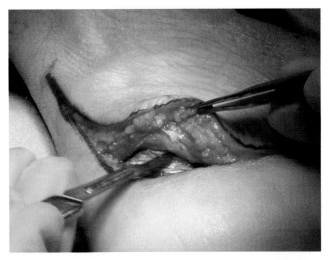

Figure 35.13. Subperiosteal development of lateral flap.

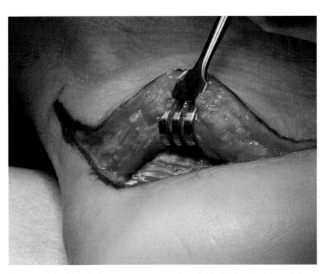

Figure 35.14. Retractor placed after full thickness flap is developed.

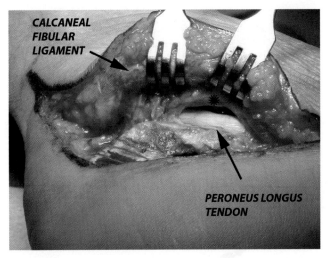

Figure 35.15. Exposure of peroneal tendons (*, peroneal brevis tendon).

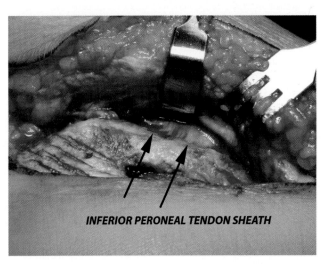

Figure 35.16. Exposure of inferior peroneal-tendon sheath.

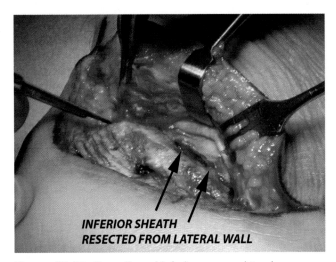

Figure 35.17. Resection of inferior peroneal-tendon sheath from lateral wall, which protects tendons and permits retraction.

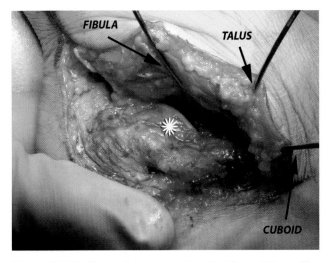

Figure 35.18. No touch technique in which three 1.6-mm K wires are used for retraction. The lateral wall is fully exposed, and the depressed lateral-joint fragment is visualized (*).

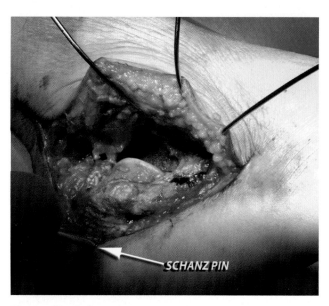

Figure 35.19. Schantz pin disimpaction of joint. The super-olateral fragment is shifted farther away from the medial joint surface than it is in Figure 35.18, which indicates that it is loose.

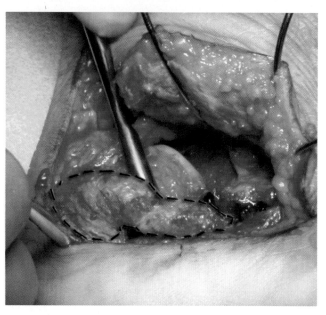

Figure 35.20. Separation of lateral wall (*dotted line*) from superolateral fragment.

The exposed corner of the calcaneal tuberosity is then predrilled and a short Schantz pin is screwed into place. Using the pin, the heel is manipulated and distracted into varus, which disimpacts the fracture and makes the edge of the fragment more visible (Fig. 35.19).

The lateral wall fragment is then carefully resected from the impacted joint fragment and placed in a container with saline (Fig. 35.20). The farthest anterior plantar edge of the depressed superolateral fragment is located and a small periosteal elevator is placed underneath it. Disimpaction of the fragment is performed gradually because sudden strong pressure may result in the fragment falling on the operating room floor (Fig. 35.21). Once lifted, it should be removed, cleaned of clot, and placed in the same container as the lateral wall.

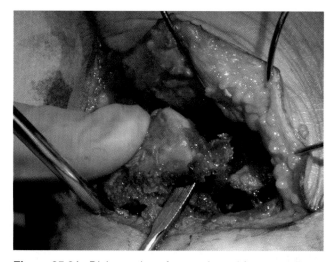

Figure 35.21. Disimpaction of superolateral fragment. The surgeon's thumb is holding the fragment laterally to maintain control during manipulation.

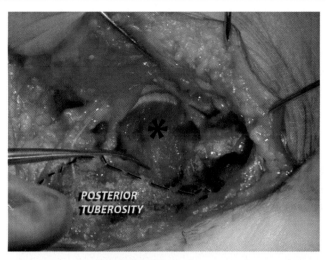

Figure 35.22. With the superolateral fragment removed, the medial sustentacular (constant) fragment (*) and the posterior tuberosity are easily seen. The primary fracture line, through the medial wall of the calcaneus (*elevator*), is identified.

Once the superolateral fragment has been removed, attention is turned to the medial sustentacular component, the posterior tuberosity, and the primary medial-fracture line (Fig. 35.22). A periosteal elevator is placed into the medial fracture line from the lateral wound, and the posterior tuberosity is disimpacted from the sustentaculum (Fig. 35.23).

The articular fragment is now evaluated. It is cleaned of clot and impacted cancellous bone (Fig. 35.24). The articular fragment should be repositioned such that height, rotation, and varus-valgus alignment are correct. This will not be possible if the fragment hits the edge of the posterior tuberosity; therefore, the posterior-inferior path for the fragment must be free of bone. This may require the surgeon to curette excess bone from the tuberosity, disimpact the tuberosity with excess varus force, or with a rongeur remove a small amount of bone that is blocking the reduction (Fig. 35.25).

The anterior process must be repositioned before the articular fragment is placed. The anterior process may be in as many as three pieces with the middle fragment pulled proximally by the interosseous ligament. A laminar spreader placed in the sinus tarsi is used to stretch the ligament thereby allowing the central piece to be more easily reduced. The surgeon should avoid ligament resection because it will destabilize the joint. In addition, a transverse fracture line may be present at the angle of Gissane. This will rotate the medial articular fragment beneath the medial-anterior tuberosity fragment. Before reduction

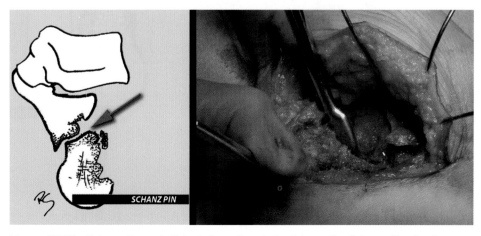

Figure 35.23. Schematic and clinical view of posterior tuberosity disimpaction (*red arrow*, direction of insertion of periosteal elevator).

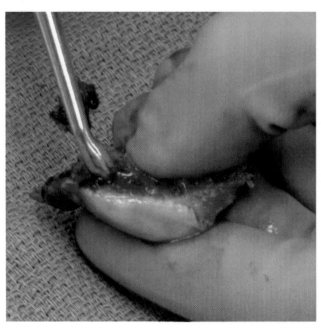

Figure 35.24. The superolateral fragment is cleaned of clot to assure perfect interposition during reduction.

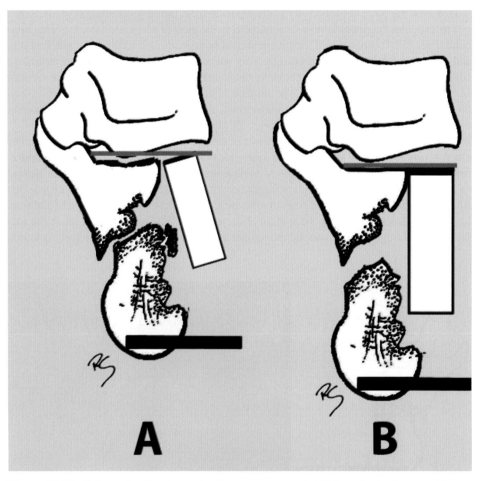

Figure 35.25. Schematic showing reduction maneuvers. **A.** While articular fragment is repositioned in height, it is still in valgus because the posterior tuberosity is blocking reduction. **B.** After the tuberosity is pulled out of the way and excess bone is rongeured off, the superolateral fragment now fits in both height and alignment (not shown is the third component of reduction, which shows rotation).

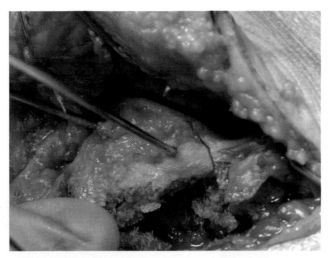

Figure 35.26. Provisional reduction of the superolateral fragment through use of two K wires to prevent rotation. The fragment is anatomically aligned at the angle of Gissane.

of the lateral articular fragment, the medial articular fragment must be repositioned, or the superolateral fragment will be reduced to a fragment that itself is not reduced.

Once the articular surface is reduced, it is provisionally held with two K wires to prevent rotation (Fig. 35.26). At this point, the anterior lateral "corner" of the articular fragment should align with the anterolateral "corner" of the medial sustentacular fragment. The anterolateral fragment should either fall in place or be manipulated back into position and held with K wires. When this reduction is anatomic, the angle of Gissane will be restored. At this point, verifying that the lateral column is anatomically reduced, the surgeon places the lateral wall back.

Once satisfied with the reduction, the surgeon should obtain intraoperative lateral, Broden's, and axial fluoroscopic views. The lateral should show a true lateral of the talus, thereby guaranteeing an accurate view of the calcaneus (Fig. 35.27). Next, with the fluoroscope in the same position, the leg is externally rotated 45 degrees and the foot is dorsiflexed. A mortise view of the ankle is then obtained; it shows the posterior facet in a Broden's view (Fig. 35.28). Finally, the leg is externally rotated 90 degrees, and the foot is maximally dorsiflexed. The fluoroscope is then angled such that the head is on the plantar aspect of the mid foot and a clear axial view of the calcaneus is obtained (Fig. 35.29).

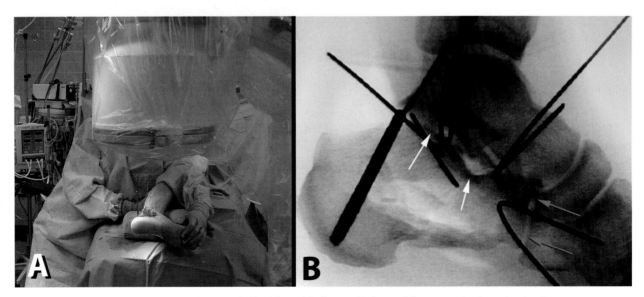

Figure 35.27. Lateral x-ray. **A.** Position with C-arm. **B.** Lateral fluoroscopic view. Anatomic reduction of calcaneal cuboid joint (*red arrows*), restoration of the angle of Gissane (*lower white arrow*), and restoration of Bohler's angle (*higher white arrow*).

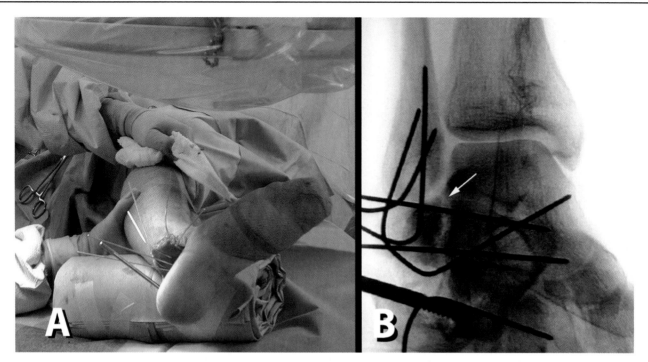

Figure 35.28. Broden's view. **A.** Positioning with the limb externally rotated 45 degrees and dorsiflexed. **B.** Mortise view of the ankle will provide best view, but the joint is still gapped and not anatomically reduced (*white arrow*).

The articular fragments should be repositioned until an anatomic reduction of the joint is accomplished. Fixation is then obtained using a 3.5-mm cortical screw placed in a lag mode. The screw should be directed from the lateral cortex and aimed slightly plantar to avoid violation of the intra-articular surface; it should extend distally toward the sustentaculum (Fig. 35.30). Once the screw is placed, the joint should be reassessed both visually and fluoroscopically.

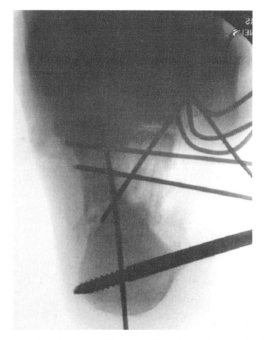

Figure 35.29. Axial view showing repositioning of posterior tuberosity through use of axial K wire to maintain position. The tuberosity is not yet completely reduced out of varus.

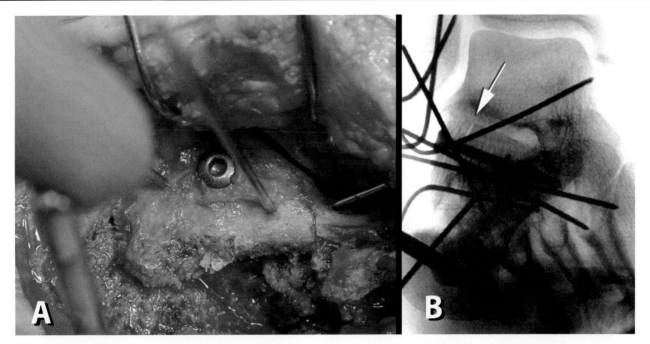

Figure 35.30. Definitive fixation of articular surface. **A.** Lag screw (3.5 mm) is placed with antirotation K wires in place. **B.** X-ray verifies anatomic joint reduction. Gap is closed and the articular surface is aligned perfectly (*white arrow*).

The calcaneal body is then definitively addressed. The anterolateral fragment and the posterior tuberosity are realigned to insure that the body is anatomically reduced. The small lateral-wall fragment is elevated so the surgeon can evaluate the cancellous defect below the joint. If a large cavity is present, the surgeon may elect to fill the void with either bone graft or a graft substitute. The lateral wall remnant is then repositioned, and a low-profile, lateral, neutralization plate is selected. One of the authors (RS) has developed a specific plate for this and uses it exclusively (Fig. 35.31). Bending of the plate is not recommended because this will throw the calcaneal tuberosity into varus.

Once plate position is acceptable, as determined by the lateral fluoroscopic view, cancellous fully threaded 4.0-mm screws are used to secure the three main components of the calcaneus: the anterior process, the posterior tuberosity, and the joint. The final reduction is verified fluoroscopically, and all K wires are removed (Fig. 35.32).

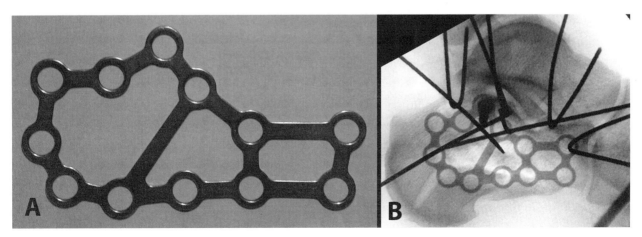

Figure 35.31. A. Low-profile, calcaneal, perimeter plate (ACE-DePuy, Warsaw, IN). **B.** Positioning of plate on lateral calcaneus and verification of size through use of fluoroscopy. In this case, a larger plate should be selected.

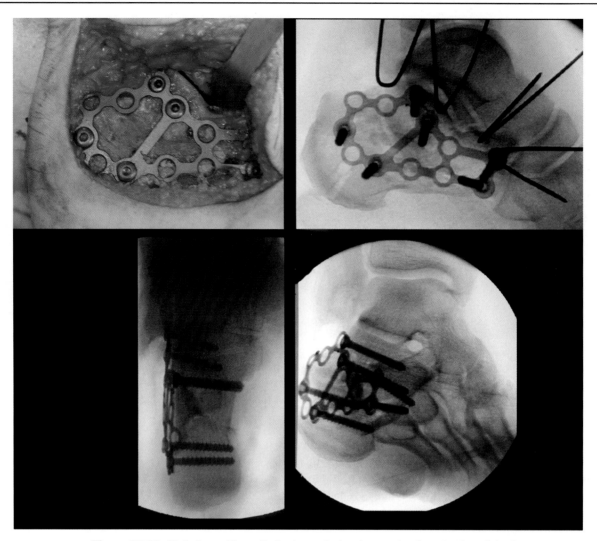

Figure 35.32. Plate in position with final x-rays showing anatomic reduction of the fracture.

Before closing the flap, the peroneal tendons should be evaluated to make sure they were not dislocated from the injury. A Freer elevator is placed into the peroneal tendon sheath at the distal inferior portion of the wound. It should advance within the sheath easily. While watching the skin, the surgeon pushes the elevator forward in an attempt to slip it over the malleolar tip. If he/she is successful, the sheath has been torn off the fibula (Fig. 35.33), and a repair must be performed. To expose the tendon sheath, a small incision (<3 cm) is made in the skin over the posterior edge of the distal tip of the fibula. Using one or two suture anchors, the sheath is secured to the bone and the repair is tested. Once completed, the tendons will no longer dislocate over the edge of the fibula.

A deep drain is placed to exit at the proximal tip of the vertical limb of the incision, and the wound is closed in a layered fashion. Deep figure-of-eight, individual, no. 0, absorbable sutures are placed in the corner of the wound. The surgeon works out to the end of each limb of the incision. The sutures are not tied but rather clamped until all deep sutures have been placed. Then, starting at the proximal and distal ends and working toward the corner of the incision, the surgeon hand ties the sutures sequentially; this technique will pull the flap and thus take tension off the corner of the wound, which is the most susceptible to wound necrosis. The skin is closed with no. 3 nylon suture using the modified Allgöwer-Donati technique: The surgeon starts again at the ends and progresses toward the apex (Fig. 35.34). Sterile dressings are applied and the tourniquet is deflated. A bulky cotton dressing and Weber splint are then placed.

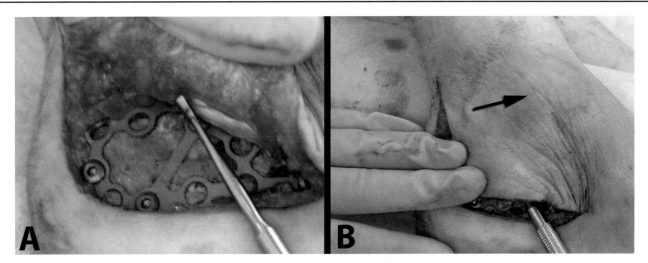

Figure 35.33. Evaluation of the peroneal tendon sheath. **A.** The insertion of an elevator into the sheath. **B.** An attempt is made to sweep the elevator over the fibula (*arrow*). This was not possible in this case.

The patient is maintained overnight in the hospital for pain control. Plain radiographs (Fig. 35.35) and CT scans (Fig. 35.36) are obtained the next day, and the drain is removed. The patient is then placed in a short-leg nonweight-bearing cast and discharged home. The patient is seen in the office for wound checks and cast exchanges. The sutures are removed only if the incision is fully sealed, usually between 4 and 6 weeks.

At 3 weeks, the patient is placed into an elastic stocking and fracture boot that is locked in neutral flexion. Early subtalar joint range-of-motion exercises out of the boot are initiated at this time; however, weight bearing is not permitted until 12 postoperative weeks have passed. If ceramic cement had been used to fill the void, weight bearing may be initiated earlier, typically at 6 weeks, but only if the wound has completely healed. In addition, we prefer that the patient sleep in the boot until weight bearing is initiated so that an equinus contracture is prevented. Once weight bearing is initiated, the patient is gradually transitioned into regular shoes as tolerated. Physical therapy, specifically for gait training and achieving balance, is also begun at this point. The patient is able to return to normal activity at 6 postoperative months.

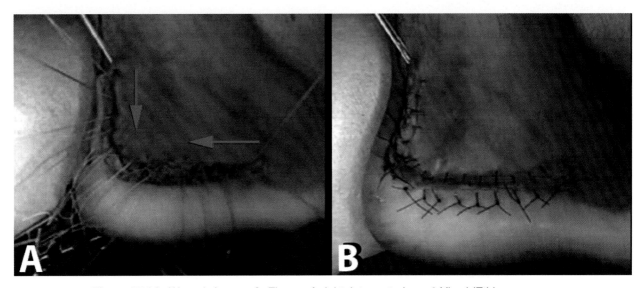

Figure 35.34. Wound closure. **A.** Figure-of-eight, interrupted, no. 0 Vicryl (Ethicon, Rutherford, NJ) are placed and tied from edges to corner (*red arrows*). **B.** Wound closure via an Allgöwer-Denoti stitch with no. 3 nylon. The knots are placed on the outside.

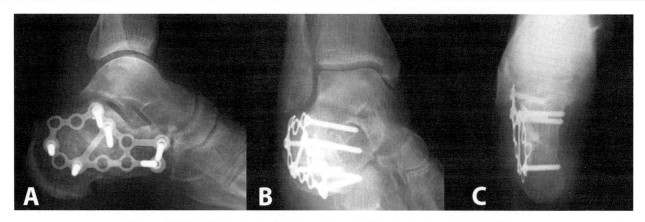

Figure 35.35. Final x-rays. **A.** Lateral view. **B.** Broden's view. **C.** Axial view.

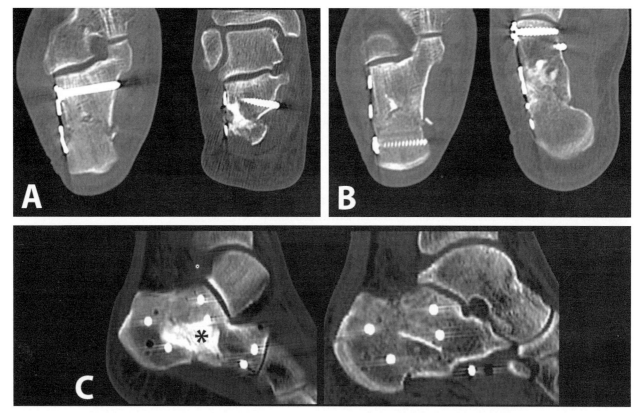

Figure 35.36. Postoperative CT scans. **A.** Coronal cuts. **B.** Transverse cuts. **C.** Sagittal reconstructions showing body reposition. Calcium phosphate cement was used as void filler (*).

RECOMMENDED READINGS

1. Buckley RE, Meek RN. Comparison of open versus closed reduction of intraarticular calcaneal fractures: a matched cohort in workmen. *J Orthop Trauma* 1992;6(1):216.
2. Sanders R, Fortin P, DiPasquale T, et al. Operative treatment in 120 displaced intraarticular calcaneal fractures: results using a prognostic computed tomography scan classification. *Clin Orthop* 1993;290:87.
3. Tornetta P III. Open reduction and internal fixation of the calcaneus using minifragment plates. *J Orthop Trauma* 1996;10(1):63–67.
4. Essex Lopresti P. The mechanism, reduction technique and results in fractures of the os calcis. *Br J Surg* 1952; 39:395.
5. Sanders R. Current concepts review: displaced intra-articular fractures of the calcaneus. *J Bone Joint Surg* 2000;82:225–250.

36

Tarsometatarsal Lisfranc Injuries: Evaluation and Management

Bruce J. Sangeorzan, Stephen K. Benirschke, and Mark T. Gould

INDICATIONS/CONTRAINDICATIONS

The primary surgical indication for treatment of an injury is the knowledge that the injury will do poorly with nonoperative treatment. Conceptually, tarsometatarsal injuries that will lead to a loss of the arch or significant deformity if treated conservatively should be treated surgically; these include both displaced injuries and subtle injuries that have instability in planes. The decision to treat a tarsometatarsal injury surgically is based on both physical examination and radiographic studies.

The transverse and longitudinal arches of the foot depend on the tarsometatarsal joints to make the foot sufficiently rigid to support the body, much as the apical blocks of ice support an igloo. Unstable tarsometatarsal injuries that compromise this structural integrity may result in deformity of the foot. In the majority of displaced injuries, the metatarsals displace dorsally and laterally on the tarsal bones, which produces pes planus with forefoot abduction. As a result, when weight is borne on the foot, it collapses. During heel lift, further deforming forces that act on the midfoot tend to exacerbate the deformity. For the metatarsals to displace in this direction, the plantar tarsometatarsal (Lisfranc) ligaments must be disrupted. Operative treatment is indicated when an ambulatory patient has an injury that renders the foot mechanically unsound, deformed, or both.

Ambulatory patients with displaced Lisfranc joints that are apparent on the plain x-rays and who have all the stabilizing ligaments disrupted are candidates for surgery. When the injuries are subtle or apparently nondisplaced, operative treatment is indicated only when two-plane instability is detected on clinical examination or stress x-rays. Because the foot functions in weight bearing, the integrity of the plantar ligaments is of greater importance than that of the dorsal ligaments.

Contraindications to surgical intervention include nonambulatory individuals, patients with serious vascular disease unlikely to heal a surgical incision but who have no significant deformity, or an injury that is unstable in only the transverse plane. Lisfranc injuries with only bone injuries can be treated by closed means or by closed reduction with percutaneous pinning. When deformity and compromised circulation is found, the surgeon faces a dilemma. Leaving a deformity puts the patient at risk for ulceration, while treating it surgically puts the patient at risk for wound-healing problems. In this circumstance, a vascular surgeon may be consulted to evaluate whether an inflow procedure would be beneficial prior to orthopedic intervention.

Neurologic impairment is also a cause for concern. The physician must decide whether sufficient energy produced the injury or whether an underlying neuropathic condition exists. Trivial injuries that cause significant displacement should stimulate an investigation into a possible neuropathic condition. A Charcot neuropathic foot has different indications for treatment and calls for different technique than does a foot without preexisting neuropathy. For treatment of a Lisfranc injury in the presence of peripheral neuropathy, more fixation will be required, and a longer period of postoperative protection is indicated.

Physical Examination Criteria

Lisfranc injury is often missed and is one of the few injuries in orthopedics in which the maxim "the eye doesn't see what the mind doesn't search for" is most appropriate. Swelling and tenderness in the midfoot with no obvious fracture should trigger a high index of suspicion. Instability should be determined by physical examination. The physician grasps the metatarsal heads and applies a dorsal force to the forefoot while the other hand palpates the tarsometatarsal joint. Dorsal subluxation or dislocation of the bases of the metatarsals suggests instability (Fig 36.1). If the first and second metatarsal can be displaced medially or laterally as well, global instability is present, and surgical treatment is needed. Low-energy injuries interrupt the medial capsule but do not disrupt the plantar ligaments. When the

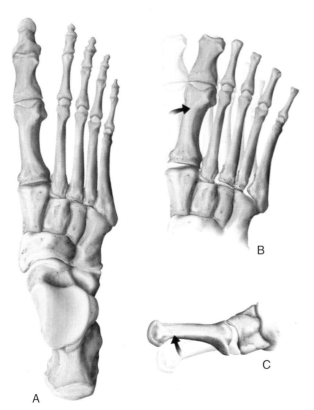

Figure 36.1. A–C. Diagrammatic representation of a dorsal view of the foot. The metatarsal bases are forced laterally and dorsally.

plantar ligaments are intact, no dorsal subluxation will occur with stress examination. These injuries may be treated nonoperatively or with less rigid fixation at the discretion of the examining surgeon.

Radiographic Criteria

With ligamentous disruption of the midfoot without fracture, x-rays made while the patient is not weight bearing may be deceptively benign. The ligaments are torn with initial displacement; however, when the deforming force is removed, the foot may spring back into a neutral position, concealing gross instability. The physician should be suspicious whenever midfoot gross swelling and pain is found.

When disruptions are found on several radiographic plane films, subtle tarsometatarsal injury is suggested. The first and most reliable image shows disruption in the continuity of a line drawn from the medial base of the second metatarsal to the medial side of intermediate cuneiform on the anteroposterior (AP) and oblique views (Fig. 36.2A).

The second most reliable type of image shows widening of the interval between the first and second ray; these x-rays should arouse suspicion. If tenderness is evident upon palpation, stress views should be obtained.

On a third most important observation, the medial side of the base of the fourth metatarsal should line up with the medial side of the cuboid on the oblique view. This is a soft sign because the cross section of the metatarsal base is not equal to the cross section of the cuboid. As a result, a step-off may be present if the angle of the beam is slightly misdirected. On the lateral view, the metatarsals are aligned with the cuneiforms at the dorsal cortex. When ligament injury is extant, the metatarsals are typically dorsally displaced in relation to the cuneiforms.

Finally, any disruption of the medial column line (MCL), a line tangential to the medial aspect of the navicular and medial cuneiform, can be found on two views. The disruption will show on the intersection of the base of the first metatarsal on an AP view taken during weight bearing. In addition, views taken during abduction stress reliably predict disruption of the Lisfranc ligamentous complex.

PREOPERATIVE PLANNING

Physical examination should document the status of the dorsalis pedis and posterior tibial pulses, the integrity of the skin, and the habitus of the foot. Tendon entrapment may be demonstrated by an altered, uncorrectable position of the toes or midfoot. Intact or altered sensation should be documented.

Preoperative imaging should include a simulated AP and lateral view of the foot under weight bearing, as well as an oblique view. Oblique views are essential in evaluating a midfoot injury and should be included in the foot trauma series. If the presence, location, or degree of injury is uncertain, stress x-rays should be taken in two planes. Typically they are done through use of fluoroscopy so the surgeon can make certain that the correct plane is achieved for the image. When the index of suspicion is high, the stress roentgenogram is performed in an operating room (OR), so that if the injury is confirmed, surgery can be done under the same anesthetic.

An appropriate anesthetic is given, and the fluoroscopy unit is brought into the OR suite. The table is bent at the knees so the foot is relatively parallel to the floor. While wearing lead gloves, the surgeon grasps the first and second metatarsal heads with one hand and the hind foot with the other. With the thumb placed over the cuboid to act as a fulcrum, the forefoot is abducted and an AP x-ray is obtained. Instability is present if a gap occurs on the medial side of the first or second tarsometatarsal joint, or disruption of the MCL is produced (see Fig. 36.2D).

Stress views in the lateral plane are performed if uncertainty exists. This is done with the surgeon grasping the midfoot with one hand and the forefoot with the other, and acutely plantarflexing through the tarsometatarsal joint. The fluoroscopy unit is oriented across the

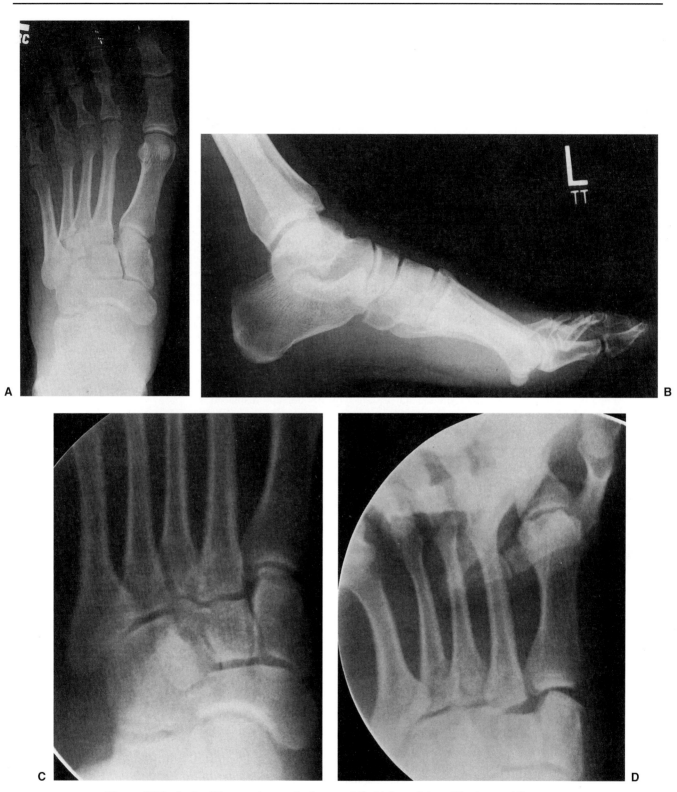

Figure 36.2. **A.** An AP x-ray demonstrating a subtle Lisfranc injury. The base of the second metatarsal is displaced laterally. **B.** This lateral x-ray, taken under nonweight-bearing conditions, shows that the dorsal cortex of the second metatarsal is subluxed dorsally relative to its cuneiform. **C.** A scout view is used to confirm that the foot is in the correct position for assessing the tarsometatarsal joints. **D.** The stress x-ray reveals instability in the first, second, and probably third tarsometatarsal joints. (*continues*)

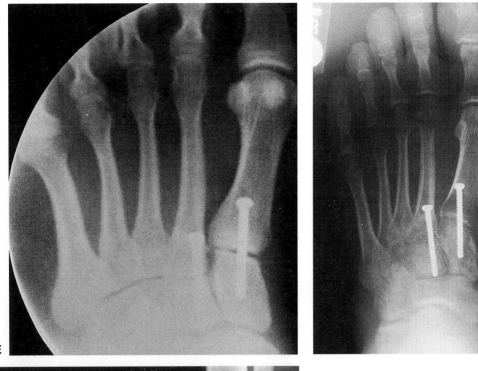

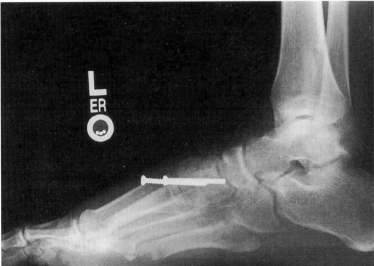

Figure 36.2. (*continued*) E. An intra-operative fluoroscopic image taken after fixation reveals that the third metatarsal is stable. F. Six weeks following surgery, the reduction appears anatomic and the clinical position of the foot is good. G. Alignment of the metatarsal bases is restored in both planes.

table and an image is obtained. Although the tarsometatarsal joints may angulate, they should not open asymmetrically. Subluxation indicates that the joints are unstable.

Possible instability should be investigated at the intercuneiform level (Fig. 36.3). These injuries are not rare, but because they are subtle, out of the plane of standard x-rays, and not well described, they are easily missed. Treatment follows the same principles as those at the Lisfranc level. Stress views in the AP plane are used to confirm the injury. Because little motion is characteristic of most of the intercuneiform joints, any significant motion is abnormal. If the instability is great enough to allow subluxation of the midfoot, it should be treated. Displacement of the intercuneiform joints leads to deformity that is poorly understood and difficult to treat.

If x-rays are done in AP, lateral, and oblique planes, and stress views are obtained when there is uncertainty, additional imaging modalities should not be necessary. Computed tomographic (CT) scans of the midfoot are difficult to interpret. The role of the magnetic resonance imaging (MRI) scan has not been established.

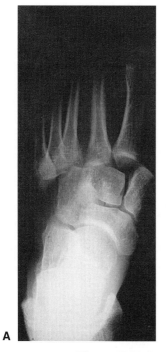

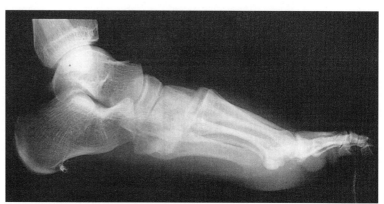

A   B

Figure 36.3. A. An AP x-ray of a left foot with severe Lisfranc injury. All five metatarsals are displaced laterally. **B.** The lateral view, taken under nonweight-bearing conditions, shows a dorsal dislocation.

SURGERY

Timing

Several factors must be considered to determine whether surgical intervention is necessary. These include the amount of soft-tissue swelling, the availability of imaging studies, and the degree of displacement. Surgery should be done emergently only in the presence of a compartment syndrome, an open injury, or a deformity that threatens the integrity of the skin. Open injuries should be stabilized as soon as possible. If emergency stabilization threatens the survival of the limb, the soft tissue may be treated and the bony stabilization performed when the safety of the soft-tissue envelope is restored. If gross instability is found, stabilizing the bone may help the soft tissue to heal, as it does in long-bone fractures.

Technique

The patient is positioned supine with a roll beneath the greater trochanter to rotate the limb internally to a neutral position. A second roll is placed beneath the popliteal fossa. Knee flexion allows plantarflexion of the foot for easier exposure and imaging.

A longitudinal incision is made in the web space between the first and second rays (Fig. 36.4B), while the surgeon takes care to avoid damage to the dorsal cutaneous nerves. The first tarsometatarsal joint is exposed between the long and short hallux-extensor tendons (see Fig. 36.4C). Typically, one finds significant hemorrhage in this area, making identification of the structures somewhat difficult. The capsule may be enfolded into the joint and should be removed and preserved for later reapproximation. A small periosteal elevator is placed along the medial side of the first tarsometatarsal joint to confirm its reduced position. The enfolded joint capsule is removed medially so that the medial edge of the joint can be seen. Because the displacement is most often dorsal and lateral, the first metatarsal usually reduces with a plantar and medial force. When the first metatarsal is reduced relative to the medial cuneiform, a Kirschner (K) wire is placed across the joint at its periphery, preventing loss of reduction before definitive fixation (see

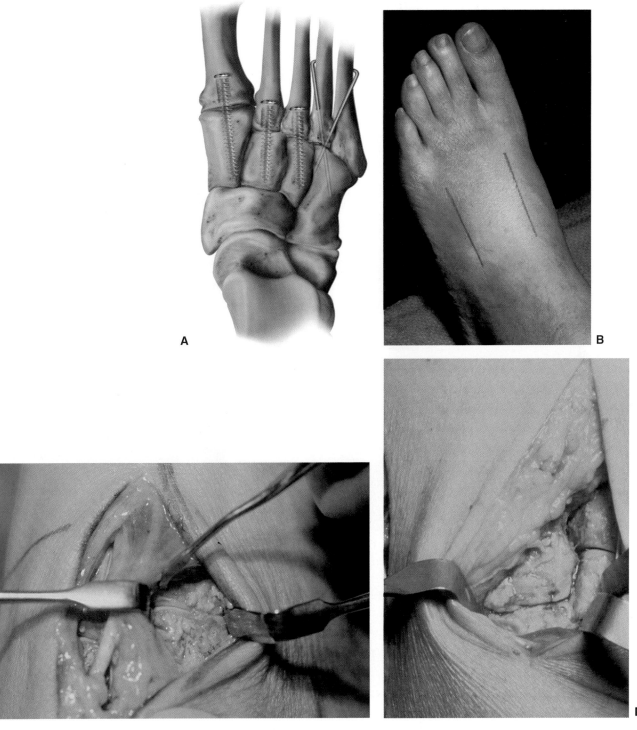

Figure 36.4. **A.** Idealized fixation. A small screw, usually 3.5 mm, transfixes the base of the metatarsal and cuneiform. The screw should be directed from distal to proximal and begin approximately 15 mm from the joint or a little farther in the first ray. If an intercuneiform injury is present, an additional screw is directed from medial to lateral. **B.** The preferred position of the two dorsal incisions. **C.** This figure shows the intraoperative exposure through the more medial of the two dorsal incisions. **D.** Intraoperative photograph showing the base of the second metatarsal reduced into its mortise. (*continues*)

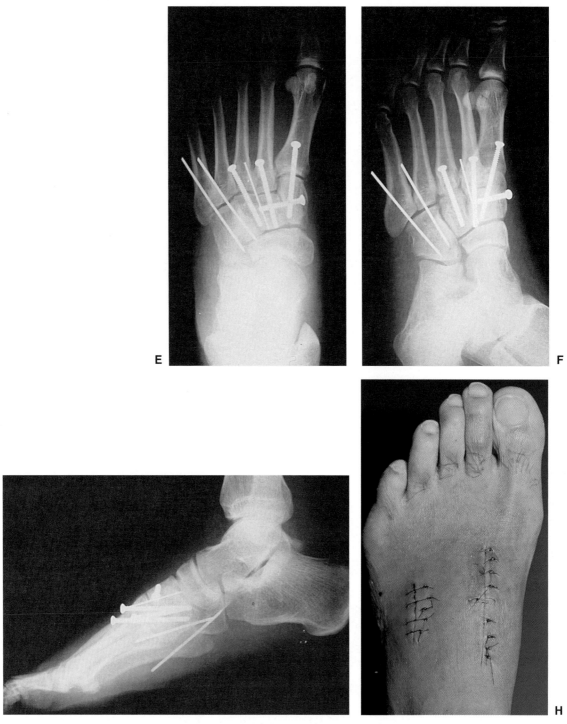

Figure 36.4. (*continued*) **E.** The 3.5-mm screws bridge the first, second, and third tar-sometatarsal joints and the joint between the medial and intermediate cuneiform. The fourth and fifth tarsometatarsal joints are transfixed by 0.062-inch K wires. **F.** This oblique view shows that the base of the fourth metatarsal, on its medial side, lines up with the me-dial side of the cuboid. **G.** A lateral x-ray of the same foot as in **(F)** shows that the dorsal cortex of the metatarsal and tarsal bones are aligned. **H.** A postoperative photograph of the operated foot at 2 weeks after surgery.

Fig. 36.4D). The K wire is placed in the area of the joint that will not be used for definitive fixation.

Before reducing the second metatarsal, the surgeon should check for injury between the medial and middle cuneiforms. Although not as common as Lisfranc-level injuries, disruption of the medial/middle cuneiform junction is the most common of the intertarsal disruptions (Fig. 36.5A). If first-second intertarsal instability is found, it should be addressed before the tarsometatarsal repair because it is difficult to secure the metatarsals to mobile tarsals. Under direct vision, the cuneiforms are reduced and held together with a pointed reduction clamp. Through a small stab wound, the surgeon drills from medial to lateral, beginning in the middle of the dorsal one third of the medial cuneiform. This starting position is necessary because the middle cuneiform is smaller in its dorsoplantar and proximal-to-distal direction than is the medial cuneiform (see Fig. 36.5F). This approach also allows the surgeon to keep the screw out of the way of the screws that will traverse the tarsometatarsal joints. The drill hole is measured, and a 3.5-mm screw is placed from medial to lateral. The screw should not be placed into the lateral cuneiform (see Fig. 36.5C,D).

Next, the second metatarsal base is reduced into its mortise between the three cuneiforms. This is accomplished by directly reducing the base of the second metatarsal against the intermediate cuneiform. If the surgeon has difficulty reducing it, interposition of bone may be found plantarly. Occasionally, part of the base of the second metatarsal is avulsed by the Lisfranc plantar ligament and blocks reduction of the second metatarsal (see Fig. 36.5A). A small elevator is used to push the fragment plantarly and medially. When it is reduced, a large, pointed, reduction clamp is placed from the base of the second metatarsal to the middle of the medial cuneiform and compressed. A K wire is placed at the periphery of the joint to maintain the position. The dorsal cortex of the second metatarsal is notched 12 to 15 mm from the joint and a hole prepared for the 3.5-mm screw with a 2.5-mm drill. Before advancing the drill, the surgeon should center it over the second toe and advance it in a position almost parallel to the plantar surface of the foot. This is necessary because the intermediate cuneiform is quite small in cross section, and if the screw is directed too plantarly, it may completely miss the cuneiform. To prevent subluxation as the screw is advanced across the joint, the drill hole should be tapped before a 3.5-mm cortical screw is inserted. When the screw has been seated, the K wire is removed.

Next, the position of the first metatarsal is reassessed relative to the medial cuneiform. If it has moved or is overreduced, it should be repositioned and a K wire placed at the edge of the joint. Again, the surgeon drills, taps, and places a 3.5-mm cortical screw. This screw should start 15 to 20 mm from the joint, but it need not be quite parallel to the plantar surface of the foot because the shape of the medial cuneiform is greater in the dorsoplantar direction. This screw should be approximately 40 mm in length. If the measured length is less than 30 mm, the starting hole was placed too close to the joint or the drill was directed obliquely out of the cuneiform. A screw this short may not provide adequate purchase in the cuneiform.

The third tarsometatarsal joint should be directly evaluated. If it requires fixation but the fourth does not, no further incision is required. A full-thickness flap is developed through the original incision until the third tarsometatarsal joint can be visualized. It will usually follow the second into a reduced position. It is held in place with a reduction clamp, and the screw is placed through a small stab wound. However, if the third and fourth metatarsal bases both require reduction and fixation, a second incision will be helpful. A longitudinal incision is made over the base of the fourth ray parallel to the first incision (see Fig. 36.4B). Depending on the size of the extensor brevis muscle, the surgeon may be able to elevate the lateral border of the muscle. If it is too large, the muscle belly is split bluntly in line with its fibers so that the tarsometatarsal joints are visualized. The third metatarsal base should be reduced first. Again, a K wire is placed as provisional fixation. Definitive fixation is provided by a 3.5-mm cortical screw.

Because the fourth and fifth tarsometatarsal joints are mobile, the goals of treatment are slightly different than for the other joints. These joints must be held in place only long enough for the surgeon to develop a scar capsule. Screws may break because of the motion in this joint. The fourth and fifth tarsometatarsals are held in place and pinned with 0.062-

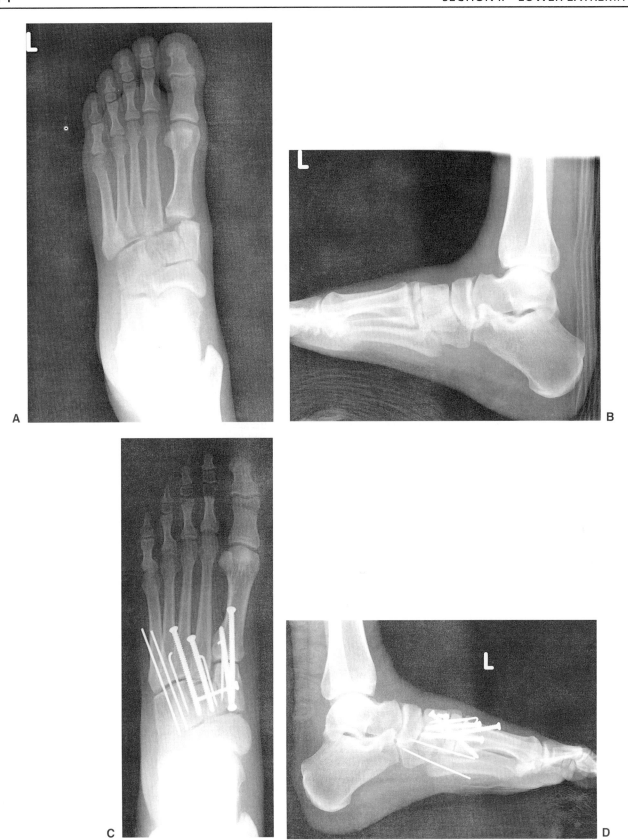

Figure 36.5. A. An AP x-ray of a left foot with Lisfranc injury and intercuneiform disruption. Note the avulsion fracture at base of second metatarsal. **B.** The lateral view, taken under nonweight-bearing conditions, shows dorsal dislocation and cuneiform fracture. **C.** A postoperative AP view with intercuneiform fixation. Tarsometatarsal fixation with 4.0-mm cortical screws and lateral K wire fixation. **D.** Postoperative lateral view, taken under non-weight-bearing conditions, shows dorsal placement of intercuneiform screw fixation, which allows adequate room for crossed 4.0-mm cortical screw fixation in the first ray. (*continues*)

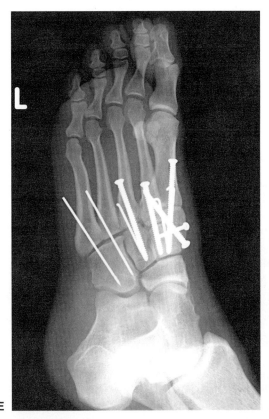
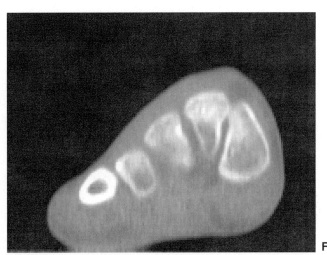

Figure 36.5. (*continued*) **E.** Oblique view confirms anatomical reduction of fourth and fifth metatarsal-cuboid joints. **F.** Coronal weight-bearing CT cut at the level of the medial and middle cuneiforms demonstrates rapid plantar tapering of the middle cuneiform. This relationship necessitates dorsal screw placement for intercuneiform fixation.

inch K wires (Figs. 36.4E–G and 36.5C–E). K wires may be used obliquely when reduction is difficult or intertarsal injuries require fixation (see Fig. 36.4A).

Lisfranc injuries may have a fracture component as well. They most commonly present as a fracture through the metaphysis of the metatarsals. When unstable, the fracture should be stabilized, and then the joint evaluated. If fractures are present without concomitant ligament injuries, reduction and pinning may be adequate, because fractures get sticky within 3 weeks and heal within 6 weeks. A common pattern includes a joint disruption at the first ray, a fracture through the second metatarsal base, and a joint injury at the third. Because the second metatarsal is recessed into a mortise between the cuneiform, it fractures and leaves the base attached to the ligaments. If the first and third rays are stabilized across the joint, the second requires only reduction and sometimes pinning for 4 weeks. When fractures pass through the metatarsal bases and the joint is intact, treatment is not so involved: Reduction and pinning with K wires may be enough. Unlike the ligaments, fractures heal reliably in 6 weeks. The K wire can be left in place until the fracture becomes stable. Once the fracture is healed, mechanical stability is restored.

ALTERNATIVE FIXATION TECHNIQUES

Persistent hardware failure and symptomatic hardware have resulted in the development of newer implant technology. The 4.0-mm cortical screw is 15% stronger in bending than the 3.5-mm cortical screw (Table 36.1). The strength advantage results primarily from the core diameter of 2.9 mm for the 4.0 mm cortical screw versus 2.4 mm for the 3.5-mm cortical screw. This newer screw has proven useful in crowded Lisfranc constructs while in theory it also reduces hardware failure (see Fig. 36.5C–E).

Table 36.1. *Comparison of 3.5-mm and 4.0-mm Cortical Screw Specifications and Bending Strength*

Specifications (mm)	3.5-mm cortical screw	4.0-mm cortical screw
Thread diameter	3.5	4.0[a]
Thread pitch	1.25	1.25
Core diameter	2.4	2.9[a]
Screw lengths	10–110	14–100
Diameter of head	6.0	6.0
Glide-hole drill bit	3.5	4.0
Pilot-hole drill bit	2.5	2.9

Screws are from Synthes (Paoli, PA).
[a]Specification results in 15% increase in bending strength of 4.0-mm screw.

In recent series, researchers have evaluated 3.5-mm absorbable screws in an attempt to minimize both the incidence of symptomatic hardware and subsequent surgical procedures for hardware removal. Results appear safe in small numbers at short-term follow-up. The efficacy of these implants has yet to be tested for maintenance of reduction in long-term follow-up.

POSTOPERATIVE MANAGEMENT

The patient is placed in a short-leg, posterior, plaster splint at the end of the operation. The patient is discharged when he or she safely masters ambulation with crutches or a walker, and pain control is achieved with oral agents. The length of stay is dependent on associated injuries, the fragility of the patient, and the degree of swelling. The range varies from outpatient surgery to 4 or 5 days as an inpatient. Sutures are removed 10 to 14 days after surgery. If the injury was isolated, the patient reliable, and fixation secure, the splint is replaced with a removable brace. If any of these three factors is absent, a short-leg non–weight-bearing cast is recommended for an additional 4 weeks.

X-rays should be taken at 6 weeks of the unplastered areas so the surgeon can document the alignment and assess fracture healing. Postoperative imaging should include a simulated weight-bearing AP and lateral as well as an oblique view. For most injuries, partial weight bearing is instituted with the patient wearing a removable protective boot at 6 weeks. Self-directed physical therapy (PT) is begun at this time. Swimming is encouraged, and riding an exercise bike is allowed. Depending on the stability and fixation, the patient is encouraged to gradually advance to full weight bearing over the 2 to 4 weeks after the protective boot is implemented. At 8 to 10 weeks, the patient can begin wearing a regular shoe if the foot is not too swollen. The screws are left in place for a minimum of 16 weeks.

If the implants are asymptomatic and transfix only the first through third tarsometatarsal joints, they may be left permanently in place. If the joint has become sufficiently stiff, the screws will not be symptomatic. However, a small amount of motion frequently occurs, which causes the screws to loosen. If this happens, the screws can often be removed under local anesthesia in the office or outpatient center.

Because swelling may persist for months, compression stockings may be beneficial. Initially the patient may begin by wearing athletic shoes. As activity level increases, a standard work shoe may replace the athletic shoe for a few hours a day in increasing amounts until normal shoes can be tolerated. The process may be facilitated by a custom-molded full-length insole of a nonrigid material such as cork or pelite.

The patients may return to work at 10 to 14 days if they work in an office. They should return to work in 3 to 4 months if they are involved in heavy labor activities. Patients should avoid jumping-type recreational activities, such as basketball and volleyball, and running for 9 to 12 months. The degree of work and recreational activities depends on the amount of trauma, the degree of articular surface injury, and the quality of the bone. Most patients will continue to have some symptoms in the foot for up to 2 years. Many will have life-long symptoms. Only 12% will need midfoot arthrodesis if bony Lisfranc injuries are anatomically reduced and held rigidly. A slightly higher trend toward midfoot arthrosis can be found in those with pure ligamentous injuries. If symptoms are mechanical (i.e., midfoot pain during heel rise), a custom, full-length, semirigid insole may be beneficial. Generally, this should be fabricated when the patient has returned to full weight bearing and the swelling has resolved.

COMPLICATIONS

Associated injuries following midfoot fractures and dislocations include inter-cuneiform injuries, tendon entrapment, and vascular injury. The interval between the medial and intermediate cuneiform is the most common, associated, intercuneiform, joint injury. The tibialis anterior is the most commonly entrapped tendon. The tibialis anterior tendon inserts in part on the base of the first metatarsal. As the first metatarsal is displaced laterally, it takes the tendon with it. As the deforming force is removed, the metatarsal moves medially, and the tendon is trapped by the medial cuneiform. This complication is treated during open reduction. At the time of surgery, the anterior tibia tendon will be in the way of reduction and can be reduced to its normal position. The most common vascular injury is to the plantar branch of the dorsalis pedis, where it is tethered between the first and second metatarsal. Damage to this vessel, however, is of little clinical significance; however, some historic references document the potential for more severe injuries that result in forefoot ischemia.

Injury to the dorsal cutaneous branches of the superficial peroneal nerve also may occur. Because the tissues are edematous and displaced and hemorrhage is significant in the subcutaneous tissue, identification of these small nerves is challenging. Care should be taken to preserve the nerves, and patients should be warned preoperatively that nerve injury is possible. If one of these nerves is divided during surgery, the proximal end can be tucked into the extensor brevis muscle belly or the two ends can be reapproximated.

Soft-tissue problems are common, particularly after direct trauma. There is little muscle to absorb the load or augment the blood flow. Patients should be warned that eschar may develop in areas that were injured and may include the surgical incision. It is uncommon for these soft-tissue problems to require free tissue transfer, but skin grafts are common in direct injuries. Full-thickness wounds are managed with dressing changes until an adequate bed of granulation tissue is generated to support a split-thickness graft.

Nonunion is uncommon in metatarsal fractures, but when it occurs and is painful or leads to instability, it must be treated. Sometimes, in spite of nonunion, "splinting" by the surrounding structures is sufficient such that symptoms are minimal and surgical treatment is unnecessary.

Incomplete reduction is a common problem that may lead to loss of the arch and abduction of the forefoot. Great care should be taken to plantarflex and adduct the metatarsals adequately. To lessen the likelihood of incomplete reduction, the surgeon must be certain that the first metatarsal is brought medially and plantarly before trying to reduce the second metatarsal. A prominent cuneiform may be observed on the dorsomedial aspect of the foot when the first metatarsal is incompletely plantarflexed and adducted. At times this deformity may also be due to unrecognized intercuneiform injury.

RECOMMENDED READING

Arntz CT, Veith RG, Hansen ST. Fractures and fracture-dislocations of the tarsometatarsal joint. *J Bone Joint Surg* 1987;70(2):173–181.

Blair WF. Irreducible tarsal metatarsal fracture dislocation. *J Trauma* 1981;21:988–990.

Cross HS, Manos RE, Buoncristiani A, et al. Abduction stress and weightbearing radiography of purely ligamentous injury in the tarsometatarsal joint. *Foot Ankle* 1998;19(8):537–541.

DeBenedetti MJ, Evanski PM, Waugh TR. The unreducible Lisfranc fracture. *Clin Orthop* 1978;136:238–240.

Foster SC, Foster RR. Lisfranc tarsal metatarsal fracture dislocation. *Radiology* 1976;120:79–83.

Kuo RS, Tejwani NC, Digiovanni CW, et al. Outcome after open reduction and internal fixation of lisfranc joint injuries. *J Bone Joint Surg* 2000;82(11):1609–1618.

Sangeorzan BJ, Veith RG, Hansen ST Jr. Fusion of Lisfranc's joint for the salvage of tarsometatarsal injuries. *Foot Ankle* 1989;10(4):193–200.

Pelvis and Acetabulum

37

Pelvic Fractures: External Fixation and C-Clamp

Enes M. Kanlic and Hector O. Pacheco

INDICATIONS/CONTRAINDICATIONS

Injuries to the pelvic ring range from simple stable fractures as the result of low-energy forces to life-threatening injuries with hemodynamic instability. The incidence of pelvic fractures in Sweden is approximately 37 per 100,000 patients per year (1). Pelvic fractures account for 3% to 8% of all fractures seen in the emergency room but are present in up to 25% of multiply injured patients. Mortality rates in patients with complex pelvic fractures and associated visceral injuries can be as high as 20% to 25%, and for patients with open pelvic fractures, the mortality rate ranges from 15% to 50% (1–6).

Of the several classification schemes for pelvic fractures, we favor the Tile classification, which is used to predict instability in the injured pelvic ring. Tile A injuries are stable fractures that can be managed nonoperatively. Tile B injuries are rotationally unstable but vertically stable. Tile C injuries are both rotationally and vertically unstable.

External fixation is utilized primarily in the management of patients with hemodynamic instability following pelvic fractures. Specific indications for anterior external fixation include selected, rotationally unstable, Tile B1 and B2 pelvic fractures. We strongly favor external fixation following fracture when the local conditions in and around the pelvis or abdomen are contaminated, such as with open fractures, diverting colostemies or a suprapubic urinary catheter must be placed. In addition, patients with concomitant visceral injuries, especially those whose injuries would be exacerbated when the abdomen is open, are often treated with pelvic external fixation. Occasionally, anterior-ring external fixation is used to augment posterior ring fixation.

The most common indication for anterior-ring external fixation is in a critically ill, unstable patient with a translationally unstable pelvic injury (Tile C). A resuscitative frame with ipsilateral supracondylar traction is used when a C-clamp is unavailable or not applicable.

Contraindications to external fixation are stable pelvic-ring injuries (Tile A) and patients with associated fractures of the iliac wing in which stable pin placement would be difficult or impossible. External fixation should be avoided when internal fixation can be performed on a stable patient in a timely fashion.

PREOPERATIVE PLANNING

Patient Stabilization

In the field or emergency room setting, emergency care workers and paramedics trained in advanced trauma life support (ATLS) often play a critical role. In patients with hemodynamic instability and a potentially unstable pelvic-ring injury, a single attempt at reduction should be considered. The responder applies traction to the unbroken lower extremity on the shortened or deformed side of the pelvis with manual lateral compression on the iliac wings or greater trochanters. The knees and ankles should be slightly flexed and internally rotated and taped together before a noninvasive external fixation device (wrapped sheet or pelvic binder) is applied (Fig. 37.1). When done at the scene of an accident, emergent transfer to an institution capable of treating pelvic trauma may be life saving (7,8).

Hemodynamically unstable patients with pelvic ring injuries require prompt evaluation and simultaneous aggressive resuscitation. Initial measures include airway control and aggressive fluid resuscitation through two 14- to 16-gauge intravenous catheters in the upper extremities. Physical examination should be directed for signs of possible mechanical instability of the pelvis. Tell-tale signs include a history of high-energy trauma from motor vehicle or motorcycle collisions, falls from a height, or rollover motor-vehicle collisions. On clinical examination, a shortened and malrotated extremity, asymmetric iliac spines, swelling or blood on genitals and perineum, contusion or ecchymosis in the lower abdomen or pelvis suggest pelvic instability. Gentle, manual, iliac-wing compression from lateral toward the midline may reveal a mobile hemipelvis and mechanical instability. A careful neurological examination to assess for leg sensation and motor function is critical. Vaginal and rectal digital exams with guaiac test for occult blood and with speculums (time permitting) help rule out an occult open fracture. If overlooked and not treated, a fracture hematoma that comes in contact with a contaminated environment may cause a life-threatening pelvic infection.

The care of a hemodynamically unstable patient with a displaced pelvic fracture is the responsibility of a multidisciplinary trauma team that includes a general surgeon, anesthesiologist, orthopedic surgeon, and invasive radiologist. Trauma protocols are helpful in evaluating and treating critically ill patients, establishing priorities, and guiding treatment. Using the algorithm (Fig. 37.2), Ertel et al (9) were able to save 15 of 20 patients (75%) who presented with multiple injuries that included unstable pelvic injuries with an average Injury Severity Score (ISS) of 41.2 ± 15.3. Fifteen patients had massive hemorrhage (14 were in extremis), and five were in hemorrhagic shock. Two of them required subdiaphragmatic clamping of the aorta to stabilize a disastrous hemodynamic situation.

As part of the primary survey, a focused abdominal sonogram for trauma (FAST) or computed tomography (CT) scan can be used to determine the presence of free fluid in in-

---

- External fixation
  - Noninvasive techniques (wrapped sheet, commercial pelvic binders, vacuum splint, or pneumatic anti-shock garment)
  - Invasive techniques
    - Anterior external fixator (w/wo skeletal traction)
      - Iliac-crest external fixation (high route)
      - Supraacetabular external fixation (low route)
    - Posterior external fixator (w/wo anterior fixator)
      - C-clamp
- Internal fixation
- Combination of external and internal fixation

Figure 37.1. Methods of pelvic fracture stabilization.

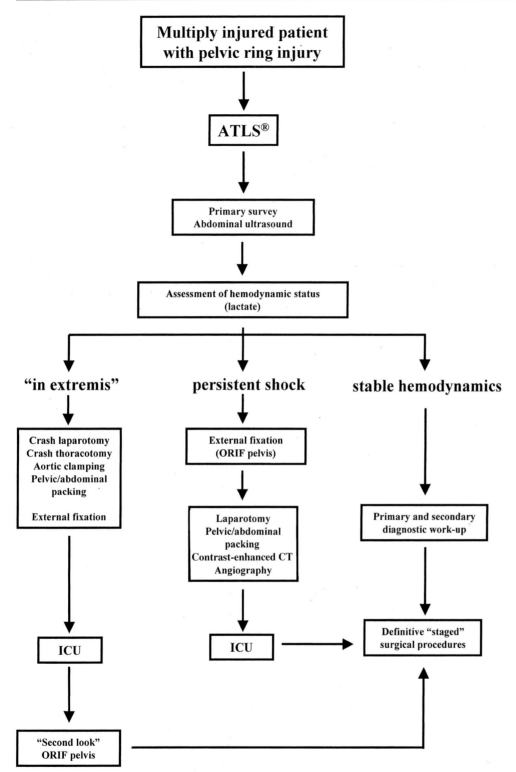

Figure 37.2. An orthopedic damage-control algorithm for patients with pelvic fracture. (From Ertel W. General assessment and management of the polytrauma patient. In: Tile M, Helfet D, Kellam J, eds. *Fractures of the pelvis and acetabulum*. 3rd ed. Philadelphia: Lippincott Williams & Wilkins; 2003:71 with permission.)

traperitoneal, retroperitoneal, or pericardial cavities. Arterial blood gas with blood lactate levels and/or base deficit analyses are good indicators of the hemorrhagic state and tissue oxygenation (9–11).

A chest x-ray is an important part of the trauma work-up because it can be used to rule out a pneumothorax, hemopneumothorax, tension pneumothorax, or flail chest. A single anteroposterior (AP) radiograph of the pelvis can be used to diagnose a pelvic fracture correctly in approximately 90% of cases. X-ray signs of instability are (a) >5-mm displacement of the sacroiliac (SI) joint in any plane (inlet and outlet views will improve accuracy if circumstances allow), (b) posterior fracture gap, and (c) avulsions of the transverse process of fifth lumbar vertebra or avulsion fractures of the sacrospinous ligament. By definition, a stable pelvic injury can withstand normal physiologic forces without abnormal deformation. The surgeon should not routinely manual test for pelvic ring stability because he/she could dislodge blood clots in a hemodynamically unstable patient. One-time manual testing, to exclude a situation in which the pelvis had been unstable but has since been reduced, may be permissible by an experienced surgeon in cases where the x-rays do not clearly demonstrate an unstable injury (12,13).

Numerous studies have shown that in patients with multiple injuries, exsanguination and closed head injury are the main causes of mortality within the first 24 hours after injury. Damage control surgeries, for hemorrhage control, decompression of body cavities such as in the chest and head, and contamination control of abdominal perforations, as well as devitalized tissue debridement in the extremities, improve survival. Determination of the patient's hemodynamic status and initial response to resuscitation measures allow placement of the patient in one of three protocol categories that dictate treatment (see Fig. 37.2).

A subset of multiply injured patients presents in extremis (i.e., without measurable vital signs). Most of these patients need a crash laparotomy, thoracotomy, and/or pelvic/abdominal packing (with or without temporary aortic cross-clamping) to survive (Fig. 37.3). While awaiting the response of the patient to aggressive resuscitation therapy, a C-clamp or an anterior, pelvic, external fixator should be applied. Subsequent, repeated, pelvic/abdominal packing against a firm stabilized pelvis will be much more effective in tamponading the bleeding.

If the patient is in a persistent shock category despite adequate fluid replacement, blood transfusions, and medications over 2 hours, an external fixator or C-clamp should replace a pelvic sheet or binder. Numerous studies have shown that in patients with unstable pelvic injuries in which ligaments and fascial planes that support the pelvic floor have been disrupted, self-tamponade rarely occurs (14). Huittinen and Slätis (15) have estimated that 80% to 90 % of bleeding following fracture and/or dislocation comes from disruption of the lumbosacral venous plexus and fracture bone surfaces and that only 10% have an arterial origin. The most common technique for stopping the diffuse bleeding (venous or arterial small vessels) is by tamponade. In patients who require abdominal exploration, la-

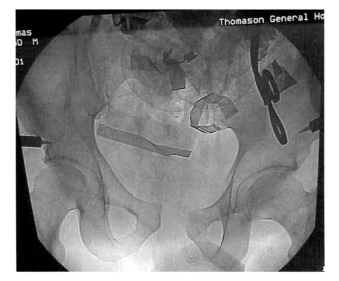

Figure 37.3. Aortic cross-clamping and C-clamp placement in a policeman, who was struck by an automobile while standing alongside a highway. On admission, he was in extremis, and crash laparotomy was conducted, and a C-clamp and pelvic packing were applied. Bleeding was controlled by temporary cross-clamping of the aorta. The patient survived the night but expired the following morning secondary to a severe closed-head injury.

parotomy will make the pelvis more unstable because the muscle forces pulling on the iliac wings are diminished (16). A correctly applied pelvic frame will improve pelvic stability yet not impede the surgeon's ability to perform either a supraumbilical laparotomy (from xiphoid process to symphysis for positive intra-abdominal fluid) (Fig. 37.4) or infraumbilical (absent intraperitoneal injury). If a patient with an unstable pelvic fracture requires a laparotomy for intraperitoneal injuries, exploration and packing to control retroperitoneal bleeding may be accomplished as well. Disruption of the soft tissues in the pelvic floor allows easy, direct access to both sides of sacrum and bladder for packing (17). Major arteries and veins (external iliac and femoral) that are damaged also require direct access and surgical hemostasis. In massive retroperitoneal bleeding caused by blunt trauma, Ertel et al (9) recommended that the hematoma in the central zone be explored. This method also allows assessment of the posterior reduction by direct manual palpation from inside the pelvis. Bleeding is better controlled when the bone surfaces or joint are directly opposed (interdigitating) and compressed. If significant displacement exists, loosening and adjusting the external fixator, previously applied to improve the fracture reduction, can be performed. To achieve firm local compression against the reduced posterior pelvis, the surgeon may need to repeat the tamponade and look quickly again for any major bleeding sources. If hemodynamic instability persists despite all measures (including partially closed distal-abdominal fascia for better support of packing), then the patient should be transferred for a contrast-enhanced CT of the abdomen. The study is fast and highly accurate in determining the presence or absence of ongoing pelvic hemorrhage (18). Patients with visualized contrast extravasation, as shown on CT scans, are candidates for angiography and embolization. Following a similar protocol, the Hannover Trauma Center was able to reduce mortality rate from 46% to 25% (8,10,15,17,19).

In most North American trauma centers, if evidence of intra-abdominal free fluid is not found on ultrasound exam or diagnostic peritoneal lavage (DPL) after noninvasive pelvis stabilization, angiography and embolization of identifiable bleeding arteries is usually the next step. Angiography does not address venous bleeding, is time consuming (which is particularly problematic for a patient in hemorrhagic shock), and may cause gluteal muscle necrosis. In addition, only 3% to 5% of patients with unstable pelvis receive major benefit from the procedure, which requires specialized personnel and equipment (13,20–22).

In a very small subgroup of patients, hemipelvectomy may be life saving (20,23). High-energy pelvic injuries that are concomitant with a major vessel injury (e.g., to the common external iliac or femoral artery), which are characterized by lack of blood flow to the extremity, and a profound neurologic deficit (and/or intraoperative finding of stretched and ruptured nerves) cause such persistent hemodynamic instability that reconstruction attempts are futile.

Open fractures with wounds in the rectal or vaginal vicinity require irrigation and de-

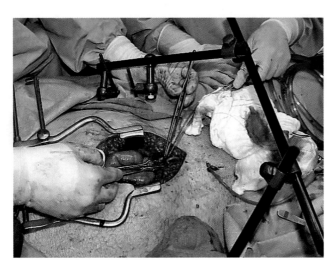

Figure 37.4. Laparotomy following application of an anterior external-fixation device. A C-clamp is covered by sheets.

bridement, a diverting colostomy placed as far as possible from subsequent surgical approaches to the pelvis, and immediate distal-colon washout. In addition, a broad spectrum of prophylactic antibiotics should be given (2–6).

Every male patient with an unstable pelvic injury (with or without blood on ureteral meatus) requires a retrograde urethrogram before bladder catheterization. In our experience, a rectal exam cannot reliably predict the position of the prostate and possible urethral injury. A urethral injury in this setting is usually treated with a suprapubic catheter inserted percutaneously or openly during laparotomy. Patients with hematuria and intact urethra must undergo a contrast study to rule out a bladder rupture. If no explanation for hematuria is identified, an abdominal CT and intravenous pyeolography is used to investigate the upper urogenital tract. In a polytrauma patient, routine CT scans without contrast will show a ruptured kidney perirenal hematoma; contrast may be contraindicated with kidney damage or poor function. If an emergent invasive radiology procedure is contemplated, contrast studies (urological and gastrointestinal) should be done after angiography (13,20).

Pelvic Stabilization

Critically ill patients with unstable pelvic injuries require early pelvic stabilization to improve fracture stability, provide a tamponade effect, improve clotting, and reduce pain. In patients with multiple injuries, including life-threatening conditions, the speed and safety of pelvic stabilization is more important than the initial accuracy of reduction or sophistication of frame constructs.

Noninvasive Methods

A bed sheet wrapped and secured with towel clamps or a hand-tied knot placed around the pelvis and greater trochanter, with the hips slightly flexed and internally rotated, can often provide short-term tamponade and stabilization (2 to 3 hours) (Fig. 37.5). This stabilization method is most effective when applied after a simple reduction maneuver using traction and pressure over the iliac wings. Unnecessary transfers should be avoided, and the patient should only be turned once for a spinal exam.

Commercially available pelvic binders are easy to apply and readjust as needed (Fig. 37.6). However, these devices limit access to the abdomen and groin. Vacuum splints and beanbag positioners, while bulky, can be helpful and allow better abdominal and inguinal access while providing pelvic immobilization (Fig. 37.7). It is unfortunate that they are not always available and do not work well in large patients.

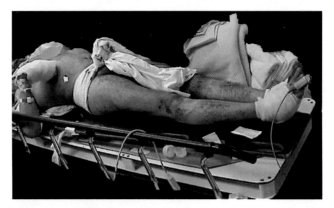

Figure 37.5. External immobilization with a sheet as a pelvic binder in a patient with an unstable pelvic injury. Sheet wrapped around the iliac-crests, ankles and lower extremities fixed in internal rotation with a gauze-roll provide rapid temporary immobilization with ongoing fluid resuscitation.

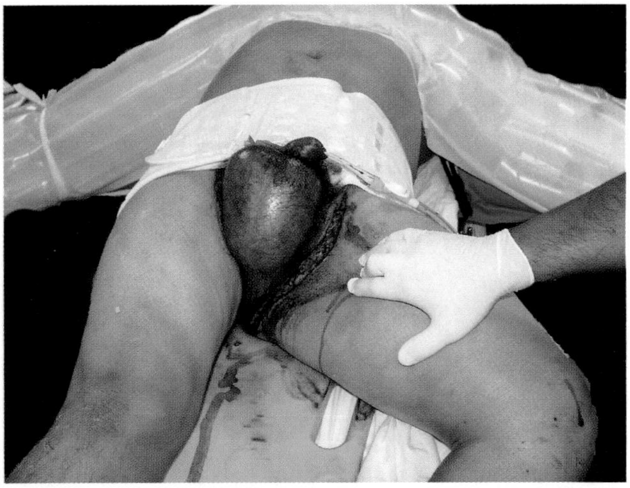

Figure 37.6. The use of a pelvic binder in a mechanically unstable, open, pelvic fracture. It is easy to apply and adjust as needed. Access to the abdomen and inguinal regions may be limited, and binder repositioning to the trochanteric regions may be necessary.

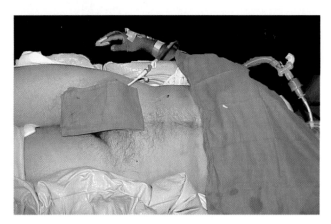

Figure 37.7. Vacuum splints apply pressure over a large area and provide good temporary fixation. They are radiolucent and allow full access to the abdomen and inguinal areas.

External Fixation

Riemer at al (24) reported a decrease in the mortality rate from 26% to 6% when external fixation was introduced as a part of resuscitation protocol at their institution. External fixation provides better bony stabilization than noninvasive methods, and the technique is minimally invasive and relatively easy and safe to apply. External fixation also helps control pain and patient mobilization. However, an anterior frame does not adequately stabilize translational, Tile C fracture patterns. Unlike the posterior C-clamp, the frame may limit access to the abdomen. With attempts to compress and immobilize the anterior pelvic ring, the fracture gap posteriorly may be increased, which may lead to greater instability and bleeding. Transfemoral skeletal traction of 25 to 30 lb, with the hip flexed, can improve the posterior fracture reduction.

In most trauma centers, external fixation is used primarily as a temporary resuscitation frame until the patient's general condition has improved and elective internal fixation can be employed. When anterior frames were used as a definitive fixation method for Tile C fractures, failure rates as high as 70% were reported. While the optimal time to convert from external to internal fixation is unknown, we prefer to wait at least 7 days to avoid "the second hit" phenomena. Earlier fixation may be feasible in patients in which percutaneously placed ilio-sacral screws can produce adequate reductions in the supine position (see Fig. 37.33). Combined posterior–internal fixation and anterior–external fixation (when anterior internal fixation is not applicable) can provide adequate stability for patient mobilization. However, discomfort, pin tract problems, and loosening limit long-term application (13,25–30). The stability of external fixation is determined by the (a) host (type of pelvis mechanical instability, patient size, and quality of bone); (b) frame characteristics (design and location, number and size of pins), and (c) application (quality of reduction and pin placement).

Anterior External Fixation

Iliac-Crest External Fixation
Procedure. The frame is applied with the patient in the supine position on a flat top radiolucent operating fracture table with traction attachments available, and if time allows, c-arm control (Fig. 37.8). Except in dire circumstances, a full prep and sterile technique is used for pin placement in either an open or percutaneous approach. With the open tech-

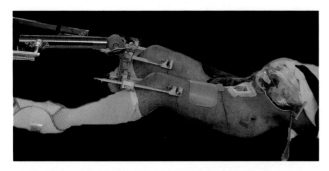

Figure 37.8. A patient with a Tile C, unstable, open, pelvis fracture as well as an avulsed rectum, liver injuries, and a right leg amputation. The previously applied C-clamp has been removed. Staged reconstruction with percutaneous IS screws on the left side and an anterior external-fixator frame is planned. Both lower extremities are secured to the traction attachments to facilitate fracture reduction.

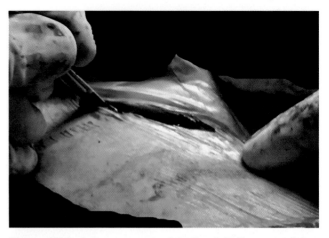

Figure 37.9. An open approach to the right iliac crest. It is started 2 to 3 cm proximal to the ASIS (surgeon's right index finger is on ASIS).

nique, an 8-cm incision in the anterior third of the iliac crest is started 2- to 3-cm posterior to the anterior–superior iliac spine (ASIS) (Figs. 37.9 and 37.10) to avoid damage to the lateral femoral cutaneous nerve. To decrease the chance of skin stretching by the fixator pins, the incision should be made after manual reduction and compression of iliac wings. This incision provides appropriate orientation for the insertion point of the pins, and it could be incorporated into an internal fixation approach as part of a staged reconstruction. Stab incisions have also been advocated if later surgical approaches might be necessary. In cases where lasting external fixation is planned, 2-cm incisions directed toward the umbilicus are less likely to cause soft-tissue necrosis and are used for a percutaneous approach after iliac wing reduction.

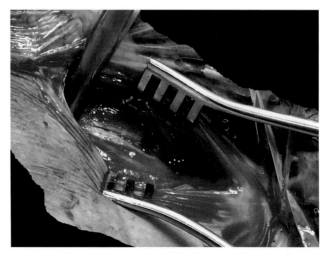

Figure 37.10. The incision is deepened. Separating the insertions of abdominal and gluteal muscles and incising the periosteum allow for good orientation of the width of the iliac crest. If the iliacus muscle is not elevated from the inner table of iliac crest, the danger of entering the retroperitoneal hematoma can be minimized.

Pin Placement. The iliac crests normally overhang the iliac wings, and to place the pins between the external and internal iliac-cortical table, the insertion of pins should be initiated between the medial third and half of iliac crest. Two pins should be placed in each ilium for a emergently used (before laparotomy) resuscitation frame, or three pins should be placed when adequate time is available. The iliac wings have a slight curvature, and the pins may not align in a straight line. The pins should be at least 1 cm apart. In the supine position, the iliac crest angles approximately 45 degrees toward the operating table, but the angle varies from patient to patient (Fig. 37.11). The outer cortex is opened with an appropriate drill bit inclined from cranial toward the greater trochanter; it is aimed for the bone stock of anterior pillar above the acetabulum. The surgeon manually advances 5-mm-diameter pins through the opening hole while trying to feel and not penetrate the internal or external tables. This procedure is not always easy, especially in obese patients.

Several techniques can be used to improve the accuracy of pin placement. The surgeon can insert Kirschner (K) wires on both sides of the iliac wing to serve as a guide. Some external fixation sets come with a special guide where a long arm is rested on the inner table. In another technique, the c-arm is used. Obturator oblique views show the iliac wing profile and pin position (Fig. 37.12). Of course, elevation of the gluteal and iliac muscles from both sides of the pelvis allows direct visual control of the iliac wing for pin placement. However, extensive soft-tissue dissection on the inside of the iliac wings can enter the retroperitoneal hematoma and should be avoided. The stability of the pins is assessed by a gentle trial of in-line traction. When secure, the pins are captured by pin-to-bar clamps and attached to a connecting bar. The same is done on the opposite side, and both independent bars can be manipulated to improve the fracture reduction.

For open book injuries (Tile B1), anterior compression alone will suffice. For bucket handle, lateral-compression injuries (Tile B2), opening and external rotation of the compressed iliac wing is required. Completely unstable, translational injuries (Tile C) require anterior pins and some type of posterior fixation. The bars are connected anteriorly with one or two transverse bars by bar-to-bar connectors that form a trapezoidal frame (Slätis type) (Fig. 37.13). The frame should be positioned to allow for laparotomy, additional soft-tissue swelling, and the patient to maintain an upright position in bed (Fig. 37.14). If any soft-tissue tension is caused by the pins (Fig. 37.15), they should be released by small relaxing incisions and sutured without tension to avoid pin-tract discomfort, necrosis, and infection (Fig. 37.16). The fracture reduction and pin placement are checked with the c-arm, and final permanent radiographs are obtained as condition permits (10,13,25).

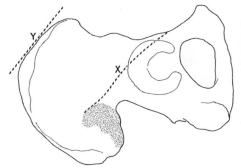
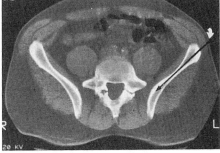

Figure 37.11. A CT scan showing the orientation of the pelvis in the supine position. The ilium lies at an angle of approximately 45 degrees. The surgeon must consider this orientation when placing the iliac crest pins. (From Rommens PM, Hesmann MH. External fixation for the injured pelvic ring. In: Tile M, Helfet DL, Kellam JF, eds. Fractures of the pelvis and acetabulum. 3rd ed. Philadelphia: Lippincott Williams & Wilkins; 2003:208 with permission).

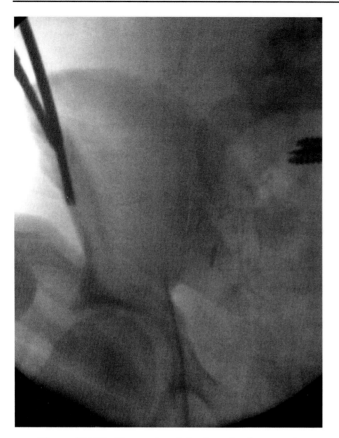

Figure 37.12. C-arm view following pin placement.

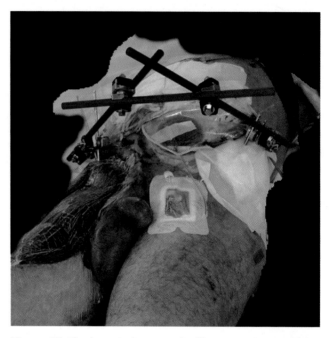

Figure 37.13. An anterior–superior iliac crest, trapezoidal frame. This patient has a diverting colostomy, suprapubic catheter, and significant soft-tissue defect on right upper thigh.

Supra-acetabular External Fixation

The bone above the acetabulum is thick and strong and holds pins well. Biomechanical studies have been shown that pins and frames in this "low route" provide better SI joint stability than "upper route" (iliac crest) frames (31,32). Some authors (20) feel that this route is ideal for emergent anterior-pelvic fixation because of the ease of palpating this thick bone, quickly putting one pin at each side, reducing the pelvis, and connecting the frame with a single anterior-transverse bar. We and others (10,33) feel that for those with limited experience with this technique, the risk of penetrating the hip joint or damaging the neurovascular structures in the greater sciatic notch, especially in the absence of the c-arm, is high.

The set-up for the low route is the same as for the iliac crest procedure. We recommend c-arm control of the surgical steps.

Procedure. A K wire is used under c-arm visualization to localize the anterior–inferior iliac spine (AIIS). Just lateral to the AIIS projection, a 2-cm, transverse, skin incision is made. This will allow less skin-pin interference when the patient is mobilized.

The soft tissues are bluntly separated down to bone in longitudinal fashion to avoid potential damage to the lateral, femoral, cutaneous nerve. A protection sleeve with an inner trocar is advanced with an oscillating motion. Through the trocar, the outer cortex is opened with a drill. A 5- or 6-mm diameter pin with threads of 50 to 70 mm and length of at least 180 mm is advanced through the trocar (Fig. 37.17). The entry point should be at the level of the AIIS, advanced toward the acetabular roof, and checked on an iliac, oblique, c-arm view (Fig. 37.18). To avoid the sciatic notch, the pin is directed toward the SI joint: 30 de-

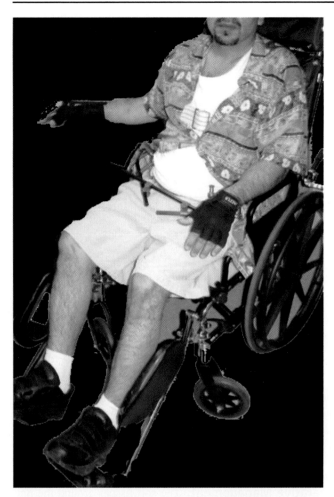

Figure 37.14. External fixation frames should be placed to allow eventual mobilization and an upright position.

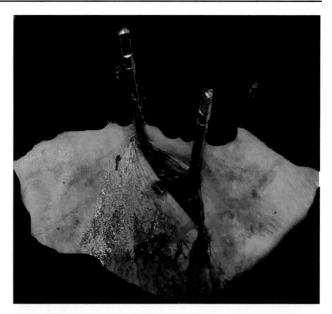

Figure 37.15. An example of soft tissues under tension around the pins. If the incision is not made in reduced iliac-wing position and it is not perfectly above the medial half of the iliac crest, the soft tissue may be compromised after pin placement. Such an outcome may cause significant discomfort, tissue necrosis, and possible infection.

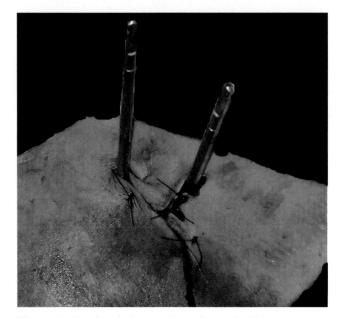

Figure 37.16. A soft-tissue release by an incision perpendicular toward the direction of tension. The incision can be closed without any undue tissue stretching.

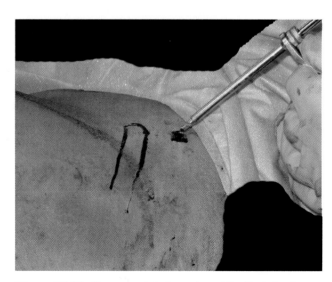

Figure 37.17. Supra-acetabular external-fixation pin placement under c-arm control. A 2-cm incision is made, and the soft tissues are spread down to the bone. The external fixation pin with soft-tissue-protecting sleeve should be utilized.

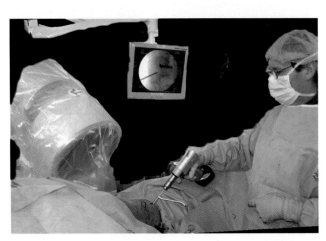

Figure 37.18. Supra-acetabular pin placement. The iliac oblique view helps the surgeon ensure that the pin does not penetrate the hip joint nor pass through the greater sciatic notch.

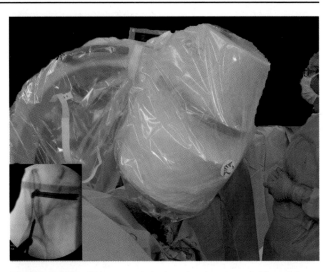

Figure 37.19. Supra-acetabular pin placement. The obturator oblique view helps the surgeon guide the drill and pin toward the SI joint.

grees medial in the sagittal direction (Fig. 37.19) and 20 degrees less than perpendicular (about 70 degrees) to the caudo-cranial axis (Fig. 37.20). Another pin is placed in the opposite side, and after additional reduction maneuvers, both pins are connected by a single bar (Figures 37.21 and 37.22). The bar should be far enough from the skin to allow for additional swelling. Correctly done, this low route will not obstruct a laparotomy approach, and patients are usually able to sit without difficulties with a frame in place (34).

Anterior Frames Postoperative Management. The soft tissues around the pins are stabilized by split gauze sponges for light compression for a day or two, and they are cleaned regularly to avoid crusting, fluid retention, and infection. Skin tension around the pins should be identified and released under local anesthesia. The frame construct should allow the patient to maintain an upright position such that pulmonary function is facilitated.

Rotationally unstable injuries with two pins in a high-frame configuration or one pin in a low-frame configuration provide enough stability for patients to bear weight. Selected, oblique, unilateral, posterior, ilium or sacral fractures with an anterior injury, if reduced well, are stabilized sufficiently with an anterior fixator to permit weight bearing. After mobilization, pelvic x-rays should be used to verify stability and assure that no reduction has been lost. An anterior frame does not provide enough stability for weight bearing on bilateral posterior injuries.

Stability may be improved with good reduction, posterior compression, several large diameter pins, a curved bars–bow fixator, a combination of iliac crest and supra-acetabular frames, and application of multiple techniques. Lateral compression injuries heal in 6 to 8 weeks; symphyseal diastasis heals in 6 to 10 weeks.

Tile C translational injuries with complete instability cannot be sufficiently controlled with an anterior frame alone. If a C-clamp is unavailable or not applicable (posterior iliac fracture), then in addition to an anterior frame, supracondylar femoral traction with 25 lb can be used with the hip slightly flexed to improve posterior and superior displacement (13,25,26).

Posterior Fixation, C-Clamp

The use of devices similar to the C-clamp were published in the German literature in 1964 and 1972, but the modern era reemerged with the reports of Ganz et al in 1991 and

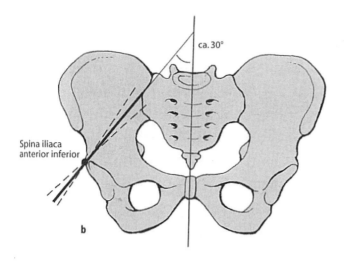

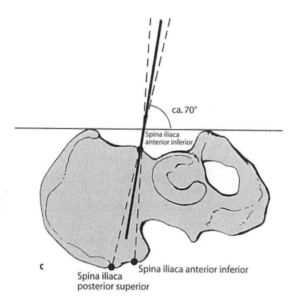

Figure 37.20. Supra-acetabular pin placement angles. (Modified from Pohlemann T, Lobenhoffer PH, Tscherne H. Therapie. In: Tscherne H, Pohleman T, eds. *Becken and acetabulum.* Berlin: Springer; 1998:143 with permission.)

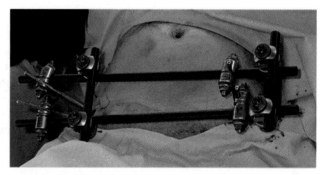

Figure 37.21. Supra-acetabular frame from the front. One pin on each side is enough for resuscitation purposes, and if longer use is planned or a higher degree of instability is present, then two pins and two connected bars will provide better stability.

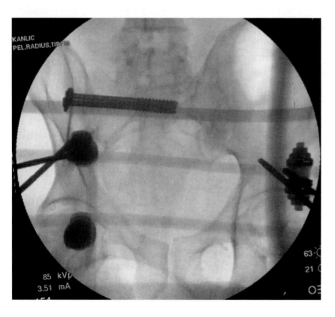

Figure 37.22. AP radiograph with right SI screws and a supra-acetabular frame. This minimally invasive combination of fixation was chosen to treat a patient with multiple injuries that include a Tile C pelvic fracture.

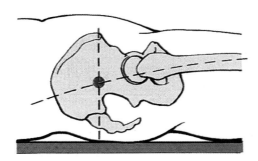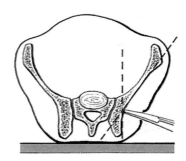

Figure 37.23. The landmarks for placement of a pelvic C-clamp. In the reduced position, the intersection of a line in the femur longitudinal axis and one that is vertical from the ASIS is the correct entry point. Palpation to effect transition of the oblique portion of iliac wing from an anterior into more vertical posterior position is helpful. (Modified from Pohlemann T, Regel G, Bosch U, et al. Notfallbehandlung und komplextrauma. In: Tscherne H, Pohleman T, eds. *Becken and acetabulum.* Berlin: Springer; 1998: 98 with permission.)

Buckle et al in 1995 (20,35,36). Biomechanical testing has shown that the C-clamp provides better fixation than any other type of pelvic external fixation in posterior, unstable, pelvic injuries (26). It improves the conditions for effective hemostasis by compressing fracture surfaces, eliminating motion and dislodgement of formed clots, decreasing pelvic volume. It also may enhance self-tamponade and provides firm support for pelvic packing when needed. Many patients show an immediate improvement of vital signs after frame application.

The C-clamp produces direct posterior compression and stabilization, yet leaves unobstructed access to the abdomen (see Fig. 37.29) and perineum (see Fig. 37.31). It is indicated only for a posteriorly unstable pelvic injury in a hemodynamically unstable patient. Contraindications are hemodynamically stable patients and those with posterior iliac-wing fractures.

The C-clamp set has a rectangular frame (Ganz) or two semicircular tubes connected by a central ratcheting gear (Browner's pelvic stabilizer). Both have large pins with sharp tips, and outside threads allow for connection with the frame and for additional dialed compression. Sets should be sterilely packed and available in emergency and operating rooms.

Figure 37.23 illustrates the position of the pin insertion at the intersection of a line along the long axis of the femur and with a vertical line angled down from the ASIS. If landmarks are missing because of deformity and swelling, the C-arm makes for a much safer procedure. The pin tip should be placed on the outside surface of the ilium at the level of the reduced, posterior, SI joint, where the bone is the thickest. The transition of the oblique and vertical portion of the iliac wings' lateral surfaces is presented in Figure 37.23. With the patient supine, the surgeon can palpate the bony landmark with a hemostat through a 2- to 3-cm longitudinal incision on the side of injury (Figs. 37.24 and 37.25). Compression pins are screwed into the threaded compression bolts and attached to the arms connected with the central ratcheted gear. The central gear is then released so the arms can be spread to accommodate patient size, and the compression pin attached to the fixator arm is "walked" on the lateral iliac wing until the vertical portion is felt (Fig. 37.26). The sharp tip is pushed into the bone and held there until the same procedure is done with other pin on opposite side.

When both pins are firmly anchored into the bone, the fracture is reduced, the arms are compressed, and central gear is tightened. Additional incremental compression is possible by screwing the pins centrally through the compression bolts (Figs. 37.27 to 37.33). Overtightening should be avoided if in cases of transforaminal sacral fracture, which can cause additional sacral-nerve damage. If the patient's condition does not improve despite aggressive resuscitation efforts and pelvic stabilization, then the patient should be taken to the operating room for laparotomy and pelvic packing (see Fig. 37.2). Otherwise, the pins are sterilely covered, the frame supported by towels, and pin care is assumed in day or two. Pelvic x-rays are obtained when possible.

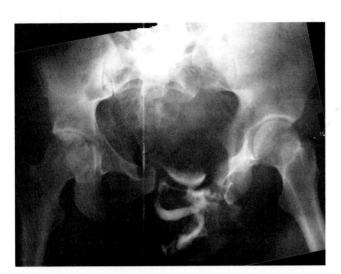

Figure 37.24. AP pelvic x-ray shows a translationally unstable, open (ruptured rectum and perirectal tissue), left-sided pelvic-ring injury with extravasation of contrast after urethrogram and right T-type acetabular fracture. The patient also had a closed head injury, chest injury, right-open-forearm fracture, and left-proximal-humerus fracture.

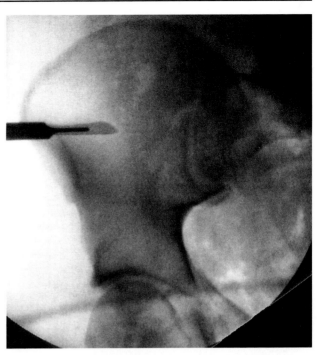

Figure 37.25. The incision location for C-clamp pin placement. If the patient's hemodynamic status allows and an operating room is available, c-arm control should be used because it will improve pin placement and the accuracy of reduction.

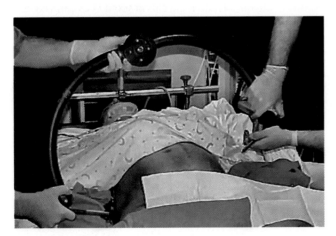

Figure 37.26. C-clamp application. Compression pins are inside of the frame, and the first pin is "walked" on the lateral wall of iliac wing on the stable side. The pin is pushed hard into the bone and held in place until reduction and the opposite pin is placed. The clamp may be applied in the emergency room, intensive care unit (ICU), or operating room.

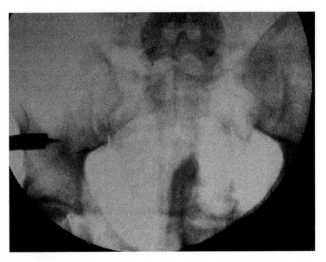

Figure 37.27. The c-arm view shows the first pin anchored on the intact side.

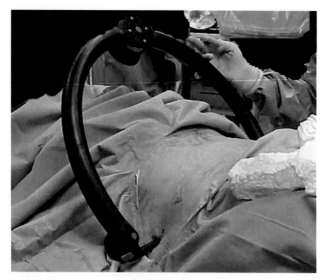

Figure 37.28. A clinical picture of the C-clamp in place. Posterior stabilization is achieved, and the frame can be rotated up or down to make space for additional procedures.

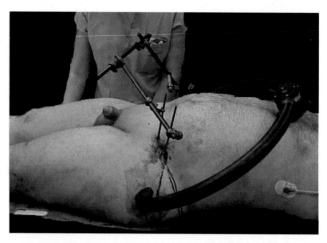

Figure 37.29. Posterior C-clamp and anterior iliac-crest frame in place. The patient's condition was stable, and enough time was available to apply an anterior frame before a laparotomy was conducted.

COMPLICATIONS

Complications include the following conditions:
- vascular or nerve damage if pins slip into greater sciatic notch,
- intrapelvic pin penetration and intestinal perforation,
- loss of reduction,
- pin loosening, and/or
- displacement of unstable hemiplevis into true pelvis.

The C-clamp is converted to the internal fixation as soon as patient condition allows, usually in 2 to 5 days. If internal fixation is impossible, then the clamp should be removed, and anterior fixation with supracondylar traction applied (9,35,36).

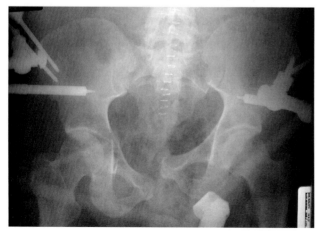

Figure 37.30. AP pelvis x-ray shows the pelvic ring temporarily reduced and fixed with the posterior C-clamp and iliac-crest anterior fixator.

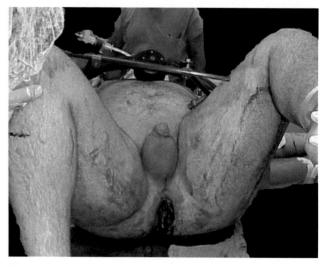

Figure 37.31. Pelvic fixation allows lithotomy position for surgery on the rectal injury.

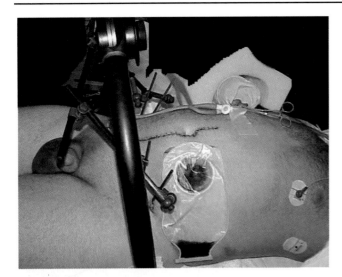

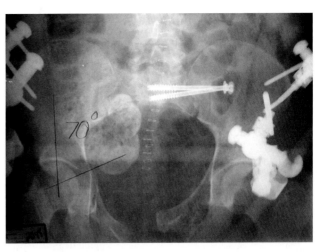

Figure 37.32. Clinical picture after primary surgeries with stable, external, posterior and anterior fixation. Rectal injury was debrided and irrigated, and a suprapubic cystotomy and diverting left-sided colostomy with distal colon irrigation were performed as well.

Figure 37.33. AP pelvic x-ray with anatomically reduced, left, SI joint and SI screws that were used to replace the C-clamp 2 days after it was employed.

RECOMMENDED READINGS

1. Ragnarsson B, Jacobsson B. Epidemiology of pelvic fractures in Swedish county. *Acta Orthop Scand* 1992;63:297–300.
2. Pohlemann T, Tscherne H, Baumgärtel, et al. Beckenverletzungen: epidemiologie, therapie und langzeitverlauf. Übersicht über die multizentrische studie der arbeitsgruppe becken. *Unfallchirurg* 1996; 99:160–167.
3. Davidson B, Simmons G, Williamson P, et al. Pelvic fractures associated with open perineal wounds: a survivable injury. *J Trauma* 1993;35(1):36–39.
4. Govender S, Sham A, Singh B. Open pelvic fractures. *Injury* 1990;21:373–376.
5. Hanson P, Milne J, Chapman M. Open fractures of the pelvis: review of 43 cases. *J Bone Joint Surg Br* 1991;73:325–329.
6. Rothenberg D, Fisher R, Strate R, et al. The mortality associated with pelvic fractures. *Surgery* 1978;84(3):356–359.
7. American College of Surgeons Committee on Trauma. *Advanced trauma life support manual.* Chicago: American College of Surgeons; 1997.
8. Pohlemann T. Pelvic ring injuries: assessment and concepts of surgical management. In: Rüedi TP, Murphy WM, eds. *AO principles of fracture management.* Stuttgart–New York: Thieme; 2000:391–412.
9. Ertel W, Keel M, Eid K, et al. Control of severe hemorrhage using C-clamp and pelvic packing in multiply injured patients with pelvic ring disruption. *J Orthop Trauma* 2001;15:468–474.
10. Ertel W. General assessment and management of the polytrauma patient. In: Tile M, Helfet D, Kellam J, eds. *Fractures of the pelvis and acetabulum.* 3rd ed. Philadelphia: Lippincott Williams & Wilkins; 2003:61–79.
11. Davis JW. The relationship of base deficit to lactate in porcine hemorrhagic shock and resuscitation. *J Trauma* 1994;36(2):168–172.
12. Dickson K. The acute management of pelvic ring injuries. In: Kellam J, Fischer T, Tornetta P III, et al, eds. *Trauma 2: orthopaedic knowledge update.* American Academy of Orthopaedic Surgeons; 2000:229–237.
13. Kellam JF, Mayo K. Pelvic ring disruptions. In: Browner BD, Levine AM, Jupiter JB, et al, eds. *Skeletal trauma;* Vol 1. 3rd ed. Philadelphia WB Saunders; 2003:1052–1108.
14. Grim MR, Vrahas MS, Thomas KA. Pressure-volume characteristics of the intact and disrupted pelvic retroperitoneum. *J Trauma* 1998;44:454–459.
15. Huittinen V, Slätis P. Postmortem angiography and dissection of the hypogastric artery in pelvic fractures. *Surgery* 1973;73:454–462.
16. Ghanayem AJ, Wilber JH, Lieberman JM, et al. The effect of laparotomy and external fixator stabilization on pelvic volume in an unstable injury. *J Trauma* 1995;38(3):396–400.
17. Pohlemann T, Gänslen A, Bosch U, et al. The technique of packing for control of hemorrhage in complex pelvic fractures. *Tech Ortho* 1995;9(4):267–270.
18. Stephens DJ, Kreder HJ, Day AC, et al. Early detection of arterial bleeding in acute pelvic trauma. *J Trauma* 1999;47(4):638–642.
19. Tscherne H, Regel G, Pape HC, et al. Internal fixation of multiple fractures in patients with polytrauma. *Clin Orthop* 1998;347:62–78.
20. Pohlemann T, Regel G, Bosch U, et al. Notfallbehandlung und komplextrauma. In: Tscherne H, Pohleman T, eds. *Becken and acetabulum.* Berlin: Springer; 1998:89–116.
21. Agolini SF, Shah K, Jaffe J, et al. Arterial embolization is a rapid and effective technique for controlling pelvic fracture hemorrhage. *J Trauma* 1997;43(3):395–399.

22. Takahira N, Shindo M, Tanaka K, et al. Gluteal muscle necrosis following transcatheter angiographic embolization for retroperitoneal hemorrhage associated with pelvic fracture. *Injury* 2001;32(1):27–32.
23. Pohlemann T, Paul C, Gansslen A, et al. Traumatic hemipelvectomy: experience with 11 cases. *Unfallchirurg* 1996;99(4):304–312.
24. Riemer BL, Butterfield SL, Diamond DL, et al. Acute mortality associated with injuries to the pelvic ring: the role of early patient mobilization and external fixation. *J Trauma* 1993;35:671–677.
25. Rommens PM, Hessmann MH. External fixation for the injured pelvic ring. In: Tile M, Helfet D, Kellam J, eds. Fractures of the pelvis and acetabulum. 3rd ed. Philadelphia: Lippincott Williams & Wilkins; 2003:203–216.
26. Pohlemann T, Krettek C, Hoffmann E, et al. Biomechanischer vergleich verschiedener notfallstabil-isierungmassnahmen am beckenring. *Unfallchirurg* 1994;97(10):503–510.
27. Kellam JF. The role of external fixation in pelvic disruptions. *Clin Orthop* 1989;241:66–82.
28. Matta JM, Saucedo T. Internal fixation of pelvic ring fractures. *Clin Otrhop* 1989;242:83–97.
29. Burgess A, Eastridge B, Young, et al. Pelvic ring disruption: effective classification systems and treatment protocols. *J Trauma* 1990;30(7): 848–856.
30. Mears DC, Fu FH. Modern concepts of external skeletal fixation of the pelvis. *Clin Orthop* 1980;151:65–72.
31. Kim WY, Hearn TC, Seleem O, et al. Effect of pin location on stability of pelvic external fixation. *Clin Orthop* 1999;361:237–244.
32. Egbers HJ, Draijer F, Haveman D, et al. Stabilisierung des beckenrings mit fixateur externe–biomehanische untersuchungen und klinische erfahrungen. *Orthopäde* 1992;21:363–372.
33. Bircher MD. Indication and techniques of external fixation of the injured pelvis. *Injury* 1996;27[Suppl 2]:B3–B19.
34. Pohlemann T, Lobenhoffer PH, Tscherne H. Therapie. In: Tscherne H, Pohleman T, eds. *Becken and acetabulum*. Berlin: Springer; 1998:136–188.
35. Ganz R, Krushell R, Jakob R, et al. The antishock pelvic clamp. *Clin Orthop* 1991;267:71–78.
36. Buckle R, Browner B, Morandi M. Emergency reduction for pelvic ring disruptions and control of associated hemorrhage using pelvic stabilizer. *Tech Ortho* 1994;4(9):258–266.

38

Diastasis of the Symphysis Pubis: Open Reduction Internal Fixation

David C. Templeman, Andrew H. Schmidt, and
S. Andrew Sems

INDICATIONS/CONTRAINDICATIONS

The pubic symphysis is a cartilaginous joint where the pubic bones meet. The articulation is composed of a fibrocartilaginous disc that is reinforced by the superior and inferior pubic ligaments. The arcuate ligament forms an arch between the two inferior pubic rami and is thought to be the major soft-tissue stabilizer of the symphysis pubis (1).

Injuries to the pubic symphysis include diastasis, fractures into the symphysis, and fracture-dislocations. Following trauma, if the pubic symphysis is not disrupted, the anterior pelvic-ring injury commonly consists of pubic rami fractures. These fractures are usually vertically oriented but may be comminuted or horizontal (2). Diastasis of the symphysis pubis rarely coexists with fractures of the pubic rami (3,4).

Open reduction and internal fixation (ORIF) is usually indicated when diastasis of the pubic symphysis exceeds 2.5 cm. Internal fixation is performed to relieve pain and improve stability of the anterior pelvic ring. The indications for surgery are based on the patient's overall condition and the stability of the entire pelvic ring.

Several different classifications can be used to characterize pelvic injuries. Early classifications were based on either the location of the fracture or the mechanism of injury. Most modern classifications, however, are based on the degree of pelvic stability (5,6). The Tile classification of pelvic ring injuries is used to predict the mechanical instability of the injured pelvic ring and are categorized as A, stable; B, rotationally unstable but vertically stable, and C, rotationally and vertically unstable. Tile B and C injuries may have associated disruption of the symphysis pubis (6).

Diastasis of the symphysis pubis and external rotation of one innominate bone results in the so-called "open-book" injury. This is a Tile B injury in which the posterior pelvic ligaments are intact and prevent cephalad displacement of the involved innominate bone.

When disruption of the symphysis pubis is greater than 2.5 cm, internal fixation is indicated. Displacement of this magnitude is thought to be accompanied by injuries to the sacrospinous ligament and the anterior sacroiliac ligaments, which are thought to allow the involved innominate bone to rotate externally. Stable fixation of the symphysis is sufficient to correct this innominate-bone instability (2).

In Tile C injuries, the symphysis pubis (or the anterior pelvic ring) is disrupted as is the posterior pelvic ring, resulting in complete instability of the pelvis. Fixation of the anterior ring alone is insufficient to restore pelvic stability and must be accompanied by reduction and fixation of the posterior pelvic injury (6,7).

Contraindications to internal fixation of the symphysis pubis include unstable, critically ill patients; severe open fractures with inadequate wound debridement; and crushing injuries in which compromised skin may not tolerate a surgical incision. Suprapubic catheters placed to treat extraperitoneal bladder ruptures may result in contamination of the retropubic space and is a relative contraindication to internal fixation of the adjacent symphysis pubis. Additional conditions that may preclude secure fixation are osteoporosis and severe fracture comminution of the anterior pelvic ring.

When the diastasis of the symphysis pubis is less than 2.5 cm, internal fixation is seldom necessary. Patients may be safely mobilized and allowed to exercise toe-touch weight bearing on the side of the externally rotated hemipelvis. Radiographs are repeated within the first few weeks to ensure further displacement has not occurred. By 8 weeks, the pelvis is usually healed enough to allow full weight bearing. Any increase in pain associated with activity must be evaluated with radiographs so hardware failure or late instability can be detected.

Chronic pelvic-ring instability may follow nonoperative treatment or unrecognized pelvic-ring injuries. This subset of patients commonly presents with pain in the symphyseal or sacroiliac region when undergoing weight-bearing activities. For this group of patients, single leg stance radiographs may be useful. The radiographs are taken as standard anteroposterior (AP) pelvis x-rays, and the three-film series should include a standing AP pelvis as well as an AP of the pelvis during left leg stance and an AP of the pelvis during right leg stance. Subtle instability may manifest as a vertical displacement at the symphysis pubis with single leg stance on the unstable side (Fig 38.1). These chronic instabilities may be approached with the same technique of fixation that one would use to treat an acute injury, but retropubic scarring of the bladder to the posterior aspect of the pubic bones and symphysis may be encountered.

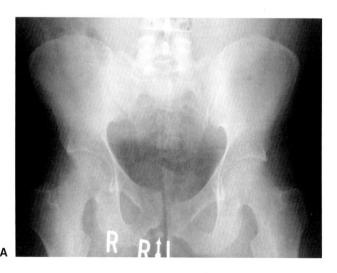
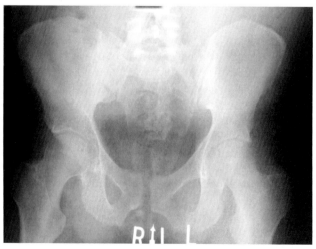

A   B

Figure 38.1. AP pelvic radiographs in single leg stance show increased vertical displacement with weight bearing on the unstable side **(A)** compared to the contralateral single-leg stance radiograph **(B)**.

PREOPERATIVE PLANNING

To determine the direction and magnitude of the symphysis pubis disruption and the relative position of the pubic bones, the surgeon should obtain AP, 40-degree caudal and 40-degree cephalad views (Fig. 38.2A-C). Differences in the height of the pubic rami usually indicate that the hemipelvis is displaced in more than one plane. The most common deformity associated with disruption of the symphysis pubis is cephalad migration, posterior displacement, and external rotation of one hemipelvis (5). This pattern indicates a posterior pelvic injury (Tile C) that requires posterior reduction and internal fixation to achieve a stable pelvis (6–8).

Patients with hemodynamic instability require immediate evaluation and resuscitation. A multidisciplinary team consisting of general surgeons, orthopedists, urologists, and interventional radiologists is frequently required to treat patients with multiple injuries (9–12).

Urologic injuries are common in patients with anterior pelvic trauma. In male patients, a retrograde urethrogram should be obtained to ensure that the urethra is intact before passing a Foley catheter. Extravasation of dye during the urethrogram is a contraindication to blind passage of a Foley catheter and requires consultation with a urologist. The presence of blood at the tip of the penile meatus is frequently cited as a sign of urethral trauma; however, it is not present in the majority of cases. When the urethra is intact, a Foley catheter is passed and a cystogram is obtained. Because the female urethra is only several centimeters in length, a retrograde urethrogram is not required before inserting a Foley catheter (10).

The bladder should be studied by cystography with an intravenous pyelogram or retrograde cystogram. External compression of the bladder is frequently caused by a pelvic hematoma.

The management of extraperitoneal bladder ruptures in patients with pelvic fractures is controversial. Traditional Foley catheter drainage of extraperitoneal ruptures avoids the need for a laparotomy and direct repair. Kotkin and Koch (10) found that patients with extraperitoneal bladder ruptures and pelvic fractures have higher rates of complications, and these authors stressed the need for adequate bladder drainage.

When an extraperitoneal bladder rupture exists, the patient is at an increased risk for infection due to seeding of the pelvic hematoma. When internal fixation of the symphysis is planned, the risk of infection from the ruptured bladder must be considered. We favor primary bladder repair, irrigation of the anterior pelvic-ring injury, and the use of antibiotics. The timing of the bladder repair is determined on an individual basis (10).

After the patient has been stabilized, radiographic studies are obtained. In addition to the plain films, a computed tomography (CT) scan is recommended to assess the posterior pelvic anatomy. The anterior structures are best studied with plain films (6,11).

SURGERY

Surgery is performed under general anesthesia. The patient is positioned supine on a radiolucent table that can accommodate a mobile C-arm image intensifier (see Fig. 38.2A). The imager permits evaluation of the reduction, placement of the hardware, and assessment of the remainder of the pelvis after the symphysis is reduced. Before prepping and draping the surgical field, the surgeon obtains AP, cephalad, and caudal (Fig. 38.2E,F) views of the pelvis with the c-arm to ensure adequate visualization; these views are particularly important if the combined fixation of the anterior and posterior pelvic-ring is required (Fig. 38.2B–D). The cephalad projection provides the best image to visualize screw length after internal fixation of the pubic symphysis.

A transverse Pfannenstiel incision is used for reduction and fixation of the symphysis (Fig. 38.3). When marked disruption of the symphysis is encountered, detachment of one head of the rectus abdominis is common. The linea alba is divided longitudinally, with lateral elevation of the insertion of the abdominis muscle laterally (Fig. 38.4). Transverse sectioning of the rectus abdominis should be avoided because it impairs subsequent repair and healing of the abdominal wall (8).

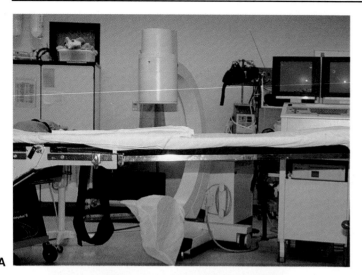

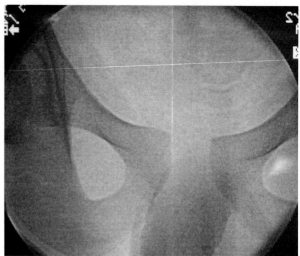

A   B

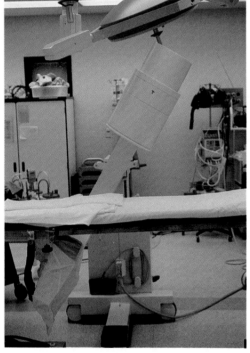

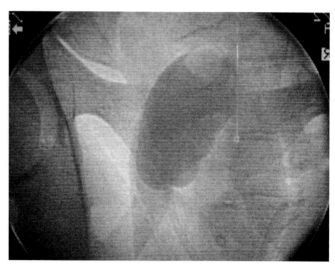

C   D

Figure 38.2. A,B. An operating room table with a radiolucent extension. This table allows tilting of the fluoroscopic unit to obtain cephalad **(C,D)** and caudad **(E,F)** images of the pelvis **(B,C)**. The cephalad view superimposes the symphysis on the sacrum; this makes the diastasis of the symphysis difficult to view. Many operating room tables do not allow enough movement of the C-arm to obtain cephalad and caudal views. (*continues*)

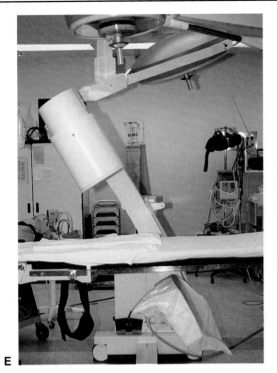

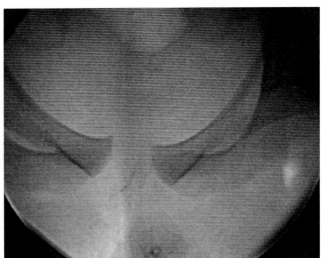

E   F

Figure 38.2. (*continued*)

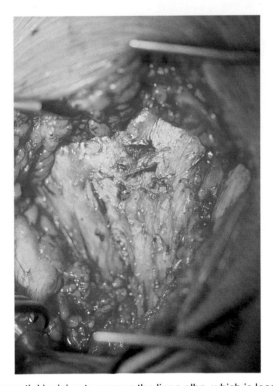

Figure 38.3. Pfannenstiel incision to expose the linea alba, which is located in the midline.

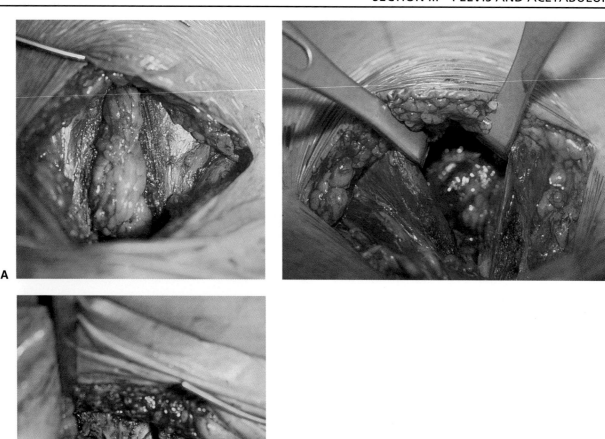

Figure 38.4. Division of the linea alba **(A)** and lateral retraction of the two heads of the rectus abdominis **(B).** Further retraction reveals disruption of the right rectus abdominis muscle. The bone of the pubic body is visible above the surgeon's hand **(C).**

Narrow Homan retractors are carefully placed in the obturator foramen, which enhances exposure and may assist in partially reducing the displaced symphysis (Fig. 38.5A). Several methods can be used to achieve reduction. The simplest method is to place large, pointed reduction clamps on each side of the symphysis (see Fig. 38.5B). Because this clamp exerts a limited amount of control and force, it works best in patients with lesser degrees of displacement.

In patients with disruption of the symphysis and the posterior pelvic ring, a three-dimensional deformity is usually present: posterior, cephalad, and external rotation of the innominate bone. Therefore, the reduction requires manipulation of the entire innominate bone. Matta (13) popularized the technique in which a pelvic-reduction clamp (Fig. 38.6A,B) is secured to the pubis with 4.5-mm screws inserted into the pubic bodies in an anterior-to-posterior direction. The screws are placed so they do not interfere with the subsequent application of the symphysis plate. For an innominate bone that is displaced in a posterior direction, placement of a plate on the inner surface of the displaced hemipelvis prevents screw pullout when the clamp is used to manipulate the innominate bone anteriorly. Reduction of the symphysis often improves alignment of the posterior injury, making its subsequent reduction and fixation easier.

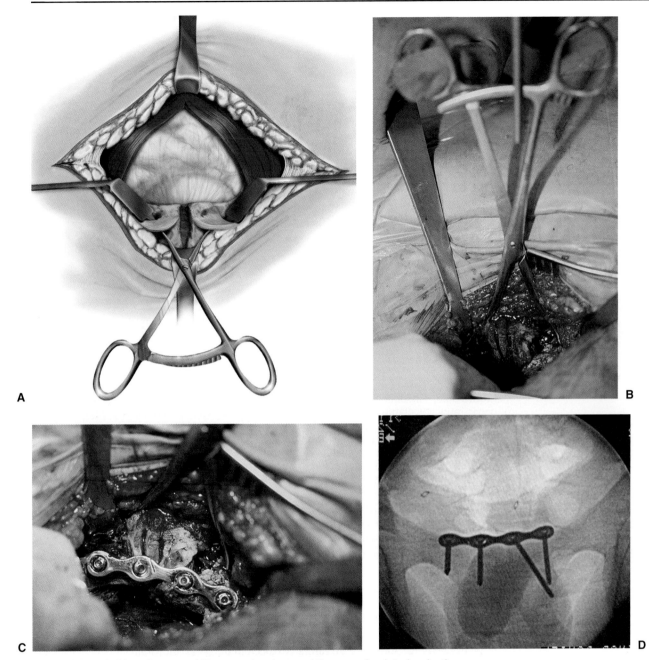

Figure 38.5. A. Line diagram of Homan retractors and the use of pointed reduction clamps to reduce the diastasis of the symphysis pubis. **B.** Intraoperative application of clamp with reduction of the pubic symphysis. **C.** Application of plate on superior aspect of the pubic bodies. **D.** Cephalad view to confirm screw length.

Several different implants may be used for fixation of the disrupted symphysis. Lange and Hansen (14) and Webb et al (15) advocated two-hole 4.5-mm plates. With this method, implant loosening may permit the return of physiologic motion of the symphysis after fixation. Thus, late problems of implant fatigue failure may be avoided.

With multiplanar displacement of the pubic symphysis, the use of a more stable implant is recommended. The most frequently used implants are pelvic reconstruction plates (Synthes, Paoli, PA) with either four or six holes. Precurved plates (which are 3.6 mm thick and unlike straight plates of 2.8 mm thickness) provide additional stability. Plates that use either 4.5- or 3.5-mm screws can be used at the discretion of the surgeon. We favor the use of the 3.5-mm implants with three screws inserted on each side of the symphysis (Fig. 38.5C).

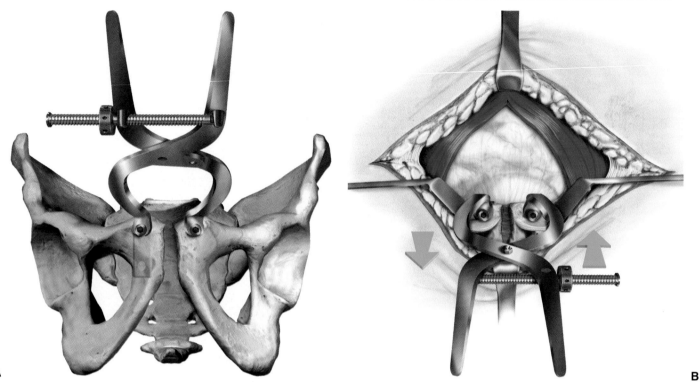

A   B

Figure 38.6. Reduction of the displaced hemipelvis as recommended by Matta. **A.** The pelvis-reduction clamp is anchored to the pubic bodies with 4.5-mm cortical screws directed in an anterior-to-posterior direction. The placement of the screws requires protection of the bladder. The clamp allows multidirectional control of the displaced hemipelvis. **B.** In addition to closing the diastasis of the pubic symphysis, posterior translation of the pelvic ring can be partially corrected (*arrows*). This will not usually obtain an anatomic reduction of displaced posterior injuries.

In addition to visualization of the reduction, palpation of the inner surface of the symphysis confirms the adequacy of the reduction. Similarly, palpation behind each pubic body assists in accurately directing screws into the distal space of the pubic body. In acute injuries, this space is readily accessible. However, when encountering chronic injuries, the surgeon should take care when developing this space to protect the bladder because it may be adherent to the posterior aspect of the pubic bones and symphysis. After fixation, the C-arm is used to verify the reduction and position of the implants (Fig. 38.5D).

The linea alba is reapproximated with interrupted sutures. The wounds are closed over a drain placed in the space of Retzius and exits proximal to the incision.

POSTOPERATIVE MANAGEMENT

The spectrum of injuries associated with disruption of the pelvic ring is diverse and prevents the use of rigid postoperative protocols. However, several principles guide patient care. Early patient mobilization improves pulmonary care and decreases the risks associated with bed rest. An upright posture is usually possible within 24 hours after surgery.

Deep venous thrombosis (DVT) occurs in 35% to 60% of patients with pelvic fractures. Proximal thromboses form in 25% to 35% of these patients and are more likely to embolize than are more distal thrombi (16,17). Based on the high incidence of DVT in patients with pelvic fractures, we strongly recommend aggressive DVT prophylaxis.

Routine screening is not helpful because of the high percentage of patients who develop DVT. Screening is considered when surgery is delayed more than 48 hours from the time of the injury. The diagnosis and treatment of thromboses that are identified preoperatively may help prevent an intraoperative pulmonary embolism (18).

The perfect form of prophylaxis and treatment for venous thrombosis remains elusive. Pharmacologic agents should be safe and easy to administer, monitor, and reverse. The use of pharmacologic anticoagulation in trauma patients is further complicated when the patient presents with associated head injuries, retroperitoneal bleeding, and thoracoabdominal injuries. Treatment cannot be started until bleeding is controlled (18). Mechanical devices that increase venous blood flow by intermittent mechanical compression offer an alternative to pharmacologic agents. However, when used as a sole form of therapy, they are ineffective. One study found that combined use of mechanical compression and low-dose heparin was effective in reducing the incidence of DVT (19).

With stable fixation, patients can be mobilized from bed to chair on the first or second day after surgery. Ambulation depends on the specific injury. For the isolated open-book injuries (Tile B), we recommend protected weight bearing on the injured side for 8 weeks. Follow-up radiographs at this time usually indicate some new bone formation in the region of the symphysis. This is interpreted as sufficient healing and stability. In patients with combined internal fixation of the anterior and posterior pelvic ring (Tile C), weight bearing should be delayed for 8 to 12 weeks.

When full weight bearing is permitted, physical therapy may be helpful. Most patients have muscle atrophy as a result of injury and inactivity. Physical therapy, directed at increasing hip abductor strength and aerobic conditioning, helps restore a normal gait. Lower back–strengthening exercises and work-increasing programs may be beneficial in patients who need to return to heavy labor.

Discharge from the hospital is dependent on the presence of associated injuries. Many patients can use crutches or are able to perform bed-to-chair transfers within a week after surgery.

Matta and Tornetta (7) reported the results of open reduction for anterior fixation of pelvic ring injuries. In a series of 127 patients with pelvic ring injuries, these authors noted that 88 of 105 fractures of the obturator ring were not internally fixed, and none required subsequent treatment for nonunion or loss of reduction.

Based on this study, Matta (13) recommended that internal fixation of the anterior pelvic ring should be reserved for symphysis pubis dislocations and only a minority of pubis rami fractures that remain widely displace after ORIF of the posterior pelvic ring.

COMPLICATIONS

Complications related to internal fixation of the symphysis pubis are uncommon. Loss of fixation is usually associated with inadequate reduction and fixation of the posterior pelvic ring. If this occurs, the entire fixation construct, in both the anterior and posterior pelvic ring, requires revision osteosynthesis.

Because of physiologic motion at the symphysis pubis, screw backout or plate failure is occasionally seen. These events seldom become symptomatic, and in our experience, late hardware removal is infrequently needed.

Wound dehiscence or infection is rare. Irrigation and debridement should include exposure of the plate and retropubic space. When a prior urologic injury has been treated, reevaluation of the urinary system is necessary. The procedure should include urinalysis, urine cultures, and may even require imaging studies. A consultation with an urologist is recommended.

Impotence may result from the initial injury. Because patients may be reluctant to discuss this issue, polite questioning in the private setting of an examination room may identify those patients with sexual dysfunction.

RECOMMENDED READINGS

1. Hollinshead WH. *Anatomy for Surgeons*. 3rd ed. Philadelphia: Harper & Row; 1982.
2. Letournel E. Surgical fixation of displaced pelvic fractures and dislocations of the symphysis pubis. *Rev Chir Orthop* 1981;67(8):771–782.

3. Gamble JG. The symphysis pubis: anatomic and pathological considerations. *Clin Orthop* 1986;203: 261–272.
4. Letournel E. Pelvic fractures. *Injury* 1978;10:145–148.
5. Bucholz RW. The pathological anatomy of Malgaigne fracture-dislocation of the pelvis. *J Bone Joint Surg Am* 1981;63:400.
6. Tile M. Pelvic ring fractures: should they be fixed? *J Bone Joint Surg Br* 1988;70(1):1.
7. Matta JM, Tornetta, P. Internal fixation of unstable pelvic ring injuries. *Clin Orthop* 1996; 329:129–140.
8. Matta JM, Saucedo T. Internal fixation of pelvic ring fractures. *Clin Orthop* 1989;242:83–97.
9. Dalai SA, Burgess AR, Siegel JH, et al. Pelvic fracture in multiple trauma: classification by mechanism is the key to pattern of organ injury: resuscitative requirements and outcome. *J Trauma* 1989;29(7):981–1000.
10. Kotkin L, Koch M. Morbidity associated with nonoperative management of extraperitoneal bladder injuries. *J Trauma* 1995;38:895.
11. Tile M, Pennal GF. Pelvic disruption: principles of management. *Clin Orthop* 1980;151:56.
12. Geerts WH, Code KI. Thrombo-prophylaxis after major trauma: a double-blind study comparing LDH and the LMWH enaparin [abstract]. *Thromb Haemost* 1985;73:284.
13. Matta JM. Indications for anterior fixation of pelvic fractures. *Clin Orthop* 1996;329:88–96.
14. Lange RH, Hansen ST Jr. Pelvic ring disruptions with symphysis diastasis. *Clin Orthop* 1985;201:130–137.
15. Webb LX, Gristina AG, Wilson JR, et al. Two-hole plate fixation for traumatic symphysis pubis diastasis. *J Trauma* 1988;28(6):813–817.
16. Geerts WH, Code K, Jay RM, et al. A prospective of DVT after major trauma. *N Engl J Med* 1994; 331(24):1601–1606.
17. Montgomery KD, Geertz WH, Potter HG, et al. Thromboembolic complications in patients with pelvic trauma. *Clin Orthop* 1996;329:68–87.
18. Montgomery KD, Potter HG, Helfet DL. Magnetic resonance venography to evaluate the deep venous system of the pelvis in patients who have acetabular fractures. *J Bone Joint Surg Am* 1995;77(11):1639–1649.
19. Stickney J, Delp SL. Deep venous thrombosis: prophylaxis. *J Orthop Trauma* 1991;227.

39

Posterior Pelvic-Ring Disruptions: Iliosacral Screws

M. L. Chip Routt, Jr.

INDICATIONS/CONTRAINDICATIONS

Iliosacral screw fixation is indicated for selected unstable fractures of the posterior pelvic ring including sacroiliac (SI) joint dislocations; sacral fractures; certain, posterior, iliac "crescent" fracture-SI disruptions; and combinations of these injuries. This technique can be used alone or in conjunction with other forms of pelvic internal or external fixation. The timing of internal fixation for displaced pelvic-ring injuries depends on numerous factors such as the fracture pattern, local skin condition, hemodynamic status, patient age and body habitus, and abdominal or urologic injuries.

The surgeon must meet certain criteria to insert iliosacral screws safely. The surgeon must completely understand normal posterior-pelvic anatomy, as well as its variations, especially the upper-sacral structure. High-quality fluoroscopic imaging of the entire pelvis must be available during surgery. The surgeon must completely understand the specific injury and the displacement patterns of the posterior pelvic ring and be able to correlate normal and altered pelvic pathologic conditions as seen on radiographic images. Based on the preoperative plain radiographs and computed tomography (CT) of the pelvis, the surgeon must be confident that the patient's upper-sacral anatomy will allow safe screw placement. Finally, the surgeon must possess the technical skill to reduce the posterior pelvic deformity accurately by closed or open techniques. Iliosacral screws should not be used unless the injured area is reduced.

Dysmorphism of the upper sacrum is a relative contraindication for insertion of iliosacral screws. The dysmorphic upper sacrum is a common anatomical variant that decreases the upper-sacral, alar, osseous area available for safe screw passage into the sacral body. Because of the complex anatomy of the pelvis, dysmorphic sacral segments can be difficult to identify predictably during surgery. Upper-sacral-segment abnormalities occur in 30% to 40% of patients and are best identified on the outlet radiograph and CT scans of the pelvis. These abnormalities are most often symmetrical but are unilateral in some patients. The radiographic outlet-image hallmarks of upper-sacral-segment dysmorphism include the following: (a) the lumbosacral disc space is colinear with the iliac crests, (b) the ventral foramen of the upper-sacral nerve root is not circular in appearance, (c) residual disc space is noted between the upper and second sacral segments; (d) the dysmorphic ala decline acutely from the upper-sacral body to the SI joints; and (e) mammillary processes are present on the dysmorphic ala. On the CT scan of the pelvis, sacral dysmorphism is noted by accentuated, undulating, SI surfaces; an obliquely oriented, anterior, alar cortex relative to the iliac cortical density (ICD); and a narrowed alar zone available for screw insertion (Fig. 39.1).

Obesity is a relative contraindication to iliosacral screw fixation for several reasons. Intraoperative fluoroscopic imaging in obese patients is compromised by the excessive abdominal panniculus, which may obstruct inlet and outlet images of the pelvis. Lateral pelvic-flank obesity limits true lateral sacral imaging. Fluoroscopic detail in obese patients may be inadequate for safe guide-screw placement. In addition, extra long instruments such as drills, taps, and screwdrivers are necessary for treating the obese patient.

Fluoroscopic imaging of the pelvis is also complicated in some polytraumatized patients because of contrast agents that were used during the initial abdominal evaluations. Therefore, it should be avoided when possible. In patients with open fractures or compromised posterior skin and soft tissues, iliosacral screw placement should be done percutaneously when possible, rather than through an open approach. In a common mistake, the surgeon enters and inadvertently decompresses a pelvic degloving injury during the process of iliosacral screw insertion. In such situations, the screw is inserted, the degloving area irrigated and debrided, and the dead space closed over suction drains. In severe cases, the dead space is packed open (Fig. 39.2).

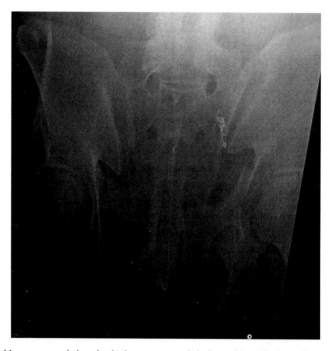

Figure 39.1. Upper-sacral dysplasia is common. It is best identified on the outlet pelvic radiograph as shown here. The hallmarks include (a) lumbosacral disc space that is nearly colinear with the iliac crests, (b) mammillary processes on the sacral ala, (c) sacral ala that are acutely and laterally sloped, (d) nonspherical ventral neuroforamen of the first-sacral nerve roots, and (e) residual disc exists between the two upper-sacral segments. Upper-sacral dysplastic segments have narrowed safe zones for iliosacral screw insertion and must be recognized. Further imaging with CT scanning of the pelvis is used to assess the safety of iliosacral screw insertion.

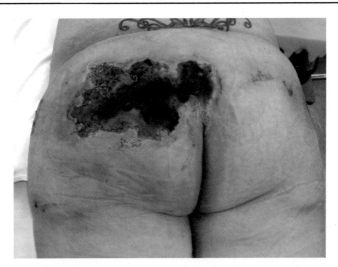

Figure 39.2. Closed or open, traumatic, degloving wounds occur when the skin and fat are separated from the underlying muscle fascia. Most often found after a crushing blow, these injuries are seen at the flank and lumbosacral areas in association with unstable pelvic-ring disruptions. This patient was crushed by an automobile and sustained pelvic ring and soft-tissue degloving injuries. On the day after her accident, she was treated with closed manipulated reduction and percutaneous iliosacral-screw fixation of her pelvic fractures. Her lumbosacral skin became necrotic 3 days after injury. The skin and local tissue necrosis evolved and was then surgically debrided 5 days after injury. Open wound management was selected for almost 2 weeks, and the area was then covered with a skin graft. The iliosacral screw fixation provided pelvic stability and allowed prone-patient positioning for easier wound management in the absence of an anterior-pelvic external fixator.

PREOPERATIVE PLANNING

In the hemodynamically unstable patient with an unstable pelvic-ring injury, resuscitation using advanced trauma life support (ATLS) protocols has been shown to reduce morbidity and mortality rates. Large-bore intravenous access allows rapid volume infusion, and the patient is kept warm. The potentially injured pelvis can be immobilized at the accident scene before patient transport through use of a variety of simple techniques. A vacuum beanbag, a large circumferential sheet, and military antishock trousers (MAST) are recommended for temporary stabilization of the pelvis. Pelvic wrapping devices are also commercially available but are costly, and they often add to an overloaded inventory. Sheets are readily available, inexpensive, and can be adjusted in width to fit any body habitus. They can be reused or discarded, require no additional inventory, and can be positioned or trimmed to allow groin, perineal, flank, abdominal, or combination access for other resuscitation or evaluation procedures. Regardless of the technique chosen, pelvic overcompression should be avoided.

The physical examination is a single mechanical and visual evaluation performed by the most experienced physician and then communicated to the rest of the treatment team. A detailed neurologic examination is documented in alert patients. During the examination of the pelvic area, the surgeon identifies abrasions, contusions, degloving injuries, or open wounds. Sterile pressure dressings are applied to open pelvic wounds to diminish ongoing bleeding. The lumbosacral palpation and visual, along with the digital rectal, examinations are performed during the posterior spine assessment after the patient has been log rolled by a team of assistants. The mechanical evaluation of the pelvis is ideally performed under fluoroscopic imaging. Pelvic ring instability is noted as gentle manual pressure is applied simultaneously toward the midline on each iliac crest. This maneuver produces significant pain in alert patients with pelvic ring instability, iliac fractures, and certain acetabular fractures. Local pain during iliac manual compression can also be due to iliac area contusions in the absence of pelvic-ring osseous injury. To prevent fracture-surface clot disruptions (among other potential consequences), vigorous and repetitive, manual, pelvic examinations are not recommended. Digital rectal, prostatic, and vaginal examinations are performed to test for both gross and occult blood. The vaginal and rectal exams are initially done with the patient supine or log rolled into the lateral position. A more thorough speculum vaginal exam is deferred until pelvic stability is achieved so the patient can be placed safely in the lithotomy position.

The radiographic assessment begins with a screening, anteroposterior (AP), plain radiograph of the pelvis. A complete radiographic series includes orthogonal views (inlet/outlet), and a lateral sacral image should be obtained especially in patients whose screening AP films show a "paradoxical inlet" of the upper-sacral area. A CT scan of the pelvis is essential to further delineate the fracture anatomy. The CT scan images of the pelvis indicate the patient's body habitus, reveal related soft-tissue abnormalities, such as hematoma, as well as degloving injuries and their extent, and also show contrast extrusions reflecting bladder, vascular, or other injuries. The pelvic CT images also show the lumbosacral nerve-root positions as well as sacral alar fractures. The iliac vessels and their relationship with displaced, superior-pubic ramus fractures are often seen clearly on the images. With similar clarity, displaced inferior-ramus fractures can be identified as they intrude on the vagina or are displaced anteriorly. The CT scan details subtle osseous injuries missed on the plain films and shows the hemipelvic displacement patterns. An ipsilateral pneumothorax can often be seen on CT scans of the pelvis because the subcutaneous air extends to the iliac area.

The timing of pelvic reduction and fixation is primarily dependent on the clinical condition of the patient, institutional capabilities, and surgeon availability and expertise. Hemodynamically unstable patients with unstable pelvic-ring injuries require some form of rapid pelvic stabilization. Anterior-pelvic external-fixation frames and posterior-pelvic antishock clamps have been advocated to stabilize the pelvic ring rapidly. When possible, the pelvic external-fixation system is applied through use of iliac crest pins inserted after a closed reduction is obtained and maintained by the circumferential pelvic wrap. Access holes are cut in the sheet overlying the iliac crest. The skin is prepped and the pins inserted between the iliac cortical tables. We recommend application of such devices using the fluoroscopy unit in the angiographic suite when possible. The circumferential wrap can also be adjusted through use of the same imaging unit to assess and adjust the pelvic closed-manipulation reduction. If the reduction has been achieved, iliosacral screws can also be inserted using access portals in the sheet (Fig. 39.3). In selected hemodynamically unstable patients, pelvic angiographic embolization is helpful in controlling pelvic arterial bleeding.

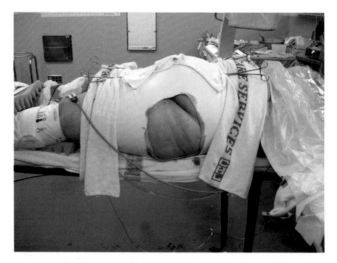

Figure 39.3. This morbidly obese adult female pedestrian was struck by a vehicle. She suffered a right-sided, pertrochanteric, closed-femur fracture and bilateral, unstable, pelvic-ring disruptions. A circumferential pelvic sheet provided an excellent closed reduction of the pelvic injuries. With the circumferential sheet in place, the physician made a surgical portal by cutting a portion of the sheet away without compromising its function. The area was prepped and draped, and iliosacral screws were inserted to stabilize definitively the left hemipelvis. The right-sided posterior-pelvic injury was stabilized next through the same technique. The sheet was removed and the reductions were maintained. Her abdominal obesity prevented anterior-pelvic external fixation.

Emergency, pelvic, open reduction and internal fixation (ORIF) induces the risk of bleeding and has a higher complication rate, but for certain patients and injury patterns, the benefits may outweigh the risks. Percutaneous, posterior-pelvic, internal fixation through use of iliosacral screws minimizes the bleeding risk, is quick, and is useful when an accurate closed-manipulated reduction of the posterior pelvic-ring injury can be accomplished. Percutaneous iliosacral screws may be used in emergency resuscitation situations in combination with standard anterior-pelvic external fixation. In patients who are hemodynamically stable, operative pelvic stabilization should be done early. Before surgery, distal femoral traction improves the reduction and provides patient comfort.

During the preoperative planning phase, the surgeon should consider the mechanism of injury, associated major-system injuries, and the local soft-tissue conditions. Special attention is given to an analysis of the plain films and CT scans. On occasion, iliac and obturator oblique radiographs of the pelvis are obtained in patients with concomitant acetabular fractures. A two-dimensional CT scan further delineates the specific sites of injury and direction of displacement (Fig. 39.4). Just as important as detailing the injury and local anatomy, the two-dimensional CT scan also is used preoperatively to determine the number of screws that can be inserted, the upper-sacral anatomy, the planned starting point on the lateral ilium, and the screw direction and length needed to achieve stable and balanced fixation (Fig. 39.5). Some clinicians prefer three-dimensional CT scans to improve their understanding of the fracture details and deformity patterns (Fig. 39.6).

Based on the mechanism of injury, the physical examination, and the radiographic studies, the surgeon formulates a plan. The preoperative plan includes all of the surgical details including timing, patient positioning, exposures, reduction strategies, clamp application sites, fixation techniques, and treatment alternatives. Even the anticipated rehabilitation goals are planned preoperatively; they are especially important for polytraumatized patients.

Not all posterior pelvic fractures are amenable to iliosacral screw fixation, and the surgeon should be familiar with various anterior-pelvic and posterior-pelvic operative

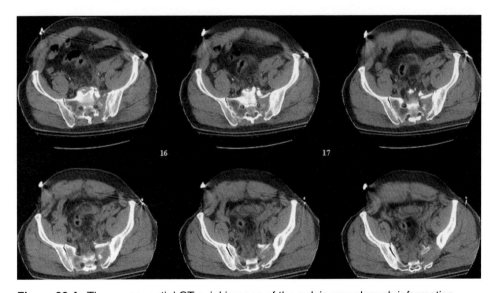

Figure 39.4. These sequential CT axial images of the pelvis reveal much information. They demonstrate patient body habitus, fracture location, fracture comminution, displacement patterns, nerve root involvement, occult injuries not previously noted on plain films, local bone quality (including that of the upper-sacral dysplasia), soft-tissue degloving injuries, hematoma, contrast extravasation, soft-tissue and/or intra-abdominal air, among other important clinical details that may impact urgent and definitive care. The anticipated reduction maneuvers, clamp application sites, and the upper-sacral safe zone for iliosacral screw(s) can be assessed on such CT images of the pelvis.

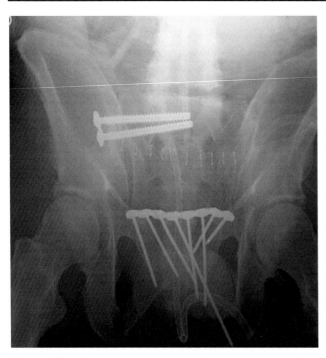

Figure 39.5. Percutaneous iliosacral screws were used to stabilize this patient's SI fracture-dislocation. The symphysis pubis was treated with open reduction and plate fixation. The local soft-tissue injury was extensive. The symphyseal reduction in combination with right-sided distal-femoral traction indirectly reduced the SI injury well. Two fully threaded, balanced iliosacral screws were inserted to stabilize the posterior pelvic injury. This postoperative plain film of the pelvis reveals the associated caudal anterior-sacral impaction fracture. This patient also had a urethral tear, which was treated with realignment of symphyseal reduction and fixation.

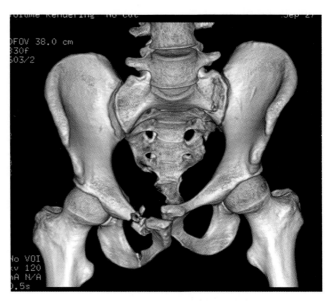

Figure 39.6. Three-dimensional CT scanning reveals the pelvic injury zones but not in sufficient detail to be used alone in planning. Just as when viewing two-dimensional CT images, the surgeon must know if the patient is wrapped in a pelvic circumferential sheet or other type of pelvic binder at the time of the CT scanning.

exposures and fixation techniques as well as percutaneous reduction and fixation strategies. The treatment plan must be tailored to the individual patient. Insertion of iliosacral screws can be performed with the patient in the supine, lateral, or prone position; each patient position has advantages and disadvantages. The lateral position complicates both anterior-pelvic and posterior-pelvic surgical exposures and is not recommended for patients with potential spinal injuries. Prone positioning allows posterior surgical exposures but denies the surgeon simultaneous anterior-pelvic surgical access. Anterior-pelvic external-fixation frames further complicate prone and lateral patient positioning for surgery.

If the supine position is selected, strict attention to detail during patient positioning, as well as skin preparation and draping, is mandatory. In polytraumatized patients, the supine position is familiar, allows several teams to work simultaneously on injured extremities, and also provides anterior pelvic access. With this approach, patient position adjustments and repeated drapings are avoided; thus valuable time is saved.

Computer guidance systems have become available and, like neurodiagnostic monitoring, are intended to simplify the procedure by making it safer. Computer navigation systems are not a substitute for the surgeon's thorough knowledge of the sacral anatomy and radiology. Current navigation systems do not accommodate fracture displacements that can occur between the time of the preoperative CT scan and the intraoperative navigation. Early results have shown that navigation systems for iliosacral screw insertion may decrease the use of fluoroscopy but not overall surgical time.

SURGERY

Positioning

A general anesthetic and a first-generation cephalosporin are administered before the patient is moved onto the operating room table. Spinal precautions protect the patient during transfer from the bed and positioning on a fluoroscopically compatible operating table. Several strong assistants are needed to elevate the patient from the operating table so the surgeon can position a soft, lumbosacral, spinal support. This support consists typically of two (or more) stacked and folded operating-room blankets. Too much elevation and the patient is in an unstable position and will lean to one side or the other. Elevating the patient's pelvis from the operating room table is necessary to allow posterior-pelvic percutaneous access. If needed, distal-femoral pin traction is continued through use of a pulley system attached to the operating table (Fig. 39.7).

Neurodiagnostic monitoring may be helpful, especially in patients with transforaminal sacral fractures undergoing closed manipulated reductions and percutaneous iliosacral-screw fixations. Neurodiagnostic monitoring is not used as a substitute for surgeon competence, a detailed preoperative plan, or adequate, intraoperative, fluoroscopic imaging. The surgeon must understand the posterior pelvic anatomy and its fluoroscopic correlations. The surgeon must not use monitoring to direct screw insertions in a random manner while hoping to find a safe area for the screw. Neurodiagnostic information also may be confusing, especially with regard to patients with preoperative neurologic abnormalities, when information is falsely positive, and when clinical correlation is lacking. Neurodiagnostic monitoring is not a safety net that will protect the surgeon from lack of knowledge regarding sacral anatomy.

Imaging

The radiology technician and fluoroscope are positioned on the side opposite from the injured posterior hemipelvis. The initial AP fluoroscopic image of the pelvis is used simply to assess proper patient positioning. Minor position corrections are made and confirmed.

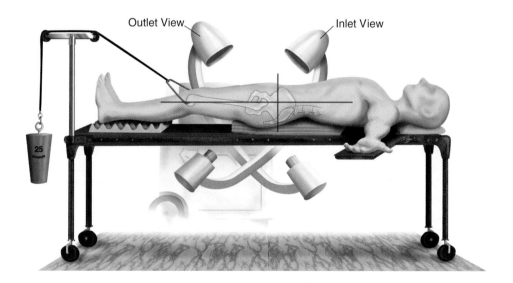

Figure 39.7. The patient is positioned supine and elevated on two folded and stacked blankets, which act as a lumbosacral support. This operating table has no central support and allows extremes of fluoroscope rotation and therefore pelvic imaging. Distal femoral traction is made possible through use of a pulley system anchored to the foot of the table.

This view can also be used if preoperative mechanical stability is to be assessed under fluoroscopy. Surprisingly, certain "nondisplaced" fracture sites thought to be previously insignificant may show impressive instability under fluoroscopy. These "nondisplaced" fractures should not be ignored.

The fluoroscope tilt is then customized for each patient until perfect inlet and outlet posterior-pelvic images are obtainable. The ideal inlet image of the pelvis superimposes the upper-sacral vertebral bodies as concentric circles, but it is the most difficult and least reliable view of the three standard images used intraoperatively. For dysmorphic upper-sacral segments, anterior, cortical, alar indentations mark the anterior cortical-alar limits and are noted on the inlet image.

The ideal outlet image is usually obtained when the superior aspect of the symphysis pubis is superimposed on the second sacral-vertebral body. The surgeon should carefully examine this outlet image, which reveals the corticated pathway of the upper-sacral nerve root. These bilateral pathways are osseous tunnels that begin posteriorly, superiorly, and centrally at the spinal canal at the same level as the lumbosacral disc space. These bilateral tunnels course anteriorly, caudally, and laterally from their spinal canal origin and end as the ventral foramen of the first-sacral nerve root. The radiographic appearance on the outlet image of these bilateral corticated pathways is like that of a small spica cast. Under the spica cast model, the body of the spica cast is the spinal canal, while the thigh components of the spica cast are the sacral nerve-root tunnels passing from the spinal canal to the ventral sacral foramen. The corticated edges of the nerve root pathways/tunnels allow their radiographic visualization in the operating room and on the plain preoperative radiographs. This spica cast analogy lends a three-dimensional quality to a two-dimensional outlet image, giving a preoperative depth perception to the surgeon of the upper-sacral nerve pathway. This is invaluable radiographic intraoperative information.

For dysmorphic upper-sacral segments, the c-arm unit tilt is adjusted to focus on the segment that will receive the iliosacral screw. In some dysmorphic patients, iliosacral screws are inserted into the narrowed upper-alar site and also into the second segment, which may be a more expansive area for screw insertions. If an upper-sacral-segment screw is chosen for a dysmorphic patient, the surgeon must understand that the anterior borders of the sacrum at S1 and S2 are different and therefore unique fluoroscopic markers highlight each specific site. The outlet view will predictably reveal the nerve root tunnels for each segment. The true lateral view will be disturbing with regard to the dysmorphic upper-segment screw insertion because the upper-sacral segment is superiorly located relative to the superimposed ICDs. Therefore, this image looks as though no lateral sacral-alar mass is safe for screw location. The preoperative plan will assure the surgeon that the screw orientation will be directed from a posterior-caudal starting point with an anterior-cephalad directional aim. Because of the unusual anatomy, these upper-sacral screws can rarely extend beyond the midline.

The inlet and outlet intraoperative fluoroscopic views of the pelvis are essential to visualize the upper sacrum. Image enhancement and alternating negative images on the fluoroscope often improve imaging of the posterior pelvis. The arc of rotation of the fluoroscope needed to obtain these "perfect" images varies for each patient and depends upon the degree of lumbosacral lordosis and deformity due to the injury. The amount of tilt needed to obtain perfect inlet and outlet views is marked on the fluoroscope arm by the technician, and the machine's wheel positions on the floor are also marked to facilitate subsequent rapid imaging. Minor rotational changes of the fluoroscope identify the tangential posterior-pelvic disruptions and may be useful in certain sacral fractures.

An "almost true" lateral sacral view is next obtained by adjusting the fluoroscope to superimpose the greater sciatic notches. On the almost-true lateral sacral image, the iliac cortical densities are identified and correlated with the preoperative CT scan once again so the surgeon understands where the anterior sacral ala are located. The ICDs mark the alar locations according to the preoperative CT scan information. The safe sacral segment for screw insertion is reconfirmed. Significant hemipelvis deformity causes this almost-true lateral sacral view to be of little use. A "true" lateral sacral image is possible only after accurate posterior-pelvic fracture reduction or in patients with minimal posterior-pelvic deformities.

Lumbosacral osteophytes are confusing and complicate orthogonal imaging, especially the inlet view of the pelvis. These osteophytes are best seen on the true-lateral sacral image. The true lateral is also used to identify transverse sacral fractures and their displacements.

Skin Preparation and Draping

The perineum, abdomen, bilateral flanks, and lower extremities are prepared with iodine solution followed by isopropyl alcohol. The scrotum, penis, and any urinary catheter are included in the operative field when combined urologic procedures are planned. Wide preparation of the posterolateral buttock skin is important and simplifies iliosacral screw insertion. Femoral vascular catheters, enteral feeding tubes, suprapubic urinary catheters, and other essential anterior-abdominal lines are prepared as skin. Ostomy sites are excluded from the surgical field. Chest tubes are positioned and isolated from the planned operative field. Sterile electrodes for neurodiagnostic monitoring are applied to the lower extremities if indicated.

Reduction

To diminish late pain and deformity, accurate reduction of the posterior pelvic ring is the goal of surgery. Reduction of pelvic ring fractures can be accomplished through use of a variety of techniques. Anatomic reduction and stable fixation of the anterior pelvic injury "indirectly" improve the posterior pelvic displacement, especially when supplementary manipulation techniques are used. Reduction forceps are used temporarily to stabilize open reductions, whereas other techniques are used to maintain closed manipulated reductions. Early surgical treatment improves the accuracy of closed, manipulated, posterior-pelvic reductions. An anterior external-fixation device [or a femoral distractor–pelvic compressor (Synthes, Paoli, PA) attached to the iliac fixator pins] can be used as a "pelvic compressor or distractor" to improve the closed reduction (Fig. 39.8).

Distal femoral traction alone often improves posterior and cephalad deformities of the posterior pelvic ring. The fluoroscopic inlet and outlet images of the pelvis confirm the

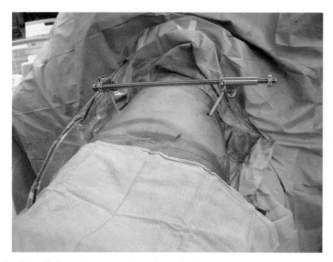

Figure 39.8. In this clinical photograph, a threaded external bar is applied between the iliac pins and functions as an external pelvic manipulator. It can be used to compress or distract pelvic displacements. Complex, multiplanar, pelvic deformities can be manipulated if the device is applied obliquely between the iliac pins. Iliosacral screws are inserted to maintain the posterior-pelvic manipulated reduction.

reduction before iliosacral screw fixation. In some situations, a perfectly placed iliosacral lag screw is used to reduce the posterior pelvic disruption. While iliosacral lag screws can be used to reduce certain distracted sacral fractures, the procedure puts nerve roots at risk for injury (Fig. 39.9). Open reductions are performed when closed manipulation techniques fail to provide an accurate posterior-pelvic reduction. Even after open reduction of the posterior pelvis, percutaneous iliosacral screws are used to provide stability whenever possible (Fig. 39.10).

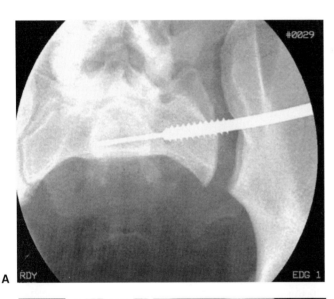

A

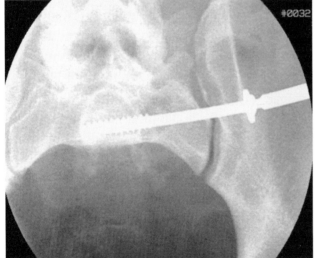

B

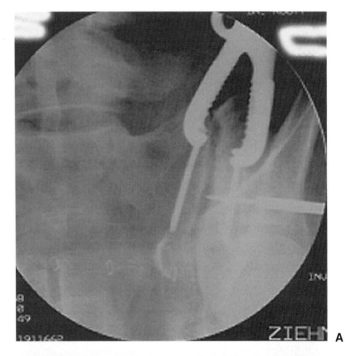

A

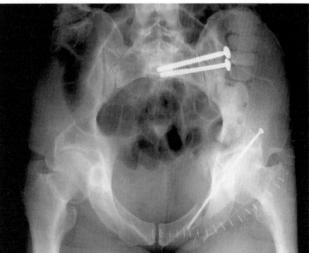

B

Figure 39.9. A. An iliosacral lag screw is targeted for reduction of a SI joint dislocation. This patient was hemodynamically unstable after appropriate resuscitation. The screw was used to achieve urgent posterior-pelvic stability. **B.** As the lag screw is tightened, the reduction is improved but is not anatomical. The SI manipulated screw reduction can be revised at a subsequent surgery through use of open reduction when the patient's clinical condition is optimized. In such situations, this lag screw functions as an internal posterior-pelvic antishock clamp.

Figure 39.10. A. Through surgeon's use of anterior exposure of the SI joint, the reduction clamp is applied between two screws across the joint and then is used to manipulate and hold the open reduction. The guide pin for a cannulated iliosacral screw is percutaneously inserted as shown on this intraoperative fluoroscopic image. **B.** Iliosacral screws were used to definitively stabilize the SI joint after open reduction. The initial lag screw compressed the joint while the subsequently inserted, fully threaded, iliosacral screw was used to fortify the SI fixation construct.

Fixation

After the reduction is accomplished, a smooth 0.62-mm Kirschner (K) wire is inserted under fluoroscopic control from the lateral buttock onto the lateral ilium. This small-diameter smooth wire resists bending during insertion, which allows accurate aiming yet causes minimal trauma to the local soft tissues. A predictable starting point on the skin is located in a posterior cephalad quadrant that is formed by intersecting lines. One line parallels the femoral shaft, whereas the perpendicular intersecting line is made from the palpable anterior–superior iliac spine (ASIS) toward the operating table. The posterior-superior quadrant marks the sacrum.

Per the preoperative plan, the inlet and outlet images of the pelvis are used to direct the orientation of the K wire. Perfect wire direction and starting point may require several skin punctures with the smooth wire. The perfect starting point and wire direction are maintained by gently tapping the wire to engage the lateral, iliac, cortical bone. The skin is then incised around the wire, and blunt deep dissection is accomplished with a narrow periosteal elevator or a drill guide. A long drill guide is placed over the wire, and a 2-mm terminally threaded guide pin is exchanged for the wire. The drill guide provides deep control of the guide pin and protects the deep soft tissues from injury. The guide pin is inserted with a power drill into the lateral iliac cortex, and its direction is confirmed through fluoroscopy. Because the guide pin is only slightly engaged in bone at this point, the surgeon can still use the drill guide to make minor directional pin corrections. Frequent inlet and outlet images of the pelvis are used as the pin is inserted from the ilium, across the SI articulation, and into the lateral aspect of the sacral ala. The guide pin is halted within the ala when its tip is located just cephalad to the upper-sacral corticated tunnel edge as seen on the outlet image. When carefully evaluated, the outlet image will identify the corticated edges of the osseous tunnel of the upper-sacral nerve root that is immediately superior and medial relative to the ventral foramen. Once identified, the nerve root path is better understood. The surgeon must know that the nerve root passes from posterior to anterior, midline to peripheral, and superior to inferior (Fig. 39.11).

As the guide pin reaches this site, the surgeon obtains a true lateral sacral image by fluoroscopically superimposing greater sciatic notches of each reduced hemipelvis. If the posterior pelvic reduction is accurate and no sacral dysmorphism had been identified in the preoperative plan, then the true lateral sacral image identifies the guide pin tip and its relation with the ICD. The preoperative CT scan reflects the relation between the ICD and the sacral ala. The correlation of this information, coupled with the intraoperative ICD, indicates whether the pin tip is safely placed. The tip of the guide pin should be caudal to the ICD and cephalad to the intraosseous path of the upper-sacral nerve root, which is also visible on the true-lateral sacral image of some patients. The true lateral image should show that the guide-pin tip is located within the midportion of the alar bone.

The guide pin is then advanced into the upper-sacral vertebral body to (but not beyond) the midline. The guide-pin depth is measured with the reverse ruler, and a cannulated drill is advanced over the guide pin. A cannulated tap is used to prepare the pathway when necessary. A 7.0-mm cannulated cancellous screw of appropriate length is inserted over the guide pin and tightened. As for SI joint disruptions, partially threaded cancellous screws with 32-mm thread lengths are chosen when compression fixation is necessary. Fully threaded 7.0-mm cancellous screws are used when compression fixation is not desired, such as after accurate reductions of transforaminal sacral fractures. Fully threaded screws also are used when needed to supplement previously applied compression-screw fixations.

During cannulated drilling, tapping, and screw insertion, the surgeon obtains frequent fluoroscopic images to assure no binding and inadvertent advancement of the guide pin. A 20- to 30-degree obturator oblique ("rollover") image is used to visualize the tangential posterior ilium as the screw is tightened. With this image, the washer is noted to flatten as it contacts the ilium. Using a washer and this rollover image, the surgeon prevents inadvertent screw penetration into the posterior ilium. He/she must be careful not to overtighten the screw and penetrate the lateral iliac cortex. This complication can occur in older patients with thin iliac-cortical bone and in young patients when the screw is forcefully tightened.

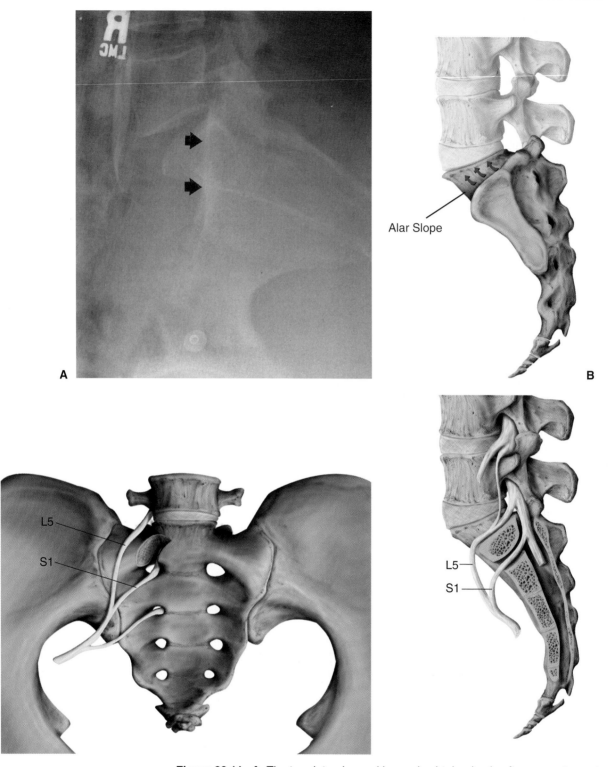

Figure 39.11. A. The true-lateral sacral image is obtained only after accurate posterior-pelvic reduction has been visualized by superimposed greater-sciatic notches. The iliac cortical density is noted by the *arrowheads*. **B.** The disarticulated SI joint and the ascending sacral-alar slope. **C.** The local nerve roots and their alar relations are demonstrated. **D.** The lateral sacral sagittal section indicates the changing structure of the alar zone and its neural relations. The fifth lumbar and first sacral nerve roots are highlighted.

Next, the guide pin is removed manually. The fixation construct is stressed under fluoroscopic imaging. Additional screws or supplementary fixation are used if residual instability is noted on the fluoroscopic stress examination. The percutaneous wound is irrigated, and the skin is closed.

Pitfalls and Tricks

A skilled radiology technician is invaluable. The technician must work diligently to provide reproducible pelvic imaging. Positioning the fluoroscopic unit in the marked position for each view saves operative time and radiation exposure. The technician, who should be preoperatively planning, should be informed about the imaging requirements. Suboptimal imaging precludes placement of percutaneous iliosacral screws.

The initial iliosacral screw is positioned strategically to allow insertion of an additional ipsilateral screw or a screw from the contralateral side if needed. The number of iliosacral screws necessary to stabilize sufficiently each posterior-pelvic disruption depends on the degree of local instability as well as the quality of supplementary fixation of the associated pelvic-ring injuries.

Screw orientation and type are very important. The "SI joint" screw is different from the "sacral" screw in several ways (Table 1). Compression lag screws are routinely used to treat SI-joint disruptions, but fully threaded screws can be used if a perfect reduction has been achieved and no further compression is needed. Sacral fractures may involve the sacral neuroforamina or alar area of the fifth lumbar nerve root; therefore, further compression with a lag screw may produce nerve root injury. For a transforaminal sacral fracture, a fully threaded noncompression cancellous screw is required.

Screws used to treat sacral fractures are usually longer than those used for SI joints because the sacral fracture is more medially located (Fig. 39.12). To obtain optimal stability through improved medial fixation, the sacral screw must be oriented more horizontally and tends to cross the chondral SI surfaces.

To increase the screw length, the screw orientation is slightly different for sacral screws than it is for SI-joint screws. SI joint screws begin caudad and posterior on the ilium and are directed cephalad and anterior to be perpendicular to the oblique SI articulation. Because of its direction, this screw usually avoids violation of the articular, SI-joint, cartilaginous surfaces.

The pathway of the fifth lumbar and first sacral nerve roots must be understood and respected. The nerves exit the spinal canal and are directed anteriorly, laterally, and caudally. Because of this nerve orientation, the "safe" zone for screw insertion becomes the

Table 39.1. *The Differences between Iliosacral Screws Used for Sacroiliac Joint Dislocations and Sacral Fractures*

Injury	Screw Type	Starting Point	Direction	Common Length	SI Cartilage
Sacroiliac	Lag or fully threaded	Caudal and posterior	Oblique	70–90 mm	Spared
Sacral	Fully threaded; rarely lag	Anterior and cephalad	Horizontal	90–150 mm	Violated

Sacroiliac (SI) screws are usually obliquely oriented in order to be perpendicular to the articular joint surfaces while sacral screws are more horizontally directed to both be perpendicular to the fracture surfaces but also to increase the screw length for balance. Lag screws are used for SI joint compression while fully threaded screws avoid over-compression of sacral fractures, particularly those involving the nerve root pathways. Sacroiliac screw lengths for most adults if oriented perpendicular to the joint surfaces range from 70 to 90 mm in length. Sacral fracture screws should be longer because the pathology is more medial than for an SI joint injury, and to achieve a balanced implant. Sacroiliac screws because of their oblique path usually avoid the SI articular surfaces, whereas sacral screws typically pass through the SI joint surfaces because of their orientation.

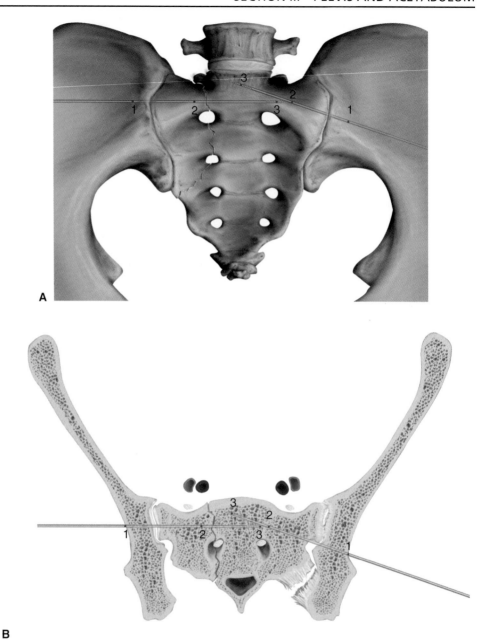

Figure 39.12. A,B. These illustrations demonstrate the screw orientations for sacral fractures (*right side*) and SI disruptions (*left side*). Critical fluoroscopic imaging intervals are numerically labeled. (*continues*)

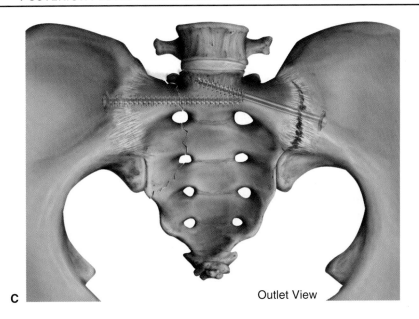

C   Outlet View

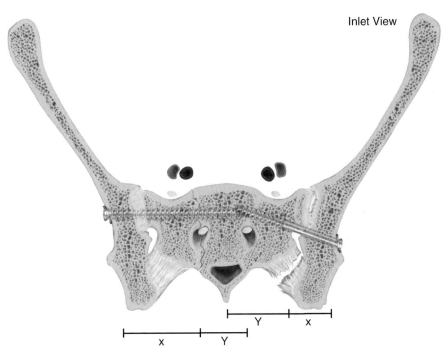

D

Figure 39.12. (*continued*) **C,D.** The screws are oriented according to the injury. The SI joint is anatomically oblique, whereas most sacral fractures occur in a sagittal plane. Sacral fractures are medially located relative to SI joint injuries. For these two reasons, screw orientation and length are different for each. The screws are inserted perpendicular to the injury; therefore, sacral and SI screws are oriented differently. Sacral-screw orientation is more horizontal, which orients the screw perpendicular to the fracture and allows longer screw length to balance the fixation. SI screws are oriented obliquely to remain perpendicular to the disrupted joint surfaces.

elliptical area within the ala below the fifth lumbar nerve-root pathway on the mid-alar cortical bone and above the first sacral nerve root tunnel. A pelvic model and preoperative drawing outlining the surgical tactic are helpful. A pelvic model also reveals the smaller area available for safe screw placement in the second sacral segment.

POSTOPERATIVE MANAGEMENT

Intravenous antibiotics are administered for 24 hours after surgery when percutaneous fixation has been used alone or in combination with anterior-pelvic external fixation. If open techniques are used, the antibiotics are continued until the surgical drains are removed. Sequential compression stockings are used to diminish the risk of deep venous thromboses. At my institution, a licensed physical therapist supervises the rehabilitation. The rehabilitation schedule is dependent on the overall condition of the patient and associated injuries. The stabilized hemipelvis is protected by partial weight bearing that the patient accomplishes with crutches or a walker for 6 weeks after the surgery. Progressive weight bearing follows, with a goal of crutch-free ambulation 3 months after surgery. Inlet and outlet radiographs of the pelvis are obtained in the recovery room and at the 6- and 12-week postoperative clinic visits. A postoperative CT scan is used to assess the reduction and implant location. Patients are seen in the clinic at 2, 6, and 12 weeks after the operation. Thereafter, patients are seen annually and as needed.

Most adult patients can return to labor employment 4 to 6 months after surgery. Some patients with less physically demanding jobs return much sooner, and others require job modifications. Heavy lifting and working at heights are avoided until the patient's strength and conditioning goals are achieved. Vocational reeducation is advocated for polytraumatized individuals with heavy job demands or those patients who are unable to return to work. Nonimpact aerobic and water activities are allowed 6 weeks after the operation.

COMPLICATIONS

Iliosacral screw complications include screw malposition, iatrogenic nerve injury, fixation failure, and infection. Screw malposition results from a poor understanding of the posterior pelvic anatomy or fluoroscopic imaging or both, or posterior pelvic malreduction. Iatrogenic nerve-root injuries occur because of erroneous reduction maneuvers, especially overcompression of transforaminal sacral fractures and screw-placement errors. The sacral alar slope, inadequate imaging, sacral dysmorphism, a surgeon's poor understanding of the posterior pelvis, and posterior pelvic malreduction (among other factors) cause screw misplacements. Surgeon knowledge of simple anatomical, imaging, and technical facts can dramatically decrease the risk of screw malposition:

1. The upper-sacral alar area is an elliptically shaped passageway bounded above by the sloping sacral ala and below by the upper-sacral nerve-root tunnel.
2. The boundaries of the upper-sacral alar area are identifiable radiographically after reduction. The outlet images demonstrate the spica cast orientation of the upper-sacral nerve-root pathway, and the true-lateral sacral image shows the superimposed ICDs, which reflect the alar orientation, and as a consequence, the fifth lumbar nerve-root path is also revealed. The true lateral image is also frequently used to visualize the corticated limit of the upper-sacral nerve-root path.
3. The iliac starting point, directional aim, and selected screw length all impact the safety of screw placement.
4. Dysmorphic upper-sacral anatomy has predictable radiographic identifiers, and the surgeon should recognize the narrowed safe zone available for screw insertion.
5. Obliquely oriented SI-joint screws must not extend beyond the midline because of the contralateral alar anatomy.

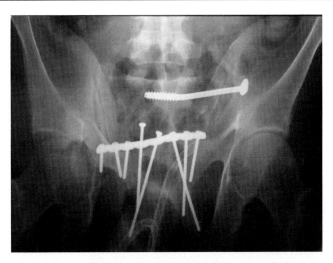

Figure 39.13. Iliosacral fixation failure occurs for a variety of reasons. In this patient with associated pelvic ring, acetabular, and urethral injuries, the anterior surgical wound was complicated with a deep infection. The complication resulted in anteriorly located implant disengagement, acetabular fracture displacement, and bending failure of the iliosacral screw.

6. On the inlet image, lumbosacral osteophytes accentuate the anterior sacrum, but they do not represent the sacral body.
7. Neurodiagnostic monitoring does not offset insufficient knowledge of sacral anatomy and its imaging. Iatrogenic nerve-root injuries occur because of screw placement errors and erroneous reduction maneuvers, especially overcompression of transforaminal sacral fractures.

Fixation failures occur in patients with highly unstable posterior-pelvic injuries, who are noncompliant or have suffered head injuries, or have an associated infection. Increased rates of fixation failure have been described in those patients treated with iliosacral screws and anterior external fixation (Fig. 39.13).

Treatment choices for fixation failure depend on numerous factors. In early failures, the unstable iliosacral screws are removed, and alternative fixations are performed after repeated reductions. The treatment of late failures is based on the amount of posterior pelvis displacement and healing. In rare situations, the overall condition of the patient or posterior pelvic soft-tissue envelope prohibits further attempts at surgical fixation, and traditional management techniques, such as traction, are chosen. Deep infection is rarely associated with percutaneous iliosacral-screw insertion.

ILLUSTRATIVE CASE FOR TECHNIQUE

A 57-year-old woman was injured in a motorcycle accident. The radiographs and CT scan of the pelvis showed a symphysis pubis disruption, a complex SI dislocation, and an ipsilateral sacral fracture (Fig. 39.14).

Her pelvis was grossly unstable to physical examination; however, her neurological status was normal. She was evaluated and resuscitated. With urgency, she was brought to the operating room and positioned supine. She was placed in 15 lb of right-sided distal-femoral traction. Through the surgeon's use of a Pfannenstiel exposure, the anterior symphyseal injury was reduced, clamped, and fixed with a plate and screws. The posterior-pelvic fracture-dislocation reduction was improved after the symphyseal open reduction and fixation along with distal femoral traction. Percutaneous iliosacral screws were used to stabilize the posterior pelvic injuries. She had an upper-sacral dysmorphism that complicated safe screw insertion. The postoperative CT scan and plain films identified the implant locations and reduction quality. Her recovery was uneventful. An attorney, she returned to work.

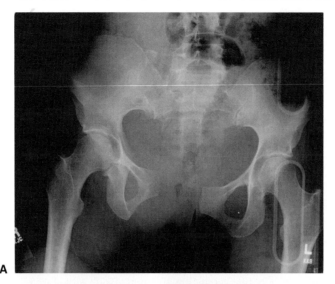

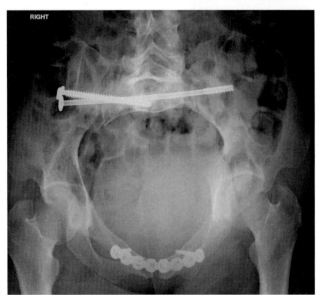

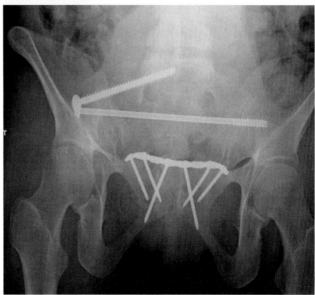

Figure 39.14. A. This female adult patient was injured while riding her motorcycle. She complained of pelvic pain and was noted to have an unstable pelvis without peripheral neurological abnormalities. The screening AP plain film of her pelvis demonstrates a complete symphysis pubis disruption and a complex right-sided posterior pelvic-ring injury including SI dislocation and sacral fracture. Upper-sacral dysplasia was noted the outlet film and was confirmed by CT scan. She was resuscitated and then taken to the operating room for pelvic stabilization. **B.** In surgery, she underwent ORIF of the symphysis pubis, but the posterior pelvic injury remained distracted despite accurate reduction of the symphysis. For that reason and accommodating the upper-sacral dysplasia, percutaneous reduction and fixation of the posterior pelvic ring was the selected technique. The second sacral-segment lag screw was inserted initially and slowly tightened under fluoroscopic imaging to prevent overcompression of the fracture. The screw was applied into the contralateral hemipelvis in an attempt to improve stability. Next, the upper-sacral fully threaded screw was inserted percutaneously to solidify further the posterior ring fixation. The postoperative inlet image of her pelvic shows the reductions of the anterior and posterior pelvic-ring injuries. **C.** The postoperative outlet image of the pelvis demonstrates the different pathways necessary for the upper-sacral and second-sacral segment screws.

RECOMMENDED READING

Arand M, Kinzl L, Gebhard F. Computer-guidance in percutaneous screw stabilization of the iliosacral joint. *Clin Orthop* 2004;422:201–207.

Burgess AR, Eastridge BJ, Young JW, et al. Pelvic ring disruptions: effective classification system and treatment protocols. *J Trauma* 1990;30:848–856.

Collinge C, Coons D, Tornetta P, et al. Standard multiplanar fluoroscopy versus a fluoroscopically based navigation system for the percutaneous insertion of iliosacral screws: a cadaver model. *J Orthop Trauma* 2005;19: 254–258.

Goldstein A, Phillips T, Sclafani, S. Early open reduction and internal fixation of the disrupted pelvic ring. *J Trauma* 1986;26:325–333.

Griffin DR, Starr AJ, Reinert CM, et al. Vertically unstable pelvic fractures fixed with percutaneous iliosacral screws: does posterior injury pattern predict fixation failure? *J Orthop Trauma* 2003;17:399–405.

Gruen GS, Leit ME, Gruen RJ, et al. The acute management of hemodynamically unstable multiple trauma patients with pelvic ring fractures. *J Trauma* 1994;36:706–713.

Helfet DL, Koval KJ, Hissa EA, et al. Intraoperative somatosensory evoked potential monitoring during acute pelvic fracture surgery. *J Orthop Trauma* 1995;9:28–34.

Kraemer W, Hearn T, Tile M, et al. The effect of thread length and location on extraction strengths of iliosacral lag screws. *Injury* 1994;25:5–9.

Latenser B, Gentilello L, Tarver A. Improved outcome with early fixation of skeletally unstable pelvic fractures. *J Trauma* 1991;31:28–31.

Matta J, Saucedo T. Internal fixation of pelvic ring fractures. *Clin Orthop* 1989;242:83–87.

Oliver CW, Twaddle B, Agel J, et al. Outcome after pelvic ring fractures: evaluation using the medical outcomes short form SF-36. *Injury* 1996;27:635–641.

Reilly MC, Bono CM, Litkouhi B, et al. The effect of sacral fracture malreduction on the safe placement of iliosacral screws: *J Orthop Trauma* 2003;17:88–94.

Routt M, Simonian P, Inaba J, et al. Iliosacral screw fixation of the disrupted sacroiliac joint. *Tech Ortho* 1994;9: 300–314.

Routt MLC Jr, Kregor PJ, Simonian PT, et al. Early results of percutaneous iliosacral screws placed with the patient in the supine position. *J Orthop Trauma* 1995;9:207–214.

Routt MLC Jr, Meier M, Kregor P. Percutaneous iliosacral screws with the patient supine-technique. *Tech Ortho* 1993;3:35–45.

Routt MLC Jr, Simonian PT, Agnew S, et al. Radiographic recognition of the sacral alar slope facilitates optimal placement of iliosacral screws: a cadaveric and clinical study. *J Orthop Trauma* 1996;10:171–177.

Routt MLC Jr, Simonian PT, Ballmer F. A rational approach to pelvic trauma: resuscitation and early definitive stabilization. *Clin Orthop* 1995;318:61–74.

Schildhauer TA, Ledoux WR, Chapman JR, et al. Triangular osteosynthesis and iliosacral screw fixation for unstable sacral fractures: a cadaveric and biomechanical evaluation under cyclic loads. *J Orthop Trauma* 2003;17: 22–31.

Shuler T, Boone D, Gruen G, et al. Percutaneous iliosacral screw fixation: early treatment for unstable posterior pelvic ring disruptions. *J Trauma* 1995;38:453–458.

Simonian PT, Routt MLC Jr, Harrington RM, et al. Anterior versus posterior provisional fixation in the unstable pelvis: a biomechanical comparison. *Clin Orthop* 1995;310:245–251.

Simonian PT, Routt MLC Jr, Harrington RM, et al. Internal fixation for the transforaminal sacral fracture. *Clin Orthop* 1996;323:202–209.

Yinger K, Scalise J, Olson SA, et al. Biomechanical comparison of posterior pelvic ring fixation. *J Orthop Trauma* 2003;17:481–487.

40

Pelvic Fractures: Sacral Fixation

Mark C. Reilly, Brent L. Norris, Michael J. Bosse,
James F. Kellam, and Stephen H. Sims

INDICATIONS/CONTRAINDICATIONS

Although sacral fractures may occur as an isolated injury, most commonly they occur as one component of a pelvic ring injury. Notoriously difficult to diagnose on plain films, a sacral injury is often found by a surgeon who displays a high index of suspicion based on the mechanism of injury and physical examination. Even nondisplaced or minimally displaced sacral fractures may be unstable and have the potential to displace prior to healing. Therefore, the orthopedic surgeon is challenged to identify and treat sacral fractures knowing that these injuries are at high risk for displacement. Information such as the pattern of the sacral fracture, its location, disruption of surrounding bone and soft-tissue structures, mechanism of injury, and the severity of the anterior pelvic-ring injury must be considered by the surgeon determining the inherent stability of a sacral fracture.

Denis et al classified sacral fractures according to their relationship to the sacral foramina. This classification system correlates with neurologic injury as well. Zone I injuries are lateral to the sacral foramina and are associated with L5 nerve-root injuries in 20% to 25% of cases. Fractures through the sacral foramina are zone II injuries, and injury to the sacral nerve roots occur in up to 50% of patients with this type of fracture. If the fracture is medial to the sacral foramina, the injury is in zone III, and neurologic injury with bowel and/or bladder dysfunction occurs in up to 70% of zone III patients.

Stable sacral fractures can be managed symptomatically with a short period of bed rest followed by mobilization and protected weight bearing until healed. Prolonged bed rest or traction is not recommended in unstable injuries because of the inherent risks of deep venous thrombosis, pressure ulceration, and aspiration or pneumonia. Frequent radiographic follow-up is mandatory to identify fractures that, although initially thought to be stable, subsequently displace following mobilization. Sacral fractures medial to the L5–S1 facet joint are more constrained by the disc and facet joint capsule and are less prone to displacement than alar or transforaminal fractures. Fractures caused by a lateral compression mechanism are also less likely to displace than anterior-posterior compression and "vertical shear" injuries.

Displaced and unstable sacral fractures require reduction and fixation. Because instability is often difficult to ascertain, displacement is more often cited as the indication for surgical treatment. Displacement of greater than 1 cm in the posterior pelvic ring is generally accepted as an indication for reduction and fixation. Complex pelvic-ring injuries that include a sacral fracture may also benefit by fixation such that patient mobilization is improved. Reduction and fixation of displaced sacral fractures that are associated with neurologic injury may help improve the chance for neurologic recovery. As with any injury, associated traumas, medical comorbidities, patient age, and preinjury functional level must be considered in determining appropriate treatment.

PREOPERATIVE PLANNING

In patients with pelvic fractures, full trauma evaluation and resuscitation with basic and advanced trauma life support (ATLS) protocols are essential. The evaluation of patients with a pelvic ring injury includes a visual examination and palpation of the back, buttocks, flank, groin, and perineum so the integrity of the skin and soft tissues can be assessed. The presence of a fluid wave, a local area of fluctuance, or a well-circumscribed area of cutaneous anesthesia may identify a Morel-Lavaleé lesion or internal degloving. To exclude the presence of an occult open fracture or an associated injury to the rectum or genitourinary tract, the surgeon must conduct thorough rectal and vaginal examinations and document the neurologic status of the limbs.

The pelvic fracture evaluation begins with the anteroposterior (AP) radiograph of the injured pelvis. Although the presence of a sacral fracture may be difficult to ascertain on this film, interruption of the arcuate lines of the sacral neural foramina, avulsions of the transverse processes of L5 and/or sacrospinous or sacrotuberous ligamentous avulsions, or asymmetry of the posterior pelvis should prompt further evaluation. The 40-degree caudad (inlet) and 40-degree cephalad (outlet) projections as well as a computed tomography (CT) scan allow the surgeon to evaluate further the integrity of the anterior and posterior pelvic ring. Occasionally, obturator and iliac oblique views give further information about a posterior pelvic injury.

The method of treatment is dependent on the condition of the soft tissues as well as the fracture pattern and stability. If operative treatment is selected, the status of the posterior soft-tissue envelope must be critically assessed. If the condition of the soft tissues is unsatisfactory, then open treatment of the sacral fracture should be deferred until an exposure can be made safely through a viable soft-tissue envelope.

For most sacral fractures, surgery is usually delayed 3 to 7 days to allow the patient's condition to stabilize, to obtain appropriate imaging studies, and to assemble the operative team. However, if the fracture is well delineated, the surgeon has all the necessary resources available, and the patient is clinically stable, surgery need not be delayed. Indications for early intervention are control of bleeding, debridement of open fractures, or a patient who requires emergent surgery for other reasons and has no contraindications to proceeding with pelvic fixation. In patients with degloving injuries, debridement of devitalized tissue or drainage of hematoma may be necessary before definitive fixation.

In general circumstances, the sacral fracture should be reduced before fixation of an associated, anterior, pelvic-ring or acetabular fracture. If only two sites of injury are found in the pelvic ring, anterior ring reduction and fixation often indirectly assists the reduction of the sacral fracture. When more than two zones of injury exist, malreduction of one component of the pelvic ring may preclude an anatomic reduction of the posterior pelvic ring or acetabulum.

For many sacral fractures, a closed reduction may be attempted because if successful, a percutaneous iliosacral-screw fixation can often be utilized. If the closed reduction is unsuccessful, however, the surgeon must be prepared to proceed with open reduction and internal fixation (ORIF), if the soft tissues allow, rather than accept a posterior pelvic-ring malreduction.

TECHNIQUE FOR OPEN REDUCTION

Surgery is performed with the patient under general anesthesia in the prone position on a radiolucent table. The thorax is supported on bolsters, and the face is appropriately positioned and padded. Pillows are placed beneath the thighs to equal the height of the bolsters. This prevents loss of lumbar lordosis and a flexed position of the pelvis, which makes obtaining and interpreting oblique radiographic projections difficult. The pelvis itself is not directly supported because bolsters pressing directly against the anterior superior spines may be a deforming force on the pelvic ring. The knees are flexed and the tibiae rest on a padded support (Fig. 40.1). Hip extension and knee flexion relax the sciatic nerve as well as improve safety when access through the greater sciatic notch is needed. The surgical field should include the entire pelvis, including the contralateral posterior–superior iliac spine (PSIS) and the ipsilateral greater trochanter, for possible placement of distractors or clamps. The patient is not routinely placed in skeletal traction because it often rotates the pelvis rather than contributes to the reduction. Likewise, the use of a perineal post may be a deforming force against the anterior pelvic ring and may result in difficulty obtaining an anatomic reduction of the posterior injury.

A vertical incision is made 2 cm lateral to the palpable PSIS (Fig. 40.2). The subcutaneous tissue is incised down to the fascia of the gluteus maximus muscle. The gluteus maximus muscle must be reflected laterally so that its neurologic and vascular supplies are preserved. The gluteus maximus originates from the posterior iliac crest, the fascia of the multifidus, and the spinous processes of the sacrum. Failure to release the maximus from its origin will result in an obligatory devascularization and denervation of any muscle left behind. Although fasciocutaneous flaps are generally preferred, elevating the gluteus fascia off the muscle belly can make repair of the maximus muscle impossible. The subcutaneous tissue is elevated medially off of the surface of the maximus fascia to the origin of the muscle, and the maximus is then elevated subperiosteally from the ilium and sharply off of the multifidus fascia (Fig. 40.3). The maximus can be elevated as far laterally as needed for

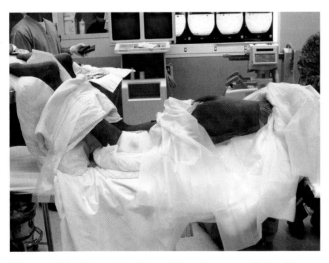

Figure 40.1. The patient is positioned prone with the hips extended and the knees flexed on the radiolucent table. The chest and thighs are supported on bolsters leaving the pelvis free for manipulation.

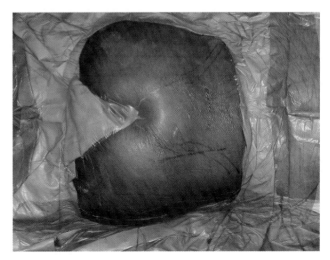

Figure 40.2. The skin incision is drawn for open reduction of a sacral fracture. The planned incision is vertical and 2 cm lateral to the palpable posterior superior iliac spine. Both hemipelvises are draped into the surgical field while the perineum is excluded.

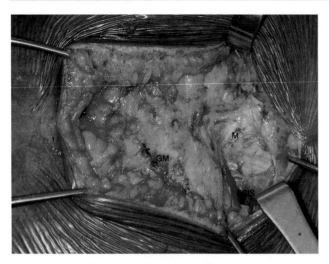

Figure 40.3. The skin and subcutaneous tissues have been elevated off the fascia of the gluteus maximus. The gluteus maximus *(GM)* is seen at the insertion onto the multifidus fascia *(M)*. The posterior superior iliac spine *(PSIS)* is exposed in the cranial portion of the wound.

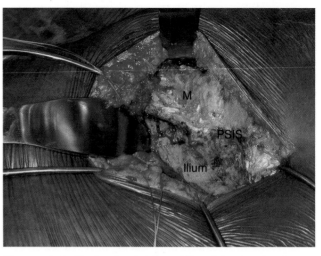

Figure 40.4. Further lateral dissection of the gluteus maximus off of the ilium has been performed. The greater sciatic notch is exposed and a cobra retractor is in place. The multifidus *(M)* fascia has not been disturbed.

exposure but in most circumstances need not be elevated much beyond the crista gluteae (Fig. 40.4).

The piriformis is then subperiosteally dissected from the anterior and lateral edge of the sacrum, and the greater sciatic notch can be cleaned from medial to lateral. The superior-gluteal neurovascular bundle will be encountered in the lateral portion of the notch. Curved elevators can be used along with manual techniques to dissect along the anterior aspect of the sacroiliac joint and as far medial as the palpable, ventral, sacral-nerve roots. The ventral, sacral, neural foraminae of S1 thorough S4 should be palpable. The erector spinae is then elevated off the dorsal surface of the sacrum as far medially as needed for fracture visualization. The dorsal cutaneous nerves emanating from the dorsal sacral foramina are visualized but are often injured, particularly in transforaminal sacral fractures. Periosteum is cleaned from the dorsal surface of the sacrum while the surgeon takes particular care to preserve fracture edges that can be used to help assess the reduction (Fig. 40.5).

The sacral fracture is now opened, either with the use of a lamina spreader or a femoral distractor, with pins placed in both PSIS. The ventral sacral-nerve roots can be visualized in zone II fractures, and any bony fragments that might impinge on the nerves can be removed at this time.

Fracture reduction is performed by placing clamps from the ilium to the spinous process of S3 or S4. The surgeon should make a careful examination of the preoperative CT scan to identify the presence of a lower-sacral spina-bifida occulta, which would prevent safe clamp placement in this location. Varying the location of the clamp position on the ilium can result in a more posterior or anterior direction of pull and can help fine-tune the reduction. A second clamp can be placed more transversely to aid in fracture compression (Fig. 40.6). To avoid damaging the ventral nerve roots, the reduction of the sacral fracture must be accurate and the nerve roots free of impinging bony fragments before significant compression is applied at the fracture site.

When treating zone III sacral fractures medial to the foramina, the surgeon may want to utilize a midline approach and place the incision directly over the spinous processes. The multifidus may be elevated subperiosteally, from medial to lateral, off of the sacral lamina. Reduction clamps may be placed from ilium to ilium or directly onto the dorsal surface of the sacrum through unicortical drill holes. Pins placed bilaterally in the PSIS can be used to distract and clean the fracture as well as assist in the reduction.

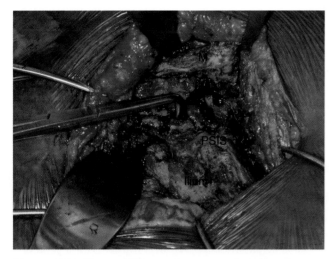

Figure 40.5. The multifidus and erector spinae have been elevated subperiosteally off of the dorsal surface of the sacrum. The comminuted sacral fracture is exposed.

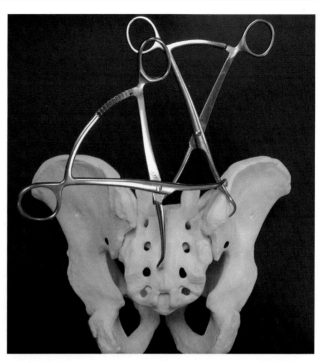

Figure 40.6. Clamp placement shown on a sawbone model of a transforaminal sacral fracture. One clamp is used to control cranial displacement of the hemipelvis. The more transversely oriented clamp helps compress the fracture.

TECHNIQUE FOR INTERNAL FIXATION

Several surgical techniques can be used to stabilize sacral fractures. They include the use of iliosacral screws, posterior iliosacral plating, dorsal sacral plating, and lumbopelvic fixation. The use of iliosacral screws is the most common method of fixation of sacral fractures. If the fracture can be reduced by closed means, insertion of percutaneous iliosacral screws can be done with the patient in either the supine or prone position.

Iliosacral Screws

Iliosacral screws are indicated for unilateral or bilateral sacral fractures in zones I or II. Fractures in zone III are also amenable to this technique, but great care must be used in screw placement so that iatrogenic nerve injury is avoided. A thorough understanding of the direction of fracture displacement improves the surgeon's chances of reducing the fracture by closed means. A closed reduction is attempted by traction to correct axial displacement. Percutaneously inserted Schantz screws, pointed pelvic-reduction clamps, a femoral distractor placed in the posterior iliac spines, or a spiked pusher to close gaps or disimpact fractures are useful instruments for adjunctive techniques of fracture reduction. Once a reduction has been obtained and confirmed fluoroscopically, provisional fixation with clamps, Kirschner (K) wires, or external fixation is useful to hold the fracture prior to definitive iliosacral-screw fixation. If a satisfactory reduction cannot be accomplished by closed means, the surgeon should proceed to open reduction.

Once the reduction has been obtained, it is checked and verified with the image intensifier. Only then can internal fixation be safely done. The height of the sacral ala should be compared bilaterally on the cephalad projection (outlet view), and the sacral neural foramina should appear bilaterally symmetric. On the caudad projection (inlet view), the contour of the posterior pelvis should appear bilaterally symmetric, and the reduction can be checked by restoration of the sacral alar line. The most common means of internal fixation for sacral fractures are iliosacral screws. Because the ideal direction of these screws should be perpendicular to the sacral fracture, the screws are inserted through a separate, small, lateral incision. Two partially threaded, large-fragment lag screws are generally placed in the first sacral segment. The length of these screws should be sufficient that the threads of the lag screw lie within the body of S1. As this bone is more dense than the alar bone, longer screws, although they may improve resistance to shear, may not have the pullout strength and interfragmental compression of screws with threads that lie within the body of S1. When closed reduction and percutaneous screws are used, some surgeons favor fully threaded screws to avoid overcompression of the fracture and impingement on the sacral nerve roots. When open reduction is performed, the reduction is directly visualized and this is less of a concern. In any case, interfragmentary compression is recommended to improve the initial fracture stability.

Posterior Iliosacral Plating: Tension Band Plating

A transiliac tension band plate is indicated for significantly displaced sacral fractures that are not adequately stabilized by iliosacral screws alone. On occasion, when iliosacral screws are tightened, gapping occurs at the caudal portion of the fracture. In our experience, this is a good indication to supplement the iliosacral screw construct with a posterior tension-band plate. The plate may also provide limited interfragmentary compression to the fracture. Although it may be utilized as a stand-alone implant, the resultant force applied when the tension band plate is secured to the bone may result in an external rotation deformity through one or both sides of the pelvis, particularly if the fracture is not already secured with iliosacral screw fixation.

A second vertical incision is placed lateral to the PSIS on the contralateral side of the pelvis, and a limited portion of the gluteus maximus is reflected off the erector spinae fascia. A straight 10- or 12-hole, 3.5- or 4.5-mm reconstruction plate is used. The optimal position of the dorsal tension band plate is just below the PSIS. This decreases plate prominence and ensures that the screws in the ilium are anchored in the strong bone of

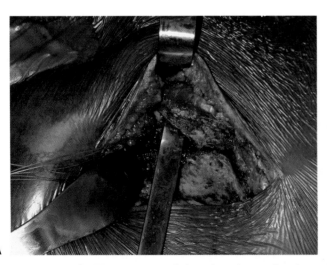
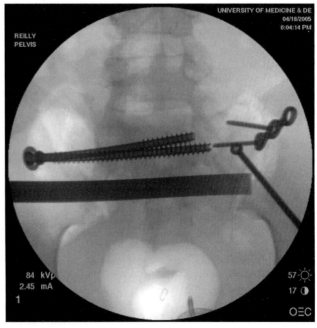

Figure 40.7. A. The osteotome is introduced ventral to the multifidus and utilized to osteotomize the spinous process of S2. **B.** Fluoroscopic image of in-place osteotome.

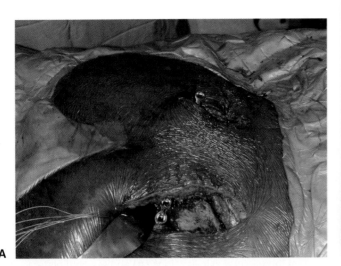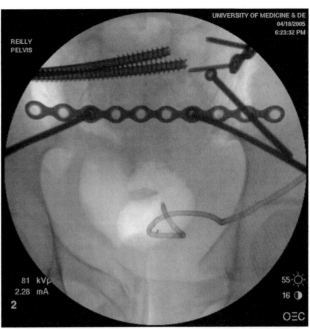

A   B

Figure 40.8. A. The osteotome has been exchanged for the straight pelvic-reconstruction plate. **B.** The plate has been secured to each posterior superior iliac spine by means of a 4.5-mm screw placed parallel to the greater sciatic notch between the tables of the iliac wings.

the sciatic buttress. The plate is typically inserted from the side of the open reduction and tunneled through to the contralateral surgical site. A 1/2-inch osteotome is passed from one incision, ventral to the erector spinae fascia, osteotomizing the sacral spinous process of S2 (Fig. 40.7). The unbent straight pelvic reconstruction plate is then passed along the same track until visualized in the second incision (Fig. 40.8). A screw is inserted bilaterally between the tables of the ilium into the sciatic buttress. Tightening these screws adds tension to the plate over the dorsum of the sacrum and causes compression of the sacral fracture. The ends of the plate are then bent to the iliac wing in situ and secured with a single screw at each end of the plate (Figs. 40.9 and 40.10).

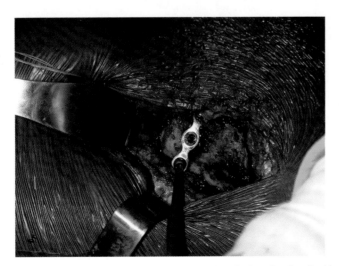

Figure 40.9. The plate is bent to the iliac wing in situ. It will then be fixed with a bicortical screw directed toward the anterior aspect of the sacroiliac joint.

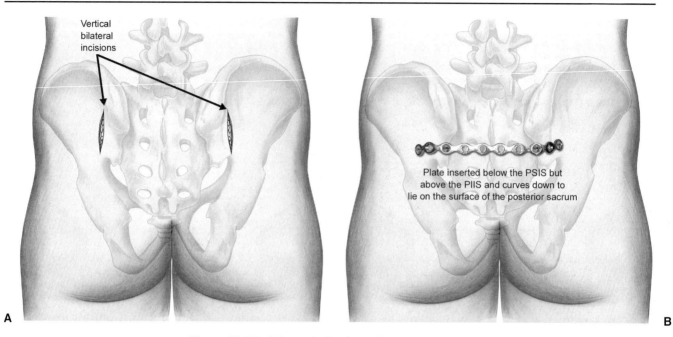

Figure 40.10. Schematic drawings of the bilateral skin incisions **(A)** and the final plate placement on the sacrum and iliac wings **(B)**.

The dorsal tension band plate may also be useful in bilateral sacral fractures. Because the body of S1 may not simultaneously accommodate the presence of multiple bilateral screws, the number of screws or the lengths of those screws may need to be compromised. In this circumstance, the plate may be utilized to augment the iliosacral screw fixation. In pelvic malunion or nonunion reconstruction, this can be a useful technique to supplement iliosacral screw fixation and improve the strength of the initial fixation construct.

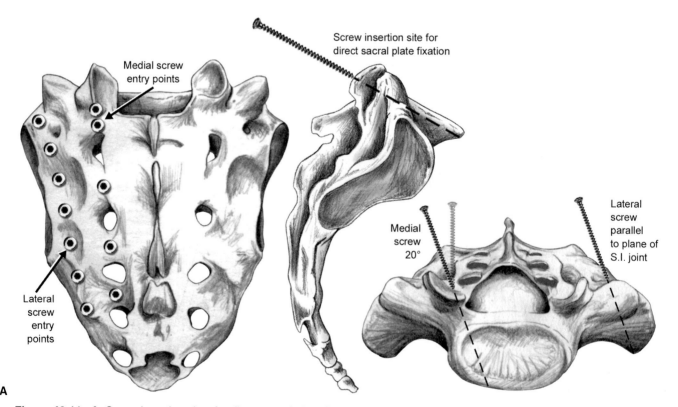

Figure 40.11. A. Screw insertion sites for direct sacral-plate fixation. Lateral entry points are adjacent to the dorsal sacroiliac-ligament insertion, while medial entry points are midway between adjacent dorsal foramina. Lateral screws are directed parallel to the plane of the sacroiliac joint, while medial screws are directed perpendicularly to the dorsal sacral lamina. (*continues*)

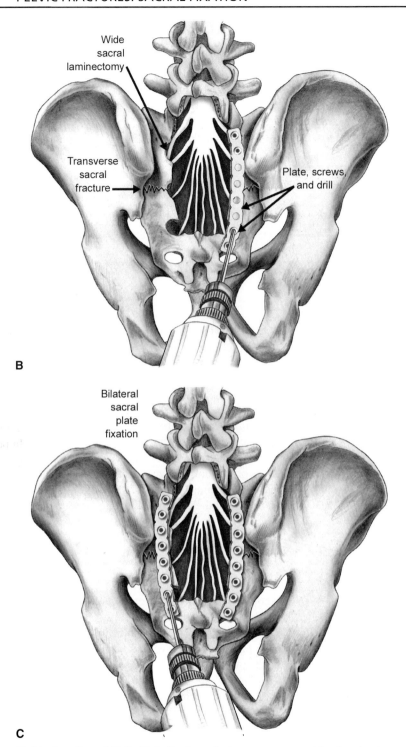

Figure 40.11. (*continued*) **B,C.** Plate fixation of a transverse sacral fracture is shown. This was performed in conjunction with a wide sacral laminectomy for nerve root decompression.

Direct Dorsal-Sacral Plating

Direct application of a plate to the dorsal surface of the sacrum may be used in the fixation of zone III and selected zone II sacral fractures. However, the plate is most commonly employed in the treatment of transverse sacral fractures. Plates may be contoured to sit lateral to the sacral foramina, and bicortical screw fixation is achieved in the ala or body of each sacral segment (Fig. 40.11). To prevent injuring the exiting ventral sacral-nerve roots, the surgeon must have a thorough understanding of the intraosseous anatomy.

In direct sacral plating, the sacroiliac joints are spared. Through a midline or lateral incision, the multifidus and erector spinae muscles are elevated to expose the sacrum. During the subperiosteal dissection, the surgeon must avoid entering the sacral canal, which is at particular risk if the lamina is fractured. Once the sacrum has been exposed, decompression of the sacral nerve roots is performed, if indicated, and the fracture is reduced. Well-contoured small-fragment plates are used to stabilize the fracture. To avoid iatrogenic injury to the important adjacent-neurovascular structures, particularly the L5 nerve root, the surgeon must have a thorough understanding of the osseous, neural, and vascular anatomy.

For some zone III fractures, fixation can be achieved with a short spanning plate with screws placed in each alar region. Usually two plates are required and should be placed over the S1 and S3 regions. Intraoperative fluoroscopy is used to avoid foraminal or central-canal hardware placement. If a displaced and/or unstable anterior-pelvic injury exists, anterior stabilization should be performed. Direct sacral plating is critical to neutralize the stress on these small, relatively weak plates.

Lumbopelvic Fixation

Certain sacral-fracture patterns result in spino-pelvic dissociation. Some H-type and U-type fractures result in the body of S1 (and sometimes S2) remaining attached to the spine while the sacral ala remain attached to the pelvis. Although iliosacral screw fixation may be successful in maintaining the reduction of the pelvis to the spine, the most common deformity is kyphosis at the transverse portion of the sacral fracture, which is caused when the pelvis flexes in relation to the spine. Because this deformity is characterized by rotation around the long axis of the iliosacral screw, the ability of screw fixation alone to resist displacement is poor. In this circumstance, lumbopelvic fixation has been shown to result in a stronger fixation construct. In typical cases, pedicle screw fixation in L5 and/or L4 can be connected to 1 or 2 screws placed between the tables of the ilia above the greater sciatic notch (Fig. 40.12). Screws should be placed within the sciatic buttress. They should be long enough to pass over the greater sciatic notch to prevent flexion of the pelvis on the lumbar spine (Fig. 40.13).

WOUND CLOSURE AND POSTOPERATIVE CARE

Regardless of the technique used to fix a sacral fracture, meticulous handling of the soft tissues is critical. The wound should be copiously irrigated and complete hemostasis obtained. In most cases, we favor the use of a suction drain deep to the fascia to prevent hematoma formation. Anatomic closure of the gluteus and thoracolumbar fascia should be accomplished (Fig. 40.14). If the gluteus maximus is not correctly repaired, the soft-tissue coverage over the sacrum may be compromised and the gluteal folds may be asymmetric.

In typical cases, intravenous antibiotics are used for 24 to 48 hours. In patients with considerable soft-tissue damage, a longer duration of antibiotics may be indicated. We strongly recommend deep venous thromboembolic prophylaxis in all patients unless specific contraindications clearly prohibit such a precaution.

Following internal fixation of a unilateral sacral fracture, mobilization and protected weight bearing on the contralateral side is continued for 8 weeks. Patients with bilateral sacral fractures are mobilized from bed to chair, but weight bearing is precluded for 8 weeks. If spino-pelvic fixation has been utilized, patients are allowed protected weight bearing with crutches or a walker and progressed to full weight bearing as tolerated.

Suture removal is performed 2 weeks after surgery. When the wound is healed, a rehabilitation program that emphasizes range-of-motion exercises, as well as progressive resistance and strengthening exercises, is begun. Radiographs are typically taken postoperatively at 6 and 12 weeks. At 6 months, the patient is critically assessed regarding pain, mobility, and general health status. The three pelvic views are obtained and fracture union is assessed. CT scans can be used to evaluate sacral fractures postoperatively, but they are

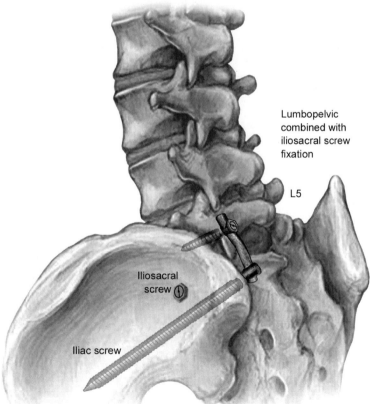

Figure 40.12. A,B. Lumbopelvic fixation is shown with pedicle screws in L5 and iliac screws placed into the sciatic buttress.

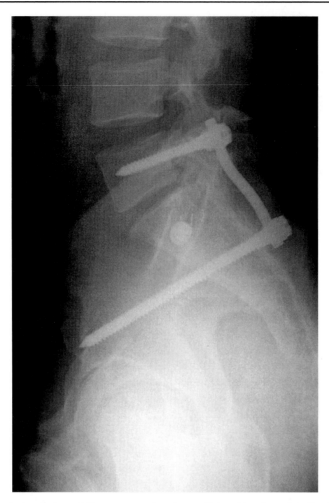

Figure 40.13. Lateral view of the sacrum showing unilateral lumbopelvic fixation augmenting iliosacral screw fixation of a comminuted sacral fracture. The iliac screw is seen to lie just cranial to the greater sciatic notch. (Courtesy of Sean Nork, MD.)

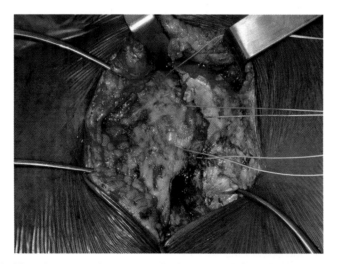

Figure 40.14. The gluteus maximus is repaired to the multifidus fascia caudally and to the lumbodorsal fascia cranially. By preserving the gluteus maximus fascia, the surgeon can soundly repair the gluteus to cover the dorsum of the sacrum and restore the contour of the posterior soft tissues of the buttock.

not as sensitive as plain radiographs at demonstrating residual cranial displacement. Patients are reviewed at 6 months, 1 year, and yearly thereafter. The patient may need up to 2 years to achieve maximal medical and functional recovery.

ILLUSTRATIVE CASE FOR TECHNIQUE

A 24-year-old woman sustained a complex pelvic-ring injury after being in a motor vehicle accident. She underwent emergent laparotomy and repair of an intestinal injury. Her abdomen was packed open. The AP, caudad, and cephalad views of the pelvis demonstrate bilateral zone II sacral fractures as well as bilateral, superior and inferior, ramus fractures; the right-sided fracture extends into the pubic body (Fig. 40.15). Cranial displacement of the right hemipelvis is found as is an adduction deformity of the left hemipelvis. An axial CT scan demonstrates comminution of the sacral fractures as well as a fracture of the PSIS that extends into the sacroiliac joint on the left (Fig. 40.16). A three-dimensional CT reconstruction was also used to evaluate the patient's condition (Fig. 40.17).

Figure 40.18 shows the postoperative radiographs taken after open reduction and iliosacral screw fixation of the right sacral fracture and lag screw fixation of the left PSIS fracture. Because of the bilateral posterior pelvic-ring injuries, dorsal tension-band plating

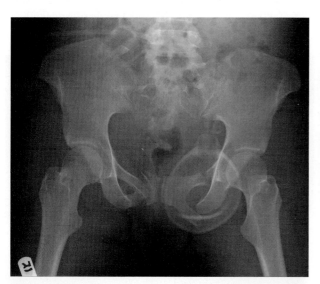

A

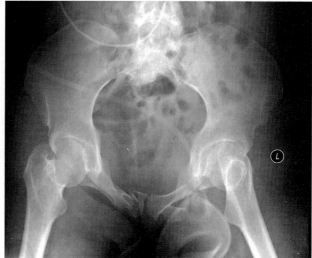

B

C

Figure 40.15. Initial radiographs demonstrate the comminuted right-sacral fracture, left sacroiliac fracture-dislocation, and comminuted, bilateral, ramus fractures. A drain is seen superimposed due to the patient's open abdomen.

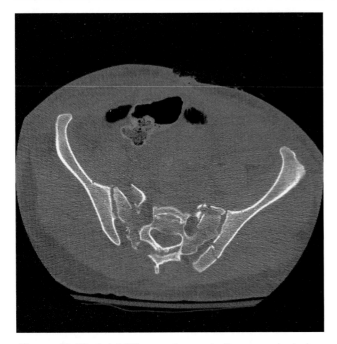

Figure 40.16. Axial CT scan demonstrating comminuted zone II sacral fractures as well as a PSIS fracture-dislocation component on the left.

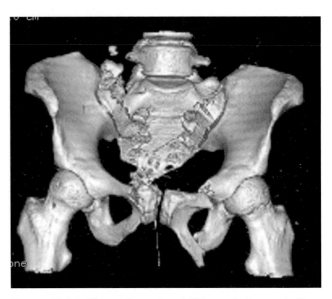

Figure 40.17. Three-dimensional CT scan helps to clarify the comminution of the sacral fractures as well as demonstrates the multiple sites of pelvic deformity.

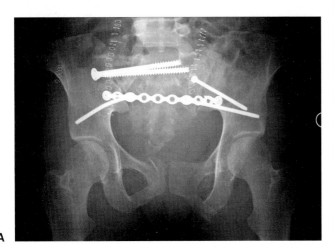

A

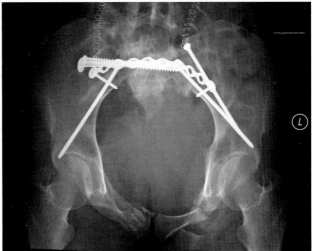

B

C

Figure 40.18. Postoperative radiographs after posterior pelvic-ring fixation. The fracture of the mammillary process of the right sacral ala may be mistaken for persistent gross cranial translation of the fracture. However, the heights of the iliac wings and the restoration of the sacral foramina seen on the cephalad view demonstrate that much of the displacement has been corrected. Persistent incongruity is seen in the left sacroiliac joint because of the comminution and impaction of the sacral side of the joint. The symphyseal fragment remains rotated.

of the sacrum was chosen to augment the screw fixation. The patient's abdomen was left open for an extended period because she experienced an abdominal compartment syndrome. The anterior pelvic-ring injuries were not operatively addressed and were allowed to heal without fixation.

RECOMMENDED READING

Denis F, Davis S, Comfort T. Sacral fractures: an important problem. *Clin Orthop* 1988;227:67–81.

Gorczyca J, Varga E, Woodside T, et al. The strength of iliosacral lag screws and transiliac bars in the fixation of vertically unstable pelvic injuries with sacral fractures. *Injury* 1996;27: 561–564.

Matta J, Saucedo T. Internal fixation of pelvic ring fractures. *Clin Orthop* 1989;242:83–97.

Reilly M, Bono C, Litkouhi B, et al. The effect of sacral fracture malreduction on the safe placement of iliosacral screws. *J Orthop Trauma* 2003;17(2):88–94.

Routt C, Simonian P, Agnew, SG, et al. Radiographic recognition of the sacral alar slope for optimal placement of iliosacral screws: a cadaveric and clinical study. *J Orthop Trauma* 1996;10(8):171.

Schildhauer T, Ledoux W, Chapman J, et al. Triangular osteosynthesis and iliosacral screw fixation for unstable sacral fractures: a cadaveric and biomechanical evaluation under cyclic loads. *J Orthop Trauma* 2003;17(1): 22–31.

Tornetta P, Matta J. Outcome of operatively treated unstable posterior pelvic ring disruptions. *Clin Orthop* 1996; 329:186–193.

41

Acetabular Fractures: The Kocher-Langenbeck Approach

Berton R. Moed

INDICATIONS/CONTRAINDICATIONS

Displaced fractures of the acetabulum resulting in joint incongruity or instability are best treated by open reduction and internal fixation (ORIF). Contraindications to surgery are ill defined and not absolute. Important concerns include preexisting patient factors, such as poor general medical status and osteopenia, and factors that relate to overall patient prognosis, such as advanced age and associated injuries. All of these conditions must be considered with the knowledge that with nonoperative treatment in the face of joint incongruity or instability or both, the prognosis for hip-joint function is poor.

In choosing the appropriate surgical approach, the surgeon has an objective to select the least extensive exposure that allows sufficient bony access for anatomic joint reconstruction. The Kocher-Langenbeck approach provides direct visualization of the entire lateral aspect of the posterior column of the acetabulum (Fig. 41.1) (1). Indirect access to the true pelvis and to the anterior column can be attained by the palpating finger or through the use of special instruments (Figs. 41.1 to 41.3) (1). Therefore, the Kocher-Langenbeck approach is applied in the treatment of fractures with the main displacement involving the posterior column. In the classification of Letournel and Judet (Table 41.1), this group consists of six fracture types: posterior wall, posterior column, posterior column and wall, transverse, transverse and posterior wall, and T-shaped. The Kocher-Langenbeck approach is the surgical exposure of choice for the first three types, in which the fracture extent is limited to the posterior wall or column or both. For the transverse, transverse and posterior wall, and T-shaped fractures, some decision making is required. All three of these fracture types have a transverse fracture line as a common component. As a general guideline, if the fracture is less than 15 days old and the transverse component is located at (juxta-) or below (infra-) the level of the roof (tectum) of the acetabulum (therefore not involving the weight-bearing area of the acetabulum), the Kocher-Langenbeck approach is indicated (1). Otherwise, an alternative exposure, such as the extended iliofemoral approach, should be used. For acute juxtatectal- and infratectal-level transverse and T-shaped fractures, in which the

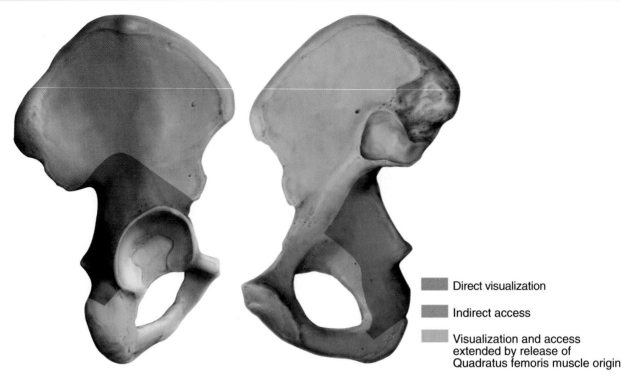

Direct visualization

Indirect access

Visualization and access
extended by release of
Quadratus femoris muscle origin

Figure 41.1. Access provided by the Kocher-Langenbeck approach.

major displacement occurs anteriorly at the pelvic brim and only minor posterior displacement, the ilioinguinal approach is perhaps the best choice.

The status of the local soft tissues is an important additional consideration. Acetabular fracture surgery through a compromised soft-tissue envelope is ill advised because of the increased risk of infection. Closed, degloving, soft-tissue injuries over the trochanteric region associated with underlying hematoma formation and fat necrosis (the Morel-Lavalle lesion) or open wounds may require debridement followed by delayed wound closure (1). The fracture pattern should be reassessed to determine whether reduction and fixation can be accomplished by using an alternative surgical approach located outside of the zone of soft-tissue injury. Another treatment option is to delay surgery until wound healing. This delay, as noted previously, may preclude use of the Kocher-Langenbeck approach.

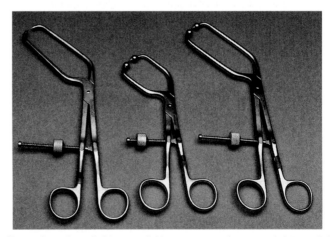

Figure 41.2. Examples of available special instruments that permit intrapelvic and anterior column access.

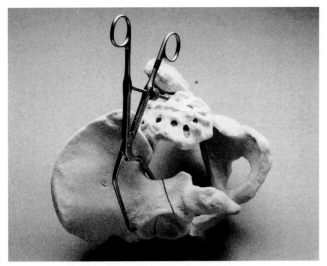
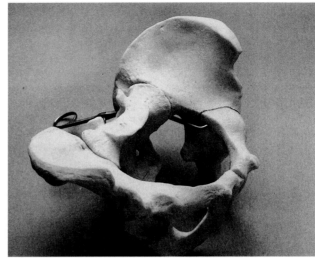

A   B

Figure 41.3. A,B. Example of clamp application for fracture reduction with a bone model.

PREOPERATIVE PLANNING

In most cases, patients with an acetabulum fracture have sustained high-energy trauma. Therefore, examination of the injured limb, even in those with an apparent isolated injury, should be just one part of a comprehensive and systematic approach. Associated injuries can be life or limb threatening. The Advanced Trauma Life Support evaluation sequence should be followed (Table 41.2). Detailed examination of the hip and lower extremity is performed during the secondary survey. As previously noted, soft-tissue injury has important implications regarding subsequent surgery; therefore, the soft tissues should be evaluated carefully. The incidence of preoperative, posttraumatic, sciatic-nerve injury was reported as being as high as 31% (2). Other peripheral nerves, such as the femoral and obturator nerves, also may be injured. A complete and clearly documented neurologic examination is extremely important both for patient prognosis and for medical-legal concerns. Preoperatively, this evaluation should be repeated periodically.

The initial anteroposterior (AP) x-ray of the pelvis is obtained during the secondary survey and can provide substantial diagnostic information regarding fracture type, as well as indicate a need for emergency treatment (Fig. 41.4). This x-ray must be supplemented by further studies to define completely the acetabular fracture pattern. The three necessary additional plain x-rays (Fig. 41.5) are centered on the affected hip and include an AP and

Table 41.1. *Acetabular Fracture Classification*

Elementary fractures
Posterior wall
Posterior column
Anterior wall
Anterior column
Transverse

Associated fractures
Posterior column and wall
Anterior column or wall and posterior hemitransverse
Transverse and posterior wall
T-shaped
Both columns

From Letournel E, Judet R. *Fractures of the acetabulum.* Berlin: Springer-Verlag; 1981, and Letournel E, Judet R: *Fractures of the acetabulum.* 2nd ed. Berlin: Springer-Verlag; 1993.

Table 41.2. *Advanced-Trauma Life-Support Evaluation Sequence*

Primary survey

Airway and cervical spine control
Breathing control
Circulation and hemorrhage control
Disability: brief neurologic evaluation
Exposure: undress the patient

Resuscitation

Secondary survey

Head-to-toes survey
Cervical spine and chest x-rays
Other procedures for patient assessment
    Peritoneal lavage
    Laboratory studies
    Extremity x-rays

Definitive care

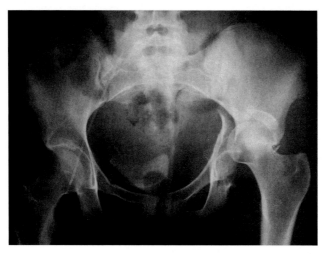

Figure 41.4. Initial AP pelvis x-ray of a 19-year-old woman involved in a motor vehicle accident. The left hip is dislocated, and there is a transverse fracture of the left acetabulum. A double density just superior to the dislocated femoral head suggests a posterior-wall fracture component.

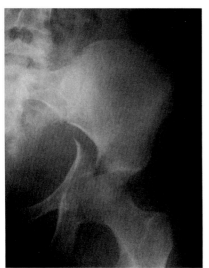 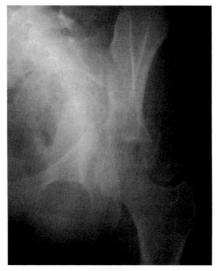 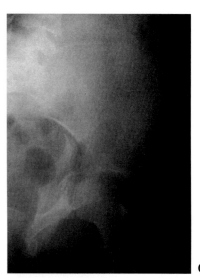

A, B   **C**

Figure 41.5. A–C. AP and 45-degree oblique hip x-rays after emergent reduction of the hip dislocation. The juxtatectal transverse-acetabular fracture with an associated posterior wall fracture is more completely delineated.

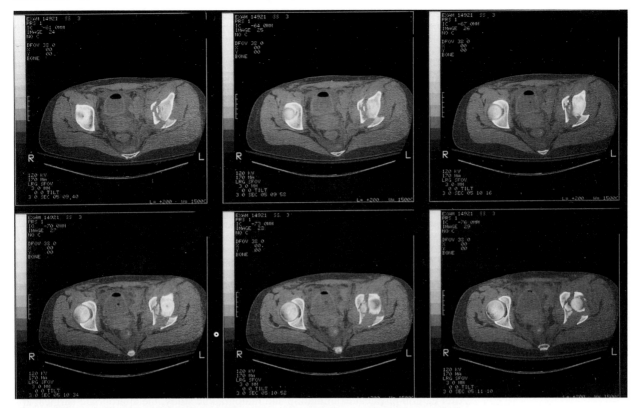

Figure 41.6. Selected two-dimensional CT sections through the dome of the acetabulum. In addition to findings consistent with a juxtatectal transverse and associated posterior-wall fracture, comminution involving the articular surface and quadrilateral plate is evident.

two 45-degree oblique views (the internal or obturator oblique view and the external or iliac oblique view) (1). Although these four plain x-rays usually provide all the information needed to define the acetabular fracture type, the standard two-dimensional computed tomography (CT) scan can supply important additional information and is indispensable for preoperative planning (Fig. 41.6). The eventual universal availability of high-quality three-dimensional CT reconstructions may eliminate much of the mystery associated with the radiographic interpretation of acetabulum fractures (Fig. 41.7). However, except for the AP

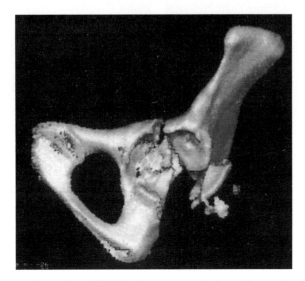

Figure 41.7. Three-dimensional CT. The fracture as deduced by evaluation of the plain x-rays and two-dimensional CT is shown fairly clearly. An overall appreciation of the fracture pattern is provided. However, there is some loss of definition, especially of the quadrilateral-plate fracture involvement.

Table 41.3. *Indications for Emergency Acetabular Fracture Fixation*

Recurrent hip dislocation after reduction despite traction
Modifier: None
Progressive sciatic-nerve deficit after closed reduction
Modifier: None
Irreducible hip dislocation
Modifier: After open reduction (stable with traction), fracture fixation may be delayed because of declining medical status of the patient or limitations of the surgical team
Associated vascular injury requiring repair
Modifier: When the fracture is directly related to the vascular injury and fracture stabilization is an important adjuvant to the vascular repair, such as an anterior-column fracture associated with laceration of the femoral artery, urgent fracture fixation is required
Open fractures
Modifier: Open-fracture treatment principles require emergency irrigation, debridement, and fracture stabilization. Fracture stabilization options include traction followed by delayed ORIF or acute ORIF

With permission from Tile M. *Fractures of the pelvis and acetabulum.* 2nd ed. Baltimore: Williams & Wilkins; 1995.

hip x-ray, which in most cases provides the same information as the AP pelvis examination, the plain and two-dimensional CT radiographic studies continue to be indispensable and should be viewed concurrently to make the definitive fracture diagnosis (1).

After careful physical examination and radiographic study, the appropriate surgical approach can be determined. The indications for emergency fracture fixation are uncommon (Table 41.3). Operative treatment is generally delayed 3 to 5 days to allow stabilization of the patient's general status and for preoperative planning. My preference is to use preoperative, skeletal, femoral-pin traction both to maintain an unstable hip in a located position and to prevent further femoral head articular-surface damage from abrasion by the raw acetabular bony fracture surfaces (Fig. 41.8). Significant intraoperative blood loss can occur.

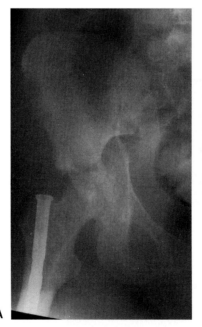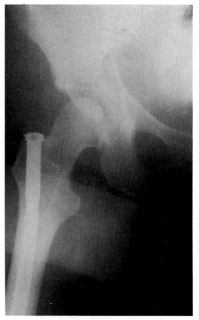

A   **B**

Figure 41.8. AP pelvis x-ray before **(A)** and after **(B)** the application of traction. The hip joint is distracted with the application of traction, pulling the articular cartilage of the femoral head a safe distance away from the acetabular fracture surface. A defect in the femoral head from the impact of the injury is evident **(B).** The femoral nail is from a previous injury.

Two to four units of blood should be made available, depending on the extent of the fracture pattern. The use of an autologous blood-transfusion system, such as the cell saver, may decrease the need for intraoperative, homologous, banked-blood transfusion.

SURGERY

Patient Positioning

Acetabular fracture fixation using the Kocher-Langenbeck approach can be performed with the patient in either the lateral or the prone position. Orthopedic surgeons from North America are more familiar with and perhaps more comfortable using lateral positioning with the affected extremity draped free, as in hip arthroplasty surgery (Fig. 41.9). However, the Kocher-Langenbeck approach is most effective with the patient placed prone on a fracture table. The benefits of the prone position are realized by maintaining the femoral head in a reduced position. Gravity becomes a help rather than a hindrance in fracture exposure and reduction. The fracture table provides controlled traction and limb positioning, further assisting in fracture reduction. Traction is applied through use of a distal femoral pin with the knee flexed to approximately 90 degrees (Fig. 41.10). This angle of knee flexion places the sciatic nerve in a relaxed position, minimizing the risk of intraoperative sciatic-nerve injury. An unscrubbed assistant is required for intraoperative adjustment of the table.

With the patient placed prone, chest rolls should be used to elevate the head and to avoid excessive abdominal pressure. The fracture table generates the added risk of injury (i.e., pudendal nerve palsy) from pressure against the perineal post. The Judet fracture table, an updated version of which is now available from Orthopedic Systems, Inc. (Union City, CA), adequately addresses these concerns (Figs. 41.10 and 41.11).

No matter what the patient position, use of a radiolucent operating table is advisable. Intraoperative c-arm fluoroscopy can then be used to assess fracture reduction and hardware location (Fig. 41.12). Before the sterile preparation and draping of the patient, the hip area should be quickly scanned with the c-arm to ensure adequate fluoroscopic visualization.

Surgical Procedure

With the patient in the lateral position and the limb draped free, the sterile field is similar to that in hip arthroplasty surgery but extended posteriorly to include the region of the posterior–superior iliac spine (Fig. 41.13). With the patient prone on the fracture table, the sterile field consists of the buttock and the posterior and lateral aspects of the thigh (Fig. 41.14).

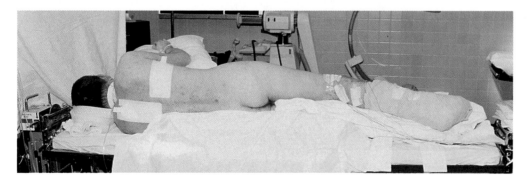

Figure 41.9. Lateral position for surgery on the right hip. The patient is supported on a beanbag on a radiolucent operating room table. The down leg is padded, and an axillary roll and head supports are in position. For this patient with an ipsilateral ankle fracture, the right leg is splinted and padded. Wires attached to the right leg are to be used for SSEP monitoring.

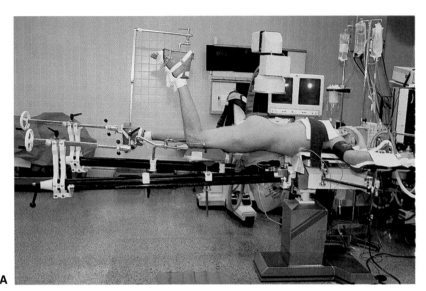

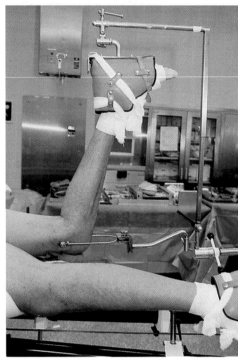

A   B

Figure 41.10. Patient in the prone position for surgery on the right hip **(A)** with a detailed view of the affected limb and femoral pin position **(B)**.

The skin incision (Fig. 41.15) is centered over the greater trochanter. The proximal branch of the incision is directed toward the posterior–superior iliac spine, ending approximately 6 cm short of this bony landmark. Distally, the incision extends approximately 15 cm along the midlateral aspect of the thigh. This skin incision is carried through the subcutaneous tissue and superficial fascia onto the fascia lata of the lateral thigh (the iliotibial tract) and the thin, deep fascia overlying the gluteus maximus muscle (Fig. 41.16).

The fascia lata is then divided in line with the skin incision, beginning at the distal aspect of the wound, continuing proximally toward the greater tuberosity, and ending at the first sighting of the gluteus maximus muscle fibers as they insert into the iliotibial tract (Fig. 41.17). The trochanteric bursa of the gluteus maximus (a large bursa between the

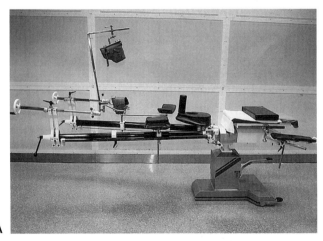

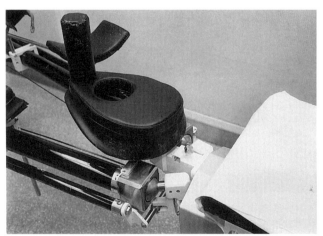

A   B

Figure 41.11. The Judet fracture table. A small pad can be used to elevate the patient's head **(A)**. A detailed view **(B)** shows the padded perineal post and the padded support with perineal cutout for male patients. The separation between the chest and padded perineal support serves to reduce abdominal pressure without requiring additional padding or chest rolls.

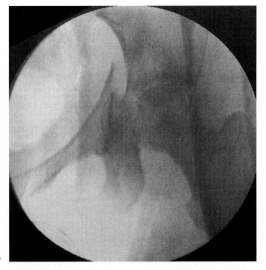

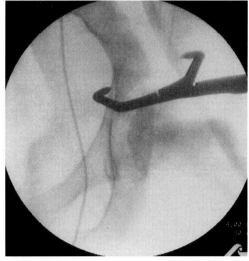

Figure 41.12. Intraoperative fluoroscopic views of a transverse with an associated posterior-wall fracture before **(A)** and after **(B)** the transverse fracture component was reduced by using a pointed reduction forceps.

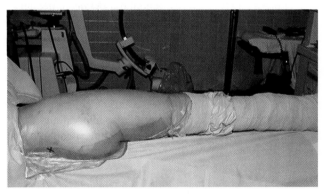

Figure 41.13. Patient from Figure 41.9 after sterile preparation and draping. The posterior–superior iliac spine is marked with an "X." The right leg is draped free. The wires for SSEP monitoring exit through a sterile plastic wrap located at the foot.

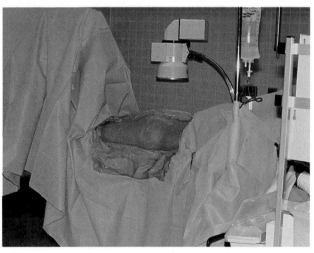

Figure 41.14. Operative field with the patient in the prone position on the Judet fracture table after sterile preparation and draping for surgery on the right hip. Please note that all subsequent intraoperative illustrations are oriented as if the patient is in this position (i.e., prone having surgery on the right hip with the anatomically superior direction on the patient located to the right and posterior located toward the top of the illustration).

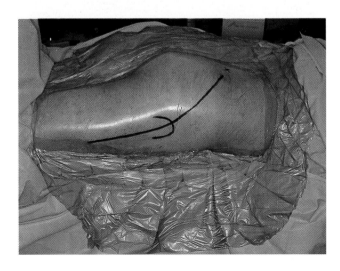

Figure 41.15. Skin incision for the Kocher-Langenbeck approach. The posterior–superior iliac spine is marked with an "X." The greater trochanter is outlined.

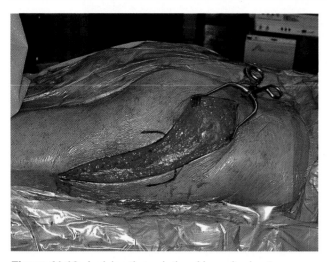

Figure 41.16. Incision through the skin and subcutaneous tissue onto the iliotibial tract and the deep fascia overlying the gluteus maximus muscle.

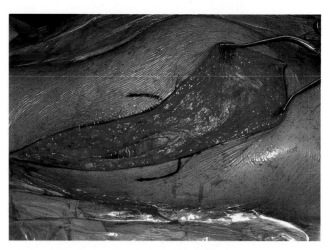

Figure 41.17. The iliotibial tract is incised, showing the underlying trochanteric bursa, and at the superiormost aspect of the fascial incision, a few muscle fibers of insertion of the gluteus maximus.

tendon of this muscle and the posterolateral surface of the greater trochanter) is incised, allowing clear visualization of the insertion area of the gluteus maximus muscle and access to the undersurface of this muscle (Figs. 41.18 and 41.19). Beginning the deep dissection in this way, at the distal branch of the Kocher-Langenbeck incision, the surgeon facilitates the next step: splitting of the gluteus maximus muscle.

The gluteus maximus muscle receives its blood supply from two major vessels: the superior gluteal artery supplying the upper one third of the muscle and the inferior gluteal artery supplying the lower two thirds. Although within the substance of the muscle multiple anastomotic connections are extant between these two arteries, the upper one-third/lower two-thirds division in the muscle is a relatively avascular interval and is the desired plane of dissection. This interval can often be identified by digital palpation of the undersurface of the gluteus maximus. In addition, inspection of the superficial surface of the muscle frequently reveals a line of fat marking the interval (Fig. 41.20). This intervascular interval may not correspond exactly with the line of the skin incision that is directed toward the posterior–superior iliac spine. Often it is oriented in a more lateral direction (as in Fig. 41.20), but it is well within the limits of the wound (see Fig. 41.20). Once the intervascular interval is identified, incision in the gluteal fascia and blunt dissection, splitting the gluteus maximus muscle fibers, can begin. Despite possessing a dual blood

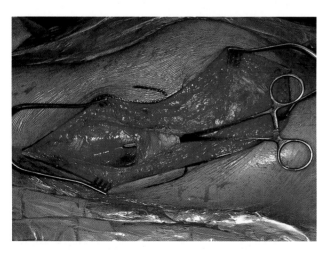

Figure 41.18. Trochanteric bursa is isolated before its incision.

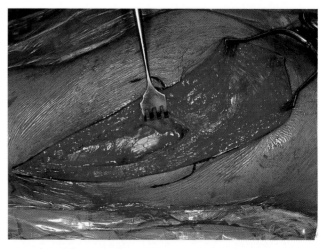

Figure 41.19. View after incision of the trochanteric bursa.

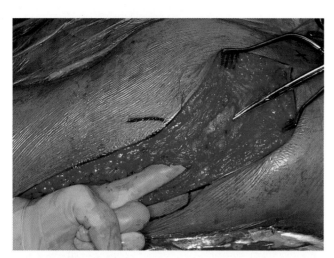

Figure 41.20. Palpation of the undersurface of the gluteus maximus muscle after incision through the trochanteric bursa. A fat line is noted at the tip of the scissors. The line of the scissors marks the upper one-third/lower two-thirds division in the gluteus maximus muscle.

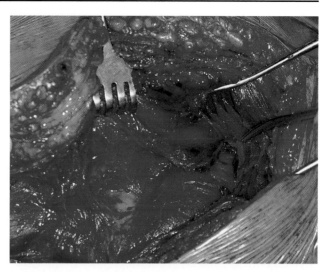

Figure 41.21. Gluteus-maximus muscle fibers are split to the first nerve branch. A self-retaining retractor holds the gluteus-maximus muscle fibers apart. The nerve (located at the tip of the scissors) is crossing the split in the gluteus-maximus muscle fibers from posterior to anterior in the surgical field.

supply and potential for an intervascular plane of dissection, the gluteus maximus muscle has innervation only from the inferior gluteal nerve. There is no internervous plane, and the nerve branches of the upper one third of the muscle cross the intended interval of dissection a little more than halfway between the level of the greater trochanter and the posterior–superior iliac spine. Therefore, splitting of the muscle fibers should stop as soon as the first nerve branch to the upper part of the muscle is encountered (Fig. 41.21).

The deep muscles are now exposed. However, an additional subgluteal bursa often must be cleared to allow visualization of the tendon of the deep, lower portion of the gluteus maximus muscle that inserts into the gluteal tuberosity of the femur (Figs. 41.22 and 41.23). Release of this gluteus maximus insertion into the femur allows adequate posteromedial retraction of the large mass of the gluteus maximus muscle without undue stretch on the inferior gluteal nerve. The tendon is released, with care taken not to injure branches of the first perforating branch of the profunda femoris artery, which run in close proximity (Fig. 41.24).

The next step is to locate the sciatic nerve. The safest way to locate the nerve is along the posterior surface of the quadratus femoris muscle. Variations in the musculature of the

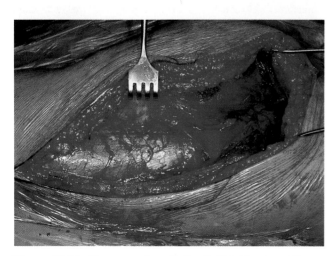

Figure 41.22. Exposure deep to the iliotibial tract and the gluteus maximus muscle. The rake retraction places tension on the gluteus maximus tendon of insertion into the femur, which is partially obscured by a subgluteal bursa.

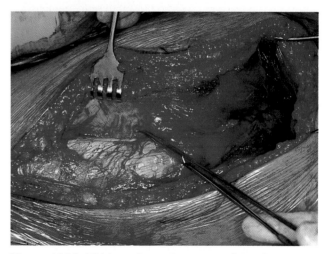

Figure 41.23. Thickened superior aspect of the gluteus maximus tendon is visualized after removal of the bursa and is isolated with a right-angle clamp.

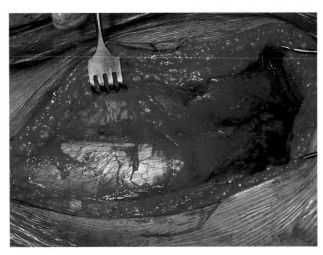

Figure 41.24. Gluteus maximus tendon has been released.

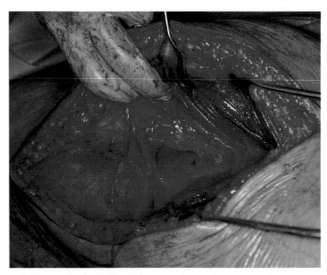

Figure 41.25. Delineation of the tissue just superior to the released gluteus maximus tendon that obscures the posterior surface of the quadratus femoris muscle. This tissue runs from posterior to anterior, covering the sciatic nerve.

buttock are fairly common (3). However, important variations in the quadratus femoris anatomy are virtually nonexistent. Furthermore, posterior injuries that may disrupt the short external-rotator anatomy generally leave the quadratus femoris muscle unscathed. Therefore, the relation between the sciatic nerve and the quadratus femoris muscle serves as a constant reference point. The posterior surface of this muscle is usually obscured by residual bursal and areolar tissue (Figs. 41.24 and 41.25). This tissue must be incised to expose the nerve (Fig. 41.26). Dissection of these tissues may be accomplished through the use of either scissors or blunt dissection. Once the nerve is visualized, it should be explored through its course to the greater sciatic notch (Fig. 41.27). Any impinging bone fragments should be removed, and any anatomic variations in the nerve noted. Direct manipulation of the nerve should be avoided.

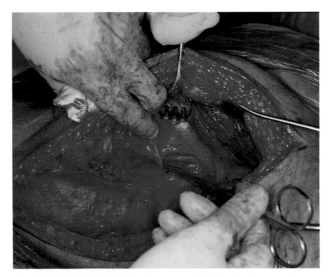

Figure 41.26. Tissue has been partially incised, revealing the sciatic nerve deep to it. The tip of the scissors points to the remaining tissue over the quadratus femoris muscle.

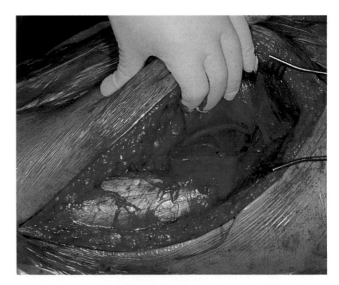

Figure 41.27. Tissue has been completely incised, and the course of the sciatic nerve can be seen. The sciatic nerve runs superficial to the obturator internus tendon and gemelli muscle bellies and then dives deep to the piriformis muscle toward the greater sciatic notch.

The dissection continues with the location of the tendons of the short external rotators of the hip. First, the piriformis tendon is identified. It can be found running alongside the gluteus minimus muscle just under the cover of the inferior aspect of the gluteus medius muscle as it inserts into the greater trochanter (Figs. 41.28 and 41.29). If one is not careful, it is possible to mistake the posterior aspect of the gluteus medius muscle and its tendon for the piriformis (Fig. 41.30) (4). Adding to the potential for confusion is the variability in the relation between the sciatic nerve and the piriformis muscle. Typically (about 84% of the time), the sciatic nerve runs deep to the piriformis muscle, appearing in the buttock at the inferior border of this muscle (see Fig. 41.27) (3). Three variations of this "normal" anatomy have been reported, and others probably exist (3). The most common variation (12%) is for one part of the nerve (the peroneal division) to pass through the muscle and the other part (the tibial division) to appear below the muscle. The entire nerve also may pass through the muscle (1%). These two variations result in a split piriformis muscle with two tendons of insertion. The third variation is passage of the peroneal division above the piriformis and the tibial division below it (3%). With enough operative cases, one will eventually encounter one of these anatomic anomalies (Fig. 41.31). Knowledge of the anatomic variability of this area and the prior identification of the sciatic nerve on the posterior surface of the quadratus femoris muscle will prevent intraoperative confusion and decrease the risk of iatrogenic sciatic nerve injury. After its identification, the piriformis tendon is isolated, tagged with a suture, and released from its insertion (Fig. 41.32). The anastomotic branch of the inferior gluteal artery (which participates in the cruciate anastomosis of the thigh) runs in proximity to the piriformis muscle almost in parallel with the piriformis tendon (5). Failure to locate this artery may result in its unintentional laceration, followed by troublesome intraoperative bleeding. This vessel does not provide an important blood supply. Formal ligation is the easiest and best course of action.

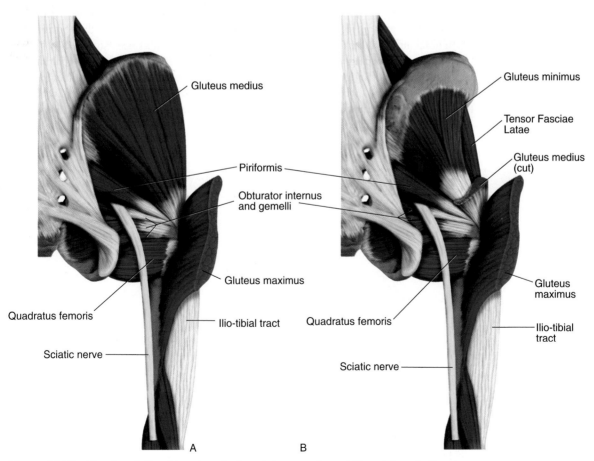

Figure 41.28. Muscle relationships deep to the gluteus maximus **(A)** and deep to the gluteus medius muscle **(B)**.

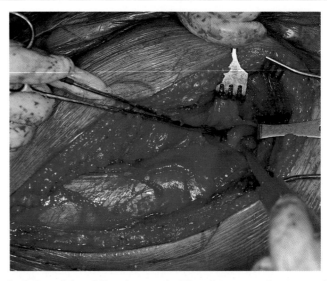

Figure 41.29. Isolation of the piriformis muscle. The gluteus maximus muscle (split) is held by the self-retaining retractor. The posterior margin of the gluteus medius muscle is reflected anterosuperiorly by an Army-Navy retractor to reveal the piriformis tendon, which is held by a right-angle clamp. The tip of the intraoperative suction points to the gluteus minimus muscle.

The obturator internus tendon, with the superior and inferior gemelli muscles on either side, can be found just inferior and slightly deep to the piriformis (see Fig. 41.28). The gemelli muscles insert onto the tendon of the obturator internus, and the bellies of these two muscles may obscure this tendon (Fig. 41.33). If this situation occurs, the tendon can be identified by palpation, with either a right-angle clamp or a finger placed deep to the tendon. External rotation of the hip will relax the tendon, allowing easier access to its deep surface. Internal rotation of the hip, placing the tendon under tension, will verify its position. In an alternative approach, the overlying gemelli muscles can be teased away to reveal the obturator internus tendon (Fig. 41.34). Once located, the obturator internus tendon is isolated, tagged with a suture, and released from its insertion. To avoid injury to the blood supply of the femoral head, both the piriformis and obturator internus tendons should be incised approximately 1.5 cm

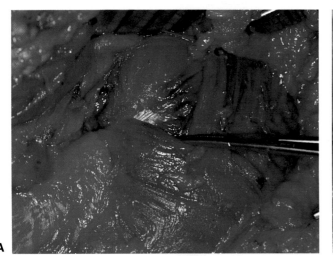

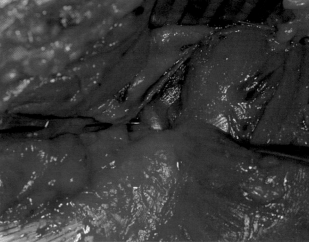

A   B

Figure 41.30. Illustration from a patient different than that shown in Figure 41.9, showing a variation of the gluteus medius muscle in which a deep fold creates an apparently separate posterior portion of the muscle and tendon of insertion. A clamp reflects the more superficial portion of the muscle, revealing a tendon that may be mistaken for the piriformis **(A).** The actual piriformis tendon has a different orientation and configuration **(B).**

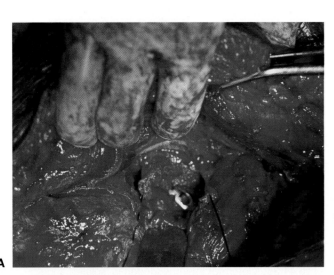

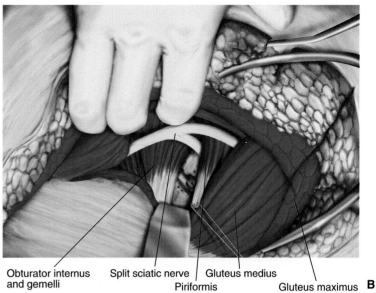

A

B

Obturator internus   Split sciatic nerve │ Gluteus medius
and gemelli   Piriformis   Gluteus maximus

Figure 41.31. Intraoperative photograph **(A)** and companion drawing **(B)** showing a split sciatic nerve with the peroneal division above the piriformis muscle and the tibial division below the piriformis muscle.

from their insertion points into the greater trochanter (Fig. 41.35). A fascial layer running from the undersurface of the gluteus maximus muscle to the posterior column of the acetabulum separates the piriformis muscle from the obturator internus and gemelli muscles. This fascia is easily visualized after the release of the piriformis and obturator internus tendons (Fig. 41.36). The sciatic nerve lies directly adjacent to the medial origin of this fascia (see Fig. 41.36). Care must be taken not to injure the sciatic nerve when this fascia is released during the clearing of the soft tissues from the posterior column (Fig. 41.37).

The obturator internus muscle arises from within the true pelvis from the internal circumference of the obturator foramen and the obturator membrane (5). The muscle fibers end in four or five tendinous bands that converge and pass through the lesser sciatic notch.

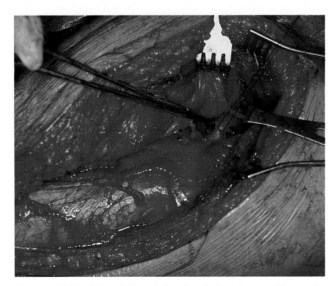

Figure 41.32. The piriformis tendon is isolated and tagged with a suture.

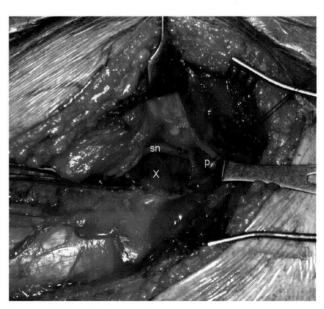

Figure 41.33. Obturator internus tendon, obscured by the muscle bellies of the gemelli (*X*), is isolated with a right-angle clamp. The sciatic nerve (*sn*) and piriformis tendon (*p*) can be seen.

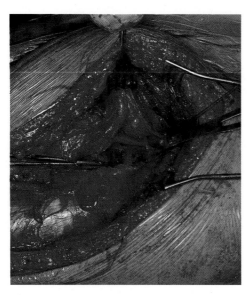

Figure 41.34. Muscle bellies of the gemelli have been dissected to reveal the obturator internus tendon.

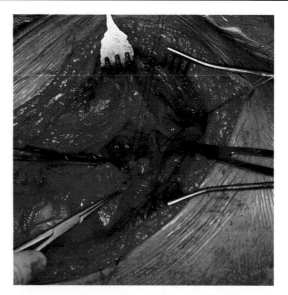

Figure 41.35. Obturator internus tendon is isolated and tagged with a suture. The stump of the previously released piriformis tendon can be seen just cephalad to the obturator internus tendon as it inserts into the greater trochanter.

These bands turn a right angle around the grooved external surface of the lesser sciatic notch, joining to form the single tendon of insertion. The bony surface is covered by cartilage and is separated from the tendon by a bursa. Once the obturator internus tendon is released from its insertion into the greater trochanter, it is elevated away from the hip capsule (along with the gemelli muscles) and followed medially toward the lesser sciatic notch. The underlying bursa is opened, permitting access to (and palpation through) the lesser sciatic notch (Fig. 41.38). A specially designed sciatic nerve retractor can now be placed with its tip anchored in the lesser sciatic notch (Fig. 41.39). Use of this instrument facilitates the bony exposure by permitting controlled retraction of the sciatic nerve and the posterior soft

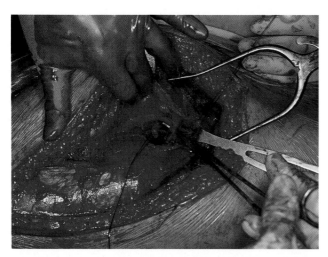

Figure 41.36. Delineation of the fascia separating the piriformis muscle from the superior gemellus muscle/obturator internus tendon/inferior gemellus muscle group. A right-angle clamp clearly shows the medial margin of this fascia and its proximity to the sciatic nerve. The sciatic nerve can be seen running superficial to the obturator internus tendon and gemelli muscles and then coursing deep to the piriformis muscle.

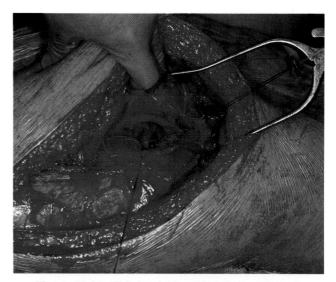

Figure 41.37. This fascial band has been released.

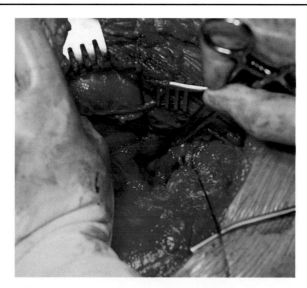

Figure 41.38. Obturator internus tendon has been elevated, allowing access to the lesser sciatic notch. In this photograph, the hemostat is directed toward, and its tip inserted into, the lesser sciatic notch.

tissues. The retractor is positioned such that at the level of the lesser sciatic notch, the obturator internus tendons and gemelli muscles lie between the retractor and the sciatic nerve, cushioning the nerve. However, the surgeon must realize that the sciatic nerve retractor extends beyond the limits of this muscle cushion and directly contacts the nerve at the superior and inferior aspects of the retractor (Fig. 41.40). The relation between the sciatic nerve and the sciatic nerve retractor must be such that the edges of the retractor do not impinge or place undue pressure on the nerve. The surgical assistant in charge of maintaining position of the retractor must be cognizant of the importance of this task. The position of the retractor should be checked frequently during the operative procedure.

Once the sciatic nerve retractor has been appropriately positioned, the posterior hip capsule and retroacetabular surface of the posterior column are explored and cleared of debris. The dissection is carried from lateral to medial, progressing from the fracture site superiorly toward the greater sciatic notch and inferiorly toward the ischial tuberosity. Superiorly, the hip abductors are elevated from the external surface of the ilium and held with a curved retractor (Fig. 41.41).

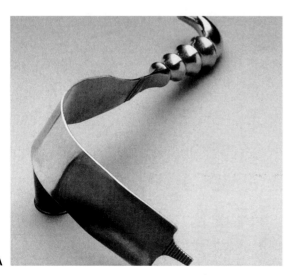

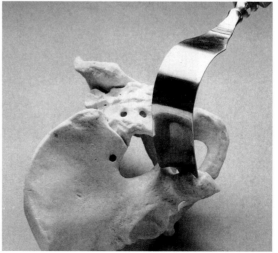

A   B

Figure 41.39. Sciatic nerve retractor **(A)** and its desired position in the lesser sciatic notch, as demonstrated in a bone model **(B)**.

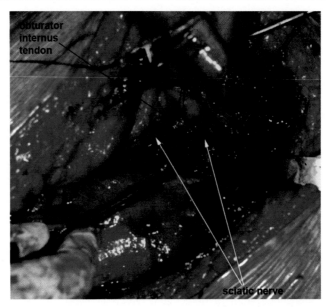

Figure 41.40. Sciatic nerve is unprotected both below and above (arrows and as marked by the tip of a hemostat) the obturator internus tendon and gemelli muscles.

As the dissection approaches the greater notch, care must be taken to prevent injury not only to the sciatic nerve that is unprotected at this level, but also to the superior-gluteal neurovascular bundle. The superior-gluteal neurovascular bundle exits the greater sciatic notch above the piriformis muscle, superior to the level of the sciatic nerve. Its position can often be assessed by palpation of the superior-gluteal arterial pulse at the level of the greater sciatic notch. The superior-gluteal neurovascular bundle tethers the abductor muscle mass. It can be injured not only by direct laceration but also by traction from excessive retraction of the abductor muscle mass. Inferiorly, the tendon of the obturator externus muscle may be encountered (Fig. 41.42). Release of this tendon usually is not necessary.

In cases with fractures involving the ischial tuberosity or others requiring increased access to this area, more extensive exposure may be obtained through the release of the quadratus femoris muscle, and infrequently, the obturator externus tendon. The quadratus femoris muscle is extremely vascular. It should be released at its origin from the ischial

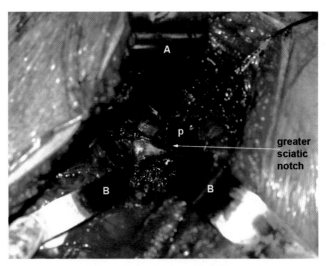

Figure 41.41. Sciatic nerve retractor **(A)** is placed in the lesser sciatic notch. Just superior to this retractor, the greater sciatic notch (*arrow*) and the overlying piriformis muscle (*p*) can be seen. Two curved retractors **(B)** reflect the hip abductors. The external surface of the posterior column, with its overlying soft-tissue debris, is well visualized.

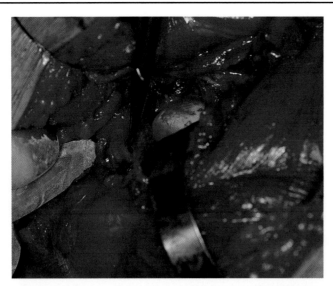

Figure 41.42. Obturator externus tendon is identified with a right-angle clamp. For orientation, sutures mark the released piriformis and obturator internus tendons, the curved retractor reflects the hip abductors, and the incised hip capsule reveals the femoral head. The surgeon's middle finger rests on the quadratus femoris muscle just inferior to the obturator externus tendon as it heads toward the greater trochanter. The posterior column and hip joint can be well visualized without release of this tendon.

tuberosity to avoid excessive bleeding and damage to the branches of the medial circumflex artery. Release of the obturator externus tendon in a manner similar to that described for the piriformis and obturator internus tendons is not required for fracture treatment. Furthermore, this release is ill advised due to the obturator externus tendon's close proximity to the blood supply of the femoral head.

The extent of the fracture pattern dictates the extent of the surgical approach. For fractures limited to the posterior wall that do not require access to the true pelvis, the dissection is basically complete, as described up to this point. Otherwise, the dissection must continue through the greater sciatic notch into the true pelvis and onto the quadrilateral surface of the acetabulum. With the careful use of digital dissection and periosteal elevators, the origin of the obturator internus muscle is elevated from the quadrilateral plate. Access is now available for digital assessment of column fracture reduction and for the use of specialized reduction clamps (see Figs. 41.2, 41.3, and 41.12). If necessary, this access can be enlarged by release of the sacrospinous ligament (1).

To visualize the hip joint, a circumferential marginal capsulotomy is performed (Figs. 41.42 and 41.43). However, for fractures involving the posterior wall, capsular attachments to the posterior-wall fracture fragment must be maintained to minimize the risk of posterior wall devascularization. Marginal capsulotomy is performed on either side of the posterior-wall fracture fragment, which is then reflected in continuity with the remainder of the hip-joint capsule. Incision of the labrum is avoided unless needed to assess fracture reduction. Radial capsular incisions also should be avoided to avoid injury to the blood supply to the femoral head.

The intra-articular surface of the hip joint is directly visualized through application of traction to the femur. This can be accomplished easily and in a controlled manner with the use of the fracture table (Figs. 41.44 and 41.45). Other methods include use of the femoral distractor (Synthes, Paoli, PA), manual distraction by a surgical assistant using a traction pin in the distal femur or a Schanz screw in the greater trochanter, or just pulling directly on the leg. Visualization of different aspects of the acetabular joint surface is often improved by movement of the hip from the neutral position. Hip flexion facilitates access to the acetabular fossa and the anteroinferior joint surface. This is helpful for the removal of loose bodies but places increased stretch on the sciatic nerve.

Greater trochanteric osteotomy in an attempt to extend the access of the Kocher-Langenbeck approach farther along the external surface of the anterior column is rarely

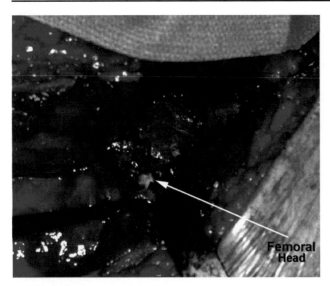

Figure 41.43. Hip capsule has been incised in a marginal, circumferential manner to reveal the femoral head (arrow) and the hip joint. Fracture of the posterior column with a displaced, intra-articular, free fragment is visualized.

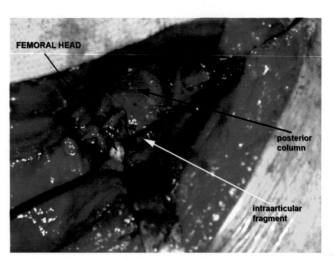

Figure 41.44. With a fracture table, the hip has been distracted to improve visualization and to unload the hip joint for the facilitation of fracture reduction. Arrows identify the femoral head, posterior column, and the displaced, intra-articular, fracture fragment.

required or indicated. The hip abductors remain tethered by the superior-gluteal neurovascular bundle, limiting the effectiveness of this method in gaining significant added exposure. Placing the hip in an abducted position, especially with the patient prone, approximates the exposure gained by trochanteric osteotomy. If sufficient anterosuperior exposure cannot be obtained by this maneuver, gluteus medius tenotomy or trochanteric osteotomy are available options. The need for adjunctive tenotomy or greater trochanteric osteotomy usually means that an alternative to the Kocher-Langenbeck approach should have been initially selected.

The closure of the Kocher-Langenbeck incision is straightforward. Released tendons of insertion of the gluteus maximus and short external-rotator muscles are reattached through use of nonabsorbable suture. After the placement of deep, closed suction drains, the fascia lata, gluteal fascia, subcutaneous tissues, and skin are closed in layers.

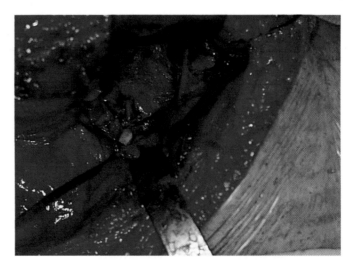

Figure 41.45. Intra-articular, osteochondral, fracture fragment is reduced.

POSTOPERATIVE MANAGEMENT

Postoperatively, the patient is mobilized as quickly as the associated injuries will allow. Out of bed on the first postoperative day, the patient subsequently begins formal physical therapy for muscle strengthening and active range-of-motion exercises. Total hip arthroplasty precautions are not needed, as internal fixation has (or should have) rendered the hip joint completely stable. Partial, toe-touch weight bearing with crutches or a walker is required for 10 to 12 weeks. However, progression to full weight bearing must be individualized. Physical therapy should continue until muscle strength and range of motion are regained or a plateau is reached. Multiple elements must be factored into the recovery equation including the magnitude of the soft-tissue injury, the fracture type, any associated injuries, and preexisting medical status. Therefore the expected recovery time is quite variable, ranging from approximately 6 to 12 months for return to a fully ambulatory status.

COMPLICATIONS

Perioperative complications of acetabular fracture surgery may occur as a direct result of the surgical approach selected for fracture fixation, or they may be related to the magnitude of the patient's overall injury pattern. Major complications associated with the Kocher-Langenbeck approach include sciatic nerve injury, infection, severe bleeding, and heterotopic bone formation. Thromboembolic disease (deep vein thrombosis [DVT]/pulmonary embolism [PE]) is a serious problem associated with the trauma of acetabular fracture as well as the subsequent surgery for fracture fixation.

The overall reported incidence of posttraumatic, iatrogenic, sciatic-nerve palsy ranges from 2% to 16% (6). Letournel (1) reported nerve palsy incidences at 10% via the Kocher-Langenbeck approach. However, he noted that one fourth of these patients had not had complete documentation of their preoperative status, leaving the actual cause of nerve injury in doubt. Whatever the actual number, risk of sciatic nerve injury is substantial with the use of the Kocher-Langenbeck approach. Intraoperative somatosensory evoked potential (SSEP) monitoring has been advocated as a method for decreasing this risk (6). Although the results of using SSEP monitoring appear promising, its actual value awaits a randomized prospective trial (7). Management of sciatic nerve injury consists of observation and the use of an ankle-foot orthosis. The prognosis for recovery of the tibial division is good despite severe initial damage. Recovery of the peroneal division is more dependent on the severity of the initial injury.

Deep infection after fracture fixation by using the Koche-Langenbeck approach has been reported in 1.5% of patients (1). Perioperative antibiotics and meticulous surgical technique are preventive measures. Once diagnosed, infection requires urgent surgical debridement. Secure internal fixation should be maintained until the fracture has united (8).

Bleeding from injury to the superior gluteal artery is a well-described complication of the Kocher-Langenbeck approach, with an incidence as high as 5% (9). Exposure and ligation of the vessel may be required but is associated with iatrogenic injury to the superior gluteal nerve. The application of topical thrombogenic agents and extended direct pressure with packing are often effective in obtaining hemostasis. Continued excessive bleeding from retraction of the artery into the pelvis, requiring retroperitoneal exposure for vessel control, is extremely rare.

Heterotopic ossification (HO) has been called the most widespread complication of acetabular fracture surgery. However, HO after the Kocher-Langenbeck approach, resulting in significant loss of hip motion, probably occurs in fewer than 10% of patients (1,10,11). Options for treatment include the use of perioperative prophylactic agents or delayed excision after the maturation of functionally significant HO or both (10). In nonrandomized retrospective studies, both indomethacin and irradiation have been shown to be effective for prophylaxis. The combination of indomethacin and irradiation appears to be extremely effective (11). The advisability of using irradiation in a young fracture-patient population to suppress HO in less than 10% is subject to debate.

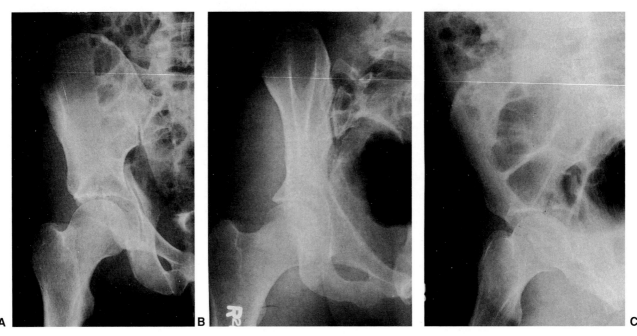

Figure 41.46. A–C. AP and 45-degree oblique x-rays. These x-rays and the figures that follow are from the same patient whose surgery supplied the foregoing intraoperative photographs used to demonstrate the Kocher-Langenbeck approach.

DVT and resultant PE are potential life-threatening complications of acetabular fracture surgery. The risk of DVT is high (34% in one series) (12). PE occurs in approximately 2% of cases. Routine perioperative anticoagulant prophylaxis is indicated. Preoperative screening by using duplex Doppler ultrasonography or magnetic resonance venography provides early diagnosis and allows identification of candidates for inferior venal-caval filter placement (12).

ILLUSTRATIVE CASE FOR TECHNIQUE

A 23-year-old man was involved in a motor-vehicle accident, sustaining an atypical T-shaped fracture of the acetabulum with intra-articular comminution (Figs. 41.46 to 41.48). ORIF was advised because of the instability and incongruency of the hip joint. Surgery was performed 4 days after injury by using the Kocher-Langenbeck approach (Figs. 41.49 to 41.52). One week later, the patient was discharged to home from the hospital with instruction to proceed with toe-touch weight bearing with crutches.

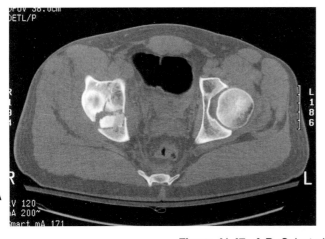
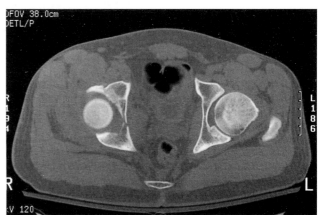

Figure 41.47. A,B. Selected preoperative two-dimensional CT sections through the dome and columns of the acetabulum.

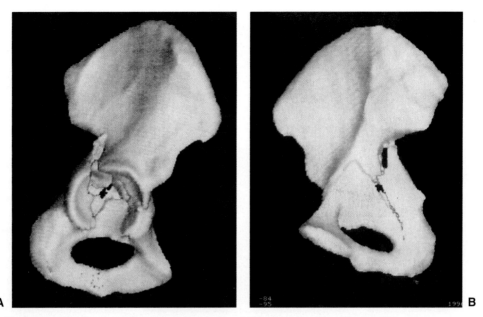

Figure 41.48. Preoperative three-dimensional CT, showing the external **(A)** and endopelvic **(B)** aspects. An atypical T-shaped pattern with intra-articular comminution is demonstrated.

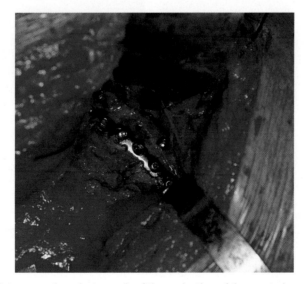

Figure 41.49. Intraoperative photograph of the reduction of the posterior column (previously seen unreduced in Figs. 41.43–41.45) and the fixation construct used.

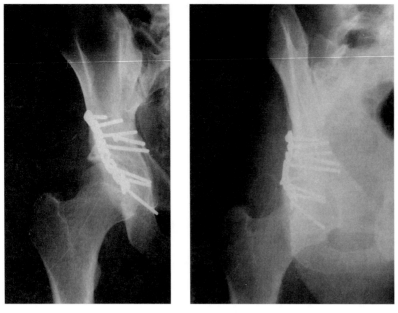
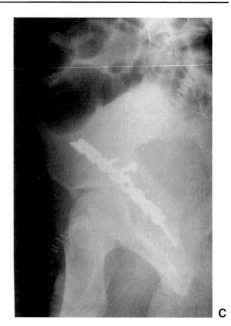
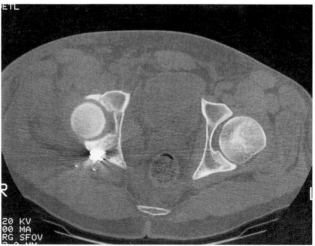

Figure 41.50. A–C. Postoperative x-rays.

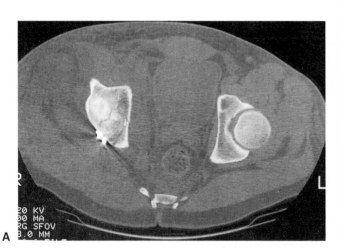

Figure 41.51. A,B. Postoperative two-dimensional CT sections corresponding to the levels of the preoperative samples shown in Figure 41.47.

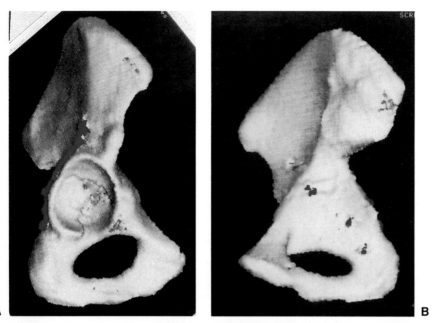

A **B**

Figure 41.52. A,B. Postoperative three-dimensional CT with fixation highlighted in red.

RECOMMENDED READINGS

1. Letournel E, Judet R. *Fractures of the acetabulum*. 2nd ed. Berlin: Springer-Verlag; 1993.
2. Tile M. *Fractures of the pelvis and acetabulum*. 2nd ed. Baltimore: Williams & Wilkins; 1995.
3. Hollinshead WH. *Anatomy for surgeons, volume 3: the back and limbs*. 3rd ed. Philadelphia: Harper & Row; 1982.
4. Henry AK. *Extensile exposure*. 2nd ed. Edinburgh: Churchill Livingstone; 1973.
5. Gray G. *Anatomy of the human body*. 28th ed. Philadelphia: Lea & Febiger; 1970.
6. Helfet DL, Schmeling GJ. Somatosensory evoked potential monitoring in the surgical treatment of acute, displaced acetabular fractures: results of a prospective study. *Clin Orthop* 1994;301:213–220.
7. Baumgaertner MR, Wegner D, Booke J. SSEP monitoring during pelvic and acetabular surgery. *J Orthop Trauma* 1994;8:127–133.
8. Matta JM. Operative treatment of acetabular fractures. In: Chapman MW, Madison M, eds. *Operative orthopaedics*. Vol. 1. Philadelphia: JB Lippincott Co; 1988:329–340.
9. Letournel E, Judet R. *Fractures of the acetabulum*. Berlin: Springer-Verlag; 1981.
10. Moed BR. Complications of acetabular fracture surgery: prevention and management. *Int J Orthop Trauma* 1992;2:68–81.
11. Moed BR, Letournel E. Low-dose irradiation and indomethacin prevent heterotopic ossification after acetabular fracture surgery. *J Bone Joint Surg Br* 1994;76:895–900.
12. Montgomery KD, Geerts WH, Hollis GP, et al. Practical management of venous thromboembolism following pelvic fractures. *Orthop Clin North Am* 1997;28:397–404.

42

Acetabular Fractures: Ilioinguinal Approach

Joel M. Matta and Mark C. Reilly

INDICATIONS/CONTRAINDICATIONS

The ilioinguinal approach was developed by Letournel as an approach to the anterior column of the acetabulum and the inner aspect of the innominate bone. It allows exposure of the entire, internal, iliac fossa and pelvic brim from the anterior aspect of the sacroiliac joint to the pubic symphysis. The quadrilateral surface of the innominate bone and the superior and inferior rami are also accessible. Access to a portion of the external aspect of the ilium also is possible (Fig. 42.1).

The ilioinguinal is the approach of choice for all fractures of the anterior wall and column. The majority of acute, associated, anterior-plus-posterior, hemitransverse fractures may also be managed with the ilioinguinal approach. If the fracture is older than 15 days, the ilioinguinal may still be used unless the posterior component of the fracture is significantly displaced. In this circumstance, an extended iliofemoral approach is more applicable.

The ilioinguinal approach may be used for the majority of associated both-column fractures. The presence of a fracture involving the posterior wall does not necessarily preclude the use of this approach. If the posterior-wall fragment contains a spike of ilium, the reduction may be possible through the exposure of the lateral ilium. The ilioinguinal approach is not recommended for an associated both-column fracture with small or comminuted posterior-wall fragments or those with fracture involvement of the sacroiliac joint.

Certain transverse fractures also may be managed with the ilioinguinal approach. Specifically, fractures with significant displacement at the pelvic brim but slight or no displacement posteriorly may be addressed in this manner. In addition, the ilioinguinal may be used as a subsequent approach when incomplete reduction of the anterior column portion of a T-shaped fracture has been obtained through a prior Kocher-Langenbeck approach (Fig. 42.2).

Access to the bone with the I.I. approach

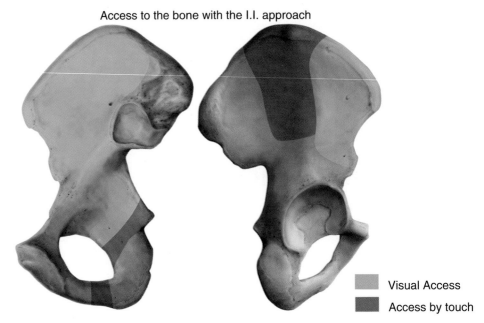

Visual Access

Access by touch

Figure 42.1. Access to the innominate bone with the ilioinguinal approach. (Redrawn with permission from J. M. Matta, *Surgical Approaches to Fractures of the Acetabulum and Pelvis.* Copyright © J. M. Matta, 1996.)

Fractures - Ilioinguinal Approach

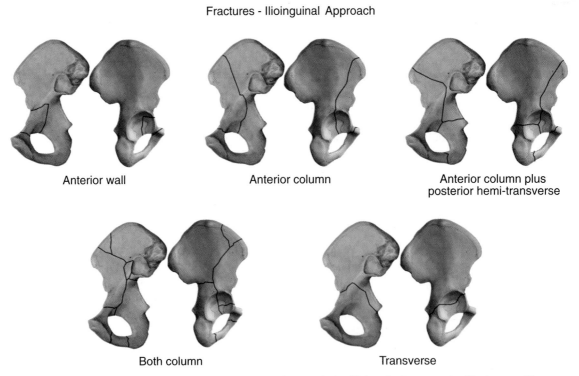

Anterior wall   Anterior column   Anterior column plus
                                                                      posterior hemi-transverse

Both column   Transverse

Figure 42.2. Fractures addressed through the ilioinguinal approach. (Redrawn with permission from J. M. Matta, *Surgical Approaches to Fractures of the Acetabulum and Pelvis.* Copyright © J. M. Matta, 1996.)

PREOPERATIVE PLANNING

Initial radiographic evaluation of a patient with an acetabulum fracture should include an anteroposterior (AP) pelvic radiograph and 45-degree oblique views of the pelvis. Although obtaining these views may be initially uncomfortable for the patient, they are vital to fully understand the fracture pattern. Adequate analgesia should be provided, and the physician may need to be on-site to ensure proper positioning. These films should be obtained in the radiology department rather than as portable radiographs and with the patient out of traction. A careful evaluation of the radiographs allows the fracture to be classified properly by determination of the exact fracture pattern.

Computed tomography (CT) may add important additional information regarding the fracture configuration and presence of incarcerated or impacted fragments within the acetabulum. Three-dimensional CT reconstructions also can assist in providing a better understanding of complicated fracture patterns. Drawing the fracture on a dry bone or pelvic model (or drawing the innominate bone) helps ensure that the surgeon understands the fracture configuration before embarking on surgical intervention.

The ilioinguinal approach proceeds through anatomic areas infrequently used by most orthopedic surgeons. In addition, reduction of the fracture and proper placement of fixation require a thorough understanding of the fracture pattern and the normal acetabular anatomy. Before undertaking the approach, the surgeon is strongly advised to practice on a cadaver and to assist a surgeon who is familiar with the exposure, reduction, and fixation of these difficult injuries.

SURGERY

Technique of Approach

The surgery is performed under general anesthesia with the patient positioned supine on the Judet–Tasserit fracture table (Fig. 42.3). The affected leg is positioned with the hip slightly flexed to relax the iliopsoas muscle, femoral nerve, and external iliac vessels. If required during the surgery, a lateral traction device may be used through a traction screw placed into the greater trochanter. Before surgery, a Foley catheter is introduced into the bladder.

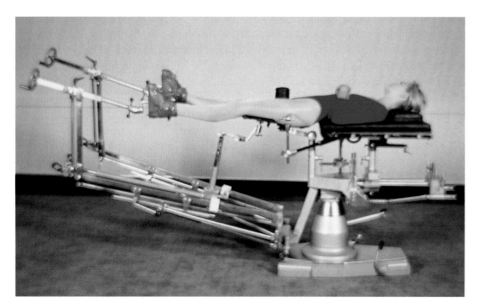

Figure 42.3. Patient positioned on the Judet–Tasserit fracture table. The hip is flexed to relax the iliopsoas and external iliac vessels. The lateral traction device is demonstrated. (Redrawn with permission from J. M. Matta, *Surgical Approaches to Fractures of the Acetabulum and Pelvis.* Copyright © J. M. Matta, 1996.)

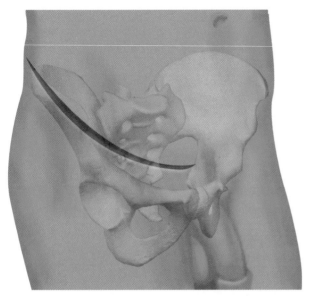

Figure 42.4. Skin incision for the ilioinguinal approach. The incision begins 3 to 4 cm above the symphysis pubis and must extend beyond the most convex portion of the ilium. (Redrawn with permission from J. M. Matta, *Surgical Approaches to Fractures of the Acetabulum and Pelvis.* Copyright © J. M. Matta, 1996.)

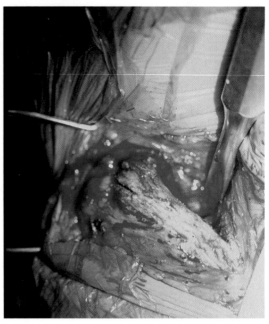

Figure 42.5. Release of the insertion of the abdominal muscles and subperiosteal dissection of the internal iliac fossa.

The incision begins at the midline, 3 to 4 cm proximal to the symphysis pubis. It proceeds laterally to the anterior, superior, iliac spine and then along the anterior two thirds of the iliac crest. The incision must extend beyond the most convex portion of the ilium (Fig. 42.4). The periosteum is incised along the iliac crest, and the attachment of the abdominal muscles and the origin of the iliacus are released. By subperiosteal dissection, the iliacus is elevated from the internal iliac fossa as far posterior as the sacroiliac joint and medially to the pelvic brim (Fig. 42.5). The internal iliac fossa is then packed for hemostasis. Through the lower portion of the incision, the aponeurosis of the external oblique muscle and the external rectus abdominis fascia are exposed. These structures are sharply incised in line with the cutaneous incision at least 1 cm proximal to the external inguinal ring. The aponeurosis of the external oblique muscle is then reflected distally. This unroofs the inguinal canal and exposes the inguinal ligament. The spermatic cord or round ligament is visualized at the medial aspect of the incision. A Penrose drain is then placed around the spermatic cord or round ligament and the adjacent ilioinguinal nerve. It may be used to facilitate retraction during the procedure (Fig. 42.6).

The inguinal ligament is sharply incised so that a 1- to 2-mm cuff of the ligament remains with the common origin of the internal oblique and transversus abdominis muscles and the transversalis fascia (Fig. 42.7). Great care must be taken to avoid injuring the underlying neurovascular structures. Immediately beneath the inguinal ligament, the lateral femoral-cutaneous nerve exits into the thigh. This nerve may be found adjacent to or up to 3 cm medial to the anterior, superior, iliac spine. It must be identified and protected throughout the operation. Directly beneath the midportion of the incision lie the external iliac vessels (Fig. 42.8). Medial to these vessels, the insertion of the conjoined tendon onto the pubis is incised. It may be necessary to incise a portion of the rectus abdominis tendon as well; it is incised just above its insertion onto the pubis. The retropubic space of Retzius is now accessible and is packed with moist sponges after evacuation of the fracture hematoma.

At this point, the anterior aspects of the femoral vessels and the surrounding lymphatics are exposed in the midportion of the incision within the lacuna vasorum. The more laterally situated lacuna musculorum contains the iliopsoas, the femoral nerve, and the lateral

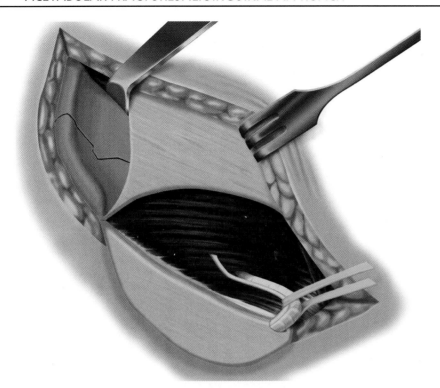

Figure 42.6. Inguinal canal has been unroofed, and the external oblique aponeurosis is reflected inferiorly. The ilioinguinal nerve and the spermatic cord are protected by a Penrose drain. The inguinal ligament is identified. (Redrawn with permission from J. M. Matta, *Surgical Approaches to Fractures of the Acetabulum and Pelvis.* Copyright © J. M. Matta, 1996.)

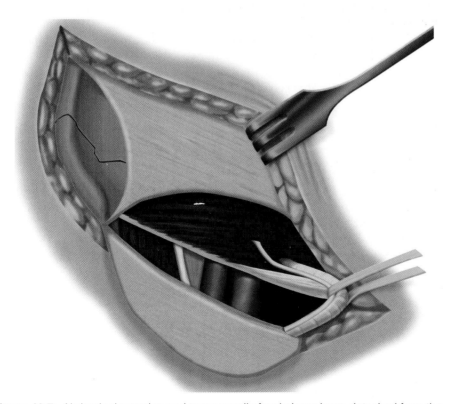

Figure 42.7. Abdominal muscles and transversalis fascia have been detached from the inguinal ligament. A 1-mm cuff of ligament remains for closure. (Redrawn with permission from J. M. Matta, *Surgical Approaches to Fractures of the Acetabulum and Pelvis.* Copyright © J. M. Matta, 1996.)

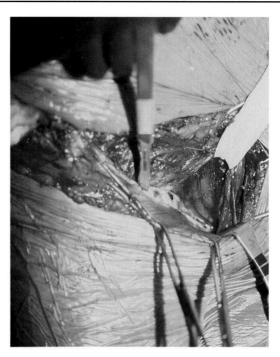

Figure 42.8. Directly beneath the inguinal ligament lie the external iliac vessels. Note how superficial the external iliac artery and vein may lie beneath the ligament.

femoral cutaneous nerve. The iliopsoas sheath, or iliopectineal fascia, separates the two lacunae (Fig. 42.9). The vessels and lymphatics are carefully dissected away and retracted from the medial aspect of the fascia, and the iliopsoas muscle and femoral nerve are retracted from the lateral aspect (Figs. 42.10 and 42.11). The iliopectineal fascia is sharply incised to the pectineal eminence (Fig. 42.12). The pulse of the external iliac artery should be palpated before this step to ensure that the vascular bundle is protected from injury. The iliopectineal fascia is sharply detached from the pelvic brim (Fig. 42.13). In certain individuals, this occasionally may be performed with finger dissection. Detaching the iliopsoas fascia allows access to the true pelvis and subsequently the quadrilateral surface and the posterior column. A second Penrose drain is placed around the iliopsoas; femoral nerve;

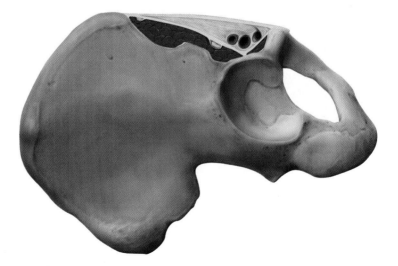

Figure 42.9. In this oblique section at the level of the inguinal ligament, the iliopectineal fascia separates the lacuna musculorum and the lacuna vasorum. (Redrawn with permission from J. M. Matta, *Surgical Approaches to Fractures of the Acetabulum and Pelvis.* Copyright © J. M. Matta, 1996.)

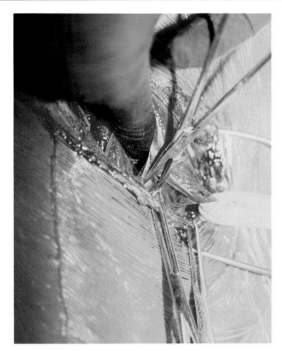

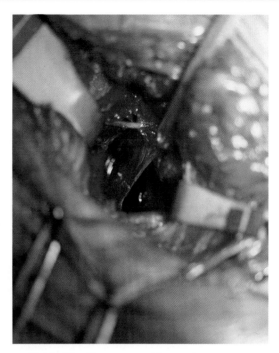

Figure 42.10. External iliac vessels and lymphatics are dissected away from the medial aspect of the iliopectineal fascia. The iliopsoas and femoral nerve have already been dissected away from the lateral aspect of the fascia and are retracted by the surgeon's finger.

Figure 42.11. The iliopsoas and femoral nerve are retracted laterally, and the external iliac vessels are retracted medially, exposing the iliopectineal fascia.

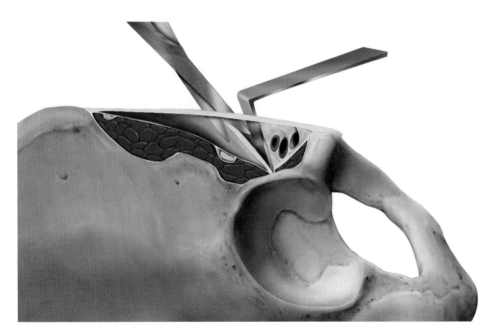

Figure 42.12. This oblique section demonstrates the division of the iliopectineal fascia from the inguinal ligament to the pectineal eminence. (Redrawn with permission from J. M. Matta, *Surgical Approaches to Fractures of the Acetabulum and Pelvis.* Copyright © J. M. Matta, 1996.)

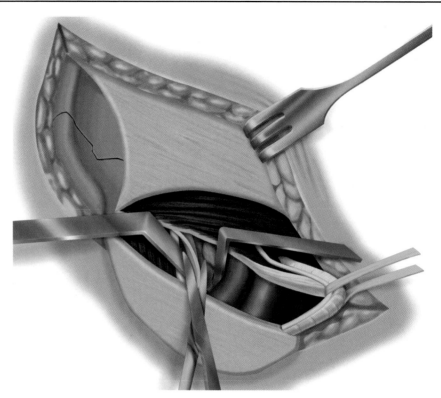

Figure 42.13. Iliopectineal fascia is dissected free from its attachment to the pelvic brim. (Redrawn with permission from J. M. Matta, *Surgical Approaches to Fractures of the Acetabulum and Pelvis.* Copyright © J. M. Matta, 1996.)

and lateral, femoral, cutaneous nerve for retraction purposes. A third Penrose is placed around the femoral vessels and lymphatics. Care should be taken to leave undisturbed the fatty areolar tissue surrounding the vessels, as this contains the lymphatic vessels. Disrupting the lymphatics may result in impaired postoperative lymphatic drainage and edema.

Before retraction of the external iliac vessels, the iliopectineal nerve and artery should be identified posteromedial to the vessels. A search is made for an anomalous origin of the obturator artery from the inferior epigastric artery or the presence of an anastomosis between the obturator and the external iliac vessels. Whereas the presence of a venous anastomosis is relatively common, an arterial anastomosis is rare. If either of these is present, the artery or vein or both should be clamped, ligated, and divided to prevent intraoperative avulsion of the vessel and hemorrhage, which may be difficult to control.

Subperiosteal dissection is used to expose the pelvic brim and superior pubic ramus. The periosteum also may be elevated from the quadrilateral surface. Care should be taken when placing retractors near the greater sciatic notch to avoid injury to the superior gluteal vein or branches of the internal iliac artery. The reduction and fixation of the fracture may now be completed by working back and forth in the three visualization windows.

Medial retraction of the iliopsoas and femoral nerves allows visualization of the entire internal iliac fossa, the sacroiliac joint, and the pelvic brim via the first window (Fig. 42.14). Lateral retraction of the iliopsoas and femoral nerve, combined with medial retraction of the external iliac vessels, opens the second window (Fig. 42.15). This window gives access to the pelvic brim, from the sacroiliac joint to the pectineal eminence, as well as access to the quadrilateral surface for reduction of posterior column fractures. The pulse of the external iliac artery should be frequently checked when working within this window. Medial retraction of the vessels gives access to the superior pubic ramus and the symphysis pubis if required (Fig. 42.16). The spermatic cord or round ligament is retracted medially or laterally as needed.

Limited access to the external aspect of the iliac wing may be obtained by detaching the sartorius and the inguinal ligament from the anterior, superior, iliac spine and elevating the

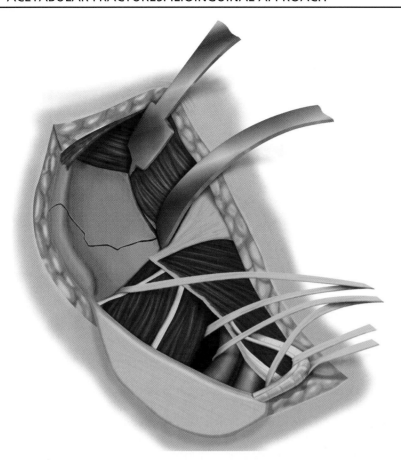

Figure 42.14. First window of the ilioinguinal approach. The internal iliac fossa is visualized. A Hohmann retractor is placed on the anterior sacroiliac joint. (Redrawn with permission from J. M. Matta, *Surgical Approaches to Fractures of the Acetabulum and Pelvis*. Copyright © J. M. Matta, 1996.)

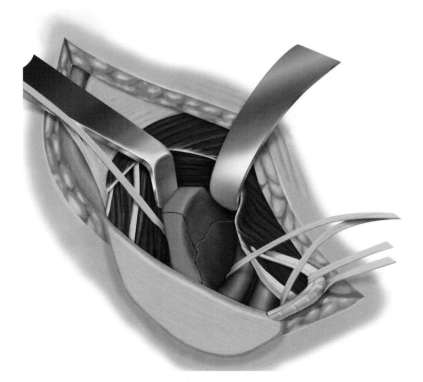

Figure 42.15. Second window of the ilioinguinal approach. The pelvic brim and quadrilateral surface are visualized.

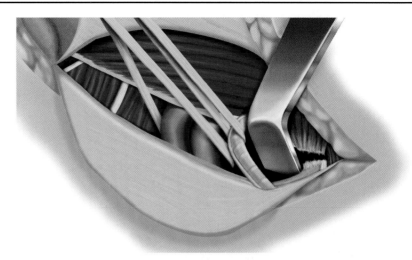

Figure 42.16. Third window of the ilioinguinal approach. The symphysis pubis and retropubic space of Retzius are exposed. The spermatic cord or round ligament may be retracted medially or laterally as needed. (Redrawn with permission from J. M. Matta, *Surgical Approaches to Fractures of the Acetabulum and Pelvis.* Copyright © J. M. Matta, 1996.)

tensor fascia-lata muscle from the ilium. This often facilitates placement of reduction clamps across the anterior innominate bone.

After internal fixation of the fracture, suction drains are placed in the retropubic space of Retzius as well as along the quadrilateral surface and internal iliac fossa. The external aspect of the bone should also be drained if it has been exposed. The abdominal fascia is sewn to the fascia lata with heavy suture. If the sartorius has been detached, it is repaired through a drill hole in the anterior, superior, iliac spine (Fig. 42.17). Muscular relaxation should be used during closure, and continuous traction is required to prevent the abdominal fascia from retracting proximally and posteriorly. If the abdominal muscles are not anatomically repaired, a sound repair of the floor and roof of the inguinal canal is not possible. The tendon of the rectus abdominis is repaired, and the transversalis fascia and the conjoined tendon of the internal oblique and transversus abdominis muscles are reattached to the inguinal ligament (Fig. 42.18). The roof of the inguinal canal is repaired by closure of the aponeurosis of the external oblique (Fig. 42.19). The iliopectineal fascia is not repaired.

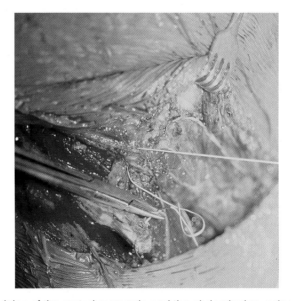

Figure 42.17. Origins of the sartorius muscle and the abdominal muscles are secured through a drill hole in the anterior, superior, iliac spine.

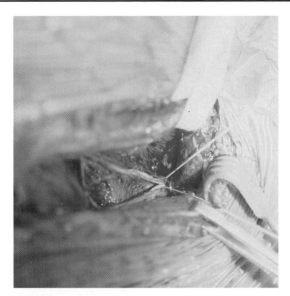

Figure 42.18. Inguinal ligament is repaired. Superior are the transversalis fascia and the conjoined tendon of the internal oblique and transversus abdominis muscles. Inferior is the inguinal ligament.

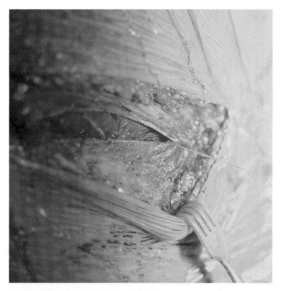

Figure 42.19. Aponeurosis of the external oblique is repaired, closing the roof of the inguinal canal.

Technique of Reduction and Fixation

The first objective in the treatment of an associated both-column injury is anatomically to reduce the fracture of the anterior column. The iliac crest and wing are reduced first. The reduction of fracture lines in the ilium must be perfect if the articular surface is to be reduced. It is important to restore the normal concavity to the internal iliac fossa, which is frequently greater than imagined. Often traction must be applied through the fracture table to allow disimpaction of the iliac wing. Frequently the iliac wing fracture bifurcates to reach the iliac crest at two points, creating a free triangular fragment of the wing (Fig. 42.20). Because it facilitates the accurate reduction of the anterior column, this fracture fragment should be anatomically reduced and fixed first. (Fig. 42.21). At the level of the iliac crest, a 3.5- or 4.5-mm screw may be inserted between the tables of the ilium, which will fix the vertical or triangular fractures (Fig. 42.22). Care must be taken when inserting these screws so reduction is not lost during the

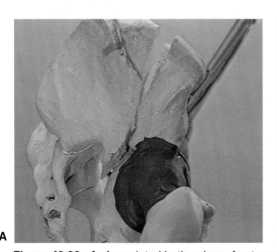

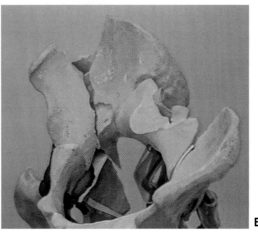

A   B

Figure 42.20. A. Associated both-column fracture of the right acetabulum. View of the lateral aspect of the ilium. **B.** Associated both-column fracture of the right acetabulum. Note the free triangular-fracture fragment at the iliac crest. There is also a free fracture fragment at the pelvic brim. (Reprinted with permission from AO/ASIF, *Both Column Fracture Through the Ilioinguinal Approach* [Video]. Copyright © AO/ASIF Video, 1991.)

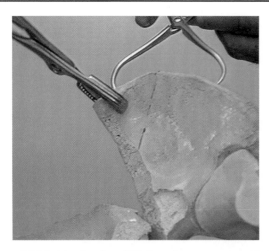

Figure 42.21. Farabeuf and Weber clamps are used in the reduction of the triangular iliac-crest fracture fragment. (Reprinted with permission from AO/ASIF, *Both Column Fracture Through the Ilioinguinal Approach* [Video]. Copyright © AO/ASIF Video, 1991.)

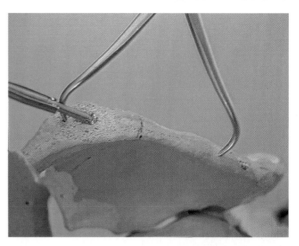

Figure 42.22. Screw is inserted between the tables of the ilium parallel to the iliac crest while the Weber clamp maintains the reduction. (Reprinted with permission from AO/ASIF, *Both Column Fracture Through the Ilioinguinal Approach* [Video]. Copyright © AO/ASIF Video, 1991.)

final tightening. Alternatively, a 3.5-mm pelvic plate applied to the iliac crest may provide more reliable fixation. This implant may be placed either in the internal iliac fossa just below the crest, or it may be located directly on the iliac crest. Plates applied directly to the iliac crest allow the placement of long screws between the two tables of the iliac wing. However, screws and plates in this location are often a source of irritation, and this may necessitate their removal.

Comminution of the anterior column fracture at the pelvic brim is common. Although these free cortical fragments are extra-articular, it is imperative that they be reduced anatomically and fixed: The reduction of the anterior column is impossible to judge without these pieces.

The anterior column fracture is then reduced. The reduction maneuver may be accomplished with the use of the Farabeuf clamp and ball spike (Fig. 42.23). Occasionally, clamps placed across the anterior border of the bone may be useful. A screw placed from just lateral to the pelvic brim and directed toward the sciatic notch will hold the reduction (Fig. 42.24). In addition, a screw may be placed between the tables of the ilium at the level of the iliac crest (Fig. 42.25). A long curved plate is then contoured to the superior aspect

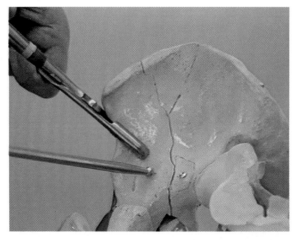

Figure 42.23. Farabeuf and Weber clamps are used to reduce the anterior column fracture. Note that the fracture fragment from the pelvic brim has been reduced and fixed with a single screw. The accurate reduction of the anterior column is not possible unless the two extra-articular fracture fragments are accurately reduced and stabilized. (Reprinted with permission from AO/ASIF, *Both Column Fracture Through the Ilioinguinal Approach* [Video]. Copyright © AO/ASIF Video, 1991.)

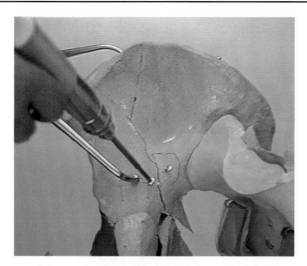

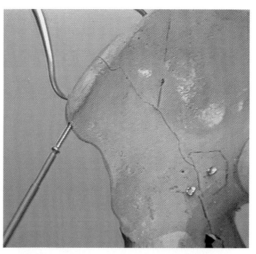

Figure 42.24. Anterior column reduction is held with a screw placed from just lateral to the pelvic brim and directed toward the sciatic notch. (Reprinted with permission from AO/ASIF, *Both Column Fracture Through the Ilioinguinal Approach* [Video]. Copyright © AO/ASIF Video, 1991.)

Figure 42.25. Additional 3.5-mm screw is placed between the tables of the ilium at the level of the iliac crest. (Reprinted with permission from AO/ASIF, *Both Column Fracture Through the Ilioinguinal Approach* [Video]. Copyright © AO/ASIF Video, 1991.)

of the pelvic brim. Specialized, precurved, pelvic plates are available with curvature radii of 88 and 108 degrees. These are designed to fit the curvature of the typical male and female pelvic brims. This plate may extend anterior from the front of the sacroiliac joint to the body of the pubis. The plate has a typical contour, which includes a concavity for the body of the pubis, a convexity over the pectineal eminence, and a concavity for the internal iliac fossa (Fig. 24.26). In addition, the plate must be twisted to match appropriately the contour of the ilium. Contouring of the plate is frequently time-consuming. It is important that the plate fit the bone as perfectly as possible to avoid loss of fracture reduction.

The posterior column is then reduced with the use of an angled reduction clamp, restoring the profile of the greater sciatic notch. The reduction clamp is usually placed entirely within the second window of the approach (Fig. 42.27), but occasionally a large clamp placed across the anterior border of the bone is helpful. In most cases, the quadrilateral surface is attached to the posterior column, and the accuracy of the posterior column reduction may be assessed by inspecting the reduction of the quadrilateral surface to the anterior

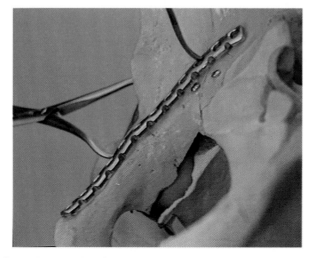

Figure 42.26. Curved pelvic plate is contoured to the innominate bone. Shown is the concavity at the superior ramus, the convexity at the pectineal eminence, and the concavity of the internal iliac fossa. (Reprinted with permission from AO/ASIF, *Both Column Fracture Through the Ilioinguinal Approach* [Video]. Copyright © AO/ASIF Video, 1991.)

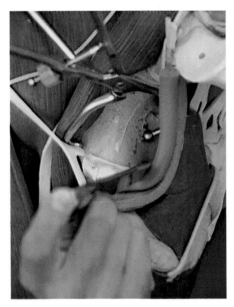

Figure 42.27. Posterior column fracture is reduced with the use of an angled reduction clamp placed entirely within the second window of the approach. The iliopsoas and femoral nerve are retracted laterally, the external iliac vessels are retracted laterally, and the external iliac vessels are retracted medially. One point of the reduction clamp is on the anterior wall and the other is on the quadrilateral surface. (Reprinted with permission from AO/ASIF, *Both Column Fracture Through the Ilioinguinal Approach* [Video]. Copyright © AO/ASIF Video, 1991.)

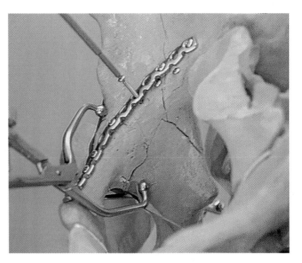

Figure 42.28. Posterior column is held reduced with an angled reduction clamp. The screw is placed through the plate and parallel with the quadrilateral surface. (Reprinted with permission from AO/ASIF, *Both Column Fracture Through the Ilioinguinal Approach* [Video]. Copyright © AO/ASIF Video, 1991.)

column. The posterior column fixation is achieved by screws placed parallel to the quadrilateral surface (Fig. 42.28). These screws may be placed either inside or separate from the pelvic-brim plate and used to achieve fixation in the retroacetabular surface (Fig. 42.29). In addition, a screw started on the anterior pillar of the lateral surface of the ilium and directed obliquely toward the quadrilateral surface may be used. This screw may also be used in situations in which a separate fragment of the quadrilateral surface requires fixation. Comminuted fragments of the quadrilateral surface are frequently encountered, but these pieces

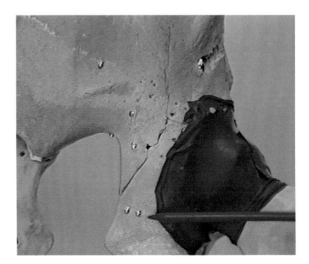

Figure 42.29. Posterior column fixation achieves purchase in the retroacetabular surface of the ilium. Tips of the two screws inserted through the pelvic brim plate (red pointer). (Reprinted with permission from AO/ASIF, *Both Column Fracture Through the Ilioinguinal Approach* [Video]. Copyright © AO/ASIF Video, 1991.)

usually make up a portion of the cotyloid fossa and do not contribute to the direct articular portion of the joint or to hip stability. Plates contoured over the pelvic brim and onto the quadrilateral surface are not routinely used.

An extended posterior-wall fracture, if present, can be addressed by developing the exposure to the lateral surface of the ilium. A large reduction clamp placed across the anterior innominate bone can be used to reduce the posterior wall. This fracture can be fixed with obliquely oriented screws placed from just lateral to the pelvic brim and directed posteriorly toward the superior extension of the ilium. However, it is imperative to use the image intensifier to confirm an extra-articular screw location.

Impacted areas of articular cartilage are frequently encountered, especially with medial displacement of the femoral head. The lateral traction device on the Judet–Tasserit table may be used to position the femoral head beneath the intact segment of articular surface. The femoral head may then be used as a mold for the reduction of the impacted segments. The disimpaction of such fragments is performed through the anterior column or quadrilateral surface fracture lines.

Technical Note

Final reduction of the articular surface of the acetabulum cannot be directly visualized but is assumed to be correct after anatomic restoration of the internal contour of the innominate bone (Fig. 42.30). The image intensifier is a valuable adjunct to ensure both the proper orientation of screws near the acetabulum and the perfect reduction of the articular surface. An AP pelvis radiograph should be obtained in the operating suite to confirm the adequacy of reduction. Before the patient is discharged from the hospital, AP and 45-degree oblique views of the pelvis are obtained to document reduction and fixation. If there is any suspicion that hardware may be intra-articular, fluoroscopic examination can be a valuable tool. The x-ray beam may be directed exactly parallel to any screw to document its location. Occasionally a postoperative CT scan may give additional information regarding the fracture reduction or hardware placement, but this is not routinely performed.

POSTOPERATIVE MANAGEMENT

Prophylactic antibiotic coverage with a first-generation cephalosporin and gentamicin is continued for 72 hours after surgery. The suction drains are generally removed at 48 hours or when drainage has ceased.

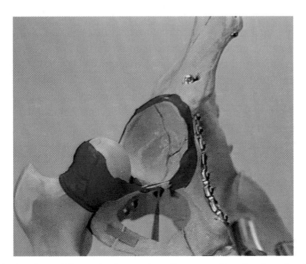

Figure 42.30. Reduction of the articular surface is never directly visualized. (Reprinted with permission from AO/ASIF, *Both Column Fracture Through the Ilioinguinal Approach* [Video]. Copyright ©AO/ASIF Video, 1991.)

Anticoagulation therapy follows a previously described protocol (1). All patients are screened with Doppler ultrasound for possible deep venous thrombosis (DVT) at the time of admission. Those positive for DVT receive a caval filter. If no DVT is present, mechanical sequential-compression devices are applied preoperatively and left continually throughout the patient's hospital course. An adjusted-dose warfarin (Coumadin) regimen is begun on the 2nd postoperative day and continued for 6 weeks.

A partial-weight-bearing gait protocol is initiated, and weight bearing is limited to 30 pounds until 8 weeks after the operation. Standing active-motion exercises of the hip are encouraged during this time. At 8 weeks after surgery, weight bearing is advanced to full, and active-motion exercises against resistance are begun. An emphasis is placed on strengthening the hip flexors and abductors. No heterotopic bone prophylaxis is necessary.

After discharge, patients are seen in follow-up at 3 weeks, 3 months, 6 months, 1 year, and yearly thereafter. An AP pelvis radiograph is obtained at each visit. If loss of reduction or early posttraumatic arthritis is suspected, then Judet obliques may be obtained as well.

Patients are generally able to return to work in 4 to 6 months; if heavy labor is involved, they may return to work in 6 months. They usually return to recreational activities by 6 months and to vigorous athletics by 1 year. Although the majority of patients with acetabular fractures will report that their hip never feels entirely normal, 70% are eventually able to return to their previous levels of function.

COMPLICATIONS

Complications with the ilioinguinal approach involve primarily neurovascular injuries. The lateral, femoral, cutaneous nerve is the most frequently injured nerve, resulting in lateral thigh paresthesia or numbness. Injuries to the femoral nerve are usually stretch injuries, attributable to vigorous retraction of the iliopsoas and femoral nerve. Sciatic nerve injuries are due either to placement of retractors in the sciatic notch or to direct nerve injury by a drill. Lymphatic complications and postoperative thigh edema are avoidable if the perivascular tissue surrounding the external iliac vessels is left undisturbed. The potential exists for direct laceration of the external iliac artery or vein. In addition, overzealous retraction of the vessels may produce an intimal injury of the external iliac artery and subsequent arterial thrombosis. Careful palpation of the arterial pulse throughout the surgery is critical. Postoperatively, the peripheral pulses should be monitored for 24 hours to identify any evolving vascular compromise.

In his early series, Letournel (2–4) found a 30% incidence of surgical wound infections. With the routine use of prophylactic antibiotics and closed suction drainage of the space of Retzius, however, surgical infection rates have significantly decreased (5,6). With restoration of the internal contours of the innominate bone, the hip joint is not immediately in direct connection with the infection. Routine exploration of the hip joint is not performed unless clinical signs and symptoms lead one to suspect an intra-articular infection. Deep wound infection, when encountered, is managed by repeated exploration of the wound, irrigation, debridement, and closure over drains. Appropriate broad-spectrum antibiotic coverage is used until culture results are obtained and directed coverage is possible.

Postoperative inguinal hernia may complicate incomplete or inadequate repair of the inguinal canal. Careful dissection of the floor of the inguinal canal during exposure should leave sufficient tissue for a sound repair. Letournel reported significant abdominal-wall hernias in only 1.1% of their patients.

ILLUSTRATIVE CASE FOR TECHNIQUE

A 24-year-old woman was involved in a motor vehicle accident, sustaining an associated both-column fracture of the acetabulum. AP pelvis and 45-degree oblique radiographs are shown in Figure 42.31. The patient underwent open reduction and internal fixation (ORIF) of her fracture through the ilioinguinal approach. An AP radiograph at the 4-year follow-up showed that the fracture healed with maintenance of the hip joint (Fig. 42.32). Her hip function was normal.

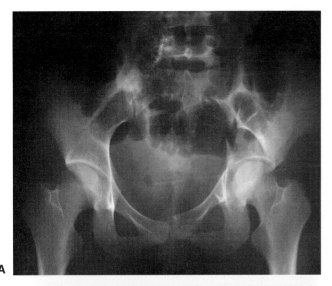

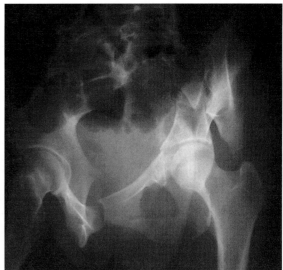

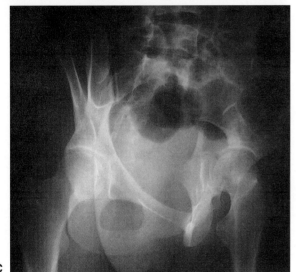

Figure 42.31. A. AP pelvis, (B) obturator oblique, and (C) iliac oblique radiographs of an associated both-column acetabulum fracture.

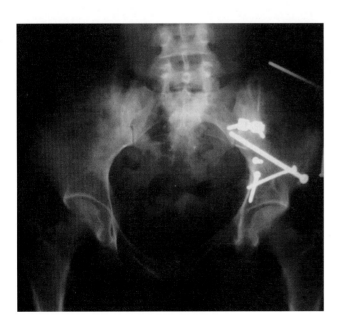

Figure 42.32. AP pelvis radiograph at 4-year follow-up. The fracture is healed, and the hip joint is rated excellent based on both radiographic and clinic examination.

RECOMMENDED READINGS

1. Matta JM, Letournel E, Browner BD. Surgical management of acetabulum fractures. *Intr Course Lect* 1986;35:
    382–397.
2. Judet R, Judet J, Letournel E. Fractures of the acetabulum: classification and surgical approaches for open re-
    duction. *J Bone Joint Surg Am* 1964;46:1615.
3. Matta JM. Operative indications and choice of surgical approach for fractures of the acetabulum. *Tech Orthop*
    1986;1:13.
4. Matta JM. Fracture of the acetabulum: accuracy of reduction and clinical results in patients managed opera-
    tively within three weeks after the injury. *J Bone Joint Surg Am* 1996:78:1632.
5. Fishman Al, Greeno RA, Brooks LR, et al. Prevention of deep venous thrombosis and pulmonary embolism in
    acetabulum and pelvic fracture surgery. *Clin Orthop* 1994;305:10–19.
6. Letournel E. The treatment of acetabular fractures through the ilioinguinal approach. *Clin Orthop* 1993;292:
    62–76.

43

Acetabular Fractures: Extended Iliofemoral Approach

Craig S. Bartlett, Arthur L. Malkani, Milan K. Sen, and David L. Helfet

INDICATIONS/CONTRAINDICATIONS

Over the past 30 years, advances in surgical approaches, reduction techniques, surgical implants, and preoperative and postoperative evaluation of acetabular fractures have resulted in a dramatic improvement in the outcomes in patients with acetabular fractures. Nevertheless, the management of these injuries continues to be a challenging problem for the orthopedic surgeon, in part, due to the complex anatomy of the pelvis and acetabulum.

The primary goal of operative treatment of acetabular fractures is an accurate reduction of the articular surface such that a congruent hip joint is obtained and normal joint mechanics are restored. This is the primary tenet in the management of all intra-articular fractures, and it is especially important in the weight bearing joints of the lower extremity. In the case of the hip joint, malreduction leads to abnormal loading of the articular cartilage and subsequent painful posttraumatic arthrosis and loss of function.

The indications for operative fixation of acetabular fractures in general include displacement of the articular surface, incongruence of the hip joint, unacceptable roof-arc measurements, incarceration of an intra-articular fragment within the joint, and subluxation of the femoral head. The timing of surgery is dependent upon several factors including the availability of an experienced surgeon; management of associated visceral, skeletal, and soft-tissue injuries; and completion of all imaging studies necessary for preoperative planning. Special situations arise such as in the case of an incarcerated intra-articular fragment, an unreducible femoral-head dislocation, or a femoral head fracture that mandate more urgent intervention to prevent further damage to the articular cartilage or minimize the risk of avascular necrosis of the femoral head. Conversely, a Morel-Lavalle lesion deserves special attention and may delay operative management of the acetabular fracture.

The selection of the proper surgical approach for acetabular exposure may not be straightforward and is largely dependent on the fracture pattern and the experience of the surgeon. Mayo identified five factors that affect the choice of surgical approach: (a) the fracture pattern; (b) the local soft-tissue conditions; (c) the presence of associated, major, systemic injuries; (d) the age and projected functional status of the patient; and (e) the delay from injury to surgery. Although elaborate, the Letournel-Judet classification system is clinically useful in this regard. Injuries to the pelvic ring must also be considered when determining the surgical approach for an acetabular fracture.

Complex fracture patterns often require exposure of both the anterior and posterior columns for adequate visualization and reduction. In these cases, an extensile approach will provide adequate access to the roof of the acetabulum for anatomic restoration of its articular surface. The extended iliofemoral approach was developed by Letournel in 1974. It is one of the three most widely used surgical approaches used to gain access to the acetabulum; the others are the Kocher-Langenbeck and the ilioinguinal approaches.

The extended iliofemoral approach allows access to both columns of the acetabulum. It includes the lateral aspect of the iliac wing, the internal iliac fossa, and the retroacetabular surface. It is an anatomic approach that follows an internervous plane in which the muscles innervated by the femoral nerve are reflected anteriorly and the muscles supplied by the superior and inferior gluteal nerves are reflected posteriorly. The posterior flap is mobilized as a unit without damaging its neurovascular bundles (Fig. 43.1).

Specific indications for the extended ilioinguinal approach include (a) high (transtectal) transverse and T-type fracture patterns with involvement of the weight bearing dome (Fig. 43.2); (b) associated anterior column and posterior hemitransverse fractures; (c) associated both-column fractures, with a posterior wall or a comminuted posterior-column lateral-dome involvement (Fig. 43.3) or extension into the sacroiliac joint; (d) transverse or associated fractures where treatment has been delayed. Matta also considered this approach in

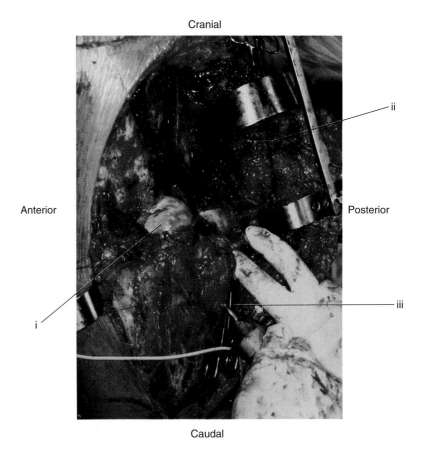

Figure 43.1. The extended iliofemoral approach for exposure of a comminuted left both-column acetabular fracture. (*i*) Femoral head. (*ii*) Abductor muscles and tensor fascia lata. (*iii*) Schanz pin in greater trochanter parallel with femoral neck.

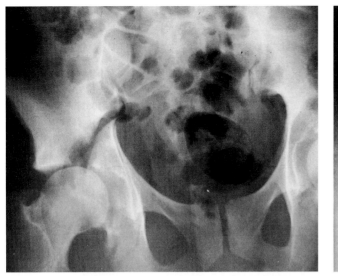

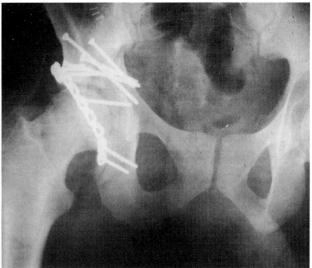

Figure 43.2. A 28-year-old man with right transtectal ischial T-type acetabular fracture.
A. Preoperative AP pelvis. **B.** Postoperative AP pelvis.

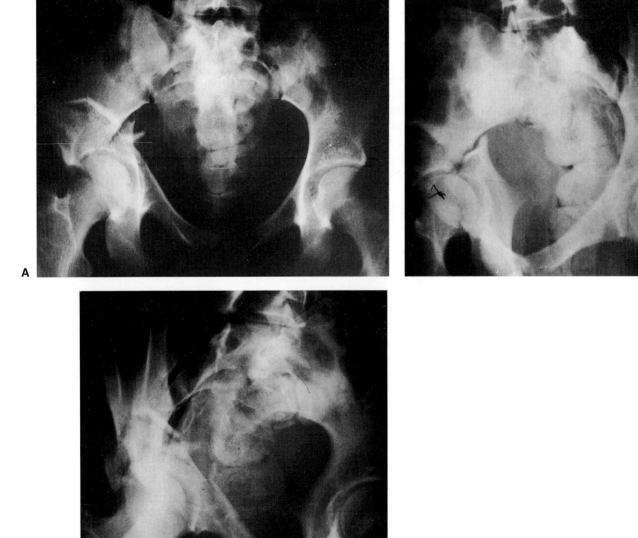

Figure 43.3. An 18-year-old woman with a both-column right acetabular fracture. **A.** AP pelvis. **B.** Iliac oblique view. **C.** Obturator oblique view.

certain transverse posterior-wall fractures, such as those involving an extended posterior-wall component where disruption of the retroacetabular surface makes difficult the assessment of reduction completed solely through a Kocher-Langenbeck approach.

When there are delays in treatment, the usefulness of approaches such as the ilioinguinal or Kocher-Langenbeck diminishes because of limited joint visualization, organization of the hematoma, increased formation and maturation of callus, and difficulty mobilizing and reducing the fracture lines. Technical problems escalate at approximately 2 weeks after injury with the ability to obtain an anatomic reduction dropping from 75% to 62% of cases by the 3rd week. This is due to the increasingly difficult task of taking down varying amounts of callus, which will progressively interfere with the anatomical reduction of all fractured segments of iliac crest and acetabulum. Even in experienced of hands, late surgical reconstruction of acetabular fractures results in excellent or good outcomes in only 65.5% of cases. Therefore, to improve the likelihood of achieving an anatomic reduction, the extended iliofemoral method is the preferred surgical approach for the most complex acetabular-fracture cases in which surgery has been delayed more than 2 to 3 weeks.

The major technical limitation of the extended iliofemoral exposure is access to the lower portion of the anterior column (Figs. 43.4 and 43.5). Dissection medial to the iliopectineal eminence becomes more difficult where the psoas muscle and iliopectineal fascia block exposure. While a psoas tenotomy can increase visualization, the risk of injury to the femoral artery and nerve must be considered.

There are some relative contraindications to the extended iliofemoral approach. Blunt trauma to the gluteal muscle mass and peritrochanteric region is probably the most common cause for concern. Contusions and abrasions in this area are often associated with the Morel-Lavalle lesion, an area of fluctuance secondary to fatty necrosis and a hematoma that develops under the degloved skin and subcutaneous tissues around the hip. The Morel-Lavalle lesion requires surgical debridement and drainage before internal fixation and is associated with a higher infection rate.

Other relative contraindications to the extended iliofemoral approach include the presence of a closed-head injury, which may lead to massive heterotopic ossification. Extensile approaches are generally avoided in the elderly because of the prolonged operative

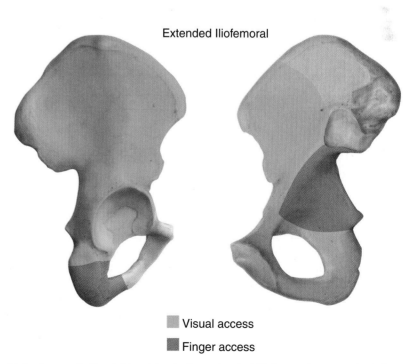

Extended Iliofemoral

■ Visual access

■ Finger access

Figure 43.4. Access to the right pelvis via the extended iliofemoral approach. **A.** Lateral (outer) bony pelvis. **B.** Medial (inner) bony pelvis.

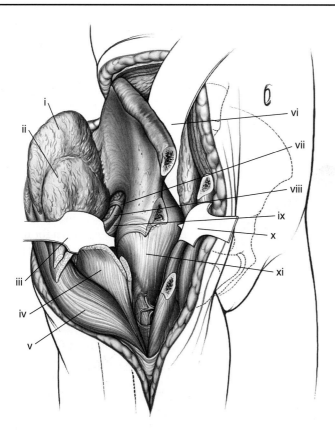

Figure 43.5. Maximal exposure of right acetabulum via the extended iliofemoral approach. (*i*) Gluteus medius muscle. (*ii*) Gluteus minimus muscle. (*iii*) Blunt Homan in lesser sciatic notch. (*iv*) Greater trochanter. (*v*) Tensor fascia-lata muscle. (*vi*) Malleable retractor under the iliacus muscle. (*vii*) Superior–gluteal neurovascular bundle. (*viii*) Piriformis muscle. (*ix*) Sciatic nerve. (*x*) Pointed Homan retractor over the anterior capsule of the hip. (*xi*) Hip-joint capsule.

time, extensive blood loss, prolonged rehabilitation, and increased risk of infection and heterotopic ossification. Finally, the presence of superior–gluteal vascular injury makes this approach less desirable because ligation of the lateral femoral-circumflex artery during the dissection removes a major source of collateral circulation to the abductor musculature; however, this stance on the procedure remains controversial.

PREOPERATIVE PLANNING

The preoperative evaluation begins with a thorough history and physical examination, as well as an appropriate trauma workup, to identify any associated skeletal and visceral injuries. An accurate neurologic examination is mandatory, as the incidence of sciatic nerve injury after acetabular fractures ranges from 12% to 38%.

An accurate diagnosis of the fracture and its subsequent classification can be accomplished with three basic roentgenograms described by Judet et al and include an anteroposterior (AP) view of the pelvis, an iliac oblique view, and an obturator oblique view of the acetabulum. These three roentgenographic views provide sufficient information to allow the surgeon to outline the fracture pattern on a pelvic model as part of the preoperative plan.

Conventional computed tomography (CT) scans with axial views provide additional information about the extent of injury to the acetabulum (Fig. 43.6A), especially identification of posterior-wall fractures, rotation of the columns, the presence of intra-articular fragments or femoral head fractures, and the assessment of articular displacement. Axial CT

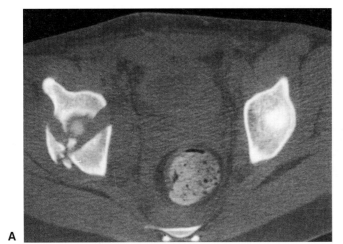

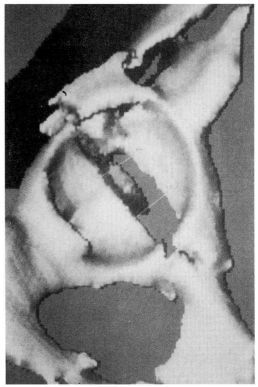

Figure 43.6. CT of pelvis of patient in Figure 43.3. **A.** Axial view revealing significant dome comminution. **B.** Three-dimensional reconstruction facilitating perception of configuration.

scans also can identify associated injuries to the posterior aspect of the pelvis, such as a sacroiliac-joint disruption and sacral fractures. Thin (1 to 2 mm) cuts should be used, along with sagittal and coronal reformatting, to evaluate thoroughly the fracture pattern preoperatively. Advances in imaging software technology have led to the development of three-dimensional CT, which provides an even better understanding of the spatial relation of the fracture pattern relative to the pelvis (see Fig. 43.6B).

Trauma patients, especially those with lower extremity or pelvic injuries, are at extremely high risk for developing deep vein thrombosis (DVT); in some series, the DVT cases are at 60%. We screen all of our acetabular fracture patients for DVT and treat them with compression boots and subcutaneous low-molecular-weight heparin if a delay in surgery is anticipated. Our preferred method of screening is magnetic resonance venography, which we have found to be extremely sensitive and reliable. Patients with an increased risk of DVT or those with documented, preoperative DVT are managed with a vena cava filter and intravenous heparin before surgery.

SURGERY

Surgical Anatomy

Three main stages characterize the dissection: (a) elevation of all the gluteal muscles with the tensor fascia lata, (b) division of the external rotators of the hip, and (c) an extended capsulotomy along the lip of the acetabulum. The end result is complete exposure of the outer aspect of the ilium and the whole posterior column inferiorly to the upper part of the ischial tuberosity. Furthermore, the approach may be extended to allow a limited exposure of the internal iliac fossa and the anterior column to the level of the iliopectineal eminence. This allows simultaneous exposure of both columns and permits direct visualization of the reduction and fixation of the anterior and posterior columns (see Fig. 43.4). The articular surface of the acetabulum along with the femoral head may also be visualized if this approach is combined with a surgical dislocation of the hip.

The physician performing an extended iliofemoral approach requires special training and a familiarity with the complex anatomy of the pelvis, particularly the many neurovascular structures that are encountered. Those structures that require identification are listed below.

Sciatic Nerve. The sciatic nerve is at risk during exposure of the posterior column and must be identified, as in the Kocher-Langenbeck approach, along the belly of the quadratus femoris muscle. Traction along the nerve should be minimized by maintaining the hip in extension with the knee flexed at all times.

Lateral Femoral Cutaneous Nerve. The lateral femoral cutaneous nerve is at risk during exposure of the anterior–superior iliac spine. It is also very susceptible to a traction injury during mobilization of the soft tissues. Patients should be warned preoperatively of the significant risk of numbness in the anterolateral thigh after this exposure.

Superior–Gluteal Neurovascular Bundle. The superior–gluteal neurovascular bundle is at risk during exposure of the greater sciatic notch. Therefore, it must be protected from undue traction or penetration by retractors.

Femoral Neurovascular Structures. The medial margin of the extended iliofemoral approach is the iliopsoas muscle and the iliopectineal eminence. Further medial dissection without an ilioinguinal incision places the femoral neurovascular structures at risk.

Pudendal Nerve. The pudendal nerve is at risk as it exits the pelvis through the greater sciatic notch, wraps around the ischial spine, and travels back into the pelvis through the lesser sciatic notch.

Operating Room Preparation

General or spinal anesthesia is administered. We prefer the continuous epidural anesthesia as it provides improved postoperative pain relief. A Foley catheter is placed in the patient's bladder. The patient is supported on a beanbag and placed in the lateral decubitus position on a radiolucent operating table or fracture table, depending on the surgeon's preference.

Vascular access in two separate sites with large-bore catheters is important for these lengthy procedures in which significant blood loss is common. The patient's age and medical condition often dictate placement of an arterial or central line.

We routinely use an intraoperative cell saver to minimize transfusion requirements. This permits recycling of about 20% to 30% of the effective blood loss and is best used when blood loss of more than 2 L is expected.

The hip is kept extended and the knee flexed throughout the procedure to minimize sciatic nerve injury. In addition, intraoperative sciatic-nerve monitoring with spontaneous electromyography (EMG) and somatosensory evoked potentials (SSEP) is used in all cases. The entire pelvis, hip, abdomen, and involved extremity are prepped free, and sterile subdermal electrodes are inserted. The sensory electrodes are inserted adjacent to the common peroneal and posterior tibial nerves and the motor adjacent to the tibialis anterior, peroneus longus, abductor hallucis, and flexor hallucis brevis. The ground is inserted in the heel.

Surgical Approach

The incision is in the form of an inverted "J" (Fig. 43.7) and begins at the posterior–superior iliac spine, extending along the iliac crest toward the anterior–superior iliac spine (ASIS). From here, the distal arm of the incision proceeds along the anterolateral aspect of the thigh for a distance of 15 to 20 cm (Fig. 43.8). The surgeon has a tendency to make this arm more medial than is desired. To avoid this, one should visualize a point 2 cm lateral to the superolateral pole of the patella. With the leg held in neutral rotation, this location is generally in line with the desired incision. Furthermore, a gentle posterior curve may be helpful in obese patients.

The fascial periosteal layer at the iliac crest is identified (Fig. 43.9) and divided sharply along its avascular "white line," where bleeding will be minimized. Often it is easiest to start in the area of the gluteus medius tubercle where landmarks are more obvious and to progress posteriorly and anteriorly from this point. Posteriorly, the strong fibrous origins of

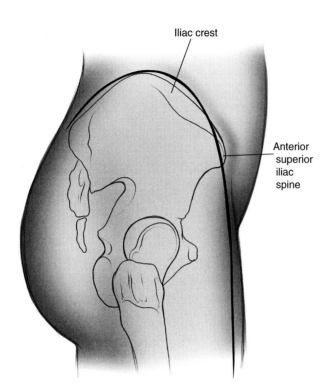

Figure 43.7. Inverted "J" skin incision, right side.

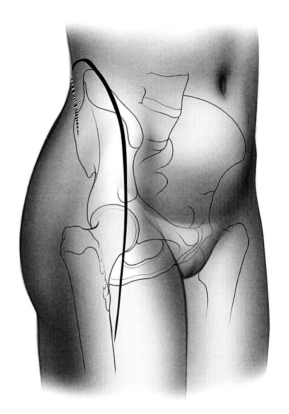

Figure 43.8. Anterolateral view, right side. The inverted-J skin incision with distal extension for the extended iliofemoral approach.

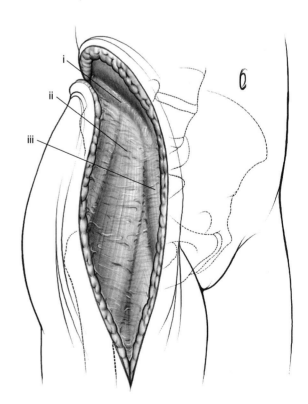

Figure 43.9. Subfascial exposure of right iliac crest and anterior distal limb. (*i*) Avascular white line. (*ii*) Fascia covering tensor fascia-lata muscle. (*iii*) Fascia covering sartorius muscle.

the gluteus maximus should be sharply released from the crista glutei. Depending on the starting location, the tensor fascia-lata muscle and the gluteus medius are subperiosteally released in a stepwise fashion from the outer aspect of the iliac crest (Fig. 43.10). Using an elevator, the musculature along the external surface of the iliac wing is released up to the superior border of the greater sciatic notch and anterosuperior aspect of the hip joint capsule (Fig. 43.11). During this segment of the exposure, care must be taken to identify the superior- gluteal neurovascular bundle, which is at risk as it exits from the notch.

Attention turns next to the anterior portion of the approach (see Fig. 43.9). The distal limb of the incision is carried over the fascia covering the tensor fascia-lata muscle, and the muscle sheath is entered. The surgeon must stay within the bounds of the sheath, as this will keep the dissection lateral to the lateral femoral-cutaneous nerve, sparing the majority of its branches. It is often helpful to open the sheath from distal to proximal.

Next, the tensor fascia muscle is reflected off its fascia and retracted laterally and upward to expose the floor of the sheath and fascia overlying the rectus femoris muscle (see Fig. 43.10). Small vessels from the superficial circumflex artery are divided and coagulated close to the bone between the superior and inferior spines. Distally, the incision must be long enough to expose the inferior aspect of the muscle belly. This facilitates further release of the gluteal muscles from the crest.

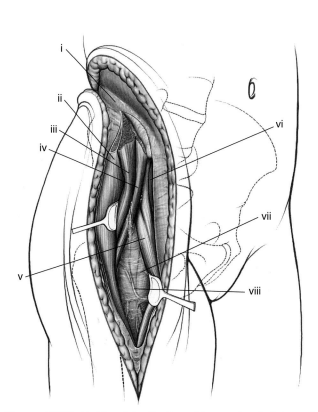

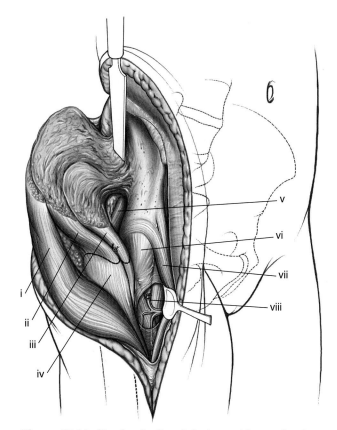

Figure 43.10. Subfascial reflection of tensor fascia lata and abductor muscle origins from right iliac crest. (*i*) Avascular white line. (*ii*) Tensor fascia-lata muscle. (*iii*) Gluteus medius muscle. (*iv*) Gluteus minimus muscle. (*v*) Rectus femoris muscle. (*vi*) Sartorius muscle. (*vii*) No-name fascia covering vastus lateralis. (*viii*) Ascending branch of the lateral, femoral, circumflex artery.

Figure 43.11. Proximally, the abductor and tensor fascia-lata muscles have been stripped subperiosteally from the outer table of the right ileum. Distally, the ascending branch of the lateral circumflex artery has been ligated. The abductor insertions have been marked for release. (*i*) Tensor fascia lata muscle. (*ii*) Gluteus medius muscle. (*iii*) Gluteus minimus muscle. (*iv*) Greater trochanter. (*v*) Piriformis muscle. (*vi*) Hip-joint capsule. (*vii*) Two heads of the rectus muscle. (*viii*) Ligated ascending branch of the lateral, femoral, circumflex artery.

The fascia overlying the rectus muscle is divided longitudinally and horizontally, and its reflected head and direct heads retracted downward and medially to expose a very strong aponeurosis (the "no name" fascia) over the vastus lateralis muscle (see Fig. 43.10). When the rectus is retracted, a constant small vascular pedicle reaching the lateral border of the muscle always requires coagulation. The aponeurosis can be divided longitudinally to expose the ascending branches of the lateral circumflex vessels, which must be isolated and ligated (see Fig. 43.11). Should the upper portion of this exposure be unnecessary, these vessels can occasionally be spared.

Next the thin sheath of the iliopsoas muscle is exposed and longitudinally incised. This allows the use of an elevator to strip the fibers of the psoas from the anterior and inferior aspects of the hip capsule. The exposure of the iliac wing is complete when the reflected head of the rectus femoris is sharply released from its insertion.

The gluteus minimus tendon is identified as it inserts into the anterior edge of the greater trochanter and tagged and transected, leaving a 3- to 5-mm cuff for repair (Figs. 43.11 and 43.12). The gluteus minimus muscle also has extensive attachments to the superior aspect of the hip capsule that may need to be released. Posteriorly and superiorly, the gluteus medius tendon, measuring 15 to 20 mm in length, is also isolated, tagged, and transected, leaving a 3- to 5-mm cuff (see Figs. 43.11 and 43.12). The surgeon must transect and tag these structures sequentially and carefully for subsequent reattachment. The tensor fascialata and gluteal muscles are held in continuity as a flap and reflected posteriorly to expose the external rotators and sciatic nerve (see Fig. 43.12).

The tendons of the piriformis muscle, obturator internus muscle, and the inferior and superior gemelli muscles are tagged and transected as in the Kocher-Langenbeck approach (Figs. 43.12 and 43.13). The tendinous femoral insertion of the gluteus maximus is identified, tagged,

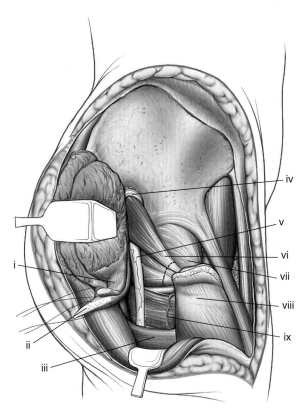

Figure 43.12. Abductors of the right hip have been tagged and their insertions into the greater trochanter released, allowing their muscle pedicle to be retracted to expose the sciatic nerve. The external rotators also have been marked for release. (*i*) Gluteus minimus tendon. (*ii*) Gluteus medius tendon. (*iii*) Gluteus maximus tendon. (*iv*) Superior–gluteal neurovascular bundle. (*v*) Sciatic nerve. (*vi*) Piriformis and conjoint tendons. (*vii*) Hip-joint capsule. (*viii*) Greater trochanter. (*ix*) Quadratus femoris.

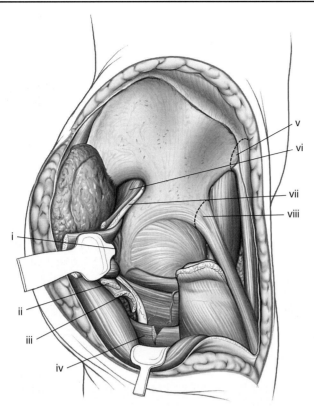

Figure 43.13. Retraction of right-hip external-rotator muscles and release of gluteus maximus insertion distally. Medially, the anterior–superior and anterior–inferior iliac spines have been marked for either release or osteotomy. (*i*) Blunt Homan in lesser sciatic notch. The conjoint tendons have been positioned between the retractor and the sciatic nerve. (*ii*) Gluteus minimus tendon. (*iii*) Gluteus medius tendon. (*iv*) Partial release of gluteus maximus tendon. (*v*) Anterior–superior iliac spine and sartorius muscle origin. (*vi*) Piriformis muscle. (*vii*) Sciatic nerve. (*viii*) Anterior–inferior iliac spine and reflected head of rectus femoris muscle.

and released with a cuff for repair (see Fig. 43.13). It cannot be overemphasized that the quadratus femoris and its blood supply to the femur via the ascending branch of the medial femoral circumflex artery must be preserved. The dissection is now complete (see Fig. 43.1).

The piriformis muscle can be followed toward the greater sciatic notch and the obturator internus muscle to the lesser sciatic notch. A Homan or sciatic nerve retractor is then placed into the lesser notch, allowing complete exposure to the posterior column of the acetabulum. The surgeon must ensure that the tendon of the obturator internus maintains its position in the lesser notch between the sciatic nerve and the retractor. Should additional retraction be required, a blunt Homan is gently placed into the greater sciatic notch, with the surgeon aware that no structure is protecting the nerve. The distal portion of the posterior column can be visualized to the ischial tuberosity through sharp dissection of the origin of the hamstring muscles proximally, if necessary.

Although medial exposure of the anterior column is limited by the iliopsoas muscle and the iliopectineal fascia (see Figs. 43.4, 43.9, and 43.13), further access to the internal iliac fossa and acetabulum is possible. This access is obtained by subperiosteal dissection beneath the sartorius and direct head of the rectus or by osteotomy of the superior and inferior iliac spines, which will, respectively, release these muscles (see Figs. 43.5 and 43.13). The insertion of the external oblique muscle onto the crest can also be subperiosteally released to reveal the inner table of the pelvis, which is further exposed by the surgeon stripping off the iliacus muscle with a periosteal elevator. However, extensile exposure of the outer and inner tables of the iliac wing, especially in the presence of local fractures, will create a risk of iliac-bone devascularization.

Cranial

Anterior

Posterior

I ——————————————————————————————————— II

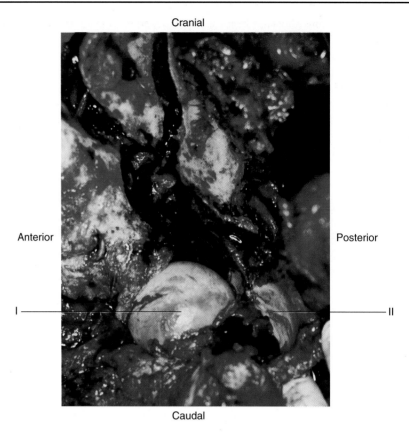

Caudal

Figure 43.14. Close-up of acetabular-joint exposure of patient in Figure 43.1. (*I*) Femoral head. (*II*) Loose articular fragments.

Although devascularization of the iliac wing is rare, Matta warned of its occurrence, especially in associated both-column fractures. To avoid devascularization of the iliac bone in this case, he suggested leaving, at a minimum, the direct head of the rectus femoris and anterior hip capsule attached to the anterior column. Also of concern with this exposure is the blood supply to the dome of the acetabulum, which is at risk during dissection of the anterior–inferior iliac spine.

Displaced acetabular fractures often tear the hip-joint capsule. If not present, exposure of the acetabular articular surface can be obtained with a marginal capsulotomy, leaving a cuff of tissue for repair. Once the hip joint is exposed, distraction with either a Schanz screw placed into the femoral head or a femoral distractor will facilitate visualization (Figs. 43.1 and 43.14). The visualization is important for evaluating the articular reduction, ruling out any intra-articular hardware, and removing any incarcerated osteochondral fragments.

Once the exposure of the extended iliofemoral approach has been completed, the fracture can be reduced according to the preoperative plan. The soft-tissue flaps must be kept moist with wet sponges and periodic irrigation throughout the procedure.

Reduction Technique

Several regions of bone are optimal for screw placement. These include the iliac crest, the superogluteal ridge, the greater sciatic buttress (above the sciatic notch and to the anterior–inferior iliac spine), the anterior column, and the posterior column. Extra-long screws, ranging from 50 to 120 mm, should be available.

In a transverse fracture, rotational malalignment of the inferior portion of the acetabulum may be found. In the T-type fracture patterns, the anterior and posterior fragments may be separate and both columns may have become displaced and malrotated. Usually, the anterior segment has medial displacement of its inferior portion so that the radius of curvature of the acetabulum is greater than that of the femoral head. In both transverse and T-type acetabular fractures, reduction is achieved with a pelvic-reduction clamp attached to 4.5-mm screws placed proximal and distal to the posterior-column fracture. The pelvic-reduction clamp initially allows distraction for debriding of the fracture surfaces, and then facilitates manipulative reduction of the fracture. A bone spreader in the fracture site can also facilitate exposure of the fracture or the joint (Fig. 43.15A). Additional control of rotation is provided by a Schanz screw placed into the ischium and a pelvic clamp in the greater sciatic notch.

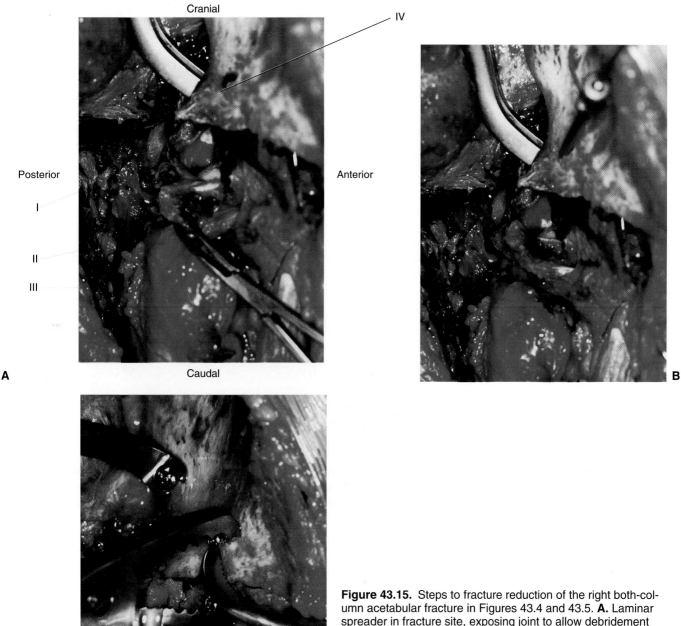

Figure 43.15. Steps to fracture reduction of the right both-column acetabular fracture in Figures 43.4 and 43.5. **A.** Laminar spreader in fracture site, exposing joint to allow debridement of loose intra-articular fragments and callus. (*I*) Femoral head in joint. (*II*) Superolateral dome fragment with capsular attachments. (*III*) Greater trochanter. (*IV*) Intact iliac wing. **B.** Predrilling the gliding hole for the anterior-to-posterior column screw. **C.** Use of a Farabeuf clamp affixed to screws to reduce the anterior column to the superolateral fragment and a pelvic-reduction clamp affixed to screws to reduce the anterior-to-posterior column (posterior-column portion not shown).

For the reduction of the T-type and more comminuted variants, the anterior column should be reduced first with respect to the residual acetabular roof portion of the ilium. The adequacy of reduction of the posterior column can be visualized by direct assessment of the articular surface and also with digital palpation through the greater and lesser sciatic notches.

Before definitive reduction, a gliding hole can be inserted into the proximal aspect of the posterior column from superior to inferior (see Fig. 43.15B). This hole helps the surgeon assure that the gliding hole is in the middle of the posterior column.

A gliding hole can also be inserted from the lateral aspect of the iliac wing into the anterior column distal and medial to the articular surface. Generally, this requires the insertion of a lag screw 6 cm proximal to the superior aspect of the articular surface and 2 cm posterior to the gluteal ridge. The lag screw is then angled from posterosuperior to anteroinferior directly down the superior pubic ramus to secure the anterior column of the acetabulum. In large individuals, this can be accomplished with a 4.5-mm cortical screw. In small individuals, including most women, a 3.5-mm cortical screw is preferred. Care must be taken to assure that this screw remains extra-articular and also does not penetrate the anterior aspect of the superior ramus in the area of the iliopectineal eminence where the femoral vessels are in close proximity. The use of intraoperative fluoroscopy for the insertion of this screw is highly recommended.

Proper placement of pelvic-reduction forceps with respect to the plane of the fracture and geometry of the osseous surfaces is crucial for an adequate reduction. A variety of instruments is available to facilitate reduction: narrow curved osteotomes, bone hooks, ball spike pushers, King-Tong and Queen-Tong forceps, and the Farabeuf and pointed reduction clamps (see Fig. 43.15C).

To ensure an anatomic reduction of the acetabulum, the surgeon should work from the periphery toward the acetabulum (Fig. 43.16) by reducing each fracture fragment sequentially. Once the iliac wing is stabilized with lag screws, by 3.5-mm laterally applied reconstruction plates, or both, the posterior column is reduced to the iliac wing as the surgeon has direct visualization of the acetabular articular surface.

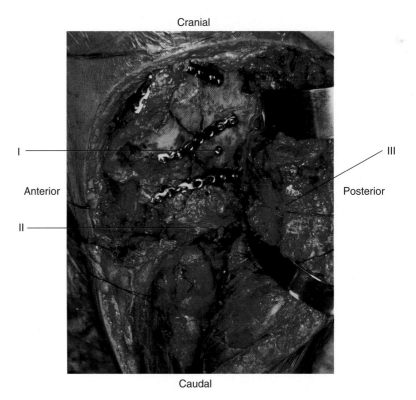

Figure 43.16. Reconstruction of comminuted left both-column acetabular fracture shown in Figures 43.1 and 43.14. Reconstruction proceeds centripetally from the periphery. (*I*) Posterior-to-anterior column lag screw. (*II*) Greater trochanter. (*III*) Abductor muscles and tensor fascia lata.

The posterior-column lag screw and 3.5-mm reconstruction plate fixation is utilized for transverse and T-type fractures. The anterior column is then reduced to the intact posterior column. This reduction can be accomplished with anterior to posterior 4.5-mm lag screws inserted from the anterior–superior spine into the sciatic buttress, or anterior-column lag screws from the lateral aspect of the iliac wing (as described previously), or both. The adequacy of the reduction is assessed, both by direct visualization of the acetabulum, with finger palpation of the greater and lesser sciatic notches and quadrilateral plate, and if necessary, in the internal iliac fossa. The use of fluoroscopy is essential to assure the adequacy of reduction and the position of the fixation (Fig. 43.17).

Closure

Because intra-articular hardware can lead to rapid chondrolysis, the surgeon must confirm hardware position before closure. This confirmation is best achieved radiographically through use of intraoperative fluoroscopic Judet views (especially the obturator oblique) and clinically by rotating the hip back and forth while a finger, to detect any crepitus, is placed along the quadrilateral surface.

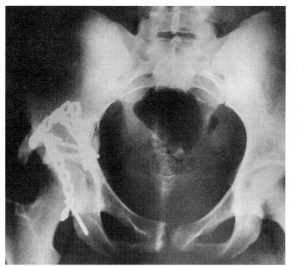

A

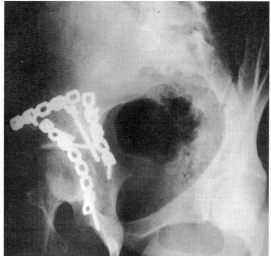

B

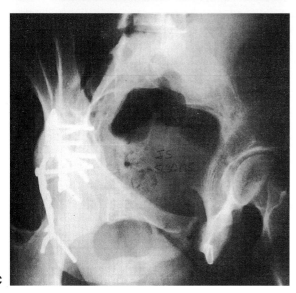

C

Figure 43.17. Patient from Figures 43.3 and 43.6 at 1-year follow-up. Congruent reduction and maintenance of joint space is shown. **A.** AP pelvis. **B.** Iliac oblique view. **C.** Obturator oblique view.

At the completion of osteosynthesis, suction drains are placed along the external surface of the iliac wing in the vicinity of the posterior column and vastus lateralis muscle. If the internal iliac fossa has been exposed, a third drain is placed here. All drains should exit anteriorly.

The hip capsule is repaired first, followed by reattachment of the tendinous insertions of the short external rotators to the greater trochanter through drill holes, and femoral insertions of the gluteus maximus. Next, the trochanteric insertions of the gluteus medius and minimus muscles are repaired, through use of five or six sutures for each tendon, as recommended by Letournel. Finally, the tensor fascia-lata and gluteal muscles are reattached to their origins on the iliac crest.

If a medial exposure has been performed, then the origins of the sartorius and direct head of the rectus femoris muscles are reattached through drill holes. If osteotomies have been performed, lag screws should be used.

Finally, the fascia overlying the tensor fascia-lata muscle is repaired. Then a subcutaneous suction drain is placed and the skin closed.

POSTOPERATIVE MANAGEMENT

Postoperatively, patients are maintained on intravenous cefazolin for 48 to 72 hours. Our postoperative anticoagulation regimen includes 6 weeks of warfarin in conjunction with compression boots. Heterotopic ossification prophylaxis is also mandatory, preferably with indomethacin 75 mg daily for 6 weeks. Drains are not removed until output has tapered to 10 to 20 ml per 8-hour shift and the patient has begun mobilizing, usually over the first 48 to 72 hours.

We stress early mobilization during the postoperative period, allowing patients to sit at the edges of their beds, dangle their legs, and progress to chairs within the first 24 to 48 hours after surgery. We do not use continuous passive motion as we have not had difficulty regaining hip motion in this patient population.

After the removal of drains, patients are allowed to undertake toe-touch weight bearing up to 20 pounds with crutches. Strengthening exercises along with gait training are initiated by the physical therapist. Weight bearing is not advanced and active abduction, any adduction, and flexion of the hip past 90 degrees are avoided for 6 to 8 weeks.

Acetabular fractures with a concomitant neurologic injury can pose a difficult rehabilitation problem because of lack of muscle activity or neurogenic pain. These frequently require consultation with a neurologist and the pain management service.

We routinely obtain postoperative roentgenograms (AP pelvis and 45-degree oblique Judet views) and a CT scan to assess critically the fracture reduction and hardware position. The CT scan is usually obtained on postoperative day 5, just before discharge. At the time of discharge, home physical therapy is arranged.

During the first follow-up visit at 2 weeks, staples or sutures are removed. At the 6-week follow-up, new roentgenograms are obtained, and generally, the abduction/adduction/flexion precautions are discontinued. The patient returns at 8 to 10 weeks, and depending on the roentgenographic findings, progression to full weight bearing is allowed, as tolerated, over the ensuing 4 weeks. An aggressive outpatient rehabilitation program should be initiated at this stage.

At 3 months postoperatively the patient is reevaluated and is expected to be weight bearing as tolerated with the assistance of a cane. In the absence of any contraindications, rehabilitation becomes more aggressive with the initiation of strengthening exercises. At 6 months follow-up the patient should be back to full activity. Additional evaluation with radiographs are done at 1 year after the surgery and then annually.

RESULTS

The most important factor responsible for successful long-term clinical outcome following surgical fixation of acetabular fractures is the quality of the reduction. Rowe and Lowell reviewed 93 acetabular fractures treated nonoperatively and noted poor results for all 10 patients in whom the weight-bearing dome was not anatomically reduced.

After the pioneering work of Letournel and others, many investigators have shown that long-term clinical outcomes correlate closely with the quality of reduction achieved during surgery. In his review of 569 acetabular fractures treated within 3 weeks of injury, Letournel achieved an anatomic reduction (a maximum of 1 mm of displacement on any of three views) in 74% of cases, with 82% of these patients having very good clinical outcomes in follow-ups that were conducted as late as 33 years after the surgery. Of the 26% with an imperfectly reduced acetabulum, very good results were obtained in 54% of cases if the femoral head was centered under the dome and in only 23% of cases where residual subluxation of the femoral head was present. In patients treated within 3 weeks of injury, Letournel noted osteoarthritis (OA) in only 10.2% of those with perfect reductions, as opposed to 35.7% with imperfect reductions. In an interesting finding, when treatment was delayed past 3 weeks, these rates were 24% and 23% respectively.

Recently, Mears et al retrospectively reviewed their results in 429 acetabular fractures. Like Letournel, they found that clinical outcomes correlated well with the quality of reduction. In their study, 89% of the patients with anatomic reductions had good or excellent clinical results based on Harris Hip Scores. In 77% of patients with fair or poor results, at least one of the following predisposing factors was present: femoral head or neck injury, acetabular impaction, marked displacement, preexisting arthritis, or delayed presentation. In their study, 53% of their patients with morbid obesity also had fair or poor clinical outcomes.

The incidence of posttraumatic OA is greatest in patients with articular surface incongruity or residual subluxation of the hip joint. In the study of Mears et al, 12% of patients underwent total hip arthroplasty or arthrodesis at an average of 5 years 2 months postoperatively.

Kebaish et al, in a retrospective review of 90 displaced acetabular fractures, showed superior long-term results in their patients when the articular surface was restored to within 4 mm. In a similar retrospective study, Matta et al demonstrated satisfactory clinical outcomes if the femoral head remained congruous within the weight-bearing dome and if articular surface incongruity did not exceed 3 mm. However, in a subsequent prospective study, Matta and Merritt suggested that 3 mm is probably unacceptable. He reported that an anatomic reduction was achieved in 71% of 262 acetabular fractures, with 83% of these patients having good or excellent outcomes at an average follow-up of 6 years. Of the 29% with an imperfectly reduced acetabulum, good or excellent results were obtained in 68% of cases if the defect measured 2 to 3 mm, but these positive results were found in only 50% of those with defects that measured more than 3 mm. The most clear, predictive, initial factor for a poor result was damage to the femoral head.

More recent results of Matta are in agreement with those of Helfet and Schmeling who previously noted that an articular step-off of more than 2 mm or a gap of more than 3 mm were associated with a fourfold increase in joint space narrowing at early follow-up. Alonso et al noted an 81% rate of good or excellent results in 21 patients treated with an extended iliofemoral approach, in which all cases achieved a reduction within 2 mm. Finally, Malkani et al and Hak et al used cadaver models to further support 2 mm or less as the appropriate criterion for an acceptable reduction.

Loss of reduction can also occur during the postoperative period. It is more likely in elderly patients with osteopenic bone where fractures must be adequately buttressed. The loss of accuracy of reduction and the increased incidence of intra-articular damage in the elderly population further compromise the outcomes in this population.

COMPLICATIONS

Complications following operative treatment of acetabular fractures are best divided in three groups: intraoperative, early, and late. Intraoperative complications include neurovascular injury, malreduction, articular penetration of hardware, and death. Early postoperative complications include DVT, pulmonary embolism (PE), skin necrosis, infection, loss of reduction, arthritis, and death. The late group includes heterotopic ossification (HO), chondrolysis, avascular necrosis, and posttraumatic arthrosis.

Sciatic Nerve Injury

Iatrogenic sciatic-nerve injury or worsening of a preexisting deficit is a significant problem. In our experience, patients at increased risk include those with preoperative sciatic nerve compromise and those with fracture patterns that involve the posterior wall or column. Other authors have identified patients treated via an ilioinguinal approach to be at increased risk, possibly related to indirect reduction of the posterior column with the hip flexed. The peroneal nerve division is most commonly involved. The most significant factor in reducing the incidence of iatrogenic sciatic-nerve injury appears to be the experience of the surgical team.

Letournel initially reported an 18.4% incidence of postoperative, iatrogenic, sciatic-nerve injury using the Kocher-Langenbeck approach, which he subsequently reduced to 3.3%. However, he also noted that none of his 114 patients treated with an extensile approach developed this complication. Matta initially reported a 9% incidence of iatrogenic nerve palsy, which he reduced to 3.5% after gaining further experience (3.4% of 59 extended iliofemoral approaches). The incidence of iatrogenic nerve palsy remained elevated, with an overall incidence rate of 12%, when open reduction and internal fixation (ORIF) was delayed longer than 3 weeks. The majority of these injuries involved the sciatic nerve. Alonso et al found postoperative sciatic-nerve palsy in only 1 of their 21 patients treated with an extended iliofemoral approach.

The use of intraoperative sciatic-nerve monitoring by use of SSEP remains controversial. In the studies of Helfet et al, intraoperative nerve monitoring reduced the incidence of iatrogenic sciatic nerve injury to 2%. However, more recent studies have questioned the value of intraoperative SSEPs because the monitoring has failed to demonstrate a reduction in the rate of iatrogenic nerve palsies. A high false-positive rate makes unclear the extent to which intraoperative SSEP changes predict functional outcome. Intraoperative monitoring of motor pathways with EMG allows for earlier detection of neurologic compromise and removal of noxious stimuli, and in theory, decreasing the risk of neurologic sequelae. In one of Helfet's studies, the addition of spontaneous EMG to intraoperative SSEP monitoring was superior to SSEP alone. Because of the significant learning curve that exists in the treatment of acetabular fractures, most authors agree that intraoperative monitoring may prove most beneficial among relatively less-experienced surgeons.

Superior–Gluteal Neurovascular Injury

Superior–gluteal vessel injury is difficult to diagnose and is caused by either the fracture or an iatrogenic insult during surgery. Letournel reported an incidence of 3.5% in his series. This potentially lethal occurrence is more likely to occur with severe displacement of the sciatic notch (e.g., in high-transverse fractures with marked medial rotation). Acutely, hemodynamic instability with an arterial injury must be addressed during the initial evaluation and resuscitation, and it is usually done with arteriography and embolization. However, once the bleeding has been stopped, concerns may arise with regard to muscle flap viability.

Because the extended iliofemoral approach completely detaches the gluteal muscles from the iliac wing (see Fig. 43.1), the superior gluteal vessels are the only blood supply to the flap. If they are compromised, then complete ischemic necrosis is, in theory, likely. Mears and Rubash developed their triradiate approach partly in response to reports of flap necrosis following the extended iliofemoral approach; however, it has not been established whether the superior gluteal artery is to blame in these cases. In fact, the incidence of this complication is relatively low. In over 400 acetabular fractures addressed with an extended iliofemoral approach by Letournel, Mast, Martimbeau, and Matta, no one reports abductor flap necrosis. Alonso et al did not observe this complication when they used either an extended iliofemoral or a triradiate approach in 59 cases of complex acetabular fracture.

Furthermore, massive abductor necrosis resulting from a superior–gluteal artery injury combined with an extended iliofemoral approach was postulated based on early animal and cadaver studies alone. Canine studies by Tabor et al showed that although necrosis of muscle and loss of mass occurs after the extended iliofemoral approach in the presence of gluteal vessel injury, it does not appear to be functionally significant. In their study, none of the gluteal muscle flaps sustained complete ischemic necrosis. Thus, some collateral flow to the abductor muscles must be present and appears to increase in the presence of superior–gluteal vessel injury.

Bosse et al had recommended that, to assess the integrity of the superior gluteal artery, a preoperative angiogram be completed prior to performing an extended iliofemoral approach. However, a more recent study, based on intraoperative Doppler examination by Reilly et al, demonstrated only a 2.3% incidence of absent flow on the superior gluteal artery. No evidence of abductor muscle ischemia was found in any patient of Reilly et al. This result does not support the use of routine preoperative angiography in the management of these injuries.

Deep Vein Thrombosis and Pulmonary Embolism

Letournel reported a 2.3% incidence of in-hospital death following operative fixation of acetabular fractures; the majority of the deaths occurred in patients older than 60 years. Although DVT probably plays a major role, its true incidence after an acetabular fracture is unknown. However, patients with lower extremity trauma are particularly a risk. By venography, Kudsk et al demonstrated a 60% incidence of silent DVT in patients with multiple trauma immobilized 10 days or more. In a prospective study, Geerts et al also demonstrated a 60% incidence of DVT in patients with primary lower-extremity orthopedic injuries. Letournel reported a 3% incidence of clinically evident DVT with four fatal and eight minor pulmonary emboli in a series of 569 patients, most of whom had received anticoagulant prophylaxis.

Using a combination of perioperative mechanical prophylaxis and postoperative anticoagulation prophylaxis, venous thrombosis and PE rates of less than 3% and 1% respectively, have been achieved. Improved detection of venous thromboembolism through use of magnetic resonance venography has also led to a lower incidence of PE because it has inspired aggressive treatment of asymptomatic DVTs in the pelvis and proximal thigh. However, other data suggest that magnetic resonance venography has a high false-positive rate for the detection of thrombi in the pelvic veins, and its usefulness as a screening tool is still debated. Borer et al recently reviewed 973 patients with pelvis or acetabular fractures and found that the overall rate of PE was 1.7%, and the overall rate of fatal PE was 0.31%. Routine preoperative screening for DVT had no effect on the incidence of PE in this study.

Infection

The incidence of infection has been reported to be as high as 19% but probably lies between 4% and 5%. Matta noted a 5% incidence of postoperative wound infection in 262 patients. Of 59 patients who received extended iliofemoral approaches, 5 (8.5%) developed deep infection. Mayo found a 4% overall infection rate, which was 19% in 26 patients who underwent an extended iliofemoral approach. Letournel reported 24 postoperative infections in 569 patients (4.2%) with nine superficial, ten early deep, and five delayed or late infections. Furthermore, he observed skin necrosis in 1.8% (10.2% of extended iliofemoral approaches) and hematomas in 6.7% of cases. To minimize wound problems, he advocated the use of prophylactic antibiotics, multiple suction drains in all recesses to prevent hematoma formation, surgical evacuation of hematomas, and if present, debridement of the Morel-Lavalle lesion over the greater trochanter. Other factors such as morbid obesity and burns must also be taken into consideration as they may render the patient more susceptible to infection.

Heterotopic Ossification

The most common complication following the operative fixation of acetabular fractures through the extended iliofemoral approach is HO (Fig. 43.18), with an incidence ranging from 18% to 90%. However, functional limitation in patients with HO occurs in only 5% to 10%

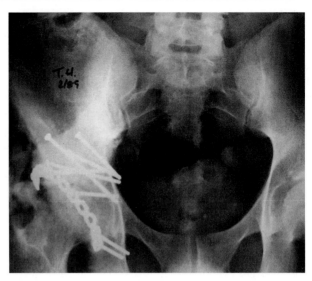

Figure 43.18. AP pelvis of patient in Figure 43.3, at 5 months after extended iliofemoral approach. Significant (Brooker grade III) HO is present in the soft tissues of the right hip.

of cases. Nevertheless, heterotopic bone formation is more common and severe with the extended iliofemoral approach because of the external surface of the iliac wing is stripped. Letournel reported its occurrence in 46% of his extended iliofemoral approaches performed within 4 months of injury; a 21% incidence was found in 635 other approaches. Prior to his use of prophylaxis, these rates were 69% and 24% respectively. Matta noted a significant loss of motion in 20% and Letournel observed severe HO (Brooker III and IV) in 35% of patients treated with this approach within 3 weeks of injury. Both indomethacin and low-dose radiation therapy (single or multiple fractions) have been shown to decrease the incidence and severity of HO in patients with acetabular fractures. However, concerns remain about the cost and the long-term effects of radiotherapy, particularly in the younger trauma population.

Despite prophylaxis with indomethacin, Alonso et al and by Johnson et al have reported rates of HO ranging from 86% to 88% in patients treated with an extended iliofemoral approach. Of these patients, Brooker class III or IV ossification was present in 14% and 13%, respectively. In the Johnson et al study, the majority of patients in the treated group had Brooker class 0-II ossification, with the untreated group having mostly Brooker III and IV ossification. A more recent study by Moed et al showed a 50% incidence of HO after extensile exposures in patients treated with indomethacin. Only one patient in the treated group had severe (Brooker III-IV) ossification. Indomethacin clearly does not eliminate the occurrence of HO, but it significantly decreases its severity.

Avascular Necrosis

The incidence of avascular necrosis (AVN) after operative treatment of acetabular fractures has generally ranged from 3% to 9%, with the majority of cases identified between 3 and 18 months after surgery. However, an increased incidence of AVN of the femoral head is found in cases presenting after 3 weeks and those associated with a posterior fracture/dislocation. In all probability, the fate of the femoral head is determined at the time of the injury.

ILLUSTRATIVE CASE FOR TECHNIQUE

A 23-year-old woman was involved in a motor vehicle accident, sustaining a right associated both-column acetabular fracture and extensive burns on the left side of her body. She also had a Morel-Lavalle degloving injury involving her right thigh and buttock and a preoperative, right, sciatic-nerve injury with a foot drop. AP pelvis and Judet view radiographs and selected CT scan images, are shown in Figure 43.19A–E. At 3 days postinjury, the patient underwent ORIF through an extended iliofemoral approach. Her postoperative course was complicated by an infection of the iliac crest wound which necessitated surgical debridement and 6 weeks of intravenous antibiotics. Postoperative radiographs are shown in Figure 43.20. Her postoperative CT scan shows congruent reduction of the hip joint (Fig. 43.21). At 5 months follow-up she has a healed acetabular fracture, is full weight bearing, and has progressively improving sciatic-nerve function.

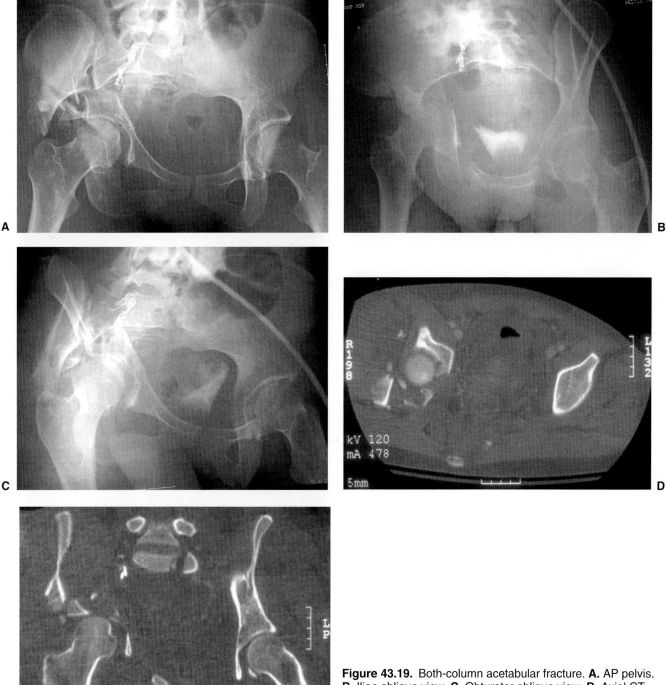

Figure 43.19. Both-column acetabular fracture. **A.** AP pelvis. **B.** Iliac oblique view. **C.** Obturator oblique view. **D.** Axial CT-scan image showing extensive comminution. **E.** Coronal CT-scan image demonstrates subluxation of the femoral head.

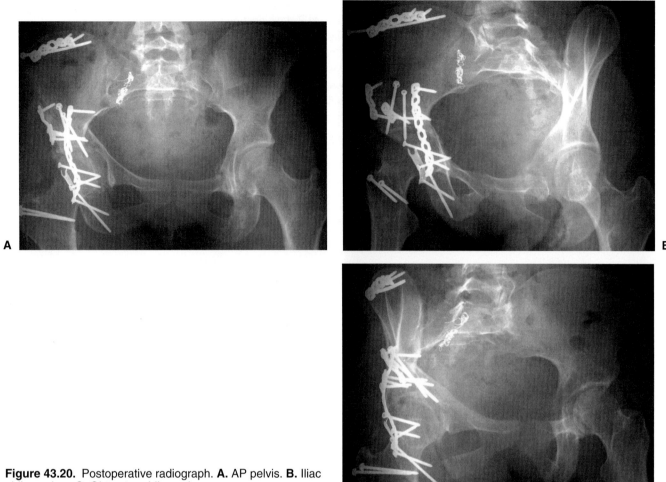

Figure 43.20. Postoperative radiograph. **A.** AP pelvis. **B.** Iliac oblique view. **C.** Obturator oblique view.

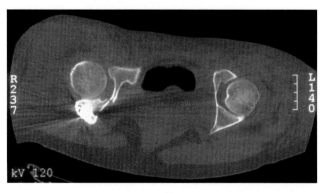

Figure 43.21. Postoperative axial CT-scan image demonstrates congruent reconstruction of the hip joint.

RECOMMENDED READING

Alonso JE, Davila R, Bradley E. Extended iliofemoral versus triradiate approaches in management of associated acetabular fractures. *Clin Orthop* 1994;305:81–87.

Baumgaertner MR, Wegner D, Booke J. SSEP monitoring during pelvic and acetabular fracture surgery. *J Orthop Trauma* 1994;8(2):127–133.

Borer DS, Starr AJ, Reinert CM, et al. The effect of screening for deep vein thrombosis on the prevalence of pulmonary embolism in patients with fractures of the pelvis or acetabulum: a review of 973 patients. *J Orthop Trauma* 2005;19(2):92–95.

Borrelli J, Goldfarb C, Catalano L, et al. Assessment of articular fragment displacement in acetabular fractures: a comparison of computerized tomography and plain radiographs. *J Orthop Trauma* 2002;16(7):449–456.

Borrelli J Jr, Koval KJ, Helfet DL. Pelvis and acetabulum. In: *Fractures in the elderly*. 1st ed. Koval KJ, Zuckerman JD, eds. Philadelphia: Lippincott-Raven Publishers; 1998:159–174.

Bosse MJ, Poka A, Reinert CM, et al. Heterotopic ossification as a complication of acetabular fracture: Prophylaxis with low-dose irradiation. *J Bone Joint Surg* 1988;70(8):1231–1237.

Bosse MJ, Poka A, Reinert CM, et al. Preoperative angiographic assessment of the superior gluteal artery in acetabular fractures requiring extensile surgical exposures. *J Orthop Trauma* 1989;2(4):303–307.

Burd TA, Lowry KJ, Anglen JO. Indomethacin compared with localized irradiation for the prevention of heterotopic ossification following surgical treatment of acetabular fractures. *J Bone Joint Surg* 2001;83(12):1783–1788.

Calder HB, Mast JW, Johnstone C. Intraoperative evoked potential monitoring in acetabular surgery. *Clin Orthop* 1994;305:160–167.

Chapman MW. Effect of surgical approaches on the blood supply to the acetabulum. Paper presented at: The First Annual International Consensus on Surgery of the Pelvis and Acetabulum; October 11–15, 1992; Pittsburgh, Pennsylvania.

Chiu FY, Chen CM, Lo WH. Surgical treatment of displaced acetabular fractures: 72 cases followed for 10 (6–14) years. *Injury* 2000;31(3):181–185.

Fishmann AJ, Greeno RA, Brooks LR, et al. Prevention of deep vein thrombosis and pulmonary embolism in acetabular and pelvic fracture surgery. *Clin Orthop* 1994;305:133–137.

Ganz R, Gill TJ, Gautier E, et al. Surgical dislocation of the adult hip: a technique with full access to the femoral head and acetabulum without the risk of avascular necrosis. *J Bone Joint Surg* 2001;83(8):1119–1124.

Garland DE. Clinical observations on fractures and heterotopic ossification in the spinal cord and traumatic brain injured populations. *Clin Orthop* 1988;233:86–101.

Garland DE, Blum CE, Waters RL. Periarticular heterotopic ossification in head-injured adults: incidence and location. *J Bone Joint Surg* 1980;62(7):1143–1146.

Geerts WH, Code KI, Jay RM, et al. A prospective study of venous thromboembolism after major trauma. *N Engl J Med* 1994;331(24):1601–1606.

Ghalambor N, Matta JM, Bernstein L. Heterotopic ossification following operative treatment of acetabular fracture: an analysis of risk factors. *Clin Orthop* 1994;305:96–105.

Haidukewych GJ, Scaduto J, Herscovici D, et al. Iatrogenic nerve injury in acetabular fracture surgery: a comparison of monitored and unmonitored procedures. *J Orthop Trauma* 2002;16(5):297–301.

Hak DJ, Olson SA, Matta JM. Diagnosis and management of closed internal degloving injuries associated with pelvic and acetabular fractures: the Morel-Lavallee lesion. *J Trauma* 1997;42(6):1046–1051.

Heeg M, Ostvogel H, Klasen H. Conservative treatment of acetabular fractures: the role of the weightbearing dome and anatomic reduction in the ultimate results. *J Trauma* 1987;27(5):555–559.

Helfet DL. Invited commentary on "incidence of sciatic nerve injury in operatively treated acetabular fractures without somatosensory evoked potential monitoring" by Middlebrooks et al. *J Orthop Trauma* 1997;11(5):329.

Helfet DL, Schmeling GJ. The management of acute, displaced complex acetabular fractures using indirect reduction techniques and limited surgical approaches. *Orthop Trans* 1991;15:833–834.

Helfet DL, Schmeling GJ. Management of complex acetabular fractures through single nonextensile exposures. *Clin Orthop* 1994;305:58–68.

Helfet DL, Schmeling GJ. Somatosensory evoked potential monitoring in the surgical treatment of acute, displaced acetabular fractures: results of a prospective study. *Clin Orthop* 1994;301:213–220.

Helfet DL, Anand N, Malkani AL, et al. Intraoperative monitoring of motor pathways during operative fixation of acute acetabular fractures. *J Orthop Trauma* 1997;11(1):2–6.

Helfet DL, Borrelli JD Jr., DiPasquale TG, et al. Stabilization of acetabular fractures in elderly patients. *J Bone Joint Surg* 1992;74(5):753–765.

Helfet DL, Hissa EA, Sergay S, et al. Somatosensory evoked potential monitoring in the surgical management of acute acetabular fractures. *J Orthop Trauma* 1991;5(2):161–166.

Johnson EE, Kay RM, Dorey FJ. Heterotopic ossification prophylaxis following operative treatment of acetabular fracture. *Clin Orthop* 1994;305:88–95.

Johnson EE, Matta JM, Mast JW, et al. Delayed reconstruction of acetabular fractures 21–120 days following injury. *Clin Orthop* 1994;305:20–30.

Judet R, Judet J, Letournel E. Fractures of the acetabulum: classification and surgical approaches for open reduction: preliminary report. *J Bone Joint Surg* 1964;46(8):1615–1646.

Kaempffe FA, Bone L, Border JR. Open reduction and internal fixation of acetabular fractures: heterotopic ossification and other complications of treatment. *J Orthop Trauma* 1991;5(4):439–445.

Kaspar S, Winemaker MJ, de VdB. Modified iliofemoral approach for major isolated acetabular revision arthroplasty. *J Arthroplasty* 2003;18(2):193–198.

Kebaish AS, Roy A, Rennie W. Displaced acetabular fractures: long-term follow-up. *J Trauma* 1991;31(11):1539–1542.

Kudsk KA, Fabian TC, Baum S, et al. Silent deep vein thrombosis in immobilized multiple trauma patients. *Am J Surg* 1989;158:515–519.

Letournel E. Acetabulum fractures: classification and management. *Clin Orthop* 1980;151:81–106.

Letournel E, Judet R. *Fractures of the acetabulum*. 2nd ed. Berlin: Springer-Verlag; 1993.

Malkani AL, Voor MJ, Rennirt G, et al. Increased peak contact stress after incongruent reduction of transverse acetabular fractures: a cadaveric model. *J Trauma* 2001;51(4):704–709.

Matta JM. Fractures of the acetabulum: accuracy of reduction and clinical results in patients managed operatively within three weeks of the injury. *J Bone Joint Surg* 1996;78(11):632–645.

Matta JM, Merritt PO. Displaced acetabular fractures. *Clin Orthop* 1988;230:83–97.

Matta JM, Anderson LM, Epstein HC, et al. Fractures of the acetabulum: a retrospective analysis. *Clin Orthop* 1986;205:241–250.

Mayo KA. Surgical approaches to the acetabulum. *Tech Orthop* 1990;4(4):24–35.

Mayo KA. Open reduction and internal fixation of fractures of the acetabulum: results in 163 fractures. *Clin Orthop* 1994;305:31–37.

Mears DC, Gordon RG. Internal fixation of acetabular fractures. *Tech Orthop* 1990;4(4):36–51.

Mears DC, Rubash HE. Extensile exposure of the pelvis. *Contemp Orthop* 1983;6:21–31.

Mears DC, Velyvis JH, Chang CP. Displaced acetabular fractures managed operatively: indicators of outcome. *Clin Orthop* 2003;407;173–186.

Middlebrooks ES, Sims SH, Kellam JF, et al. Incidence of sciatic nerve injury in operatively treated acetabular fractures without somatosensory evoked potential monitoring. *J Orthop Trauma* 1997;11(5):327–329.

Moed BR, Karges DE. Prophylactic indomethacin for the prevention of heterotopic ossification after acetabular fracture surgery in high risk patients. *J Orthop Trauma* 1994;8(1):34–39.

Moed BR, Maxey JW. The effect of indomethacin on heterotopic ossification following acetabular fracture surgery. *J Orthop Trauma* 1993;7(1):33–38.

Montgomery KD, Potter HG, Helfet DL. Magnetic resonance venography to evaluate the deep venous system of the pelvis in patients who have an acetabular fracture. *J Bone Joint Surg* 1995;77(11):1639–1649.

Montgomery KD, Potter HG, Helfet DL. The detection and management of proximal deep venous thrombosis in patients with acute acetabular fractures: a follow-up report. *J Orthop Trauma* 1997;11(5):330–336.

Moore KD, Goss K, Anglen JO. Indomethacin versus radiation therapy for prophylaxis against heterotopic ossification in acetabular fractures: a randomised, prospective study. *J Bone Joint Surg* 1998;80(2):259–263.

Pennal GF, Davidson J, Garside H. Results of treatment of acetabular fractures. *Clin Orthop* 1980;151:115–123.

Perkins R, Skirving AP. Callus formation and the rate of healing of femoral fractures in patients with head injuries. *J Bone Joint Surg* 1987;69(4):521–524.

Reilly MC, Olson SA, Tornetta P, et al. Superior gluteal artery in the extended iliofemoral approach. *J Orthop Trauma* 2000;14(4):259–263.

Reinert CM, Bosse MJ, Poka A, et al. A modified extensile exposure for the treatment of complex or malunited acetabular fractures. *J Bone Joint Surg* 1988;70(3):329–337.

Routt ML Jr, Swiontkowski MF. Operative treatment of complex acetabular fractures: combined anterior and posterior exposures during the same procedure. *J Bone Joint Surg* 1990;72(6):897–904.

Rowe CR, Lowell JD. Prognosis of fractures of the acetabulum. *J Bone Joint Surg* 1961;43(1):30–59.

Sazbon L, Najenson T, Tartakovsky M, et al. Widespread periarticular new-bone formation in long-term comatose patients. *J Bone Joint Surg* 1981;63(1):120–125.

Senegas J, Liorzou G, Yates M. Complex acetabular fractures: a transtrochanteric lateral surgical approach. *Clin Orthop* 1980;151:107–114.

Stickney JL, Helfet DL. Deep vein thrombosis prevention in orthopaedic trauma patients [abstract]. *J Orthop Trauma* 1991;5(2):227–228.

Stockle U, Hoffmann R, Sudkamp NP, et al. Treatment of complex acetabular fractures through a modified extended iliofemoral approach. *J Orthop Trauma* 2002;16(4):220–230.

Stover MD, Kellam JF. Articular fractures: principles. In: *AO principles of fracture management*. 1st ed. Ruedi TP, Murphy WM, Colton CL, et al, eds. New York: Thieme; 2000:104–119.

Stover MD, Morgan SJ, Bosse MJ, et al. Prospective comparison of contrast-enhanced computed tomography versus magnetic resonance venography in the detection of occult deep pelvic vein thrombosis in patients with pelvic and acetabular fractures. *J Orthop Trauma* 2002;16(9):613–621.

Tabor OB, Bosse MJ, Greene KG, et al. Effects of surgical approaches for acetabular fractures with associated gluteal vascular injury. *J Orthop Trauma* 1998;12(2):78–84.

Tornetta P, Reilly M, Matta J. Acetabular fracture/dislocation. *J Orthop Trauma* 2002;16(2):139–142.

Vrahas M, Gordon RG, Mears DC, et al. Intraoperative somatosensory evoked potential monitoring of pelvic and acetabular fractures. *J Orthop Trauma* 1992;6(1):50–58.

SECTION IV

Miscellaneous Topics

44

Surgical Dislocation of the Hip for Fractures of the Femoral Head

Milan K. Sen and David L. Helfet

INDICATIONS/CONTRAINDICATIONS

Fractures of the femoral head are commonly seen in association with traumatic hip dislocations (1–6). Hip dislocations are usually the result of high-energy injuries and are posterior in 82% to 94% of cases (3,7,8). They are typically the result of a dashboard injury with an axial load transmitted through the flexed hip (5,8–10). The reported incidence of femoral head fractures in patients with posterior dislocations of the hip ranges from 7% to 16% (1,4,10,11). Anterior hip dislocations are less common but can also be associated with femoral head fractures; according to one series, femoral head fractures were seen in 15% of anterior hip dislocations (12), and in another, up to 77% of anterior hip dislocations involved femoral head fractures (3).

Emergent reduction of the femoral head is undertaken to decrease the risk of avascular necrosis, which is secondary to ischemia caused by tension on the blood supply of the femoral head (13–16). This treatment is preferably done within 6 to 12 hours from the time of injury (4,13,17). Prior to attempting a closed reduction, the surgeon should exclude the presence of a concomitant femoral-neck fracture. Postreduction, an axial computed tomography (CT) scan with 2-mm cuts is necessary to ensure concentric reduction (5,18,19). Typically, open reduction and internal fixation (ORIF) is required for definitive management of the femoral head fracture (4). At the same time, the surgeon can address other associated musculoskeletal injuries, which commonly include fractures of the acetabulum as well as the femoral neck and shaft (4). As these injuries are often seen in the setting of high-energy trauma, the patient must be evaluated appropriately for associated abdominal, thoracic, and craniofacial injuries (8).

Urgent ORIF of the fragments is warranted in the presence of femoral neck fracture, postreduction hip-joint asymmetry, progressive sciatic-nerve injury, or an intra-articular fragment displacement of at least 2 mm or that renders the hip unstable (1,20–22). For

Pipkin type I or II femoral-head fractures, free or nonreduced fragments that remain after reduction must be excised or reduced and stabilized to avoid early posttraumatic arthrosis (5,11,14,17). Historically, recommendations have included excision of large fragments, including those that measure up to one third of the femoral head (2,4,5,21). However, because the entire acetabulum is involved in weight bearing (23), any fragment that is amenable to fixation should be rigidly fixed. Smaller fragments may be excised (6,14, 22–28), and avulsion fractures of the ligamentum teres can be treated conservatively.

In the past, much controversy existed with regard to the optimal surgical approach for fixation of femoral head fractures. Initially, the Kocher-Langenbeck approach was used. Through the Kocher-Langenbeck approach, surgeons can address fractures of the posterior acetabular wall but had only limited access to the articular surface of the femoral head for fracture reduction and fixation. In addition, some studies identified an increased incidence of avascular necrosis of the femoral head when Kocher-Langenbeck was used instead of the Smith-Peterson approach (26,27).

Through the Smith-Petersen method, the surgeon has access to the anterior portion of the femoral head for debridement of intra-articular debris. However, this approach does not allow complete visualization of the femoral head, nor can the surgeon address posterior acetabular-wall fractures. In addition, heterotopic ossification has been shown to be a significant risk with the anterior approach (24,27). While combined anterior and posterior approaches would improve visualization in the case of extensive femoral-head fractures, the risk of complication is increased with such extensive dissection.

In 2001, Ganz et al (29) described a technique for surgical dislocation of the hip. It involves a Kocher-Langenbeck approach with a trochanteric flip and anterior dislocation of the hip. This approach allows visualization of the entire femoral head as well as the full circumference of the acetabulum. Using this exposure, the surgeon can obtain anatomic reduction and rigid fixation of the femoral head fragments, as well as a thorough debridement of the joint, without compromising the blood supply to the femoral head (29–31).

PREOPERATIVE PLANNING

The preoperative evaluation and operating room preparation for this procedure is described in Chapter 43.

SURGERY

The patient is placed in a lateral decubitus position. A standard Kocher-Langenbeck incision is made through the skin, subcutaneous tissue, and tensor fascia lata (Fig. 44.1). The leg is then internally rotated to expose the posterior border of the gluteus medius. Unlike the approach used in total hip arthroplasty, no attempt is made to mobilize the gluteus medius or expose the piriformis tendon. Electrocautery is used to mark the gluteus medius at the posterior edge of the greater trochanter. The posterior border of gluteus medius is then traced distally to the posterior ridge of the vastus lateralis muscle, which is the point at which the deep branch of the medial femoral-circumflex artery becomes intracapsular.

A 1.5-cm thick trochanteric osteotomy, following the line traced by the electrocautery, is then performed with an oscillating saw (Fig. 44.2). To protect the deep branch of the medial femoral-circumflex artery, the surgeon is careful to work anterior to the most posterior insertion of the gluteus medius. In addition, the surgeon must keep a posterior shelf of bone just behind the osteotomy to protect the insertion of the short external rotators. At its distal end, the osteotomy should exit at the level of the vastus ridge. The vastus lateralis is then released along its posterior edge to the level of the gluteus maximus tendon, and the greater trochanter is everted anteriorly. Release of the remaining posterior fibers of gluteus medius allows free mobilization of the trochanteric segment. Additional exposure can be obtained by the elevation of the vastus lateralis and intermedius from the lateral and anterior aspects of the femur respectively. With anterior retraction of gluteus medius, the trochanteric

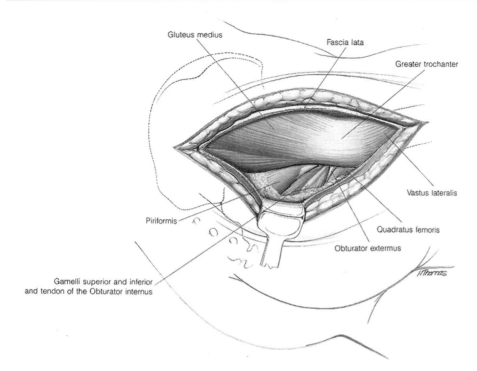

Figure 44.1. Incision and division of the tensor fascia lata.

fragment, and vastus lateralis, the tendon of the piriformis and the gluteus minimus muscle should be visible. The gluteus minimus is then carefully elevated off of the hip capsule. Gentle flexion and external rotation of the hip allows visualization of the anterior, superior, and posterosuperior hip capsule.

Attention must be paid at all times to the position and location of the sciatic nerve as it passes inferior to the piriformis tendon. Flexion of the knee releases some of the tension on

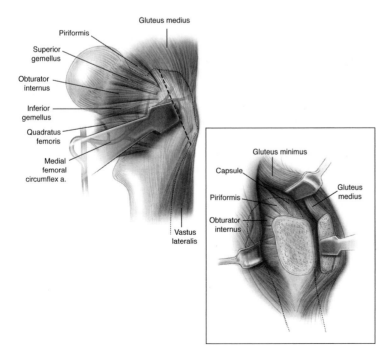

Figure 44.2. A. Sliding trochanteric osteotomy. **B.** Retraction of trochanter, gluteus medius, and gluteus minimus with exposure of joint capsule.

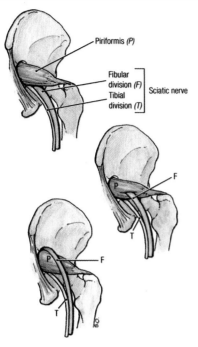

Figure 44.3. Variations in relationship of the sciatic nerve to the piriformis muscle. (From Agur AMR, Lee MJ. In: Kelly PJ, ed. *Grant's atlas of anatomy*, 10th ed. Philadelphia: Lippincott Williams & Wilkins; 1999:329, with permission.)

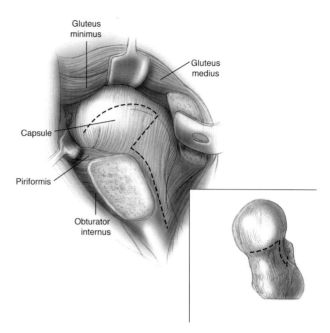

Figure 44.4. Outline of capsular incision.

the nerve. In 12.7% of individuals, the peroneal branch of the sciatic nerve passes either through the piriformis or superior to it (Fig. 44.3) (32). In these individuals, the piriformis tendon should be released to prevent stretching of the nerve during dislocation of the hip. To protect the ascending branch of the medial femoral-circumflex artery, the tendon should be released 1.5 cm from its insertion rather then at its attachment to the femur.

The incision of the capsule should be initiated on its anterolateral surface parallel to the long axis of the neck. At the base of the neck, the incision curves anteriorly and inferiorly along the reflection of the anterior capsule (Fig. 44.4). The main branch of the medial femoral- circumflex artery lies superior and posterior to the lesser trochanter; therefore, to avoid injury, the capsular incision must remain anterior to the trochanter. The proximal end of the anterolateral capsular incision is extended to the acetabular rim. It then curves posteriorly, remaining parallel to the labrum, until the surgeon encounters the retracted piriformis tendon. Care must be taken not to damage the labrum when doing the capsulotomy.

With flexion and external rotation, the hip can now be dislocated anteriorly. The leg is placed in a sterile bag over the front of the table (Fig. 44.5). This positioning allows visualization of the entire femoral head (Fig. 44.6). It also allows for inspection of the labrum, and with carefully placed retractors, the entire articular surface of the acetabulum (Fig. 44.7).

At the point when visualization is optimized, the surgeon may do a thorough irrigation and debridement of the femoral head and acetabulum. The labrum and articular surfaces should be inspected. Small comminuted fragments that are not amenable to fixation may be excised. If a stump of the ligamentum teres remains attached to the femoral head, or if it has avulsed a small fragment of the head, it is also excised.

Sizable fragments of the femoral head should be fixed (Fig. 44.8). The aim of fixation is to achieve rigid subarticular fixation while leaving a smooth articular surface on the femoral head. Common strategies include burying pins or screws or capturing the fragment by lag effect from a nonarticular entry point (25). Methods of fixation have included countersinking screws (33), using headless screws (34,35), utilizing bioabsorbable pins or screws (36), or completing suture fixation (21,22,27). Screws with threaded washers are contraindicated because a significant number have backed out of the hardware (26).

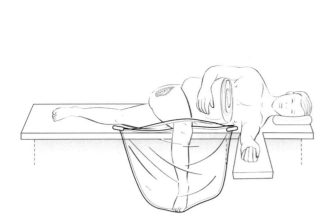

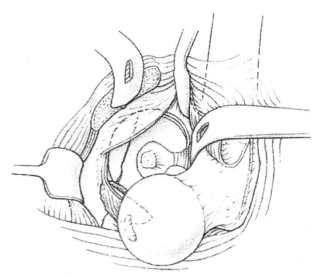

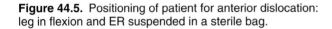

Figure 44.5. Positioning of patient for anterior dislocation: leg in flexion and ER suspended in a sterile bag.

Figure 44.6. Dislocation of the hip with exposure of the articular surface of the acetabulum.

Headless screws provide less compressive force across the cancellous bone of the femoral head than do standard, small, fragment screws (34). Therefore, we prefer to countersink bioabsorbable or small fragment screws with heads (Synthes, Paoli, PA) into the fragment. We often augment the fracture fixation with the addition of a lag screw that is entered from nonarticular regions.

While the articular surfaces are exposed, regular irrigation with saline can be used to prevent desiccation. Prior to reduction of the hip, a 2.0-mm drill hole is made in the femoral head to document preservation of the blood supply. Previous studies have shown a high correlation between adequate blood supply and the presence of a viable head (see Fig. 44.8) (37). Laser Doppler flowmetry is another proven method of documenting the vascularity of the femoral head prior to reduction (30). The hip is then reduced with manual traction on the flexed knee followed by internal rotation and extension.

The wound is irrigated with 3 L of normal saline, and meticulous hemostasis is achieved. The capsulotomy is then closed with 1-0 vicryl suture. The greater trochanter is secured us-

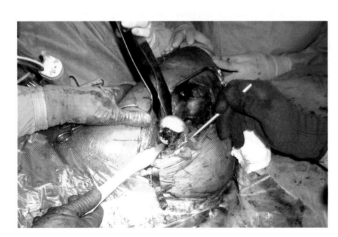

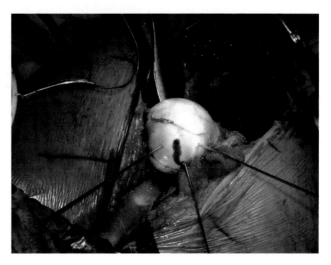

Figure 44.7. Dislocation of hip with exposure of femoral head and Pipkin fragment.

Figure 44.8. Dislocation of femoral head and temporary fixation of Pipkin fragment with Kirschner (K) wires. Active bleeding from the dislocated femoral head demonstrates that the blood supply remains intact.

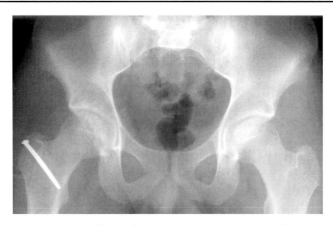

Figure 44.9. Postoperative x-ray illustrating placement of screws for fixation of trochanteric osteotomy.

ing two 3.5-mm cortical screws directed toward the lesser trochanter. Two large Hemovac drains are placed deep to the tensor fascia lata.

POSTOPERATIVE MANAGEMENT

Postoperatively, the patient is mobilized immediately. Crutch ambulation training with touch-down weight bearing of 20 pounds is instituted for 6 to 8 weeks. Strengthening and motion exercises are instituted and encouraged (22,38).

X-rays and a CT scan are taken postoperatively. These images are used to confirm fracture reduction, hardware placement, and concentric hip reduction (Fig. 44.9).

Drains are not discontinued until output has tapered to 10 to 20 ml per 8-hour shift. In the hospital, patients are maintained on intravenous cefazolin for 48 to 72 hours. Our postoperative anticoagulation regimen includes 6 weeks of warfarin in conjunction with compression boots.

Heterotopic ossification prophylaxis is also mandatory (39). It is preferably accompanied with oral indomethacin SR at a dose of 75 mg daily for 6 weeks.

RESULTS

A recent study by Gardner et al (40) looked at three patients with Pipkin II fractures of the femoral head. All three were treated with ORIF of the femoral head fractures through the surgical dislocation technique. Follow-up ranged from 11 to 24 months. At the time of their latest follow-up, all three patients were ambulating without difficulty and without a limp. None have pain with ambulation or range of motion of the hip, nor do they have any radiographic evidence of avascular necrosis or degenerative changes.

COMPLICATIONS

Avascular Necrosis

The most significant potential complication related to the hip-dislocation approach to fracture fixation is avascular necrosis of the femoral head. The femoral head receives the majority of its blood supply from the deep branch of the medial femoral-circumflex artery (4,41–45). This branch of the medial femoral circumflex artery (MFCA) is located at the proximal border of the quadratus femoris muscle. It then courses superiorly, crossing anterior to the conjoined tendon of the obturator internus and the superior and inferior gemelli

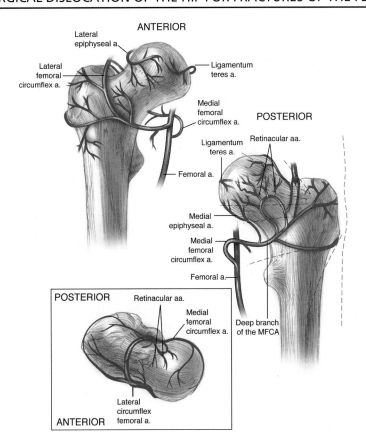

Figure 44.10. Blood supply to the femoral head and its relationship to the short external rotators.

muscles (Fig. 44.10). It then perforates the hip capsule to supply the femoral head. Preservation of the quadratus femoris and the short external rotators of the hip protect this branch of the medial femoral-circumflex artery, maintaining the critical blood supply to the femoral head.

Avascular necrosis is a well-described consequence of traumatic dislocation of the hip; incidences range from 8.3% to 26.3% of those treated for traumatic hip dislocation (8,10,14). When the dislocation is endured longer than 6 hours, the risk of avascular necrosis greatly increases (13). The Ganz approach calls for use of a controlled anterior dislocation of the hip for a short duration, minimizing the risk of injury to the nutrient vessels. Ganz et al (29) looked at 213 patients treated with surgical dislocation of the hip for a variety of pathologies. At 2 to 7 years follow-up, no evidence of avascular necrosis of the hip has been found.

In additional studies, Ganz et al (30) used a high-powered, laser, Doppler flowmeter to evaluate the changes in blood flow to the head. They found that the dislocation resulted in some impairment of blood flow, but it reversed completely with reduction of the hip. They also found that the anterior capsulotomy used in this approach did not alter the blood flow to the head despite the disruption of the anterior intracapsular and extracapsular anastomoses and the capsular branches of the lateral circumflex artery. This result indicates that the vessels on the anterior aspect of the femoral head are not critical to circulation to the femoral head. Rather, preservation of the posterior extracapsular vessels is the paramount concern.

Neurologic Injury

Neurapraxia of the sciatic nerve was seen in two patients in the study of Ganz et al (29). Both patients recovered within 6 months. Of note, both of these patients had undergone previous surgery, and scarring around the sciatic nerve is thought to have contributed to the neurapraxia.

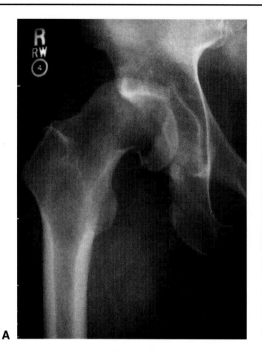
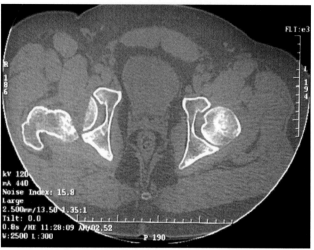

A   B

Figure 44.11. Anteroposterior (AP) pelvis radiograph **(A)** and axial CT scan image **(B)** show fracture dislocation of the femoral head with large Pipkin-II fragment.

Trochanteric Nonunion

Three patients (1.4%) required a second operation for failure of trochanteric fixation. These results compare favorably with the 98% union rate described in the literature for the extended, trochanteric, slide osteotomy in total hip arthroplasty (46).

Heterotopic Ossification

The incidence of heterotopic ossification at one year was 37%. Most of the ectopic bone formation occurred at the tip of the greater trochanter, and 86% were classified as Brooker grade I. Two patients required excision of the ectopic bone to improve their range of motion.

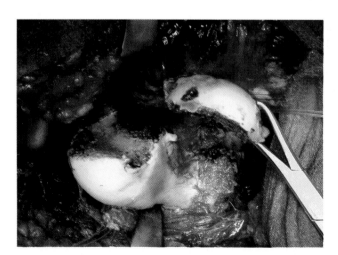

Figure 44.12. Intraoperative photo of femoral head fracture.

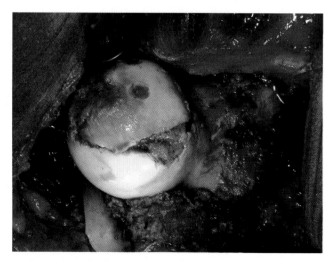

Figure 44.13. ORIF of femoral head fracture. The two bioabsorbable screws are well visualized.

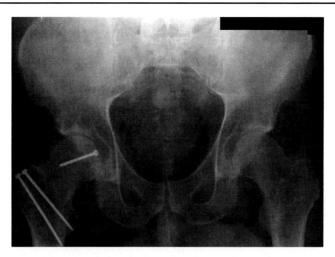

Figure 44.14. Postoperative AP radiograph.

Cosmesis

Seven of the patients in the Ganz et al study had "saddleback" deformities of the subcutaneous fat due to insufficiency of the subcutaneous sutures. Five of these patients underwent plastic surgery to improve the cosmetic appearance.

ILLUSTRATIVE CASE FOR TECHNIQUE

A 32-year-old male presents 36 hours after a motor vehicle accident. He was riding a bicycle and was struck by a sports utility vehicle traveling at approximately 45 mph. He rolled over the hood of the vehicle and onto the ground. He was initially evaluated at an outside hospital and found to have an isolated, right, femoral-head fracture dislocation. At the time of presentation, the hip remained hinged on the posterosuperior wall of the acetabulum (Fig. 44.11).

He was taken to the operating room for ORIF of the femoral head. A surgical dislocation was performed. He was found to have a sagittal split involving one third of the weight-bearing surface of the femoral head (Fig. 44.12). The incarcerated fragment remained attached to the ligamentum teres. This surgical approach provided excellent visualization of the femoral head and allowed for anatomic reduction of the Pipkin fragment. Fixation was obtained using a 3.5-mm cortical screw in the fovea and two countersunk bioabsorbable screws placed anteriorly and posteriorly (Fig. 44.13).

The patient did well postoperatively. The x-ray demonstrates excellent reduction of the femoral-head fracture and a congruent hip joint (Fig. 44.14). At the 3-month follow-up, the fracture was healed, and the patient was full weight bearing on the affected leg. At the 6-month follow-up, the patient remained pain free with excellent range of motion in his hip. No radiographic evidence of avascular necrosis was found at latest follow-up.

RECOMMENDED READINGS

1. Brumback RJ, Kenzora JE, Levitt LE, et al. Fractures of the femoral head. *Hip* 1987:181–206.
2. Butler JE. Pipkin type-II fractures of the femoral head. *J Bone Joint Surg* 1981;63(8):1292–1296.
3. DeLee JC, Evans JA, Thomas J. Anterior dislocation of the hip and associated femoral-head fractures. *J Bone Joint Surg* 1980;62(6):960–964.
4. Epstein HC. Posterior fracture-dislocations of the hip: long-term follow-up. *J Bone Joint Surg* 1974;56(6):1103–1127.
5. Epstein HC, Wiss DA, Cozen L. Posterior fracture dislocation of the hip with fractures of the femoral head. *Clin Orthop* 1985;201:9–17.
6. Mostafa MM. Femoral head fractures. *Int Orthop* 2001;25(1):51–54.
7. Thompson VPE. Traumatic dislocation of the hip. *J Bone Joint Surg* 1951;33(3):746–778.
8. Yang RS, Tsuang YH, Hang YS, et al. Traumatic dislocation of the hip. *Clin Orthop* 1991;265:218–227.

9. Alonso JE, Volgas DA, Giordano V, et al. A review of the treatment of hip dislocations associated with acetabular fractures. *Clin Orthop* 2000;377:32–43.

10. Brav EA. Traumatic dislocation of the hip: army experience over a twelve-year period. *J Bone Joint Surg* 1962;44:1115–1134.

11. Lang-Stevenson A, Getty CJ. The Pipkin fracture-dislocation of the hip. *Injury* 1987;18(4):264–269.

12. Epstein HC, Harvey JPJ. Traumatic anterior dislocations of the hip: management and results. An analysis of fifty-five cases. *J Bone Joint Surg* 1972;54(7):1561–1562.

13. Hougaard K, Thomsen PB. Traumatic posterior dislocation of the hip: prognostic factors influencing the incidence of avascular necrosis of the femoral head. *Arch Orthop Trauma Surg* 1986;106(1):32–35.

14. Sahin V, Karakas ES, Aksu S, et al. Traumatic dislocation and fracture-dislocation of the hip: a long-term follow-up study. *J Trauma* 2003;54(3):520–529.

15. Tornetta P. Hip dislocations and fractures of the femoral head. In: Rockwood CA, Bucholz RW, Heckman JD, et al, eds, *Rockwood and Green's fractures in adults*. 5th ed. Philadelphia: Lippincott Williams & Wilkins; 2001.

16. Yue JJ, Wilber JH, Lipuma JP, et al. Posterior hip dislocations: a cadaveric angiographic study. *J Orthop Trauma* 1996;10(7):447–454.

17. Jaskulka RA, Fischer G, Fenzl G. Dislocation and fracture-dislocation of the hip. *J Bone Joint Surg* 1991;73(3):465–469.

18. Hougaard K, Lindequist S, Nielsen LB. Computerised tomography after posterior dislocation of the hip. *J Bone Joint Surg* 1987;69(4):556–557.

19. Ordway CB, Xeller CF. Transverse computerized axial tomography of patients with posterior dislocation of the hip. *J Trauma* 1984;24(1):76–79.

20. Pape HC, Rice J, Wolfram K, et al. Hip dislocation in patients with multiple injuries: a follow-up investigation. *Clin Orthop* 2000;377:99–105.

21. Roeder LF Jr, DeLee JC. Femoral head fractures associated with posterior hip dislocation. *Clin Orthop* 1980;147:121–130.

22. Swiontkowski MF. Intracapsular hip fractures. In: Browner B, Jupiter J, Levine A, et al, eds, *Skeletal trauma: basic science, management, and reconstruction*. 3rd ed. Philadelphia: Saunders; 2003.

23. Greenwald AS, Haynes DW. Weight-bearing areas in the human hip joint. *J Bone Joint Surg* 1972;54(1):157–163.

24. Marchetti ME, Steinberg GG, Coumas JM. Intermediate-term experience of Pipkin fracture-dislocations of the hip. *J Orthop Trauma* 1996;10(7):455–461.

25. Sarmiento A, Laird CA. Posterior fracture-dislocation of the femoral head: report of a case. *Clin Orthop* 1973;92:143–146.

26. Stannard JP, Harris HW, Volgas DA, et al. Functional outcome of patients with femoral head fractures associated with hip dislocations. *Clin Orthop* 2000;377:44–56.

27. Swiontkowski MF, Thorpe M, Seiler JG, et al. Operative management of displaced femoral head fractures: case-matched comparison of anterior versus posterior approaches for Pipkin I and Pipkin II fractures. *J Orthop Trauma* 1992;6(4):437–442.

28. Yoon TR, Rowe SM, Chung JY, et al. Clinical and radiographic outcome of femoral head fractures: 30 patients followed for 3–10 years. *Acta Orthop Scand* 2001;72(4):348–353.

29. Ganz R, Gill TJ, Gautier E, et al. Surgical dislocation of the adult hip: a technique with full access to the femoral head and acetabulum without the risk of avascular necrosis. *J Bone Joint Surg* 2001;83(8):1119–1124.

30. Notzli HP, Siebenrock KA, Hempfing A, et al. Perfusion of the femoral head during surgical dislocation of the hip: monitoring by laser Doppler flowmetry. *J Bone Joint Surg* 2002;84(2):300–304.

31. Siebenrock KA, Gautier E, Woo AK, et al. Surgical dislocation of the femoral head for joint debridement and accurate reduction of fractures of the acetabulum. *J Orthop Trauma* 2002;16(8):543–552.

32. Agur AMR, Lee MJ. In: Kelly PJ, ed, *Grant's atlas of anatomy*. 10th ed. Philadelphia: Lippincott Williams & Wilkins; 1999:329.

33. Swiontkowski MFT. Operative management of femoral head fractures. *Orthop Trans* 1989;13:51.

34. Lange RH, Engber WD, Clancy WG. Expanding applications for the Herbert scaphoid screw. *Orthopedics* 1986;9(10):1393–1397.

35. Murray P, McGee HM, Mulvihill N. Fixation of femoral head fractures using the Herbert screw. *Injury* 1988;19(3):220–221.

36. Jukkala-Partio K, Partio EK, Hirvensalo E, et al. Absorbable fixation of femoral head fractures: a prospective study of six cases. *Ann Chir Gynaecol* 1998;87(1):44–48.

37. Gill TJ, Sledge JB, Ekkernkamp A, et al. Intraoperative assessment of femoral head vascularity after femoral neck fracture. *J Orthop Trauma* 1998;12(7):474–478.

38. Salter RB, Simmonds DF, Malcolm BW, et al. The biological effect of continuous passive motion on the healing of full-thickness defects in articular cartilage: an experimental investigation in the rabbit. *J Bone Joint Surg* 1980;62(8):1232–1251.

39. Burd TA, Lowry KJ, Anglen JO. Indomethacin compared with localized irradiation for the prevention of heterotopic ossification following surgical treatment of acetabular fractures. *J Bone Joint Surg* 2001;83(12):1783–1788.

40. Gardner MJ, Suk M, Pearle A, et al. Surgical dislocation of the hip for fractures of the femoral head. *J Orthop Trauma* 2005. In press.

41. Chung SM. The arterial supply of the developing proximal end of the human femur. *J Bone Joint Surg* 1976;58(7):961–970.

42. Crock HV. An atlas of the arterial supply of the head and neck of the femur in man. *Clin Orthop* 1980;152:17–27.

43. Gautier E, Ganz K, Krugel N, et al. Anatomy of the medial femoral circumflex artery and its surgical implications. *J Bone Joint Surg* 2000;82(5):679–683.

44. Sevitt S, Thompson RG. The distribution and anastomoses of arteries supplying the head and neck of the femur. *J Bone Joint Surg* 1965;47(3):560–573.

45. Trueta JHM. The normal vascular anatomy of the femoral head in adult man. *J Bone Joint Surg* 1953;35(3):442–460.

46. Chen WM, McAuley JP, Engh CA, et al. Extended slide trochanteric osteotomy for revision total hip arthroplasty. *J Bone Joint Surg* 2000;82(9):1215–1219.

45

Periprosthetic Femur Fractures

Richard F. Kyle, Jonathan C. Haas, and Patrick Yoon

PERIPROSTHETIC FRACTURE FOLLOWING TOTAL HIP ARTHROPLASTY

Indications/Contraindications

Periprosthetic fractures around total joint replacements are becoming an increasingly common problem encountered by orthopedic surgeons. Not only is the number of total joint replacements performed increasing annually, but the expected longevity of patients who undergo these procedures is also increasing. These fractures may occur intraoperatively or postoperatively. The incidence of periprosthetic hip fractures is generally higher in uncemented (4.1% to 27.8%) than in cemented (<3%) prosthesis. Risk factors for intraoperative fractures include rheumatoid arthritis, cementless arthroplasty, metabolic bone disease, complex deformity, and revision surgery. Risk factors for postoperative fractures include weakened bone secondary to osteoporosis, stress risers, empty screw holes, eccentric reaming, cortical perforations, stem tip protrusion, loose implants, and osteolysis.

While periprosthetic fractures may occur on either the acetabular or femoral side, most of the literature discusses fractures on the femoral side of a total hip arthroplasty (THA) or around the femoral side of a total knee arthroplasty (TKA). In the first section of the chapter, we describe techniques for repairing periprosthetic fractures adjacent to the femoral component of a total hip arthroplasty. We address fractures associated with TKA in the second part of this chapter.

Several classification schemes are useful in guiding treatment of THA. Johannson classified periprosthetic femur fractures into type I (proximal to the stem tip), type II (around the tip), and type III (distal to the tip) categories. In a primary cementless implant the majority of intraoperative fractures are type I with the minority being types II or III. Duncan and Masri's classification roughly correlates with Johannson's classification: type A (peritrochanteric), B (tip), and C (distal) fractures. The incidence of these is reported to be 4%, 87%, and 9% respectively for types A, B, and C. Type A fractures are subdivided into A(G) (greater trochanteric) and A(L) (lesser trochanteric) fractures, which are generally treated nonoperatively. B fractures are divided among B1 (stable prosthesis, 18%), B2 (loose prosthesis requiring stem revision, 45%), and B3 (marked osteopenia, 37%). Types I and A are the most common intraoperative fracture and can be treated with cerclage wiring. Types II and B generally require a plate, allograft, and cables. Types III and C can generally be treated without regard to the prosthesis if they are sufficiently distal.

Prevention of periprosthetic fractures includes correcting risk factors that are reversible; avoiding intraoperative techniques that create stress risers, such as eccentric reaming; performing routine surveillance x-rays to check for osteolysis; and revising prostheses when progressive osteolysis is presented. It also calls for aggressive treatment for patients with osteoporosis.

Our main goal is to restore the patient to prefracture level of function. In general, surgical treatment is preferred except for the high-risk surgical patient. Although nonoperative treatment is associated with high union rates, it exposes the patient to risks associated with prolonged bed rest and greater rates of malunion. Nonoperative treatment may be appropriate for the stable type I or A fracture noted postoperatively or perhaps for a minimally displaced type II or III fracture.

The vast majority of displaced fractures are treated operatively. Treatment options for an intact prosthesis include cerclage wiring in high fractures and the use of plating and cortical struts in low fractures. Occasionally, only wires or cables are used for a very long spiral fracture that is minimally displaced. In general, however, some combination of cables, plates, and strut allografts is used. We have found that either two struts or a combination of one plate and one strut have proven to be the strongest constructs tested in torsion and bending. Any defects or stress risers created (tip of stem, cortical perforation, etc.) should be bypassed by a strut or plate by at least two cortical diameters because this strategy restores 84% of the original strength of the bone. With loose implants, treatment options include removal of the implant while maintaining as much bone stock as possible. A loose implant should then be revised with a longer stem and cortical strut grafts.

Acetabular fractures during or after THA are uncommon. Lewallen et al classified these into type I (stable cup) and type II (unstable cup). Type I fractures may be treated nonoperatively with good healing rates through use of a brace or spica cast. Type II fractures should be treated with cup revision.

Preoperative Planning

Adequate radiographs are needed to identify the extent of the fracture, stability of the prosthesis, and the quality of the bone. The standard radiographs include a low anteroposterior (AP) pelvis x-ray centered about the pubis, as well as an AP and frog or cross-table lateral of the affected limb. If acetabular osteolysis is seen or suspected, then Judet films should be obtained to assess the area and extent of bony peri-acetabular deficiency. In some patients, additional information can be gained from scanograms to assess leg lengths. Identification of prosthesis type is necessary if special femoral-extraction devices may be needed. The preoperative assessment also includes range-of-motion and neurovascular statuses so that any preoperative deficiencies and the patient's leg lengths can be documented. If a plate is to be used, we template the fracture and determine the length of side plate needed to bridge the fracture site adequately; we will always err on using a plate that is too long. Occasionally a plate must span the entire length of the femur.

Previous operative reports are important so the surgeon can identify the surgical approach used and the type, size, and modularity of the prosthesis implanted. Preoperative templating is necessary to assess the length and diameter of the prosthesis when revision arthroplasty is needed. As a general rule, the surgeon should make sure that all stress risers, such as cortical windows and holes in the diaphysis, are bypassed with a stem that is at least two times the shaft diameter. Areas of transition between stem tips and plates or stem tips and stem tips should be avoided. Cortical strut grafts over holes, windows, fractures, and in areas of transition are beneficial. Most nonmodular stems are less than 265 cm, so the use of longer modular stems may be needed. The stem diameter should be large enough so the fit helps splint the fracture and allows an adequate surface for bone ingrowth and good rotational control of the prosthesis. Preoperative templating is crucial because it allows the surgeon to anticipate the need for all implants.

If infection is suspected, a complete blood count (CBC), differential C-reactive protein (CRP), and erythrocyte sedimentation rate (ESR) should be obtained. If any of these parameters are elevated, then a hip aspiration under fluoroscopic guidance should be preformed. Because revision surgery generally entails a relatively high blood loss, patients should be typed and cross matched for blood replacement in case it is needed. We do not routinely have patients predonate blood and frequently use a cell saver.

Surgery

Patient Positioning.   Because surgery may take several hours, a Foley catheter is routinely inserted, particularly if an epidural anesthetic is administered. The patient is placed in the lateral decubitus position, affected side up, on a radiolucent table with the affected hip and leg draped free. A lateral positioner is used, and all bony prominences are padded. The wider posterior portion of the holder abuts the posterior iliac crest, and the narrow anterior portion should come up directly against the anterior–superior iliac spine. The common error is to place the anterior positioner too distal, impeding full-hip flexion. The knees and the feet are lined up to use as a gauge for leg lengths. The entire lower extremity, hip, and pelvis are prepped and draped.

Technique

Nondisplaced Intraoperative Proximal Femur (Type I)   As prophylaxis against propagating a crack in the proximal femur, a Verbrugge clamp is placed around the proximal femur just prior to surgeon impact on an uncemented femoral stem. Should a fracture occur, it will likely be nondisplaced, and evidence has shown that it is unlikely to influence the long-term outcome of the joint replacement. When the fracture is recognized, one or more cerclage wires or cables are sufficient. If it is displaced, then it is reduced and cerclage wires are used (Fig. 45.1).

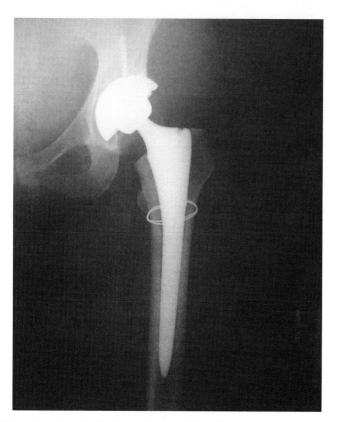

Figure 45.1.   Type I periprosthetic femur fracture (nondisplaced calcar crack) treated with a single Luque wire.

Fracture at the Tip of the Femoral Component (Type II with Loose Prosthesis)
If the prosthesis is loose in a femoral tip fracture (Fig. 45.2), a long-stem revision with allograft struts is used to bridge the tip of the stem and fracture site. Cortical perforations are used as needed to extract the old prosthesis.

The surgeon begins with the proximal part of the incision to minimize blood loss and define the plane between the iliotibial band and the vastus lateralis. This incision can be difficult to make due to scarring, but developing this layer will allow easier placement of retractors and facilitate closure. Electrocautery is used while the surgeon works to stay on bone until the neck of the prosthesis is identified.

Once joint fluid is encountered, it is sent off for culture and gram stain. Multiple fluid and tissue cultures are obtained and sent to the laboratory with every hip revision surgery. Infection can be a cause of prosthesis loosening and subsequent fracture.

Usually abundant pseudocapsule is excised until the acetabulum can be adequately visualized. The proximal femur is skeletonized to allow sufficient mobility for stem extraction and adequate acetabular exposure. A saw or osteotome is used to remove any bone from the greater trochanter that overhangs the lateral aspect of the prosthesis. Failing to remove the bone will result in a greater trochanteric fracture when the stem is removed.

Once the stem is removed, the femoral fracture is addressed. The goal is to reduce and stabilize the fracture. The midlateral incision should be extended distally past the fracture. The vastus split is facilitated by blunt dissection in line with its fibers, and care is taken to clamp and cauterize the perforators. The fracture is identified and reduced with minimal stripping, and multiple Verbrugge clamps are carefully placed. The femur may then be reamed and broached, and the femoral component tried at this time. The legs are assessed for length and stability.

Prior to dislocating the hip, the surgeon first places a suture in the skin just superior to the incision and a second marker stitch in the greater trochanter. Second, both knees and feet are aligned and checked for any length discrepancies. Third, with the trial component in place, the knee is flexed so the surgeon can check for quadriceps tightness. Occasionally, fluoroscopy is used to check the fracture reduction, the stem for length, and the percentage of canal fill. One or two cortical struts should be contoured to the femur through use of a

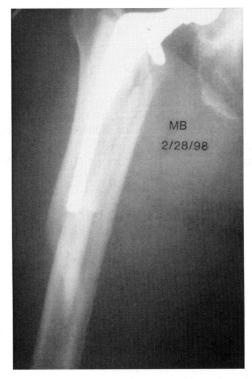

Figure 45.2. Type II periprosthetic femur fracture originating around the tip of a loose stem.

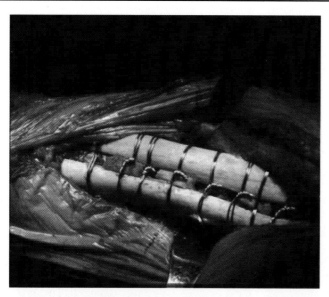

Figure 45.3. Allograft cortical struts around the proximal femur secured with multiple Luque wires.

high-speed burr. The goal is to minimize the concavity of the graft so the fit between the graft and the femur is intimate. Wires or cables are passed first before the struts to facilitate ease of passing the wires. With the femoral trial still in place, a cortical strut graft is applied laterally to the anterior on the femur, and if needed, it is applied medially to the anterior on the femur; the graft location is dependent on the fracture pattern and the quality of bone. The allograft struts are secured with multiple wires or cables spaced at least 3.0 cm apart (Fig. 45.3). The strut should extend distal to the fracture at least 2.5 times the shaft diameter to enhance fixation and prevent propagation of the fracture. Securing the cortical struts will help prevent fracture displacement and propagation with seating of the final implant. In most cases, it is best to reduce the fracture and use the long-stem implant like an intramedullary nail to fix the fracture. Bone struts are applied after implanting to reinforce fracture fixation and rebuild bone stock. We prefer Luque wires because they are relatively inexpensive and will not cut through the bone like cables. The twist of the Luque wire should be directed posteriorly where its prominence cannot be felt. If there are risk factors for delayed union or nonunion, bank bone graft is placed at the fracture site. The final prosthesis is then seated. (Fig. 45.4), and leg lengths and stability are once again checked.

A Hemovac drain is placed deep and the incision closed. Dressings are placed with compression around the thigh. Thromboembolic devices and sequential compression devises are placed in the operation room. An abduction pillow is used. Postoperatively, AP pelvic as well as AP and lateral femur films are obtained.

Fracture Distal to the Femoral Component (Type III with Stable Prosthesis)
After the prep and drape, as described above, is complete, a standard lateral approach to the femur is performed on a type III fracture with stable prosthesis (Fig. 45.5). The vastus lateralis is dissected in line with the skin incision, and the perforating vessels are identified. The fracture site is identified while great care is taken to minimize stripping. The medial soft tissues must not be disturbed. The fracture is reduced and provisionally stabilized with clamps. For most fractures distal to an implant, plate fixation is preferred. In very distal fractures, a dynamic condylar screw and side plate are often chosen.

Using the 95-degree guide (Fig. 45.6), the guide pin for the screw is drilled into the lateral condyle such that it is parallel with the trochlear notch in the axial plane (Fig. 45.7) and parallel with the distal tips of the femoral condyles in the AP plane. This guide wire is 2 cm proximal to the distal ends of the condyles and slightly anterior to the midline on the lateral view (Fig. 45.8). The guide pin is overdrilled with the cannulated reamer and the screw is inserted. To keep the side plate aligned with the lateral cortex, a Kirschner (K) wire is placed into a screw hole proximally during the early part of this process. The side plate is

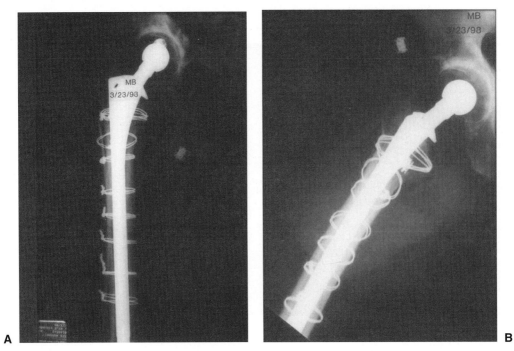

Figure 45.4. AP **(A)** and lateral **(B)** radiographs of final revision construct with long-stem implant, struts, and multiple Luque wires.

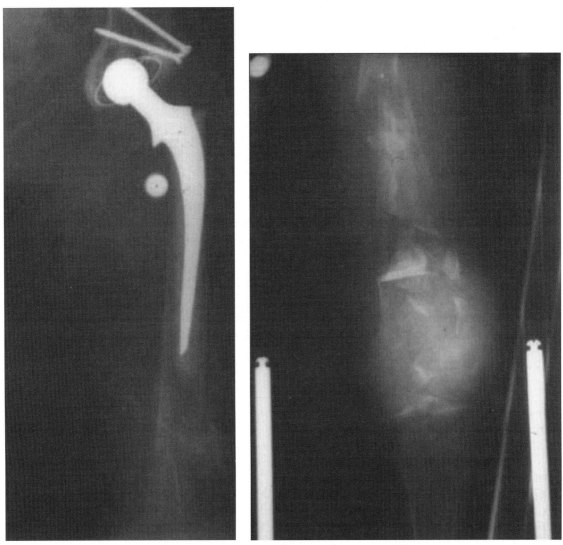

Figure 45.5. Proximal AP **(A)** and distal AP **(B)** radiographs of a type III (distal fracture with a stable prosthesis).

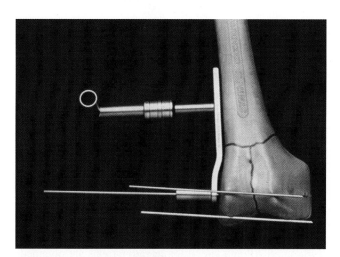

Figure 45.6. The 95-degree guide is placed on the lateral distal femur with one pin placed in front of the condyles and one pin placed at the distal tips of the condyles. This indicates the correct guide pin direction in two planes.

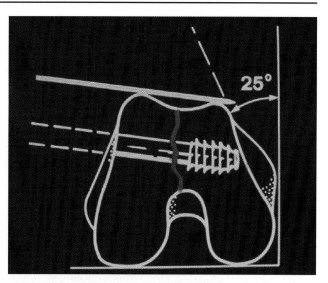

Figure 45.7. The anterior pin indicates the orientation of the trochlear notch. Central guide pin and screw placement should parallel this pin.

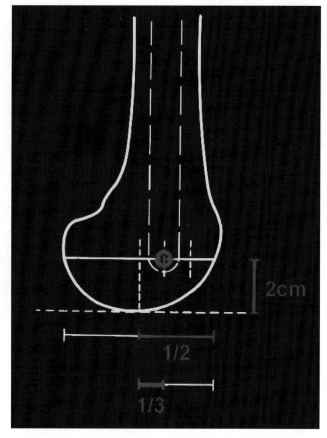

Figure 45.8. In the lateral view, the guide pin should be 2 cm proximal to the distal tips of the condyles and slightly anterior to midline on the lateral fluoroscopic view.

attached and the shaft screws are inserted distal to the fracture site. An allograft strut is applied to the anterior cortex with minimal stripping and held in place with cerclage wires rather than cables. Proximal to the fracture site, these cables will also hold the end of the side plate onto the bone (Fig. 45.9).

These fractures can also be treated with a locking plate through a bridge technique or indirect reduction to avoid stripping of the comminuted fracture fragments. It is amenable for those situations where the stem is solidly fixed and one simply needs to fix the fracture site (Fig. 45.10). The goal is to place multiple screws in the distal fragment to maximize purchase in the short distal fragment with fixation proximally through use of either cables or unicortical, short, locking screws placed through the bone and around the stem (Fig. 45.11).

Postoperative Management

In patients who have had a prosthesis revised, an abduction pillow is utilized. Thromboembolic devices are placed while the patient is in the operating room. In the recovery room, an AP pelvis as well as full-length AP and lateral femur radiographs are obtained. Patients are mobilized out of bed on the first postoperative day to facilitate rehabilitation and to minimize the risk of deep venous thrombosis (DVT).

Postoperatively the patients are allowed toe-touch weight bearing, overseen initially by a physical therapist, for the first 6 to 12 weeks, followed by progressive weight bearing as tolerated. Knee range of motion is encouraged. Drains are usually removed on the second

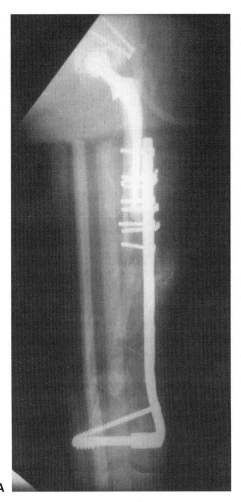
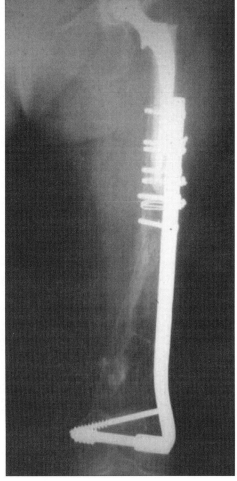

A   B

Figure 45.9. AP radiographs immediately postoperative **(A)** and after final healing of the fracture **(B)**.

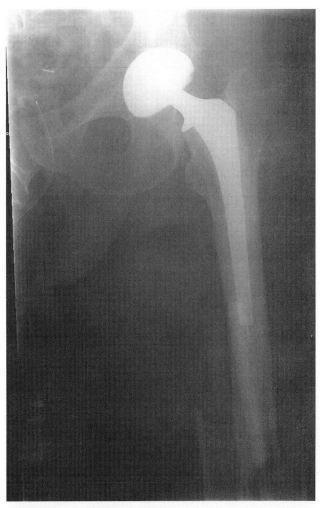
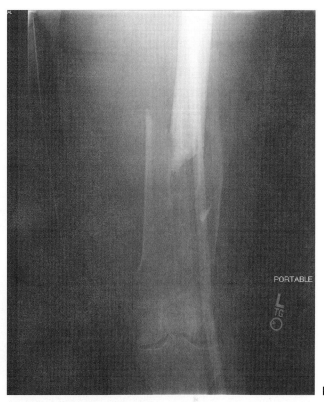

Figure 45.10. AP radiographs of the proximal **(A)** and distal **(B)** femur indicating a periprosthetic, distal, femur fracture with a stable-appearing stem.

postoperative day or when the drainage falls below 30 cc per 8-hour shift. Broad spectrum antibiotics are used for 5 days or until the cultures are negative. Patients are placed on both mechanical and pharmacologic prophylaxis for DVT. Sequential compression devices (SCDs) and an enoxaparin are used postoperatively, followed by 4 to 6 weeks of daily aspirin upon discharge.

After hospital discharge, patients are followed at 6 weeks, 3 months, 6 months, and 1 year. AP pelvis as well as AP and lateral radiographs of the femur are taken at each follow-up visit.

Complications

Complications include nonunion, malunion, hardware failure, infection, instability, and DVT.

PERIPROSTHETIC FRACTURES FOLLOWING TOTAL KNEE ARTHROPLASTY

Supracondylar femur fracture after TKA is a growing concern. The incidences range from 0.3% to 2.5% of patients. Risk factors include osteopenia, anterior femoral-cortex notching during implantation, the use of a constrained prosthesis, and neurologic disorders.

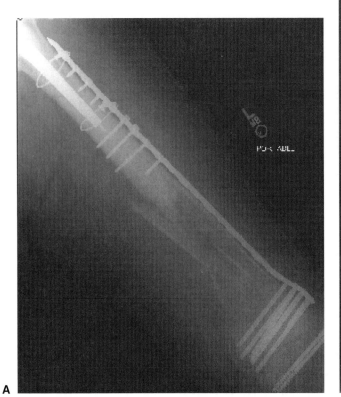

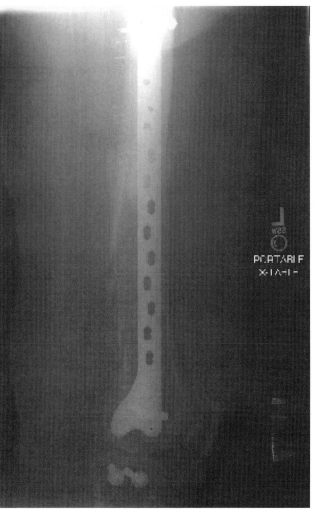

A   B

Figure 45.11. AP **(A)** and lateral **(B)** radiographs depicting the final construct with locking, distal, femur plate with proximal, unicortical, locking screws through one cortex and the cement mantle.

Radiographs of periprosthetic femur fractures above a TKA indicate a notched, anterior, femoral cortex in 40% to 52% of cases. Although no classification system is widely used, Rorabeck has classified these injuries into type I (nondisplaced, intact TKA), type II (displaced, intact TKA), and type III (prosthesis loose/failed).

Early studies reported complication rates as high as 30% with a 16% nonunion rate. With the use of retrograde nails and locked plates, success rates have dramatically improved. Treatment options include closed immobilization, plating, intramedullary (IM) nailing, and revision to a stemmed prosthesis. Nonoperative treatment is reserved for nondisplaced fractures and the debilitated elderly patient. However, there is a 50% decrease in ambulatory status and a high incidence of varus malunion. Plate fixation traditionally required that bone stock be sufficient for screw placement. With the introduction of locked plating, stable fixation in poor bone stock can be achieved. With comminuted supracondylar fractures, indirect reduction is recommended, and the fracture site is bridged with screws out of the zone of injury.

In an alternative, a retrograde nail through a semiconstrained femoral component works well. It is minimally invasive, load sharing, and less expensive; however, sufficient distal bone is necessary. In general, if the prosthesis is solidly fixed, one may fix the fracture by plates or nails. However, if the prosthesis is loose or comminution is extensive, revision arthroplasty is indicated. This requires careful prosthesis removal to avoid excess bone loss and use of a long-stemmed prosthesis as well as bone graft.

Periprosthetic fractures on the tibial side are less common and can be treated nonoperatively with patella tendon bearing (PTB) casting and bracing when nondisplaced. Open

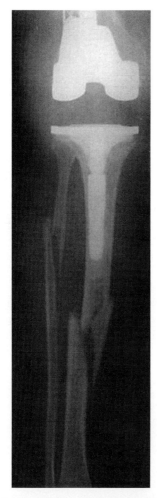

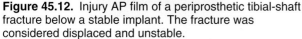

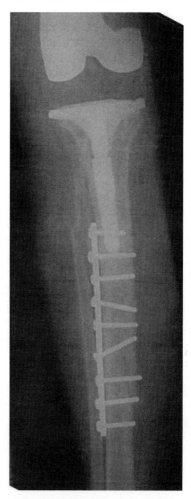

Figure 45.12. Injury AP film of a periprosthetic tibial-shaft fracture below a stable implant. The fracture was considered displaced and unstable.

Figure 45.13. Postoperative AP film depicting plate and screw osteosynthesis of the fracture.

reduction and internal fixation (ORIF) with plate and screws is used with displaced, unstable, periprosthetic, tibial-shaft fractures (Figs. 45.12 and 45.13).

Preoperative Planning

Full-length AP and lateral radiographs should be taken of the affected side. The presence of a femoral stem of a THA proximal to the knee replacement, severe bowing or other deformity of the femoral shaft, fracture pattern, and location may influence treatment. Furthermore, the configuration of the femoral component of the total knee must be ascertained. In general, the space between the flanges of a cruciate-retaining femoral component will allow reamers and placement of a retrograde nail of adequate diameter to pass. For most "boxed" or posterior-stabilized femoral components, IM fixation is impossible and instead plate fixation should be used. Some boxed femoral components, however, have a removable cover to allow insertion of the reamers and nail.

Surgery

Patient Positioning. Whether performing ORIF, IM nailing, or revision TKA, the surgeon places the patient supine on a radiolucent table. An image intensifier (for ORIF or IM nailing) and a radiolucent triangle (for IM nailing) are also necessary. A sterile tourniquet can be helpful.

Submuscular Plating Technique. For submuscular plating (Fig. 45.14), a large bump or a radiolucent triangle is used to elevate the leg and aid in reduction. In this way, the sagittal angulation of the fracture can be adjusted by moving the position of the bump. Through a small, distal, longitudinal incision over the lateral femoral condyle, a locking plate is passed from distal to proximal and slid submuscularly. A clamp or K wire is passed through a screw or pin hole at the proximal tip of the plate to maintain alignment of the plate on the femoral shaft. Although the surgeon may be tempted to use a shorter plate, if the segment is extensively comminuted, longer plates are recommended. A guide wire is passed through the central screw hole in the distal portion of the plate and passed into the condyles such that it is parallel to the trochlear notch in the axial plane and parallel to the distal tips of the condyles in the AP plane (Fig. 45.15). A Verbrugge clamp can be placed around the plate and condyles distally when necessary (Fig. 45.16). Image intensification is utilized as is direct visualization for proper rotational alignment of the plate on the lateral condyle (Fig. 45.17). For rotational control, the plate should be secured to the condyles with several wires prior to insertion of the first screw (Fig. 45.18).

Once proper position is confirmed, multiple locking screws are inserted. The fracture reduction is fine-tuned with the assistance of a bump or triangle to adjust sagittal and coronal alignment. Once satisfactory reduction is confirmed, multiple (percutaneous) proximal screws are placed. Locking screws do not influence fracture reduction; therefore, the re-

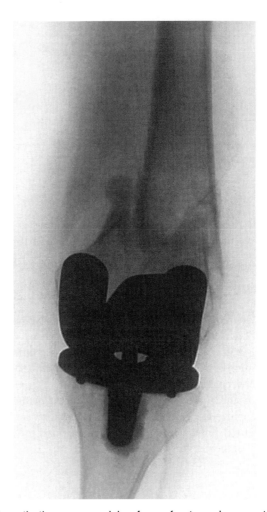

Figure 45.14. Periprosthetic, supracondylar, femur fracture above a stable total knee arthroplasty.

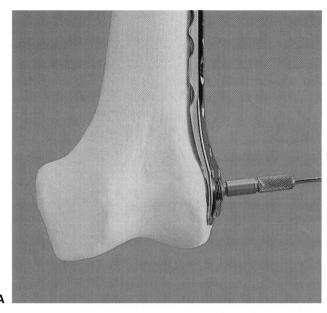

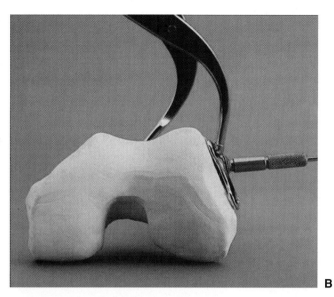

A
B

Figure 45.15. The central guide wire should be parallel to both the distal tips of the condyles in the AP plane **(A)** as well as the anterior tips of the condyles in the axial plane **(B)**.

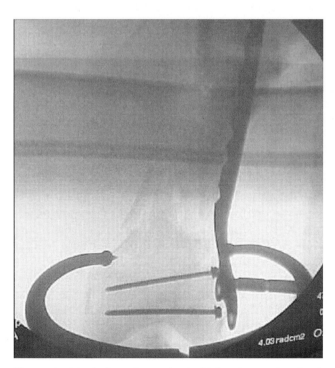

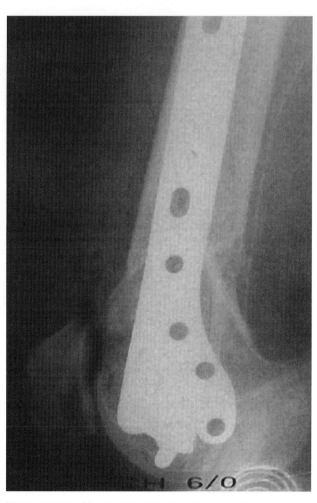

Figure 45.16. A clamp is used to hold the plate to the distal femur.

Figure 45.17. The lateral view should be checked to ascertain that the plate is aligned with the femoral shaft.

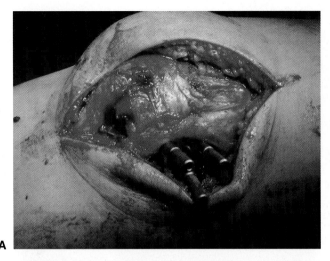

A

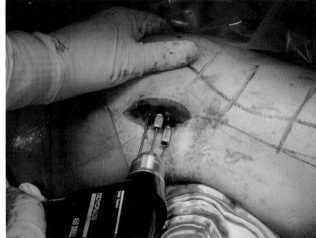

B

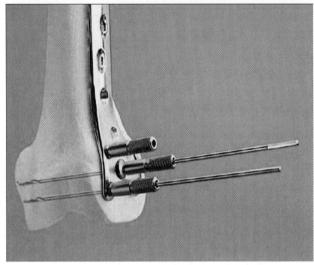

C

Figure 45.18. A–C. Three wires are inserted into the distal femur through locking guides threaded into the plate.

duction must be obtained before placement of locking screws, which can be placed through small percutaneous incisions along the shaft or through the small proximal incision made earlier to hold the alignment of the plate on the shaft (Fig. 45.19). The clamps and K wires are removed, and final position is checked with fluoroscopy. Postoperative long cassette films are necessary to show limb alignment (Fig. 45.20).

Retrograde Nailing Technique. If the prosthesis is cruciate retaining and sufficient, distal, bone stock is present, retrograde nailing is an attractive alternative technique (Fig. 24.21). The surgeon must first determine if the opening in the femoral component of the total knee is large enough for a nail to be safely inserted. Also, full-length femur films should be obtained so that the surgeon can identify whether an implant in the proximal femur or hip is also present. The knee is flexed over a radiolucent triangle. A 3-cm incision just medial to the patellar tendon is made, and a small arthrotomy is made. Under fluoroscopic control, a small, threaded, guide pin is inserted at the anterior edge of the intercondylar notch at the tip of Blumensaat's line on the lateral view and slightly medial to the midline on the AP view (Figs. 45.22 and 45.23). With a large-diameter cannulated drill, the distal femur is opened with the surgeon taking care to protect the patellar tendon during the process.

The fracture is reduced prior to reaming and nail insertion. The typical deformity is extension of the distal fragment, which can be corrected by shifting the apex of the triangle slightly proximal to let gravity pull the distal fragment downward into flexion. A ball-tipped guide wire is inserted and the femoral canal is reamed (see Fig. 45.21B). Once sufficient

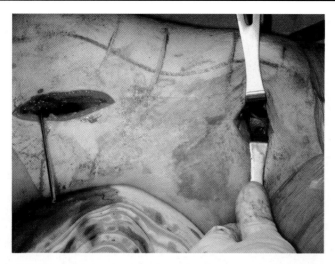

Figure 45.19. A small incision may be made at the tip of the plate to hold the plate onto the bone for rotational control or to place a standard nonlocking screw to approximate the bone and plate.

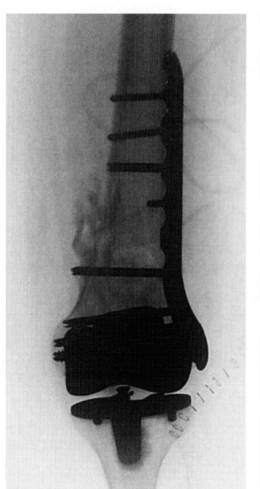
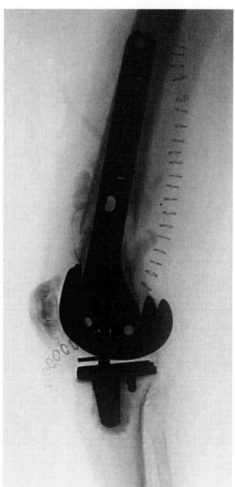

A   B

Figure 45.20. AP **(A)** and lateral **(B)** radiographs of the final construct with proximal and distal screws; the middle portion around the fracture is undisturbed.

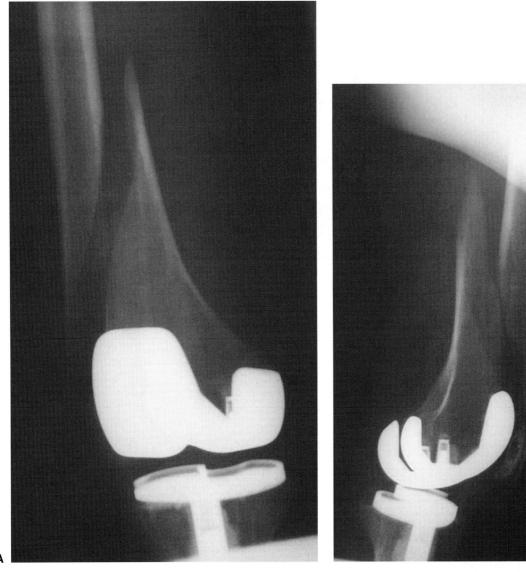

A   B

Figure 45.21. AP **(A)** and lateral **(B)** views of a periprosthetic femur fracture with poor bone stock.

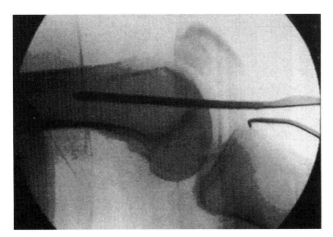

Figure 45.22. This lateral c-arm view of guide pin placement for a different patient's fracture indicates correct placement at the tip of Blumensaat's line.

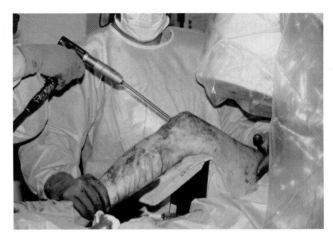

Figure 45.23. After guide pin placement and overdrilling for entry, a ball-tipped guide wire is placed across the fracture. This is left in place as the fracture is reamed.

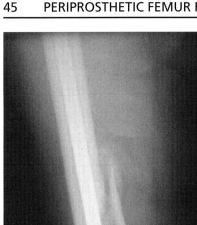

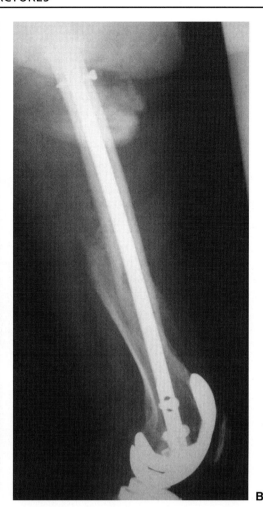

A   B

Figure 45.24. AP **(A)** and lateral **(B)** views of the fracture treated with retrograde intramedullary rodding.

cortical chatter is encountered, a nail 1 mm smaller than the last reamer is selected, and the proper nail length is determined. The proximal tip of the nail must extend at or just above the lesser trochanter. The distal interlocking screws are inserted first with the surgeon achieving as many points of fixation distal to the fracture site as possible. The fracture reduction is checked again with fluoroscopy. The proximal anterior-to-posterior interlocking screws are inserted using a freehand technique. The final result is shown in Figure 45.24.

Postoperative Management

Patients are kept from weight bearing on the affected side for 6 weeks postoperatively or until callus formation is seen on the radiographs, at which time partial weight bearing can be initiated. Routine DVT prophylaxis, including both mechanical and (if no epidural is present or no specific reason is indicated, do not use it) pharmacologic agents are used. A knee immobilizer is used for comfort, and patients are mobilized on the first postoperative day.

Complications

Complications of plate fixation include screw pull-out, stress riser, stress shielding, and poor alignment.

RECOMMENDED READING

Chen F, Mont MA, Bachner RS. Management of ipsilateral supracondylar femur fractures following total knee arthroplasty. *J Arthroplasty* 1994;9(5):521–526.

Dennis DA. Periprosthetic fractures following total knee arthroplasty. *Instr Course Lect* 2001;50:379–389.

Duncan CP, Masri BA. Fractures of the femur after hip replacement. *Instr Course Lect* 1995;44:293–304.

Duwelius PJ, Schmidt AH, Kyle RF, et al. A prospective, modernized treatment protocol for periprosthetic femur fractures. *Orthop Clin North Am* 2004;35(4):485–492.

Kyle RF, Bookout JD. The extended femoral slot: an alternative method for cemented stem failure. *Orthopedics* 2003;26(1):29,48.

Peterson CA, Lewallen DG. Periprosthetic fracture of the acetabulum after total hip arthroplasty. *J Bone Joint Surg Am* 1996;78(8):1206–1213.

Rorabeck CH, Smith PN. Fractures of the femur, tibia, and patella after total knee arthroplasty: decision making and principles of management. *Instr Course Lect* 1998;47:449–458.

Schmidt AH, Kyle RF. Periprosthetic fractures of the femur. *Orthop Clin North Am* 2002;33(1):143–152.

46

Gastrocnemius and Soleus Rotational Muscle Flaps: Soft-Tissue Coverage

Randy Sherman and Sharad Rhaban

INDICATIONS/CONTRAINDICATIONS

A muscle flap is indicated when vital structures such as bones, joints, tendons, or hardware are exposed and require coverage. In the lower leg and particularly the tibia, a muscle flap must be well vascularized and durable. Of all the local rotational flaps, the gastrocnemius is one of the most reliable. The gastrocnemius is a broad muscle with a single proximal vascular pedicle, which is well protected in the popliteal fossa. The gastrocnemius muscle or myocutaneous rotational flap is used for the procedure of choice for soft-tissue coverage of complex open wounds about the knee and proximal third of the tibia and fibula. The use of this flap is indicated in the following circumstances: (a) coverage of acute, grade IIIB, open, tibial fractures with or without hardware involving exposure of the knee joint, capsule, fracture site, or exposed cortex (Fig. 46.1); (b) obliteration of dead space and wound closure after radical debridement of osteomyelitic wounds in this region as well as infected nonunions (Fig. 46.2); (c) coverage of exposed total-knee arthroplasties or pre-arthroplasty tissue augmentation in densely scarred wound beds (Fig. 46.3); and (d) limb salvage and coverage of endoprostheses or allograft material after resection of musculoskeletal neoplasms (Fig. 46.4).

The soleus muscle, without a myocutaneous correlate, has a much more limited area of rotation and is used primarily for small, medially based, open wounds in the middle third of the leg. Indications include coverage of acute open fractures and chronic osteomyelitic wounds (Fig. 46.5).

Contraindications to the use of a gastrocnemius flap include vascular compromise of the muscle itself by disruption of the sural artery pedicle, compromise of the popliteal artery from which it emanates, or occlusion of the proximal arterial tree. Significant local trauma to the muscle itself, although rare, prevents its successful rotation.

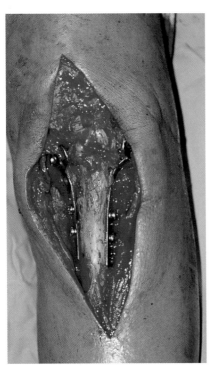

Figure 46.1. Grade IIIB open tibial-plateau fracture with exposed knee joint after internal fixation and unsuccessful attempt at primary wound closure.

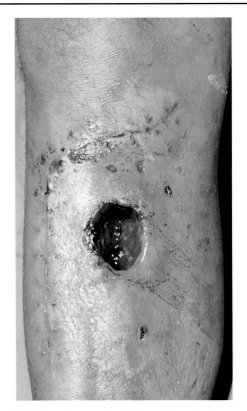

Figure 46.2. Dead space involving skin, subcutaneous tissue, muscle, and bone in a proximal-third infected nonunion.

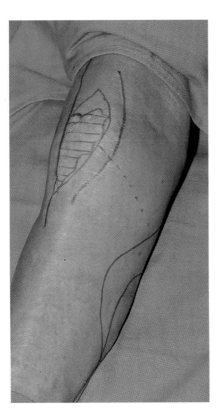

Figure 46.3. Scarred, atrophic, prepatella skin in an elderly patient after removal of an infected total-knee arthroplasty.

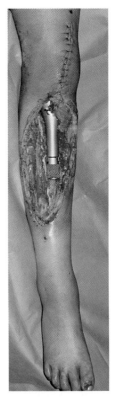

Figure 46.4. A 10-year-old girl immediately after tumor extirpation of a proximal tibial osteosarcoma and placement of endoprosthesis after loss of anterior skin.

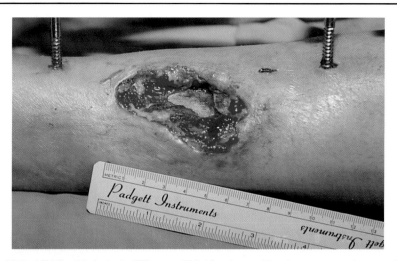

Figure 46.5. Middle-third grade IIIB open-tibial fracture with a bony sequestrum and loss of overlying soft tissue.

Recipient-site contraindications include a wound in the proximal third region in which its size and dimension are too large for coverage by the gastrocnemius muscle. Similarly, injury to the substance of the soleus muscle will hinder its ability to be transposed. Vascular compromise to the soleus muscle is extremely rare because of its segmental inflow. Because of minor perforators that exit from the posterior tibial artery distally, the surgeon must take great care to assure adequate vascularity to the most distal aspect of the soleus muscle when a large transposition is undertaken. As with the gastrocnemius, a large anterior or laterally located wound in the middle third of the leg may not be completely covered by the soleus muscle (Fig. 46.6), and free tissue transfer may be a better option.

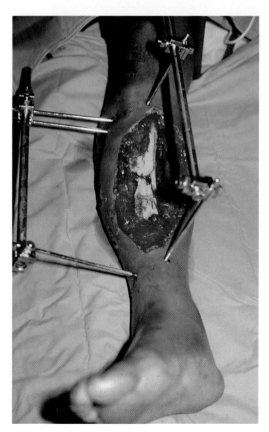

Figure 46.6. Large, grade IIIB, open, middle-third tibial fracture cannot be closed by a local soleus flap and requires free tissue transfer.

As with any muscle-coverage procedure, infection or tumor recurrence is best avoided by thorough debridement or excision before wound closure. No muscle flap will successfully combat retained sequestrum or loose infected hardware, which act as nidi for continued infection.

PREOPERATIVE PLANNING

A thorough examination of the patient is crucial when planning either a gastrocnemius or soleus muscle flap for coverage of a complex open wound. Radiographs should be viewed with particular attention paid to fracture location and the presence or absence of internal fixation devices. For acute fractures, if an external fixator is indicated, the surgeon should anticipate the need for subsequent soft-tissue closure and construct the frame to allow unrestricted transposition of the muscles from the posterior to a medial or anterior plane. The zone of injury around the fracture site should be recognized because aggressive or radical debridement may significantly alter the dimensions of the wound (Fig. 46.7). Clinical examination of the leg should be made, with particular attention paid to would length, width, and depth. Other factors such as induration, discoloration, ecchymosis, and cellulitis must be considered.

A detailed vascular examination with palpation of the dorsalis pedis and posterior tibial pulses for arterial inflow, as well as Doppler examination for venous outflow, should be documented. Arteriography may be indicated if pulses are absent or diminished (Fig. 46.8). The function of the posterior compartment muscles should be assessed whenever possible. Sensory examination of the foot must be documented, with particular attention given to the posterior tibial, sural, and saphenous nerves. The surgical incisions can be planned in conjunction with the need for additional debridement and internal or external fixation of the fracture.

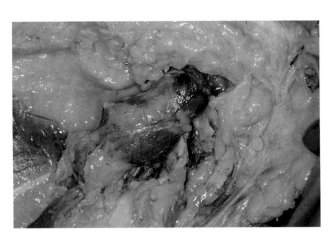

Figure 46.7. Large amount of retained titanium from a previously removed, infected, total-knee arthroplasty.

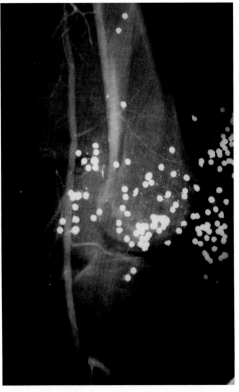

Figure 46.8. Angiogram demonstrating patency of the popliteal artery and continuity of the sural arteries despite the fracture comminution and retained gunshot pellets.

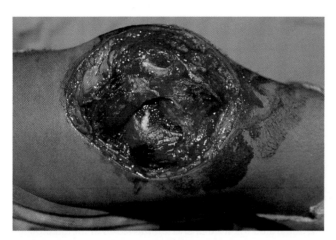

Figure 46.9. Completed debridement of infected fracture of the knee with removal of all nonviable soft tissue and bony sequestrum.

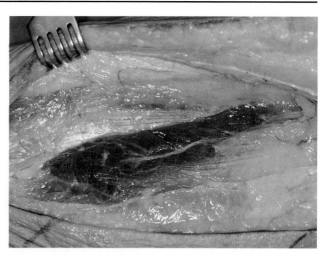

Figure 46.10. The gastrocnemius muscle is visible when the deep investing fascia is incised longitudinally.

SURGERY

Gastrocnemius

A muscle flap procedure is undertaken only after complete and definitive debridement of a traumatic or infected wound has been completed or a tumor has been extirpated (Fig. 46.9). A tourniquet is placed on the thigh, and the entire leg is prepped and draped. The approach to the gastrocnemius muscle can be made through perpendicular, oblique, or parallel incisions.

If a parallel incision is used, the gastrocnemius muscle must be tunneled beneath the resulting bipedicled fasciocutaneous flap. The gastrocnemius muscle is identified by incising the deep investing fascia of the leg longitudinally along the anterior border of the muscle (Fig. 46.10).

The fascia can be opened proximally toward the origin of the muscle and distally to its insertion on the Achilles tendon if necessary. The fatty plane between the gastrocnemius and soleus is developed by either sharp or digital dissection. This areolar plane is confirmed by visualization of the plantaris longus tendon, which lies adjacent to the soleus at or near its medial border (Fig. 46.11). The white investing fascia on the posterior border of the

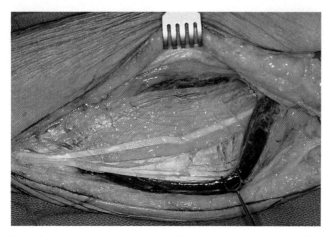

Figure 46.11. The plantaris longus tendon confirms the plane between the gastrocnemius and soleus muscles.

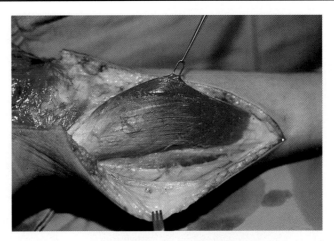

Figure 46.12. The median raphe separates the medial and lateral heads of the gastrocnemius and carries the neurovascular structures, which must be protected.

soleus and the deep border of the gastrocnemius make recognition of this plane unmistakable. Occasionally perforators between the soleus and gastrocnemius exist and must be divided. As the surgeon works posteriorly (superficial), the muscle is easily separated from the deep investing fascia. One or two myocutaneous perforators must be saved if a myocutaneous flap is planned; otherwise, they are divided. The gastrocnemius is separated along its median raphe into a medial and a lateral head. The raphe is easier to identify and more prominent in the distal portion of the muscle (Fig. 46.12). The sural nerve and lesser saphenous vein run along the raphe and should be preserved. These are constant landmarks and facilitate separation of the medial from the lateral head. When the median raphe has been identified, dissection proceeds from distal to proximal, with the surgeon working along the posterior midline while protecting the neurovascular structures at all times. When both the posterior and anterior surfaces are freed, the gastrocnemius can be released from its attachment to the Achilles tendon. The dissection continues proximally to the origin of the gastrocnemius muscle from the femoral condyle (Fig. 46.13).

With proximal dissection in the popliteal space, care must be taken to visualize and protect the vascular pedicle (Fig. 46.14). The muscle can be released from the condyle by

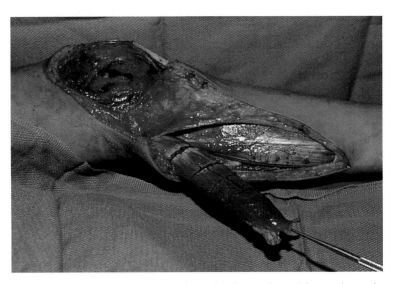

Figure 46.13. Exposure of the muscle origin on the femoral condyle requires adequate muscle retraction and sufficient proximal exposure.

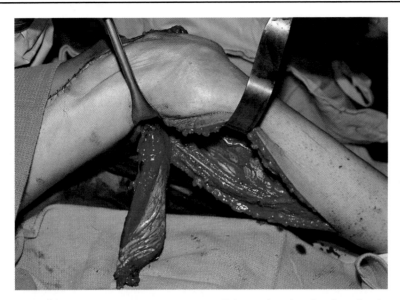

Figure 46.14. When needed, the sural artery pedicle can be visualized on the deep surface of the gastrocnemius in the popliteal fossa.

resecting its tendinous attachments, resulting in a 2- to 3-cm increase in the length for arc of rotation. The muscle can also be expanded significantly in both the transverse and longitudinal planes by crisscross incisions made both anteriorly and posteriorly through its heavily fused bilaminar myofascia (Fig. 46.15). Furthermore, the gastrocnemius muscle can be split longitudinally in the distal portion so that part of the muscle can be used to obliterate deep dead space, while the remainder of the muscle can be used for superficial coverage.

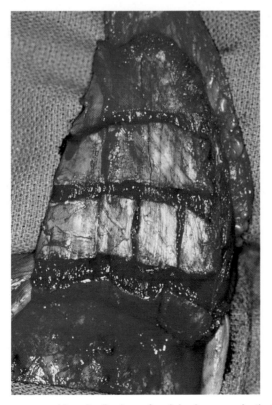

Figure 46.15. Transverse and longitudinal myofascial release on both deep and superficial surfaces allows significant expansion of muscle area to be used for coverage.

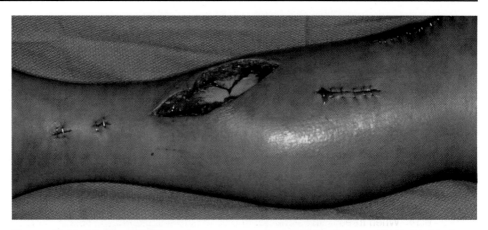

Figure 46.16. Ideal wounds for soleus coverage are small medial wounds located in the middle third of the leg.

The lateral gastrocnemius flap is raised in a similar fashion from a lateral cutaneous approach by using one of the three incisions described. Of paramount importance is the identification and protection of the peroneal nerve just below the head of the fibula as it penetrates from superficial to deep into the lateral compartment. After the safety of this nerve is assured, raising the lateral gastrocnemius muscle is done in a fashion similar to that described for the medial head. It should be noted, however, that the lateral gastrocnemius muscle is smaller than the medial head and will not provide the same quantity of muscle for laterally based lesions.

Soleus

The soleus is almost always raised from a medial approach and is used to cover small medial and anterior-based middle-third wounds (Fig. 46.16). A curvilinear incision is made over the medial aspect of the calf. The plane between the gastrocnemius and soleus muscles is easily identified and serves as an excellent starting point. When raising the soleus, the gastrocnemius–Achilles musculotendinous unit must be preserved at all times. Alice clamps are placed on the edge of the Achilles tendon to better demonstrate the area where the two merge. The fascia that fuses the posterior soleus to the Achilles is divided (Fig. 46.17). Proceeding from proximal to distal, the surgeon dissects the muscle off the Achilles

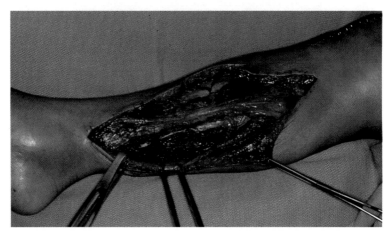

Figure 46.17. The anterior border of the Achilles is identified and retracted with Alice clamps to aid dissection of the posterior surface of the soleus from the tendon.

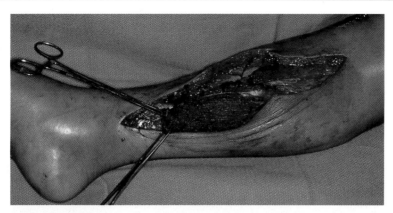

Figure 46.18. When freed from its anterior and posterior attachments, the soleus muscle is transected distally.

tendon with either a knife or Metzenbaum scissors from medial to lateral. A pseudoraphe is encountered approximately three fourths of the way through the dissection. It is important to separate this and continue the dissection both posteriorly and then laterally to include the entire soleus muscle. The muscle is released distally to include as much length as possible (Fig. 46.18). The plane between the deep side of the soleus and the deep flexor compartment is identified and can be digitally dissected. Care must be taken to identify the distal perforators arising from the posterior tibial artery and vein. These can be very short, and if inadvertently injured or cut, they may retract beneath the deep fascia, making them difficult to ligate. When these distal perforators have been identified, ligated, and divided, the soleus attachments on the lateral side are dissected free under direct visualization. The muscle must be freed quite proximally, especially on its lateral side, to achieve any significant rotation of the muscle into the wound (Fig. 46.19). Crisscross release of the soleus myofascia can be done on the deep or anterior surface of the muscle to expand the size and the dimensions of the flap (Fig. 46.20).

Each muscle, when transferred, is secured into place with absorbable sutures. It is worth emphasizing that the muscle, particularly the gastrocnemius, can be split longitudinally, with one slip obliterating dead space and the remainder addressing the requirements of the open wound. Finally, a skin graft over the flap is necessary and can be harvested from the ipsilateral calf, thigh, or buttock after application of aerosolized thrombin. The thickness of the graft is usually 0.015 to 0.018 inches (Fig. 46.21).

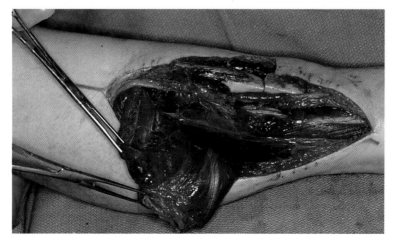

Figure 46.19. Because of the broad attachments on both the tibial and fibular sides, dissection must continue proximally for any significant transposition to be achieved.

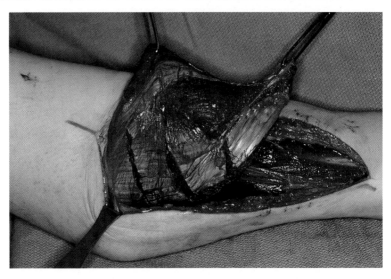

Figure 46.20. Scoring of the myofascia on the anterior surface of the soleus allows great dimensions for coverage.

Alternatively, a myocutaneous flap can be designed, based on perforators from the gastrocnemius, to include skin and subjacent subcutaneous tissue (Fig. 46.22). The skin overlying the muscle is used and can extend 5 cm proximal to the medial malleolus. The ability to close the donor site must be considered before executing this myocutaneous flap. This possibility does not exist with the soleus. Before wound closure, a Jackson–Pratt drain is placed in the wound. A well-padded short-leg posterior splint is applied with the foot and ankle in neutral dorsiflexion (Fig. 46.23).

POSTOPERATIVE MANAGEMENT

The Jackson–Pratt drain is removed when drainage is less than 30 mL per day. The dressings are changed between 3 and 5 days, and the skin grafts are inspected. At 1 week, the patient is allowed to place the leg in a dependent position for a short period and the area is trained to increase the tolerance over the course of the subsequent 3 to 5 weeks. Prolonged dependency is avoided for 6 to 8 weeks to avoid venous congestion. The timing of weight-bearing ambulation depends primarily on the orthopedic injury, rather than on the muscle

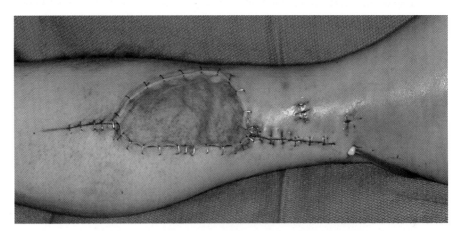

Figure 46.21. A split-thickness skin graft measuring between .015 and .018 inches can be placed immediately after successful flap transposition. To improve recipient-site aesthetics, we use sheet grafts as opposed and with equal success to meshed grafts.

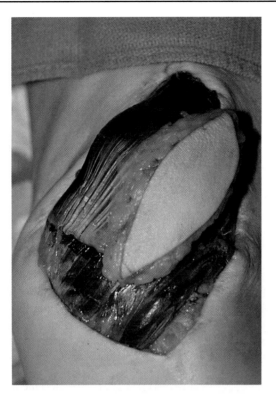

Figure 46.22. A cutaneous paddle can be reliably transferred with the gastrocnemius muscle if it contains at least one myocutaneous perforator.

flap. The patient is seen weekly in the office until the wound is completely closed and dry. Patients must be counseled preoperatively about the deformity caused by muscle rotation, including loss of natural convexity in the proximal and middle third of the leg caused by rotation of the gastrocnemius muscle. It is well documented that both the gastrocnemius and soleus muscles will atrophy over time after transposition. After a gastrocnemius or soleus muscle flap is completed, range of motion of the knee and ankle are usually started during the first week.

COMPLICATIONS

Because of the rich blood supply and durability of both the gastrocnemius and soleus muscles, flap death is rare. More common, however, is the development of a postoperative

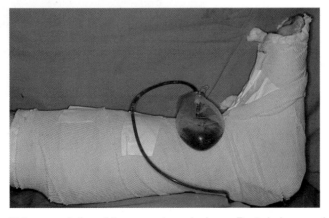

Figure 46.23. At the completion of the procedure, Jackson–Pratt drains are placed on suction, and the extremity is secured in a well-padded posterior splint with the foot plantigrade.

hematoma, which requires surgical evacuation, irrigation, and control of the bleeding site. Loss of power with plantar flexion is rarely a problem if the gastrocnemius or the soleus muscle is used alone. A combined gastrocnemius and soleus flap can lead to a greater incidence of muscle weakness and gait abnormalities. Pain and dysesthesias at the donor site resulting from flap transposition should be expected during the first 6 to 8 weeks and should not be considered a complication.

Occasionally, with dissection of the soleus muscle and loss of its middle and distal perforators, the distal end of the soleus may become devascularized, and if this complication is recognized, it should be resected. If unrecognized, it can lead to partial flap necrosis and subsequent wound infection with bone or hardware exposure or both. Reversed or distally based soleus flaps, although described, should not be considered reliable alternatives for muscle transposition.

ILLUSTRATIVE CASE FOR TECHNIQUE

A 36-year-old man sustained a grade IIIB open, comminuted, tibial plateau and proximal third fracture (Fig. 46.24). After open reduction and internal fixation (ORIF), the wound broke down. The gastrocnemius muscle was harvested from the medial side through a transverse skin incision (Fig. 46.25). The muscle was rotated into place (Fig. 46.26) with release of its investing fascia, allowing the hardware to be entirely covered. A split-thickness skin graft was placed. The wound healed without incident (Fig. 46.27).

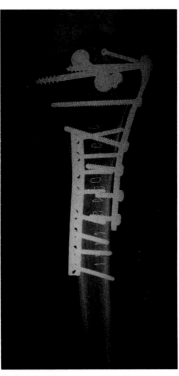

Figure 46.24. Grade IIIB, open, tibial-plateau, and proximal-third fracture after ORIF.

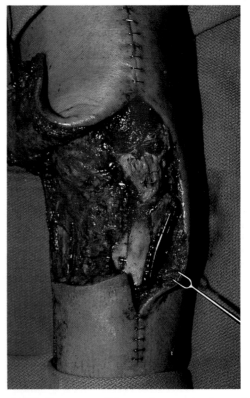

Figure 46.25. Exposure of the gastrocnemius is made through a transverse posterior incision from the wound.

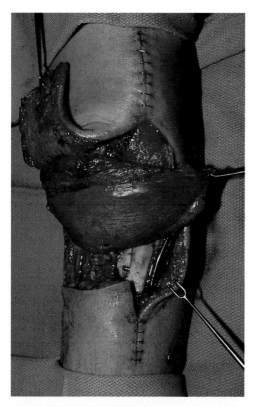

Figure 46.26. When the muscle is freed, it is transposed into place for complete wound coverage.

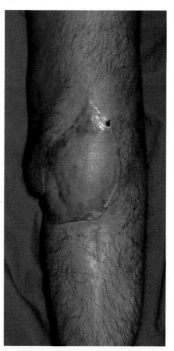

Figure 46.27. A well-healed skin graft over the muscle completes the healing process allowing the fracture to unite.

RECOMMENDED READING

Arnold PG, Mixter RC. Making the most of the gastrocnemius muscle. *Plast Reconstr Surg* 1983;72:38.

Chandrasekhar B, Brien W. Coverage strategies in total joint replacement. *Orthop Clin North Am* 1993;24:3.

Feldman SJ, Cohen BE, Mayo SW Jr. The medial gastrocnemius myocutaneous flap. *Plast Reconstr Surg* 1978;61:531.

Guzman-Stein G, Fix RJ, Vasconez LO. Muscle flap coverage for the lower extremity. *Clin Plast Surg* 1991;18:545.

Lesavoy MA, Dubrow TJ, Wackym PA, et al. Muscle flap coverage of exposed endoprostheses. *Plast Reconst Surg* 1989;83:90.

Malawar MM, Price WM. Gastrocnemius transposition flap in conjunction with limb sparing surgery for primary bone sarcomas around the knee. *Plast Reconst Surg* 1984;73:741.

Mathes SJ, McCraw JB, Vasconez LO. Muscle transposition flaps for coverage of lower extremity defects: anatomic considerations. *Surg Clin North Am* 1974;54:1337.

Mathes SJ, Nahai F. *Clinical application for muscle and musculocutaneous flaps.* St. Louis: Mosby; 1982.

McCraw JB, Fishman JH, Sharzer LA. The versatile gastrocnemius myocutaneous flap. *Plast Reconstr Surg* 1978;62:15.

Stark W. The use of pedicled muscle flaps in the treatment of chronic osteomyelitis resulting from compound fractures. *J Bone Joint Surg* 28:343, 1946.

Tobin GF. Hemisoleus and reversed hemisoleus flaps. *Plast Reconstr Surg* 1985;76:87.

Yaremchuck MV. Acute management of severe soft tissue damage accompanying open fractures of the lower extremity. *Clin Plast Surg* 1986;13:621.

Index